Essentials of the Adult Neurogenic Bladder

Essentials of the Adult Neurogenic Bladder

Edited by

Jacques Corcos
Professor of Surgery (Urology)
McGill University
Montreal, Canada

Gilles Karsenty
Professor of Surgery (Urology)
Department of Urology and Kidney Transplantation
La Conception Hospital
Aix-Marseille University
Marseille, France

Thomas Kessler
Professor of Urology
Department of Neuro-Urology
Balgrist University Hospital
University of Zürich
Zürich, Switzerland

David Ginsberg
Professor of Clinical Urology
Keck School of Medicine
University of Southern California
Los Angeles, California

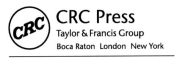

CRC Press
Taylor & Francis Group
Boca Raton London New York

CRC Press is an imprint of the
Taylor & Francis Group, an **informa** business

First edition published 2021
by CRC Press
6000 Broken Sound Parkway NW, Suite 300, Boca Raton, FL 33487-2742

and by CRC Press
2 Park Square, Milton Park, Abingdon, Oxon, OX14 4RN

Library of Congress Cataloging-in-Publication Data

Names: Corcos, Jacques, editor. | Karsenty, Gilles, editor. | Kessler, Thomas (Thomas M.), editor. | Ginsberg, David (David A.), editor.
Title: Essentials of the adult neurogenic bladder / edited by Jacques Corcos, Gilles Karsenty, Thomas Kessler, David Ginsberg.
Description: First edition. | Boca Raton : CRC Press, 2020. | Includes bibliographical references and index. | Summary: "Blurb This book summarises the entire field of adult neuro-urology in a concise, well-illustrated, and practical style. A selection of the most knowledgeable clinician and basic scientists have been included to cover the most recent development in the field. It's ideal for students, residents, physicians, continence specialists, and other health care professionals involved in the diagnosis and management of patients who have lost normal bladder/sexual function because of a neurological insult. About the Editors Jacques Corcos Professor of Surgery (Urology), McGill University, Montreal, Canada Gilles Karsenty Professor of Urology and MD, Aix-Marseille University, Marseille, France Thomas Kessler Professor of Urology and MD, Department of Neuro-Urology, Balgrist University Hospital, University of Zürich, Switzerland David Ginsberg Professor of Clinical Urology Kecks School of Medicine of University of South California, USA"-- Provided by publisher.
Identifiers: LCCN 2020009457 (print) | LCCN 2020009458 (ebook) | ISBN 9780367335809 (hbk) | ISBN 9780367278014 (pbk) | ISBN 9780429320675 (ebk)
Subjects: MESH: Urinary Bladder, Neurogenic
Classification: LCC RC919 (print) | LCC RC919 (ebook) | NLM WJ 500 | DDC 616.6/2--dc23
LC record available at https://lccn.loc.gov/2020009457
LC ebook record available at https://lccn.loc.gov/2020009458

ISBN: 9780367335809 (hbk)
ISBN: 9780367278014 (pbk)
ISBN: 9780429320675 (ebk)

Typeset in Minion Pro
by Nova Techset Private Limited, Bengaluru & Chennai, India

CONTENTS

PART I
Epidemiology and Pathophysiology of Neurogenic Bladders

PART II
Neurologic Pathologies Responsible for the Development of the Neurogenic Bladder

Section A: Peripheral Neuropathies

Section G: Other Neurologic Pathologies Responsible for Neurogenic Bladder Dysfunction

PART III
Evaluation of Neurogenic Bladder Dysfunction

PART IV
Classification

PART V
Treatment

PART VI
Synthesis of Treatment

PART VII
Complications

PART VIII
Sexual dysfunction and reproduction in neurologic disorders

PART IX
Prognosis and Follow-up

PART X
Neurogenic Bladders in Developing Countries

PART XI
References for Reports and guidelines

FOREWORD

The book you are opening today is not just another new book about neurogenic bladders. This is the most comprehensive, referenced and updated piece of literature on this topic presently on the book market. Essential in Neurogenic Bladders has been developed by international experts from five continents, all clinicians and researchers dealing with this complicated topic on a daily basis. These experts each have shared their own experience, reviewed and analyzed the most recent literature, and summarized and extracted the most important information, to write these chapters representing what any interested professional must know about neurogenic bladders.

Thanks to their availability and hard work, putting all of this work together to build this book has been a very interesting and painless experience for the four editors who warmly thank all contributors, residents, fellows and staff for their excellent work and communication.

CONTRIBUTORS

Christina W. Agudelo
Department of Urology
SUNY Downstate Medical Center
Brooklyn, New York

Ali Alsulihem
Department of Urology
Prince Sultan Military Medical City
Riad, Saudi Arabia

Jacques Corcos
Department of Urology
McGill University
Montreal, Canada

Juan José Andino
Department of Urology
Michigan Medicine
Ann Arbor, Michigan

Marcio Augusto Averbeck
Department of Urology
Moinhos de Vento Hospital
Porto Allegre, Brazil

Bertil F.M. Blok
Department of Urology
Erasmus Medical Center
Rotterdam, The Netherlands

Anne Cameron
Department of Urology
University of Michigan
Ann Arbor, Michigan

Lysanne Campeau
Department of Urology
McGill University
Montreal, Canada

Romain Caremel
Department of Urology
McGill University
Montreal, Canada

Jehane H. Dagher
Department of Medicine
Université de Montréal
Montreal, Canada

Pierre Denys
Department of PMR
Neuro Urology Unit
Hopital Raymond Poincaré APHP Garches
Paris, France

Roger R. Dmochowski
Department of Urology
Vanderbilt Medical Center
Nashville, Tennessee

Christopher S. Elliott
Division of Urology
Department of Urology
Santa Clara Valley Medical Center
Stanford University Medical School
Stanford, California

Jairam R. Eswara
Division of Urology
Brigham and Women's Hospital
Boston, Massachusetts

Karel Everaert
Department of Urology
Ghent University Hospital
Ghent, Belgium

Michele Fascelli
Department of Urology
Cleveland Clinic Foundation
Cleveland, Ohio

Nishant Garg
Department of Urology
University of California
San Diego Health
Dan Diego, California

Gamal Ghoniem
Department of Urology
University of California
Irvine, California

David Ginsberg
Department of Urology
Keck School of Medicine
University of Southern California
Los Angeles, California

Laura L. Giusto
Lerner College of Medicine
Cleveland Clinic
Cleveland, Ohio

Kenneth I. Glassberg
Department of Urology
Given Foundation
Columbia University Medical Center
New York, New York

Howard B. Goldman
Glickman Urologic and Kidney Institute
Lerner College of Medicine
Cleveland Clinic
Cleveland, Ohio

Reynaldo G. Gomez
Urology Service
Hospital del Trabajador
Universidad Andres Bello School of Medicine
Santiago, Chile

Jan Groen
Department of Urology
Erasmus Medical Center
Rotterdam, the Netherlands

Akhlil Hamid
Fiona Stanley Hospital
Perth Urology Clinic
Perth, Australia

Siobhán M. Hartigan
Department of Urology
Vanderbilt University Medical Center
Nashville, Tennessee

François Hervé
Department of Urology
Cliniques Universitaires Saint-Luc
Brussels, Belgium

Ahmed Ibrahim
Department of Urology
McGill University Health Centre
Montreal, Canada

Charles Joussain
Department of Medical Rehabilitation
University of Versailles
Paris, France

Gilles Karsenty
 Department of Urology and Kidney
  Transplantation
La Conception Hospital
Aix-Marseille University
Marseille, France

Michael J. Kennelly
Depatment of Urology
Carolinas Medical Center
Atrium Health
Charlotte, North Carolina

Thomas M. Kessler
Department of Neuro-Urology
Balgrist University Hospital
University of Zürich
Zürich, Switzerland

Carlotte Kiekens
Montecatone Rehabilitation Institute
Spinal Unit
Bologna, Italy

Stephanie Kielb
Depatment of Urology
Northwestern University Feinberg School of Medicine
Chicago, Illinois

Evgeniy I. Kreydin
Depatment of Urology
Keck School of Medicine
University of Southern California
California

Jeremy Lai
Department of Urology
Northwestern University Feinberg School of Medicine
Chicago, Illinois

John P. Lavelle
Department of Veterans Affairs
Palo Alto Health Care System
Stanford University
Palo Alto, California

Frank C. Lin
Division of FPMRS
Department of Urology
David Geffen School of Medicine at UCLA
Los Angeles, California

Helmut Madersbacher
Department of Urology
Neuro-Urology Unit Innsbruck
Innsbruck, Austria

Sachin Malde
Department of Urology
Guy's Hospital
London, UK

Ulrich Mehnert
Department of Urology
Faculty of Medicine
University of Zürich
Zürich, Switzerland

Floriane Michel
Department of Urology
Aix-Marseille Université
Marseille, France

M. Louis Moy
Department of Urology
Thomas Jefferson University
University of Florida
Gainesville, Florida

Victor W. Nitti
Depatment of Urology
David Geffen School of Medicine at UCLA
Los Angeles, California

Teruyuki Ogawa
Department of Urology
Shinshu University
School of Medicine
Matsumoto, Japan

Janine L. Oliver
Depatment of Urology
University of Colorado School of Medicine
Aurora, Colorado

Jalesh N. Panicker
Department of Uro-Neurology
The National Hospital for Neurology and
    Neurosurgery and UCL Queen Square
Institute of Neurology
London, UK

Jeanne Perrin
Laboratory of Reproductive Medicine-CECOS
La Conception University Hospital
Hopitaux Universitaires de Marseille
and
Aix Marseille University
and
Avignon Université
CNRS, IRD, IMBE
Marseille, France

Véronique Phé
Department of Urology
Hôpital La Pitié Salpêtrière
Paris, France

Dayron Rodríguez
Department of Urology
University of Texas Southwestern Medical Center
Dallas, Texas

Melita Rotar
Institute of Clinical Neurophysiology
Division of Neurology
University Medical Center Ljubljana
Ljubljana, Slovenia

Elizabeth A. Rourke
Department of Urology
Vanderbilt University Medical Center
Nashville, Tennessee

Temitope Rude
Department of Urology
University of Southern California
Los Angeles, California

Ryuji Sakakibara
Neurology, Internal Medicine
Sakura Medical Center
Toho University
Tokyo, Japan

Yahir Santiago-Lastra
Department of Urology
University of California San Diego Health
San Diego, California

Fernando Segura
Urology Service
Hospital Regional Valdivia
Universidad Austral de Chile School of Medicin
Valdivia, Chile

Samer Shamout
Division of Urology
McGill University
Montreal, Canada

Patrick J. Shenot
Department of Urology
Thomas Jefferson University
Philadelphia, Pennsylvania

Karl-Dietrich Sievert
Department of Urology
Klinikum Lippe
Klinik für Urologie
Detmold, Germany

John T. Stoffel
Department of Urology
Michigan University
Ann Arbor, Michigan

Jeffrey Thavaseelan
Notre Dame University
Perth Urology Clinic
Perth, Australia

W. Blair Townsend
Department of Urology
Carolinas Medical Center
Charlotte, North Carolina

David B. Vodušek
Institute of Clinical Neurophysiology
Division of Neurology
University Medical Center
Ljubljana, Slovenia

Blayne Welk
Department of Surgery and Epidemiology and
    Biostatistics
Western University
Ontario, Canada

Jean-Jacques Wyndaele
Department of Urology
University Antwerp
Antwerp, Belgium
and
Aix-Marseille University
La Conception University Hospital
Marseille, France

Chuan-Guo Xiao
Department of Urology
C. G. Xiao Hospital
Shenzhen, China

Claire C. Yang
Department of Urology
University of Washington
Seattle, Washington

René Yiou
Service d'Urologie
CHU Henri Mondor
Créteil, France

Naoki Yoshimura
Department of Urology
University of Pittsburgh
School of Medicine
Pittsburgh, Pennsylvania

Patricia M. Zahner
Comprehensive Urologic Specialists
Department of Surgery and Epidemiology and
    Biostatistics (Urologist)
Western University
London, UK

Philippe E. Zimmern
Department of Urology
University of Texas Southwestern Medical Center
Dallas, Texas

Voiding dysfunctions secondary to degenerative processes, traumas, or neoplasia of the central or peripheral nervous system have had and continue to have a deleterious effect on patients' life and quality of life. For centuries, the prognosis of these pathologies on patient survival was considered as bad. We know from the Edwin Smith papyrus that, as far back as 1600 BC, the ancient Egyptians were aware of the relationship between the nervous system and urinary bladder function.[1] They considered spinal cord trauma as a *disease not to be treated*.[2]

Statistics on spinal cord injury are available since World War I. At the time, the mortality rate was extremely high, greater than 90%, mainly due to urinary complications such as urosepsis and renal insufficiency. Dramatic improvements in prognosis came during World War II when Sir Ludwig Guttmann, in England, established specialized units to care for these patients and introduced the use of intermittent catheterization for lower urinary tract management.[3] During the 1970s, the use of urodynamics became more widespread, allowing a better understanding of the physiology and pathophysiology of the lower urinary tract. In the meantime, better understanding and management of bacterial colonization of the bladder, biofilms, pathophysiology of bacterial infections, and new antibiotics led to a significant decrease in morbidity and mortality due to infections. Furthermore, rehabilitation and surgical and reanimation refinements have recently contributed to improvement of neurogenic bladder (NB) prognosis. Finally, the most recent "revolutionary discovery" in the field was implemented by Schurch in early 2000. Introducing botulinum toxin A intradetrusor injection in the treatment of NB has been called, by Clare Fowler, a renowned English neurologist, "the penicillin of the 20th century," reflecting the major impact that this technique has nowadays on NB management.

The main goals in treating patients with NB dysfunction are threefold:

1. Preserve upper urinary tract integrity
2. Ensure adequate continence
3. Minimize potential complications secondary to neurogenic bladder such as stone formation and urinary infection

Achieving all these goals is not easy without extensive knowledge of anatomy, physiology, pathophysiology, evaluation techniques, various treatments, and a good understanding of the association between NB dysfunctions and other conditions such as pregnancy, benign prostatic hypertrophy, infertility, etc. Summarizing this knowledge is the purpose of this book.

In the last 20 years, as the main editor and instigator of these projects, I have directed and organized the publication of four editions of NB textbooks. The first one in 1996 was in French with a limited diffusion; it was followed in 2003 by the first extensive edition in English. In 2008 and 2016, successive updated editions were published and served as a reference to many health professionals involved in the care of neurogenic patients. Several coeditors shared with me the privilege of spreading wide this knowledge in our medical community. Eric Shick was the coeditor of the first two editions. He is now retired, but I keep the memory of his rigor and extensive understanding of these complex mechanisms—two of many of his qualities but so important in the hard task of editing a textbook. David Ginsberg and Gilles Karsenty helped me with the 2016 edition of the textbook. They are, in my opinion, the best representatives of the present and the future of neuro-urology in North America and Europe.

This edition has changed in many ways. First, and at the request of our publisher who, following market imperatives, we aimed to produce a book that is at least half as thick as our previous editions. We achieved this by asking our authors to limit their writing to the "essentials" of their topics. The second change that we made in this book is the addition of a fourth editor. Thomas M. Kessler has shown leadership and authority with the International Neuro-Urology Society, bringing together everyone interested in the field at a well-organized annual meeting.

The team we formed has worked hard for the success of this new edition. We hope that readers, whatever their level of training or specialty, easily find the answers to their questions.

Thank you to my coeditors, to all authors for their collaboration, respect of deadlines, hard work, and patience. We have together published a piece of art that will be, for the next few years, the reference in neuro-urology, linking all interested health professionals anywhere in the world. Finally, a special thank you goes to my family for having, once again, tolerated me for so many hours in front of the computer, reading, correcting, and editing.

Jacques Corcos MD

Part 1

EPIDEMIOLOGY AND PATHOPHYSIOLOGY OF NEUROGENIC BLADDERS

Chapter 1

EPIDEMIOLOGY OF NEUROGENIC BLADDER

Janine L. Oliver and Evgeniy I. Kreydin

INTRODUCTION

The epidemiology of neurogenic bladder disorders is as diverse as the patients and spectrum of neurologic conditions that cause dysfunction of the lower urinary tract (LUT). It is this diversity and heterogeneity, even within a defined disorder, that make the incidence and prevalence of symptoms, and their impact on patients and society, difficult to describe.

What follows is not an exhaustive list of all neurologic conditions associated with LUT dysfunction, but rather a primer on the epidemiology of neurogenic bladder and common causative neurologic diseases. The reader is encouraged to seek more in-depth information about LUT effects of individual neurologic disorders within this text and elsewhere.

HEALTHCARE UTILIZATION AND ECONOMIC BURDEN

An observation insurance claim–based study by Manah et al. found high healthcare utilization among patients with neurogenic bladder; in the 1-year postindex period, 39% of neurogenic bladder patients visited a urologist, 33.3% were hospitalized, and 23.4% visited an emergency room.[1] Urologic causes accounted for 50% of hospital admissions in this population. Sepsis, obstructive uropathy, and acute renal failure accounted for 7.8%, 5.4%, and 4.2% of hospital admissions, respectively.

Palma-Zamora and Atiemo attempted to quantify the economic impact of such high healthcare utilization. Although concluding that expenditures were difficult to estimate due to the heterogeneity of patients, the authors highlighted that many factors contribute to the high healthcare costs in this condition, including care for the underlying neurological disability, loss of productivity for the patient and family caregivers, and need for specialized and costly therapies.[2] In a

cross-sectional study and cost analysis of the 2006–2015 National Inpatient Sample and Nationwide Emergency Department Sample, the costs of urologic healthcare use in persons with spinal cord injury (SCI) were greater than $4 billion over the study period.[3] Based on these estimates, annual healthcare costs for neurogenic bladder are likely to be in the hundreds of millions of dollars.[2,3]

In addition, neurogenic bladder has significant impacts on the quality of life and psychological well-being of patients. For example, Itoh et al. found that stroke patients with overactive bladder (OAB) symptoms scored significantly lower on the mental well-being of the Short Form Health Survey (SF-8).[4] In a similar study by Pyo et al., stroke patients with OAB failed to show an improvement in their vitality and mental health scores during rehabilitation as compared to their non-OAB counterparts.[5] The impact of neurogenic bladder on mental health in other conditions is less well-understood and probably underappreciated. As a result, the true financial and societal costs of neurogenic bladder are likely to be significantly higher than the estimates.

DISEASES OF THE BRAIN

PARKINSON'S DISEASE AND MULTISYSTEM ATROPHY

Parkinson's disease (PD) and multisystem atrophy (MSA) are both neurodegenerative disorders that affect the substantia nigra of the basal ganglia. Whereas the effects of PD are usually limited to this portion of the central nervous system, MSA can lead to the destruction of a much wider range of neurons, including nuclei in the sacral spinal cord, that control the LUT and sexual function. PD affects nearly 1% of the population above age 60 years, and the prevalence steadily increases with age, where 1 in 40 individuals suffer from PD by age 90 years.[6,7] The prevalence of LUT symptoms (LUTS) among PD patients ranges from 27% to 64%.[8-10] The severity of LUTS in PD tends to correlate with motor dysfunction and progresses with the natural progression of the disease. MSA is a much less common condition and affects 3 per 100,000 persons aged over 50 years in the United States.[11] However, LUTS in MSA tend to be significantly more severe and arise earlier in the course of the disease.

STROKE

Approximately 800,000 cerebrovascular accidents (CVAs or strokes) occur annually in the United States; one-third of stroke victims die as a result, one-third regain a prestroke level of functionality, and one-third remain with a long-term disability.[12] Both urinary incontinence and retention can occur, but storage symptoms tend to be more common. Incontinence is present in 35%–40% of patients 1 week after a stroke, and although some patients show improvement in their voiding dysfunction within a year, 25%–35% remain incontinent.[13]

CEREBRAL PALSY

Cerebral palsy (CP) is the most common cause of childhood-onset, lifelong physical disability in most countries. Primarily a disorder of movement and posture, this condition arises secondary to a permanent, nonprogressive disturbance (such as birth asphyxia) of fetal or infant brain development. The prevalence of CP ranges from 1.5 to slightly above 3 per 100,000 live births.[14] A systematic review found that an average 55.5% of CP patients over a wide range of ages reported one or more LUTS. Storage symptoms were most commonly reported and present in 20%–90% of patients.[15]

OTHER BRAIN DISORDERS

Several other brain disorders can cause or are associated with LUT dysfunction. Normal pressure hydrocephalus (NPH) is a pathological enlargement of the lateral ventricles and can be idiopathic or secondary to an identifiable cause such as a stroke. It is generally a geriatric condition with prevalence of about 6% in those 80 years and older and consists of the classic triad of dementia, gait disturbance, and incontinence.[16] LUTS are very common with more than 90% of NPH subjects reporting incontinence and storage symptoms in two recent studies.[17,18] Cerebral tumors can lead to LUTS when they involve the frontal lobe, the hypothalamus, or the pons. In two older series of frontal lobe tumors, 14% and 28% of respondents reported OAB symptoms with and without incontinence.[19,20]

patients with SCI. Approximately 50% of injuries are functionally complete, and 33% result in tetraplegia. The effect of SCI on the lower urinary tract generally follows a suprasacral/infrasacral pattern, where the former results in detrusor and sphincter overactivity and detrusor-sphincter dyssynergia (DSD), and the latter in detrusor and sphincter underactivity. However, these relationships are far from universal: Weld and Dmochowski assessed urodynamic findings in 243 patients with SCI and found that detrusor overactivity was present in 14% of infrasacral injuries and detrusor areflexia in 21% of suprasacral injuries.[23]

MULTIPLE SCLEROSIS

Multiple sclerosis (MS) is a demyelinating disease that afflicts females two to three times more often than males and has a predilection for Caucasian ancestry.[24] The disease is widespread and accounts for the third most common cause of disability among Americans between 15 and 50 years of age. MS can affect the brain and the spinal cord; thus, symptomatology in MS can be variable. Storage symptoms are common, occurring in 34%–99% of patients. However, voiding symptoms were found in 20% of patients in one study.[25] Several authors have reported on urodynamic findings in MS patients. In the largest meta-analysis published in 1999, Litwiller et al. examined over 1500 patients in 22 studies, finding detrusor overactivity, DSD, and detrusor hypocontractility in 62%, 25%, and 20% of patients, respectively.[26]

OPEN NEURAL TUBE DEFECTS/SPINA BIFIDA AND SACRAL AGENESIS

The incidence of open neural tube defects (ONTDs), also known as spina bifida, has fallen significantly in countries where dietary folic acid fortification was mandated in the 1990s and 2000s. Prevalence in those countries is estimated to be under 40 per 100,000 live births, whereas countries that have not mandated folic acid fortification experience rates as high as 80 per 100,000 live births.[27,28] Urological manifestations of ONTD are variable and the end physiology of the LUT is unpredictable. However, patients with ONTD tend to suffer from urinary incontinence with fewer than 50% reporting being continent.[29] By the time individuals are 16 years old, over 20% have undergone bladder continence surgery, and the majority do not void spontaneously.[30]

DISEASES OF THE SPINAL CORD

DISK DISEASE, SPINAL STENOSIS, AND SPINE SURGERY

SPINAL CORD INJURY

Global prevalence for SCI ranges from 10.4 to 83 cases per million with significant variation among geographic regions.[21,22] Males account for 80% of

The incidence of herniated disk is about 5 to 20 cases per 1000 adults annually. The average age of patients with a herniated disk is around 41 years, and males are slightly more affected than females.[31] The prevalence of myelopathy due to degeneration of the spine is estimated at a minimum of 605 per million in North America.[32] The true incidence of LUT dysfunction associated with disk disease is unknown. Normal urodynamic findings, detrusor overactivity, and detrusor areflexia can be observed.[33,34] Cauda equina syndrome occurs in approximately 1%–5% of cases of lumbar disk herniation. Lumbar spinal stenosis in a severe form can also cause cauda equina compression. Patient symptoms and urodynamic findings vary.[35] In patients with cervical spondylotic myelopathy, poor compliance and detrusor sphincter dyssynergia are common findings.[36]

RADICAL PELVIC SURGERY

LUT dysfunction is not uncommon following surgical treatment of rectal cancer. In a contemporary cohort with median follow-up greater than 2 years, rates of urinary retention were 10.5%, 8.2%, 10.4%, and 8.0% in patients undergoing abdominoperineal resection only, low anterior resection only, surgery with postoperative radiation therapy, and surgery with preoperative radiation therapy, respectively.[37]

Similarly, radical gynecologic surgery is associated with high rates of LUT dysfunction, and greater LUT dysfunction is associated with more radical surgery.[38,39]

DIABETES

Approximately 30 million adults in the United States have diabetes, and diabetic polyneuropathy is the most common neuropathy in developed countries. Clinical neuropathy occurs in approximately 10% of diabetic patients.[40]

LUTS are common in diabetics, and diabetic bladder dysfunction includes a range of LUTS from storage symptoms to complete urinary retention.[41]

INFECTIOUS DISEASE

A variety of infectious diseases can cause neurologic dysfunction and thus neurogenic LUT dysfunction. The overall prevalence of such symptoms is not described well. Many of these infections are geographically focal or may preferentially afflict certain at-risk populations. The authors encourage interested readers to seek information beyond the scope of this text to familiarize themselves with conditions affecting the population they treat.

GUILLAIN-BARRÉ SYNDROME

Guillain-Barré syndrome (GBS) is a rare inflammatory demyelinating disorder of the peripheral somatic and autonomic nervous system. It affects between 1 and 2/100,000 individuals a year.[42] The exact cause is unknown but is postulated to develop after infection. The incidence increases with age, with people older than 50 years at greatest risk. LUT dysfunction occurs in approximately one-third, with underactive detrusor being a common abnormality.[43,44]

HUMAN IMMUNODEFICIENCY VIRUS/ ACQUIRED IMMUNODEFICIENCY SYNDROME

Approximately 1.1 million people are living with human immunodeficiency virus (HIV) in the United States.[45] New HIV diagnoses are relatively stable in the United States. Men who have sex with men are the population most affected by HIV. HIV also disproportionately affects black/African American populations and Hispanic/Latino populations. Voiding dysfunction in patients with acquired immunodeficiency syndrome (AIDS) is usually a result of neurologic complications (such as HIV encephalitis, demyelination disorders, and AIDS-related dementia), including opportunistic infections (such as cerebral toxoplasmosis and cytomegalovirus [CMV] polyradiculopathy), and generally herald a poor prognosis.[46] Urodynamic abnormalities are often identified.[47,48]

LYME DISEASE

Lyme disease is associated with a variety of neurologic abnormalities (termed *neuroborreliosis*), including encephalopathy, polyneuropathy, and leukoencephalitis.[49] Between 2008 and 2015, 275,589 cases of Lyme disease were reported to the Centers for Disease Control and Prevention (CDC), with the majority of cases occurring in the Northeast, mid-Atlantic, and upper Midwest regions of the United States.[50] Presenting symptoms are typically urinary retention or storage symptoms, and urodynamic findings of detrusor overactivity and detrusor areflexia have been described. Of note, these symptoms may be associated with acute radiculitis.[51,52] Neurologic manifestations often improve with antibiotic therapy.[49,53]

HERPES

Herpes zoster and anogenital herpes simplex are known to cause urinary retention.[54,55] This is uncommon and typically transient. Almost one out of three people in the United States will develop herpes zoster during their lifetime. People who are immunosuppressed or immunocompromised and those over the age of 50 years are at increased risk of developing herpes zoster and at increased risk of complications. Herpes zoster rates are increasing among adults gradually. The effects of varicella vaccination are being studied.[56]

SYPHILIS

Since 2000, syphilis rates in the United States have been rising.[57] The rise is attributed to increased cases among men, specifically men who have sex with men. Roughly 10% of patients develop neurosyphilis, which can occur at any stage of the disease and cause voiding dysfunction. Neurosyphilis can present as several clinical syndromes, including meningitis and tabes dorsalis (due to involvement of the dorsal columns of the spinal cord and the dorsal root ganglia), as a late complication. Urodynamic findings include detrusor areflexia, detrusor overactivity, poor compliance, and DSD.[58-60]

REFERENCES

1. Manack, A., S.P. Motsko, C. Haag-Molkenteller et al., Epidemiology and healthcare utilization of neurogenic bladder patients in a us claims database. *Neurourology and Urodynamics*, 2011. 30: p. 395–401.
2. Palma-Zamora, I.D. and H.O. Atiemo, Understanding the Economic Impact of Neurogenic Lower Urinary Tract Dysfunction. *Urologic Clinics of North America*, 2017. 44: p. 333–343.
3. Skelton, F., J.L. Salemi, L. Akpati, et al., Genitourinary Complications Are a Leading and Expensive Cause of Emergency Department and Inpatient Encounters for Persons With Spinal Cord Injury. *Archives of Physical Medicine and Rehabilitation*, 2019.
4. Itoh, Y., S. Yamada, F. Konoeda, et al., Burden of overactive bladder symptom on quality of life in stroke patients. *Neurourol Urodyn*, 2013. 32(5): p. 428–34.
5. Pyo, H., B.R. Kim, M. Park, et al., Effects of Overactive Bladder Symptoms in Stroke Patients' Health Related Quality of Life and Their Performance Scale. *Ann Rehabil Med*, 2017. 41(6): p. 935–943.
6. de Rijk, M.C., L.J. Launer, K. Berger, et al., Prevalence of Parkinson's disease in Europe: A collaborative study of population-based cohorts. Neurologic Diseases in the Elderly Research Group. *Neurology*, 2000. 54(11 Suppl 5): p. S21–3.
7. Gelb, D.J., E. Oliver, and S. Gilman, Diagnostic criteria for Parkinson disease. *Arch Neurol*, 1999. 56(1): p. 33–9.
8. Araki, I. and S. Kuno, Assessment of voiding dysfunction in Parkinson's disease by the international prostate symptom score. *J Neurol Neurosurg Psychiatry*, 2000. 68(4): p. 429–33.
9. Sakakibara, R., F. Tateno, M. Kishi, et al., Pathophysiology of bladder dysfunction in Parkinson's disease. *Neurobiol Dis*, 2012. 46(3): p. 565–71.
10. Siegl, E., B. Lassen, and S. Saxer, [Incontinence--a common issue for people with Parkinson's disease. A systematic literature review]. *Pflege Z*, 2013. 66(9): p. 540–4.
11. Ogawa, T., R. Sakakibara, S. Kuno, et al., Prevalence and treatment of LUTS in patients with Parkinson disease or multiple system atrophy. *Nat Rev Urol*, 2017. 14(2): p. 79–89.
12. Panfili, Z., M. Metcalf, and T.L. Griebling, Contemporary Evaluation and Treatment of Poststroke Lower Urinary Tract Dysfunction. *Urol Clin North Am*, 2017. 44(3): p. 403–414.
13. Brittain, K.R., S.M. Peet, and C.M. Castleden, Stroke and incontinence. *Stroke*, 1998. 29(2): p. 524–8.
14. Graham, H.K., P. Rosenbaum, N. Paneth, et al., Cerebral palsy. *Nat Rev Dis Primers*, 2016. 2: p. 15082.
15. Samijn, B., E. Van Laecke, C. Renson, et al., Lower urinary tract symptoms and urodynamic findings in children and adults with cerebral palsy: A systematic review. *Neurourol Urodyn*, 2017. 36(3): p. 541–549.
16. Jaraj, D., K. Rabiei, T. Marlow, et al., Prevalence of idiopathic normal-pressure hydrocephalus. *Neurology*, 2014. 82(16): p. 1449–54.
17. Krzastek, S.C., W.M. Bruch, S.P. Robinson, et al., Characterization of lower urinary tract symptoms in patients with idiopathic normal pressure hydrocephalus. *Neurourol Urodyn*, 2017. 36(4): p. 1167–1173.
18. Sakakibara, R., T. Kanda, T. Sekido, et al., Mechanism of bladder dysfunction in idiopathic normal pressure hydrocephalus. *Neurourol Urodyn*, 2008. 27(6): p. 507–10.
19. Maurice-Williams, R.S., Micturition symptoms in frontal tumours. *J Neurol Neurosurg Psychiatry*, 1974. 37(4): p. 431–6.
20. Direkze, M., S.G. Bayliss, and J.C. Cutting, Primary tumours of the frontal lobe. *Br J Clin Pract*, 1971. 25(5): p. 207–13.
21. Witiw, C.D. and M.G. Fehlings, Acute Spinal Cord Injury. *J Spinal Disord Tech*, 2015. 28(6): p. 202–10.
22. Jain, N.B., G.D. Ayers, E.N. Peterson, et al., Traumatic spinal cord injury in the United States, 1993-2012. *JAMA*, 2015. 313(22): p. 2236–43.
23. Weld, K.J. and R.R. Dmochowski, Association of level of injury and bladder behavior in patients with post-traumatic spinal cord injury. *Urology*, 2000. 55(4): p. 490–4.
24. Howard, J., S. Trevick, and D.S. Younger, Epidemiology of Multiple Sclerosis. *Neurol Clin*, 2016. 34(4): p. 919–939.
25. Wang, T., W. Huang, and Y. Zhang, Clinical Characteristics and Urodynamic Analysis of Urinary Dysfunction in Multiple Sclerosis. *Chin Med J (Engl)*, 2016. 129(6): p. 645–50.
26. Litwiller, S.E., E.M. Frohman, and P.E. Zimmern, Multiple sclerosis and the urologist. *J Urol*, 1999. 161(3): p. 743–57.
27. Atta, C.A., K.M. Fiest, A.D. Frolkis, et al., Global Birth Prevalence of Spina Bifida by Folic Acid Fortification Status: A Systematic Review and Meta-Analysis. *Am J Public Health*, 2016. 106(1): p. e24–34.
28. Kancherla, V., K. Wagh, Q. Johnson, et al., A 2017 global update on folic acid-preventable spina bifida and anencephaly. *Birth Defects Res*, 2018. 110(14): p. 1139–1147.
29. Freeman, K.A., H. Castillo, J. Castillo, et al., Variation in bowel and bladder continence across US spina bifida programs: A descriptive study. *J Pediatr Rehabil Med*, 2017. 10(3-4): p. 231–241.
30. Liu, T., L. Ouyang, J. Thibadeau, et al., Longitudinal Study of Bladder Continence in Patients with Spina Bifida in the National Spina Bifida Patient Registry. *J Urol*, 2018. 199(3): p. 837–843.

31. Cummins, J., J.D. Lurie, T.D. Tosteson, et al., Descriptive epidemiology and prior healthcare utilization of patients in the Spine Patient Outcomes Research Trial's (SPORT) three observational cohorts: disc herniation, spinal stenosis, and degenerative spondylolisthesis. *Spine*, 2006. 31: p. 806–14.

32. Nouri, A., L. Tetreault, A. Singh, et al., Degenerative Cervical Myelopathy. *Spine*, 2015. 40: p. E675–E693.

33. Bartolin, Z., I. Gilja, G. Bedalov, et al., Bladder function in patients with lumbar intervertebral disk protrusion. *The Journal of urology*, 1998. 159: p. 969–71.

34. Dong, D., Z. Xu, B. Shi, et al., Clinical significance of urodynamic studies in neurogenic bladder dysfunction caused by intervertebral disk hernia. *Neurourology and Urodynamics*, 2006. 25: p. 446–450.

35. Kim, S.-Y., H.C. Kwon, and J.K. Hyun, Detrusor Overactivity in Patients With Cauda Equina Syndrome. *Spine*, 2014. 39: p. E955–E961.

36. Kim, I.S., Y.I. Kim, J.T. Hong, et al., Rationales for a Urodynamic Study in Patients with Cervical Spondylotic Myelopathy. *World Neurosurgery*, 2019. 124: p. e147–e155.

37. Kwaan, M.R., Y. Fan, S. Jarosek, et al., Long-term Risk of Urinary Adverse Events in Curatively Treated Patients With Rectal Cancer: A Population-Based Analysis. *Dis Colon Rectum*, 2017. 60(7): p. 682–690.

38. Derks, M., J. van der Velden, M.M. Frijstein, et al., Long-term Pelvic Floor Function and Quality of Life After Radical Surgery for Cervical Cancer: A Multicenter Comparison Between Different Techniques for Radical Hysterectomy With Pelvic Lymphadenectomy. *Int J Gynecol Cancer*, 2016. 26(8): p. 1538–43.

39. Nantasupha, C. and K. Charoenkwan, Predicting factors for resumption of spontaneous voiding following nerve-sparing radical hysterectomy. *J Gynecol Oncol*, 2018. 29(4): p. e59.

40. Dyck, P.J., K.M. Kratz, J.L. Karnes, et al., The prevalence by staged severity of various types of diabetic neuropathy, retinopathy, and nephropathy in a population-based cohort: the Rochester Diabetic Neuropathy Study. *Neurology*, 1993. 43(4): p. 817–24.

41. Brown, J.S., H. Wessells, M.B. Chancellor, et al., Urologic complications of diabetes. *Diabetes Care*, 2005. 28(1): p. 177–85.

42. McGrogan, A., G.C. Madle, H.E. Seaman, et al., The epidemiology of Guillain-Barre syndrome worldwide. A systematic literature review. *Neuroepidemiology*, 2009. 32(2): p. 150–63.

43. Naphade, P.U., R. Verma, R.K. Garg, et al., Prevalence of bladder dysfunction, urodynamic findings, and their correlation with outcome in Guillain-Barre syndrome. *Neurourology and Urodynamics*, 2012. 31: p. 1135–1140.

44. Sakakibara, R., T. Uchiyama, S. Kuwabara, et al., Prevalence and mechanism of bladder dysfunction in Guillain-Barré Syndrome. *Neurourology and Urodynamics*, 2009. 28: p. 432–437.

45. Linley, L., A.S. Johnson, R. Song, et al. Estimated HIV incidence and prevalence in the United States, 2010-2016. in *HIV Surveillance Supplemental Report*. 2010.

46. Lee, L.K., M.D. Dinneen, and S. Ahmad, The urologist and the patient infected with human immunodeficiency virus or with acquired immunodeficiency syndrome. *BJU international*, 2001. 88: p. 500–10.

47. Kane, C.J., D.M. Bolton, J.A. Connolly, et al., Voiding dysfunction in human immunodeficiency virus infections. *J Urol*, 1996. 155(2): p. 523–6.

48. Khan, Z., V.K. Singh, and W.C. Yang, Neurogenic bladder in acquired immune deficiency syndrome (AIDS). *Urology*, 1992. 40: p. 289–291.

49. Logigian, E.L., R.F. Kaplan, and A.C. Steere, Chronic Neurologic Manifestations of Lyme Disease. *New England Journal of Medicine*, 1990. 323: p. 1438–1444.

50. Schwartz, A.M., A.F. Hinckley, P.S. Mead, et al., Surveillance for Lyme Disease - United States, 2008-2015. *Morbidity and mortality weekly report. Surveillance summaries (Washington, D.C. : 2002)*, 2017. 66: p. 1–12.

51. Dupeyron, A., J. Lecocq, B. Jaulhac, et al., Sciatica, disk herniation, and neuroborreliosis. A report of four cases. *Joint Bone Spine*, 2004. 71: p. 433–437.

52. Finsterer, J., J. Dauth, K. Angel, et al., Dysuria, Urinary Retention, and Inguinal Pain as Manifestation of Sacral Bannwarth Syndrome. *Case Reports in Medicine, 2015*. 2015: p. 1–4.

53. Chancellor, M.B., D.E. McGinnis, P.J. Shenot, et al., Urinary dysfunction in Lyme disease. *The Journal of urology*, 1993. 149: p. 26–30.

54. Caplan, L.R., F.J. Kleeman, and S. Berg, Urinary Retention Probably Secondary to Herpes Genitalis. *New England Journal of Medicine*, 1977. 297: p. 920–921.

55. Yamanishi, T., K. Yasuda, R. Sakakibara, et al., Urinary retention due to herpes virus infections. *Neurourology and urodynamics*, 1998. 17: p. 613–9.

56. Wolfson, L.J., V.J. Daniels, A. Altland, et al., The Impact of Varicella Vaccination on the Incidence of Varicella and Herpes Zoster in the United States: Updated Evidence From Observational Databases, 1991-2016. *Clinical Infectious Diseases*, 2019.

57. Peterman, T.A., J. Su, K.T. Bernstein, et al., Syphilis in the United States: on the rise? *Expert Review of Anti-infective Therapy*, 2015. 13: p. 161–168.

58. Garber, S.J., T.J. Christmas, and D. Rickards, Voiding dysfunction due to neurosyphilis. *British journal of urology*, 1990. 66: p. 19–21.

59. Hattori, T., K. Yasuda, K. Kita, et al., Disorders of micturition in tabes dorsalis. *British journal of urology*, 1990. 65: p. 497–9.

60. Wheeler, J.S., D.J. Culkin, R.J. O'Hara, et al., Bladder dysfunction and neurosyphilis. *The Journal of urology*, 1986. 136: p. 903–5.

Chapter 2

PATHOPHYSIOLOGY OF DETRUSOR OVERACTIVITY

Sachin Malde and Jalesh N. Panicker

INTRODUCTION

The two principal functions of the lower urinary tract (LUT) are to act as a continent, low-pressure reservoir for the storage of urine, followed by periodic, voluntary, complete bladder emptying (voiding) also at low pressure. This is achieved through coordinated activity of the bladder and bladder outlet, controlled by a complex neural network distributed centrally (central nervous system [CNS]) and peripherally (peripheral nervous system [PNS]). Therefore, LUT functions are susceptible to different neurologic disorders, with potential symptoms ranging from urinary incontinence (storage dysfunction) to urinary retention (voiding dysfunction).[1] The manifestations of LUT dysfunction depend on the site, extent, and nature of the neurologic lesion.

Overactive bladder (OAB) is a symptom syndrome defined as urinary urgency, with or without urgency incontinence, usually with increased daytime frequency and nocturia.[2] OAB symptoms can arise in a patient with neurologic disease, when it is called neurogenic OAB, or can arise in a patient without neurologic disease where the etiology is uncertain, when called idiopathic OAB. Often, but not always, OAB is associated with the urodynamic observation of detrusor overactivity (DO), whatever the etiology of OAB is (neurogenic or idiopathic). Urgency (and OAB syndrome) can exist without urodynamically demonstrable DO, and DO can also exist in patients without any symptoms. This may occur in patients with a neurological disease that impairs sensory pathways (i.e., complete thoracic spinal cord lesion).

The pathologic mechanisms underlying neurogenic detrusor overactivity (NDO) may be classified into (1) abnormally increased afferent activity from the bladder and urethra, or (2) abnormal handling of afferent signals in the brain.[3] Two hypotheses have been proposed to explain increased afferent activity and therefore OAB symptoms—the urothelium-based hypothesis and the myogenic hypothesis. Abnormal handling of afferent signals in the brain is thought to be the result of damage to central inhibitory pathways leading to activation of voiding reflexes, resulting in DO (neurogenic hypothesis). These pathophysiologic mechanisms are discussed further in this chapter.

UROTHELIUM-BASED HYPOTHESIS

The urothelium and suburothelium is a metabolically active integrated functional unit that plays an important role in modulating bladder activity. The urothelium consists of an apical layer (in contact with the urine) and a basal layer (in contact with suburothelium/lamina propria) that lie in close proximity to the suburothelial myofibroblasts and afferent nerve fibers located in the lamina propria (Figure 2.1). The urothelium has been shown to express numerous sensory receptors and ion channels, including receptors for bradykinin, neurotrophins, cholinergic, adrenergic and purinergic receptors, epithelial sodium channels (ENaC), and transient receptor potential channels. These receptors allow the urothelium to respond to local chemical and mechanical stimuli resulting in neurotransmitter release and changes in the sensitivity of suburothelial fibroblasts, leading to increased afferent nerve activity.[4]

ATP has been shown to be an important excitatory transmitter resulting in urgency and/or NDO. A significantly higher amount of ATP was shown to be released from the bladder tissue of patients with NDO compared to control bladder tissue in vitro, in response to both mechanical stretch and electric field stimulation.[5] Although ATP was released from urothelial cells and myofibroblasts, the application of tetradotoxin (TTx) (a sodium channel blocker that prevents release of neurotransmitters) resulted in a reduction in the amount of ATP released, suggesting that in patients with NDO most ATP release originates from afferent nerves. Immunohistochemical analysis of bladder tissue from patients with NDO revealed increased numbers of suburothelial nerve fibers immunoreactive to P2X3 in patients with NDO

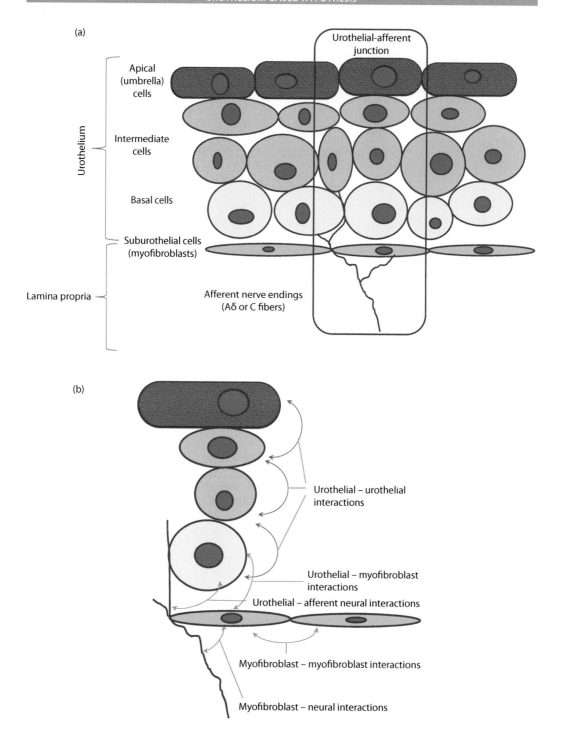

Figure 2.1 (a) Structure of bladder urothelium/suburothelium; (b) urothelial-afferent junction interactions.

compared to controls,[6] suggesting that the action of ATP on P2X receptors leads to excitability of adjacent afferent nerves. In a rat model of chronic spinal cord injury (SCI), urothelial ATP release was significantly higher compared to controls[7]; in a rat model of early SCI, intravesical application of a P2X2/3R antagonist attenuated electrical bladder activity.[8] Pharmacologic agents that are known to improve OAB symptoms in humans may also act via inhibition of ATP. Abnormally elevated levels of ATP in SCI rats were reduced after treatment with botulinum toxin,[9] and recently sildenafil was shown to suppress neuronal ATP release and nerve-mediated contractions in the bladders of spinal cord transected mice, further demonstrating the role of ATP in the pathophysiology of NDO and OAB.[10]

Suburothelial myofibroblasts are in close proximity to afferent C-fibers and have also been shown to contribute to NDO. Myofibroblasts form a functional syncytium with intercellular communication via connexin 43 (Cx43) gap junctions. Increased Cx43 immunoreactivity was found in bladder biopsies from patients with NDO compared to controls,[11] and inhibitors of Cx43 and Cx45 significantly inhibited carbachol-induced contractions of bladder strips from patients with NDO.[12] Furthermore, myofibroblasts have also been shown to generate an intracellular Ca^{2+} transient in response to ATP, and this may be another mechanism by which afferent activity is amplified in response to ATP or other transmitters.[13]

In summary, upregulation of sensory receptors and increased release of neurotransmitters may result in increased afferent activity, and afferent nerve sensitization, resulting in urgency and/or NDO.

MYOGENIC HYPOTHESIS

It is thought that patchy denervation of the detrusor smooth muscle may also contribute to NDO through increased excitability and coupling between myocytes, and thereby propagation of electrical activity across the bladder resulting in a coordinated contraction of the whole bladder.[14] Furthermore, physiologic "micromotions" (local bladder contractions) have been shown to occur in the human bladder, but in patients with DO it is thought that these micromotions are exaggerated and become synchronized into an active contraction.[15] These local contractions in the bladder wall have been shown to generate afferent discharge.[16] Patchy postjunctional denervation has been detected in the detrusor muscle of patients with NDO[17] compared to controls, and NDO muscle strips were found to have a heightened sensitivity to muscarinic agonists.[18]

NEUROGENIC HYPOTHESIS

According to the neurogenic hypothesis, abnormal handling of afferent signals in the brain can lead to OAB and NDO. Functional brain imaging has recently emerged as a useful tool for understanding neural activity in different brain cortical regions and has been used to study the control of LUT functions. Functional magnetic resonance imaging (MRI) studies with simultaneous urodynamics performed in elderly women with urgency incontinence have shown weaker activity in the prefrontal cortex, and those who had DO showed in the scanner less deactivation in the parahippocampal complex and stronger activation in supplementary motor area and adjacent regions, suggesting a compensatory response to failure of control elsewhere.[19]

In health, storage of urine is dependent on spinal reflex mechanisms that activate sympathetic and somatic pathways to the urethral outlet, and tonic inhibitory systems in the brain that suppress the parasympathetic excitatory outflow to the urinary bladder. Damage to central inhibitory pathways or sensitization of peripheral afferent terminals in the bladder can unmask primitive voiding reflexes and be expressed as spontaneous involuntary contractions of the detrusor.[20] Different pathophysiologic mechanisms underpin DO according to the level of neurologic lesion (Figure 2.2).[21,22]

SUPRAPONTINE DAMAGE

The results of brain transection studies in experimental animals suggest that suprapontine centers exert a tonic inhibitory influence on the pontine micturition center.[23] In humans, a working model of LUT control has been proposed based on the results of different functional brain imaging studies.[24] A network of key higher brain centers including the insular cortex, anterior cingulate gyrus, and prefrontal cortex provides a level of control of the LUT, which is responsible for conscious perception of sensations of bladder fullness, volitional control of storage, and voiding and emotional responses.[25,26] The suppression of the micturition reflex is compromised following damage to central inhibitory pathways, and reduced suprapontine inhibition results in the emergence of DO. In the rat cerebral infarction model, bladder overactivity has been shown to be mediated by N-methyl-D-aspartate (NMDA) receptor-mediated glutamatergic and D2 receptor-mediated excitatory activity. An alteration in dopaminergic-glutamatergic activity results in upregulation of excitatory pathways and downregulation of tonic inhibitory pathways.[27]

Alteration in dopaminergic activity has been shown to be responsible for DO in Parkinson's disease (PD). In health, the micturition reflex is under tonic dopaminergic regulation through D1 receptors, and depletion of neurons in the substantia nigra results in loss of D1-mediated inhibition and thereby DO.[28] A γ-aminobutyric acid (GABA)-ergic mechanism is also involved in the tonic dopaminergic regulation of the micturition reflex, and studies in 6-OHDA-lesioned rats, suggesting that dysfunction of GABAergic regulation underlying the micturition reflex results in bladder overactivity.[29] The adenosine A2A receptor-mediated excitatory mechanism is

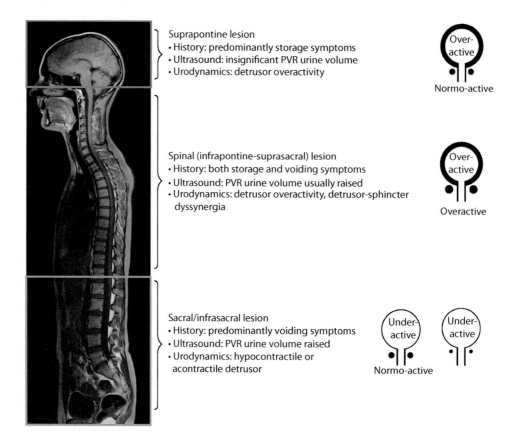

Suprapontine lesion
• History: predominantly storage symptoms
• Ultrasound: insignificant PVR urine volume
• Urodynamics: detrusor overactivity

Over-active

Normo-active

Spinal (infrapontine-suprasacral) lesion
• History: both storage and voiding symptoms
• Ultrasound: PVR urine volume usually raised
• Urodynamics: detrusor overactivity, detrusor-sphincter dyssynergia

Over-active

Overactive

Sacral/infrasacral lesion
• History: predominantly voiding symptoms
• Ultrasound: PVR urine volume raised
• Urodynamics: hypocontractile or acontractile detrusor

Under-active Under-active

Normo-active

Figure 2.2 The pattern of lower urinary tract dysfunction following neurologic disease is influenced by the site of lesion. PVR, postvoid residual. (From Panicker JN et al. *Lancet Neurol.* 2015;14[7]:720–32.)

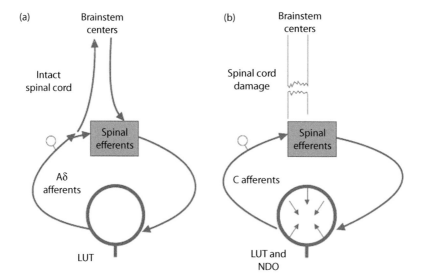

Figure 2.3 Two types of afferent nerves convey sensations of bladder filling. (a) In health, thinly myelinated Ad fibers have a lower threshold for activation and are responsible for conveying sensations of bladder filling. Whereas, unmyelinated C-fibers have a greater threshold for activation and are thought to be quiescent. (b) Following spinal cord damage, C-fibers become sensitized and are mechanosensitive at lower bladder volumes. A segmental spinal reflex emerges that is mediated by C-fiber afferent nerves and results in involuntary detrusor contractions, the basis for NDO. LUT, lower urinary tract; NDO, neurogenic detrusor overactivity. (From Panicker JN and Seth JH. *BJU Int.* 2013;112[1]:129–30.)

enhanced at a supraspinal site to induce bladder overactivity, and A2A receptor inhibition effectively suppresses bladder overactivity in rats with PD.[30] In positron emission tomography (PET), brain regions that are activated during DO following bladder filling tasks in patients with PD include the cerebellum, periaqueductal gray, supplementary motor area, insula, putamen, and thalamus. This pattern is different from healthy controls, and the alteration in brain activation sites in response to bladder filling suggests that different cortical and subcortical regions are involved in the pathogenesis of OAB and DO in PD.[31]

SPINAL CORD LESIONS

Spinal reflex pathways emerge following damage to the suprasacral spinal cord that trigger bladder overactivity. Afferent nerves conveying sensations from the LUT to the spinal cord contain unmyelinated C-fibers that have a much greater threshold for activation and are therefore quiescent in health (Figure 2.3). Following SCI, C-fibers become sensitized and are mechanosensitive at lower bladder volumes.[1] It has been shown in experimental animal models of SCI that a C-fiber afferent mediated segmental spinal reflex emerges, resulting in involuntary detrusor contractions at low bladder volumes (Figure 2.2).[32,33] The density of expression of capsaicin-sensitive TRPV1 receptors and P2X3 is increased in suburothelial nerves and basal layers of the urothelium and is thought to play a critical role in the pathogenesis of DO following SCI.[34] Clinical trials have shown the efficacy of capsaicin[35] and its ultrapotent analog resiniferatoxin[36] in managing DO. Upregulation of TRPA1 protein and mRNA levels has also been demonstrated in rat SCI models.[37]

CONCLUSION

The lower urinary tract is susceptible to different neurologic conditions, and clinical manifestations are dependent upon the location, nature, and extent of the lesion. Evidence from animal and human studies suggests that the pathophysiologic mechanisms underlying OAB and/or detrusor overactivity are multifactorial and complex. Increased afferent activity and abnormal handling of afferent signals are the two predominant pathologic mechanisms that may lead to OAB and/or DO. Increased afferent activity may be the result of changes in urothelial, suburothelial, and myocyte function, whereas damage to central inhibitory pathways may lead to activation of primitive voiding reflexes, resulting in DO. It is likely that multiple factors contribute to varying degrees.

ACKNOWLEDGMENTS

JNP is supported by the National Institute for Health Research University College London Hospitals Biomedical Research Centre (NIHR BRC UCLH/UCL).

REFERENCES

1. Fowler CJ, Griffiths D, and de Groat WC. The neural control of micturition. *Nat Rev Neurosci.* 2008;9(6):453–66.
2. Abrams P, Cardozo L, Fall M et al. The standardisation of terminology of lower urinary tract function: Report from the Standardisation Sub-committee of the International Continence Society. *Neurourol Urodyn.* 2002;21(2):167–78.
3. Chapple C. Chapter 2: Pathophysiology of neurogenic detrusor overactivity and the symptom complex of "overactive bladder". *Neurourol Urodyn.* 2014;33(Suppl 3):S6–13.
4. Birder LA. Urinary bladder urothelium: Molecular sensors of chemical/thermal/mechanical stimuli. *Vascul Pharmacol.* 2006;45(4):221–6.
5. Kumar V, Chapple CR, Rosario D, Tophill PR, and Chess-Williams R. *In vitro* release of adenosine triphosphate from the urothelium of human bladders with detrusor overactivity, both neurogenic and idiopathic. *Eur Urol.* 2010;57(6):1087–92.
6. Brady CM, Apostolidis A, Yiangou Y et al. P2X3-immunoreactive nerve fibres in neurogenic detrusor overactivity and the effect of intravesical resiniferatoxin. *Eur Urol.* 2004;46(2):247–53.
7. Smith CP, Gangitano DA, Munoz A et al. Botulinum toxin type A normalizes alterations in urothelial ATP and NO release induced by chronic spinal cord injury. *Neurochem Int.* 2008;52(6):1068–75.
8. Salazar BH, Hoffman KA, Zhang C et al. Modulatory effects of intravesical P2X2/3 purinergic receptor inhibition on lower urinary tract electromyographic properties and voiding function of female rats with moderate or severe spinal cord injury. *BJU Int.* 2019;123(3):538–47.
9. Khera M, Somogyi GT, Kiss S, Boone TB, and Smith CP. Botulinum toxin A inhibits ATP release from bladder urothelium after chronic spinal cord injury. *Neurochem Int.* 2004;45(7):987–93.
10. Chakrabarty B, Ito H, Ximenes M et al. Influence of sildenafil on the purinergic components of nerve-mediated and urothelial ATP release from the bladder of normal and spinal cord injured mice. *Br J Pharmacol.* 2019;176(13):2227–37.
11. Roosen A, Datta SN, Chowdhury RA et al. Suburothelial myofibroblasts in the human overactive bladder and the effect of botulinum neurotoxin type A treatment. *Eur Urol.* 2009;55(6):1440–8.
12. Phe V, Behr-Roussel D, Oger-Roussel S et al. Involvement of connexins 43 and 45 in functional mechanism of human detrusor overactivity in neurogenic bladder. *Urology.* 2013;81(5):1108.e1–6.
13. Fry CH, Sui GP, Kanai AJ, and Wu C. The function of suburothelial myofibroblasts in the bladder. *Neurourol Urodyn.* 2007;26(6 Suppl):914–9.

14. Brading AF. A myogenic basis for the overactive bladder. *Urology*. 1997;50(6A Suppl):57–67; discussion 8–73.

15. Drake MJ, Mills IW, and Gillespie JI. Model of peripheral autonomous modules and a myovesical plexus in normal and overactive bladder function. *Lancet (London, England)*. 2001;358(9279):401–3.

16. Coolsaet BL, Van Duyl WA, Van Os-Bossagh P, and De Bakker HV. New concepts in relation to urge and detrusor activity. *Neurourol Urodyn*. 1993;12(5):463–71.

17. Drake MJ, Gardner BP, and Brading AF. Innervation of the detrusor muscle bundle in neurogenic detrusor overactivity. *BJU Int*. 2003;91(7):702–10.

18. Stevens LA, Chapple CR, and Chess-Williams R. Human idiopathic and neurogenic overactive bladders and the role of M2 muscarinic receptors in contraction. *Eur Urol*. 2007;52(2):531–8.

19. Tadic SD, Griffiths D, Schaefer W, Murrin A, Clarkson B, and Resnick NM. Brain activity underlying impaired continence control in older women with overactive bladder. *Neurourol Urodyn*. 2012;31(5):652–8.

20. de Groat WC. A neurologic basis for the overactive bladder. *Urology*. 1997;50(6A Suppl):36–52; discussion 3–6.

21. Panicker JN, Fowler CJ, and Kessler TM. Lower urinary tract dysfunction in the neurological patient: Clinical assessment and management. *Lancet Neurol*. 2015;14(7):720–32.

22. Panicker JN, de Sèze M, and Fowler CJ. Rehabilitation in practice: Neurogenic lower urinary tract dysfunction and its management. *Clin Rehabil*. 2010;24(7):579–89.

23. Ruch TC and Tang PC. Localization of brain stem and diencephalic areas controlling the micturation reflex. *J Comp Neurol*. 1956;106(1):213–45.

24. Griffiths D. Functional imaging of structures involved in neural control of the lower urinary tract. *Handb Clin Neurol*. 2015;130:121–33.

25. Fowler CJ and Griffiths DJ. A decade of functional brain imaging applied to bladder control. *Neurourol Urodyn*. 2010;29(1):49–55.

26. Griffiths D and Tadic SD. Bladder control, urgency, and urge incontinence: Evidence from functional brain imaging. *Neurourol Urodyn*. 2008;27(6):466–74.

27. Yokoyama O, Yoshiyama M, Namiki M, and de Groat WC. Changes in dopaminergic and glutamatergic excitatory mechanisms of micturition reflex after middle cerebral artery occlusion in conscious rats. *Exp Neurol*. 2002;173(1):129–35.

28. Yoshimura N, Kuno S, Chancellor MB, De Groat WC, and Seki S. Dopaminergic mechanisms underlying bladder hyperactivity in rats with a unilateral 6-hydroxydopamine (6-OHDA) lesion of the nigrostriatal pathway. *Br J Pharmacol*. 2003;139(8):1425–32.

29. Kitta T, Matsumoto M, Tanaka H, Mitsui T, Yoshioka M, and Nonomura K. GABAergic mechanism mediated via D receptors in the rat periaqueductal gray participates in the micturition reflex: An *in vivo* microdialysis study. *Eur J Neurosci*. 2008;27(12):3216–25.

30. Kitta T, Chancellor MB, de Groat WC, Kuno S, Nonomura K, and Yoshimura N. Suppression of bladder overactivity by adenosine A2A receptor antagonist in a rat model of Parkinson disease. *J Urol*. 2012;187(5):1890–7.

31. Kitta T, Kakizaki H, Furuno T et al. Brain activation during detrusor overactivity in patients with Parkinson's disease: A positron emission tomography study. *J Urol*. 2006;175(3 Pt 1):994–8.

32. Panicker JN and Seth JH. C-fibre sensory nerves— Not so silent as we think? *BJU Int*. 2013;112(1):129–30.

33. de Groat WC, Kawatani M, Hisamitsu T et al. Mechanisms underlying the recovery of urinary bladder function following spinal cord injury. *J Auton Nerv Syst*. 1990;30(Suppl):S71–7.

34. Birder LA and de Groat WC. Mechanisms of disease: Involvement of the urothelium in bladder dysfunction. *Nat Clin Pract Urol*. 2007;4(1):46–54.

35. Fowler CJ, Beck RO, Gerrard S, Betts CD, and Fowler CG. Intravesical capsaicin for treatment of detrusor hyperreflexia. *J Neurol Neurosurg Psychiatry*. 1994;57(2):169–73.

36. de Seze M, Wiart L, de Seze MP et al. Intravesical capsaicin versus resiniferatoxin for the treatment of detrusor hyperreflexia in spinal cord injured patients: A double-blind, randomized, controlled study. *J Urol*. 2004;171(1):251–5.

37. Andrade EL, Forner S, Bento AF et al. TRPA1 receptor modulation attenuates bladder overactivity induced by spinal cord injury. *Am J Physiol Renal Physiol*. 2011;300(5):F1223–34.

Chapter 3

PATHOPHYSIOLOGY OF DETRUSOR UNDERACTIVITY/ACONTRACTILE DETRUSOR

Juan José Andino and John T. Stoffel

INTRODUCTION

According to the standardization of terminology from the International Continence Society, detrusor underactivity (DU) is urodynamically defined as a contraction of reduced strength and/or duration, resulting in prolonged bladder emptying and/or a failure to achieve complete bladder emptying within a normal time span. Acontractile detrusor (AD) is one that cannot be demonstrated to contract during urodynamic studies.[1]

PHYSIOLOGY OF UNDERACTIVE/ ACONTRACTILE BLADDER

The detrusor is made up of overlapping layers of smooth muscle that require parasympathetic stimulation to initiate detrusor contractions and generate the pressure necessary for micturition. In addition to muscle, the bladder has an extracellular matrix that is composed of approximately 50% collagen (type I and III) and 2% elastin. This matrix provides the viscoelastic properties that allow the bladder to stretch and accommodate urine at low pressures.[2] The importance of this matrix in bladder physiology is understood by studying the changes that occur to it through both normal aging and pathologic conditions. In poorly compliant bladders, the extracellular matrix becomes less elastic due to an increase in the ratio of type III versus type I collagen. These changes result in a more rigid bladder wall with decreased capacity and contractility, which may contribute in some patients to detrusor underactivity.[3,4]

Detrusor underactivity may also be related to loss of neurologic signaling mechanisms. Explanations for decreased detrusor activity require an understanding of the connections between the bladder, peripheral nervous system, and central nervous system. Bladder afferents connect the detrusor to the spinal cord through myelinated A-delta and unmyelinated C fibers at the level of S2-S4, relaying information regarding pressure, wall tension (A), and pain/temperature (C).

This information is carried through the spinothalamic tract in the spinal cord to the periaqueductal gray (PAG) region in the brain. After processing multiple inputs from the frontal cortex, limbic system, and other key areas, the PAG removes inhibition of the pontine micturition center (PMC) when it is an appropriate time to void. The PMC can then drive efferent signaling at the S2-S4 level, resulting in parasympathetic stimulation of the detrusor through the pelvic nerve. When inhibition of the PMC is intact, sympathetic stimulation maintains the bladder in a relaxed, storage state. Lesions along any aspect of these neurologic pathways can result in urinary retention from an underactive bladder due to loss of appropriate coordination between parasympathetic and sympathetic stimulation.[5,6] Table 3.1 lists some neurologic conditions associated with DU/AD.

Alternatively, or even in conjunction with neurologic causes, detrusor underactivity physiology could develop after long-standing bladder outlet obstruction. It is thought that bladder outlet obstruction can cause injury to detrusor smooth muscle or afferent neurologic signaling that then results in decreased detrusor activity. Models suggest that chronic strain from obstruction results in stiffening of the extracellular matrix due to an increase in type III collagen and the ratio of collagen to smooth muscle, thereby limiting bladder contractility. Concomitantly, increased bladder pressures can result in ischemia and reperfusion that injure intramural neurons and result in patchy denervation.[2,3,7] Table 3.2 lists some bladder outlet conditions associated with DU/AD.

EVALUATION OF UNDERACTIVE/ ACONTRACTILE BLADDER

The overarching themes when evaluating patients for DU/AD are focused on safety and quality of life. Safety issues, such as hydronephrosis and urinary tract infections (UTIs), are generally addressed first. Quality of life issues, such as urinary symptoms, are treated for improvement while maintaining good patient safety (Figure 3.1).

Table 3.1 Neurogenic Conditions Associated with Underactive/Acontractile Bladder

Cerebrovascular accident (CVA)	Urinary retention is common after the initial episode, most commonly due to AD. All cerebellar infarcts result in AD, reinforcing the importance of an intact PAG to PMC signaling pathway.[8–10]
Parkinson's disease	DU/AD was reported in up to 16% of patients.[11] This could relate to the use of antiparkinsonian drugs that can affect bladder function or involvement of the autonomic nervous system in advanced Parkinson's disease, possibly resulting in loss of parasympathetic stimulation of the bladder.[12,13]
Injury to spinal cord	Lumbosacral spinal cord injury and herniated lumbar intervertebral disk are the two most common etiologic factors that are associated with underactive bladder and urinary retention. Patients with more caudal spinal cord injuries have a higher probability of demonstrating an acontractile detrusor on urodynamics and those with cranial injuries more likely to have detrusor overactivity.[14]
Injury to pelvic plexus	Usually iatrogenic, most often occurring after major abdominal and pelvic surgery such as abdominoperineal resection or hysterectomy.[15,16] Up to 80% of patients resume normal voiding within 6 months.[17–19]
Spina bifida	More than 90% of children have bladder dysfunction, and up to 35% of patients have DU.[20] Bladder physiology is not stable, and lower urinary tract dysfunction can occur later in life. Evaluation is needed when patients develop new urinary retention or incontinence.[5,21]
Diabetic cystopathy	Most common cause of peripheral neuropathy in North America and Europe and up to 59% of patients report lower urinary tract symptoms, including DU/DA, due to sensory and motor neuropathy.[22–32]
Multiple sclerosis	Urinary involvement may be a part of the presenting symptom complex in up to 15% of patients, with acute retention or onset of urgency and frequency.[35] DU/AD was reported up to 30% in cases when plaques involve lumbosacral lesions.[23,24]
Herpes zoster and herpes simplex	Viral infection of the sacral nerve roots may be associated with DU/AD . This is temporary and spontaneously resolves over several months.[25,26]
Guillain-Barré syndrome	25% of patients have urinary symptoms with retention of urine occurring in the early stages of the disease due to DU.[27]
Acquired immune deficiency syndrome (AIDS)	Neurologic involvement occurs in as many as 40% of patients with AIDS; the most common urologic manifestation is urinary retention from suspected DU/AD.[28]

Table 3.2 Bladder Outlet Obstruction Associated with Development of Underactive/Acontractile Bladder

Long-standing bladder outlet obstruction can result in detrusor underactivity because of extracellular matrix changes and ischemic neuropathy within the bladder	
Benign prostatic enlargement/ prostate cancer	Nodules of benign prostatic tissue result in benign prostatic enlargement (BPE), causing urethral compression and therefore bladder outlet obstruction (BOO). Less commonly, obstruction may be attributed to locally advance prostate cancer.[29–31]
Stricture/bladder neck contracture	Occurs most commonly due to trauma, infections such as urethritis and lichen sclerosis, or changes associated with radiation therapy.[32]
Urinary retention in the populations below usually does not result in detrusor acontractility because the degree of obstruction is not as severe.	
Pelvic organ prolapse (POP)	Protrusion of the pelvic organs (uterus, bladder, and bowel) into or past the vaginal introitus.[33] In women with POP extending beyond the hymen, voiding dysfunction symptoms may be reported due to kinking of the urethra when prolapse is maximally everted.[34]
Dysfunctional voiding	Defined as intermittent and/or fluctuating flow rate due to involuntary intermittent contractions of the periurethral striated muscle during voiding in neurologically normal individuals..[1]
Fowler's syndrome	Failure of urethral sphincter relaxation, most typically seen in young women.[35]

Abbreviations: AD, acontractile detrusor; DU, detrusor underactivity; PAG, periaqueductal gray; PMC, pontine micturition center.

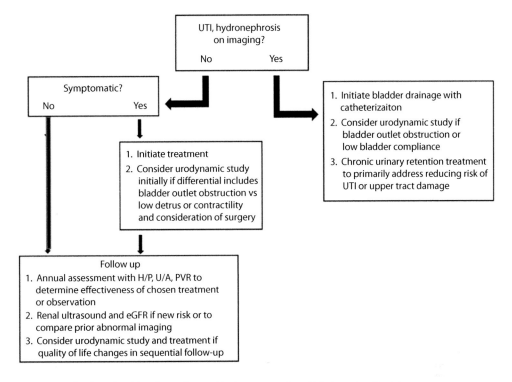

Figure 3.1   Evaluation algorithm for patients with detrusor underactivity/acontractile detrusor.

Patients who present with morbidity from DU/AD urinary retention, such as urinary tract infection or renal failure, should have the bladder drained as the initial step.[7,36,37] After the patient is stabilized and safety issues are addressed, evaluation should focus on identifying underlying physiology and any associated urinary symptoms. Clear categories of patients who may benefit from UDS studies include (1) those in whom additional information is necessary in order to make an accurate diagnosis and direct therapeutic decisions and (2) those whose lower urinary tract (LUT) condition may have the potential to cause deleterious and irreversible effects on the upper urinary tracts.[38] To this end, urodynamics are a vital tool in the evaluation of DU/AD-related urinary retention.

Classically, AD is demonstrated on urodynamics when a patient attempts to initiate voiding and no changes in detrusor pressure occur (Figure 3.2).

Detrusor underactivity requires an assessment of detrusor strength during contraction versus flow of urine. For example, a patient who generates 10 cm

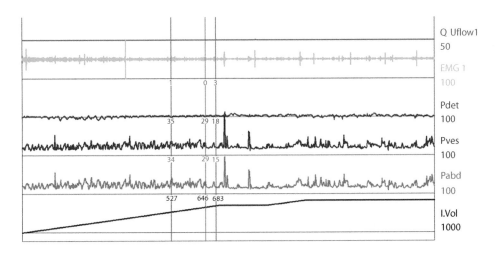

Figure 3.2   Example of an acontractile detrusor with a "flat" cystometrogram (CMG).[39] Once permission to void is given, Pves does not increase, and there is no visible detrusor contraction.

H_2O detrusor pressure during contraction but who voids to completion and reports no urinary symptoms should not be treated for detrusor underactivity. However, patients with low detrusor contractility and urinary symptoms fall under the detrusor underactivity umbrella. Urodynamic nomograms using pressure flow measurements can be helpful in differentiating obstruction from underactivity. For example, the Bladder Outlet Obstruction Index (BOOI: P_{det} @ $Q_{max} - 2 Q_{max}$) can be used. In this nomogram, BOOI less than 20 generally rules out urinary obstruction, and BOOI greater than 40 is suggestive of obstruction.[40]

In addition to urodynamics, imaging can help identify high-risk features of urinary retention including hydronephrosis, hydroureter, and/or bladder stones.[37]

MANAGEMENT OF UNDERACTIVE/ ACONTRACTILE BLADDER

There is no established pathway for the treatment of symptomatic DU/AD. Patients should be counseled that treatment is usually a step-wise progression that focuses on improvement of symptoms, not numerical changes in postvoid residual or increase in detrusor contractility (Figure 3.3).

BEHAVIORAL THERAPY
Scheduling voiding and double voiding may be a suitable conservative option in patients with low risk or asymptomatic chronic urinary retention. There is no conclusive data that demonstrate effectiveness of pelvic floor exercises, but a referral to physical therapy is reasonable if the patient reports previous pelvic floor dysfunction or pain.

MEDICATIONS
Despite the existence of muscarinic agonists and cholinesterase inhibitors, very few studies have shown efficacy of these agents in DU/AD.[41] Bethanechol has been studied and showed no improvement in patients with detrusor underactivity.[42,43] These medications also have undesirable side effects including nausea, vomiting, diarrhea, visual impairment, headaches, bronchospasms, and even severe cardiovascular events that limit their use. Alpha-1 blockers may have some benefit if concomitant BOO is present.[44]

CATHETERIZATION
Bladder drainage may be achieved with clean intermittent catheterization or an indwelling catheter. Although there are no data-based recommendations on how often to catheterize, the authors recommend a catheterization schedule that focuses on improvement of symptoms while preserving patient safety. For example, if a patient is bothered by nocturia only, catheterization before bed may result in significant improvement in quality of life. It is important to consider potential complications from starting catheterization when prescribing this treatment. In a retrospective study of 308 patients with spinal cord injury followed over 18 years, upper tract changes were more frequent in patients with indwelling catheters (18%) compared to those using intermittent catheterization (IC) (6.5%) and fewer long-term complications were associated with IC.[45,46] In patients with indwelling catheters, suprapubic placement often provides a more feasible option and prevents urethral damage. The risk of stones and symptomatic infections is likely unchanged with suprapubic location compared to urethral catheters. The risk of malignancy secondary to indwelling catheters should be discussed prior to committing to this management strategy.[47] Continent stoma may be an option for patients unable to perform intermittent catheterization per urethra. Common

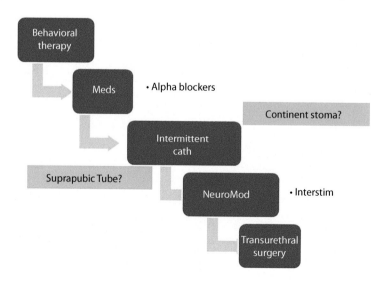

Figure 3.3   General treatment algorithm for DU/AD. (Adapted from AUA Chronic Urinary Retention white paper.[37])

stoma techniques employ appendix, small bowel, or bladder flaps.[48] Ultimately, bladder management has to be individualized based on the patient's mobility, dexterity, and impact on quality of life.

NEUROMODULATION

Sacral neuromodulation (SNM) was U.S. Food and Drug Administration approved for treatment of nonobstructive urinary retention (NOUR) in 1999. The exact mechanism of action is unknown, but it is postulated that SNM inhibits the inappropriate activation of the "guarding reflex," thus facilitating voiding.[49,50] A meta-analysis showed that sacral neuromodulation can potentially facilitate emptying in patients with NOUR. In this study, neuromodulation improved PVR by a mean 236 mL and voided volume by 299 mL.[51]

In neurogenic lower urinary tract dysfunction, efficacy and safety of SNM appear to be similar. A different meta-analysis demonstrated 68% success rate for test phase and 92% for permanent SNM with reassuring safety profile. The adverse event rate was 0% during test phase and 24% for permanent implantation.[52] While randomized, controlled trials are lacking, SNM can be considered in appropriate patients with neurogenic bladder, or patients with DU/AD, unless their neurogenic condition may require ongoing MRI surveillance. The current device models are MRI incompatible, but compatible devices are on the horizon and may be available when this chapter is published.

SURGICAL TREATMENT

TRANSURETHRAL RESECTION OF THE PROSTATE (TURP)

While multiple transurethral options are now available, electrosurgical transurethral resection of the prostate (TURP) remains the gold standard in endoscopic treatment of lower urinary tract symptoms (LUTS)/benign prostatic hyperplasia (BPH).[53] There are little data demonstrating TURP efficacy for treatment of neurogenic DA. Extrapolating from the nonneurogenic BPH/LUTS literature, there is some evidence to suggest that neurogenic male patients with DU could potentially benefit from an outlet ablative procedure.[50,54] Potts et al. performed bladder outlet procedures in 21 of their 139 patients with DU and without BOO. They defined success as no future retention, need for catheterizations, or surgery. At 6 months after TURP, 86% of patients had improved.[55] In a similar study, patients were followed for 12 years after TURP, and patients with DU showed an improvement in International Prostate Symptom Score (IPSS) up to 7 years.[56] These studies will need to be better validated in neurogenic DU/DA patients.[57] Sphincterotomy has been reported in some case series for management of urinary retention in neurogenic patients with DSD, although the efficacy of

the procedure in patients with pure neurogenic DA is not well studied.[58,59]

BLADDER DIVERTICULECTOMY

A diverticulum is a herniation of bladder mucosa between fibers of detrusor and may contribute to poor detrusor contraction, chronic retention of urine and recurrent UTIs.[50] Surgical management of the bladder diverticula is only necessary when the patient is symptomatic or has a recurrent infection, stones, urinary obstruction and vesicoureteral reflux.[60-62]

FOLLOW-UP CONSIDERATIONS

If a patient with neurogenic DU/DA is voiding, follow-up should include at least a yearly interval history and physical exam, PVR measurements, and assessment of symptoms over time, preferably with standardized questionnaires that assess outlet obstruction such as IPSS. Patients can be followed at shorter intervals if practitioners believe closer surveillance is warranted, for instance if there are worsening urinary symptoms including retention, new or changing urinary leakage, or recurrent UTIs. Follow-up for those with previous high-risk factors of altered glomerular filtration rate or upper tract findings on imaging should include serum electrolyte measures, renal ultrasound, and potentially repeat urodynamics to assess the effects of interventions.[37]

SUMMARY

Neurogenic DU and AD can be observed in a myriad of conditions and are dependent on urodynamic studies for diagnosis. Evaluation is focused on appropriate diagnosis of the etiology of LUTS and urinary retention, while management is tailored to address bladder pathophysiology to prevent injury of the upper tracts, symptomatic urinary tract infections, and/or calculi. Evidence regarding best management of these patients is lacking and must be extrapolated in some cases from the DU/AD in the nonneurogenic population. Despite this, bladder management should follow the underlying goals of protecting patient safety and maximizing quality of life.

REFERENCES

1. Abrams P, Cardozo L, Fall M et al. The standardisation of terminology in lower urinary tract function: Report from the standardisation sub-committee of the International Continence Society. *Urology*. 2003;61(1):37–49. doi:10.1016/S0090-4295(02)02243-4

2. Chai TC and Birder LA. Physiology and pharmacology of the bladder and urethra. In: W. McDougal, Alan Wein, Louis Kavoussi, Andrew Novick, Alan Partin, Craig Peters, Parvati Ramchandani (eds.), *Campbell-Walsh Urology*,. 10th ed. Elsevier; 2016.

3. Miyazato M, Yoshimura N, and Chancellor MB. The other bladder syndrome: Underactive bladder. *Rev Urol*. 2013;15(1):11–22. http://www.ncbi.nlm.nih.gov/pubmed/23671401

4. Aitken KJ and Bägli DJ. The bladder extracellular matrix. Part I: Architecture, development and disease. *Nat Rev Urol*. 2009;6(11):596–611. doi:10.1038/nrurol.2009.201

5. Panicker JN and Fowler CJ. The bare essentials: Uro-Neurology. *Pract Neurol*. 2010;10(3):178–85. doi:10.1136/jnnp.2010.213892

6. Clemens JQ. Basic bladder neurophysiology. *Urol Clin North Am*. 2010;37(4):487–94. doi:10.1016/j.ucl.2010.06.006

7. Stoffel JT. Non-neurogenic chronic urinary retention: What are we treating? *Curr Urol Rep*. 2017;18(9):1–7. doi:10.1007/s11934-017-0719-2

8. Khan Z, Starer P, Yang WC, and Bhola A. Analysis of voiding disorders in patients with cerebrovascular accidents. *Urology*. 1990;35(3):265–70. http://www.ncbi.nlm.nih.gov/pubmed/2316094

9. Gelber DA, Good DC, Laven LJ, and Verhulst SJ. Causes of urinary incontinence after acute hemispheric stroke. *Stroke*. 1993;24(3):378–82. http://www.ncbi.nlm.nih.gov/pubmed/8446973

10. Tsuchida S, Noto H, Yamaguchi O, and Itoh M. Urodynamic studies on hemiplegic patients after cerebrovascular accident. *Urology*. 1983;21(3):315–8. http://www.ncbi.nlm.nih.gov/pubmed/6836813

11. Araki I, Kitahara M, Oida T, and Kuno S. Voiding dysfunction and Parkinson's disease: Urodynamic abnormalities and urinary symptoms. *J Urol*. 2000;164(5):1640–3. http://www.ncbi.nlm.nih.gov/pubmed/11025724

12. Bethlem J and Jager WADH. The incidence and characteristics of Lewy bodies in idiopathic paralysis agitans (Parkinson's disease). *J Neurol Neurosurg Psychiatry*. 1960;23(1):74–80. doi:10.1136/jnnp.23.1.74

13. Araki I and Kuno S. Assessment of voiding dysfunction in Parkinson's disease by the international prostate symptom score. *J Neurol Neurosurg Psychiatry*. 2000;68(4):429–33. doi:10.1136/jnnp.68.4.429

14. Jeong SJ, Cho SY, and Oh S-J. Spinal cord/brain injury and the neurogenic bladder. *Urol Clin North Am*. 2010;37(4):537–46. doi:10.1016/j.ucl.2010.06.005

15. Smith PH and Ballantyne B. The neuroanatomical basis for denervation of the urinary bladder following major pelvic surgery. *Br J Surg*. 1968;55(12):929–33. doi:10.1002/bjs.1800551212

16. Mundy AR. An anatomical explanation for bladder dysfunction following rectal and uterine surgery. *Br J Urol*. 1982;54(5):501–4. http://www.ncbi.nlm.nih.gov/pubmed/7171956

17. McGuire EJ. Urodynamic evaluation after abdominal-perineal resection and lumbar intervertebral disk herniation. *Urology*. 1975;6(1):63–70. http://www.ncbi.nlm.nih.gov/pubmed/1145924

18. Blaas JG and Barbalias GA. Characteristics of neural injury after abdominoperineal resection. *J Urol*. 1983;129(1):84–7. doi:10.1016/S0022-5347(17)51931-X

19. Seski JC and Diokno AC. Bladder dysfunction after radical abdominal hysterectomy. *Am J Obstet Gynecol*. 1977;128(6):643–51. doi:10.1016/0002-9378(77)90211-3

20. Van Gool JD. Non-neuropathic and neuropathic bladder-sphincter dysfunction in children. *J Pediatr Adolesc Med*. 1994;5:178–92.

21. van Gool JD, Dik P, and de Jong TPVM. Bladder-sphincter dysfunction in myelomeningocele. *Eur J Pediatr*. 2001;160(7):414–20. doi:10.1007/s004310100741

22. Wein A and Dmochowski R. Neuromuscular dysfunction of the lower urinary tract. In: W. McDougal, Alan Wein, Louis Kavoussi, Andrew Novick, Alan Partin, Craig Peters, Parvati Ramchandani (eds.), *Campbell-Walsh Urology*. 2016.

23. Krane R and Sirosky M. Multiple sclerosis. *Clinical NeuroUrology*. Litte Brown; 1991:353–63.

24. Barbalias GA, Nikiforidis G, and Liatsikos EN. Vesicourethral dysfunction associated with multiple sclerosis: Clinical and urodynamic perspectives. *J Urol*. 1998;160(1):106–11. http://www.ncbi.nlm.nih.gov/pubmed/9628615

25. Cohen LM, Fowler JF, Owen LG, and Callen JP. Urinary retention associated with herpes zoster infection. *Int J Dermatol*. 1993;32(1):24–6. http://www.ncbi.nlm.nih.gov/pubmed/8425796

26. Yamanishi T, Yasuda K, Sakakibara R et al. Urinary retention due to herpes virus infections. *Neurourol Urodyn*. 1998;17(6):613–9. http://www.ncbi.nlm.nih.gov/pubmed/9829425

27. Kogan BA, Solomon MH, and Diokno AC. Urinary retention secondary to Landry-Guillain-Barré syndrome. *J Urol*. 1981;126(5):643–4. doi:10.1016/S0022-5347(17)54668-6

28. Khan Z, Singh VK, and Yang WC. Neurogenic bladder in acquired immune deficiency syndrome (AIDS). *Urology*. 1992;40(3):289–91. http://www.ncbi.nlm.nih.gov/pubmed/1523760

29. Berry SJ, Coffey DS, Walsh PC, and Ewing LL. The development of human benign prostatic hyperplasia with age. *J Urol*. 1984;132(3):474–9. doi:10.1016/S0022-5347(17)49698-4

30. Dhingra N and Bhagwat D. Benign prostatic hyperplasia: An overview of existing treatment. *Indian J Pharmacol*. 2011;43(1):6. doi:10.4103/0253-7613.75657

31. Cooperberg M, Presti J, Shinohara K, and Carroll P. Neoplasms of the prostate gland. In: J. McAnnich and T. Lue, (eds.), *Smith & Tanagho's General Urology*. 18th ed. 2013:350–7.

32. McCammon K, Zuckerman J, and Jordan G. Urethral stricture disease. In W. McDougal, Alan Wein, Louis Kavoussi, Andrew Novick, Alan Partin, Craig Peters, Parvati Ramchandani (eds.),: *Campbell-Walsh Urology*, 11th ed. 2016.

33. Deng D and Shindel A. Female Urology and Sexual Dysfunction. In: *Smith & Tanagho's General Urology*.18th ed. 2013:617.

34. Mueller ER, Kenton K, Mahajan S, FitzGerald MP, and Brubaker L. Urodynamic prolapse reduction alters urethral pressure but not filling or pressure flow parameters. *J Urol*. 2007;177(2):600–3. doi:10.1016/j.juro.2006.09.060

35. Osman NI and Chapple CR. Fowler's syndrome—A cause of unexplained urinary retention in young women? *Nat Rev Urol*. 2014;11(2):87–98. doi:10.1038/nrurol.2013.277

36. Dorsher PT and McIntosh PM. Neurogenic bladder. *Adv Urol*. 2012;2012:816274. doi:10.1155/2012/816274

37. Stoffel JT, Peterson AC, Sandhu JS, Suskind AM, Wei JT, and Lightner DJ. AUA White Paper on Nonneurogenic Chronic Urinary Retention: Consensus Definition, Treatment Algorithm, and Outcome End Points. *J Urol*. 2017;198(1):153–60. doi:10.1016/j.juro.2017.01.075

38. Winters JC, Dmochowski RR, Goldman HB et al. Urodynamic studies in adults: AUA/SUFU guideline. *J Urol*. 2012;188(6 Suppl):2464–72. doi:10.1016/j.juro.2012.09.081

39. Allio BA and Peterson AC. Urodynamic and physiologic patterns associated with the common causes of neurogenic bladder in adults. *Transl Androl Urol*. 2016;5(1):31–8. doi:10.3978/j.issn.2223-4683.2016.01.05

40. Abrams P. Bladder outlet obstruction index, bladder contractility index and bladder voiding efficiency: Three simple indices to define bladder voiding function. *BJU Int*. 1999;84(1):14–5. http://www.ncbi.nlm.nih.gov/pubmed/10444116

41. Chai TC and Kudze T. New therapeutic directions to treat underactive bladder. *Investig Clin Urol*. 2017;58(Suppl 2):S99–S106. doi:10.4111/icu.2017.58.S2.S99

42. Finkbeiner AE. Is bethanechol chloride clinically effective in promoting bladder emptying? A literature review. *J Urol*. 1985;134(3):443–9. doi:10.1016/s0022-5347(17)47234-x

43. Barendrecht MM, Oelke M, Laguna MP, and Michel MC. Is the use of parasympathomimetics for treating an underactive urinary bladder evidence-based? *BJU Int*. 2007;99(4):749–52. doi:10.1111/j.1464-410X.2006.06742.x

44. Yamanishi T, Yasuda K, Kamai T et al. Combination of a cholinergic drug and an alpha-blocker is more effective than monotherapy for the treatment of voiding difficulty in patients with underactive detrusor. *Int J Urol*. 2004;11(2):88–96. http://www.ncbi.nlm.nih.gov/pubmed/14706012

45. Weld K and Dmochowski R. Effect of Bladder Management on Urological Complications in Spinal Cord Injured Patients. *J Urol*. 2000;163(3):768–72. doi:10.1016/S0022-5347(05)67800-7

46. Weld KJ, Wall BM, Mangold TA, Steere EL, and Dmochowski RR. Influences on renal function in chronic spinal cord injured patients. *J Urol*. 2000;164(5):1490–3. http://www.ncbi.nlm.nih.gov/pubmed/11025689

47. Stonehill WH, Dmochowski RR, Patterson AL, and Cox CE. Risk factors for bladder tumors in spinal cord injury patients. *J Urol*. 1996;155(4):1248–50. http://www.ncbi.nlm.nih.gov/pubmed/8632542

48. Baumgart E and Stoffel JT. The Boari bladder flap: An effective continent stoma for the high-compliance neurogenic bladder. *BJU Int*. 2010;105(9):1291–4. doi:10.1111/j.1464-410X.2009.09004.x

49. Leng WW and Chancellor MB. How sacral nerve stimulation neuromodulation works. *Urol Clin North Am*. 2005;32(1):1–8. doi:10.1016/j.ucl.2004.09.004

50. Gani J and Hennessey D. The underactive bladder: Diagnosis and surgical treatment options. *Transl Androl Urol*. 2017;6(Suppl 2):S186–95. doi:10.21037/tau.2017.04.07

51. Gross C, Habli M, Lindsell C, and South M. Sacral neuromodulation for nonobstructive urinary retention: A meta-analysis. *Female Pelvic Med Reconstr Surg*. 2010;16(4):249–53. doi:10.1097/SPV.0b013e3181df9b3f

52. Kessler TM, La Framboise D, Trelle S et al. Sacral neuromodulation for neurogenic lower urinary tract dysfunction: Systematic review and meta-analysis. *Eur Urol*. 2010;58(6):865–74. doi:10.1016/j.eururo.2010.09.024

53. Foster HE, Barry MJ, Dahm P et al. Surgical management of lower urinary tract symptoms attributed to benign prostatic hyperplasia: AUA Guideline. *J Urol*. 2018;200(3):612–9. doi:10.1016/j.juro.2018.05.048

54. Tanaka Y, Masumori N, Itoh N, Furuya S, Ogura H, and Tsukamoto T. Is the short-term outcome of transurethral resection of the prostate affected by preoperative degree of bladder outlet obstruction, status of detrusor contractility or detrusor overactivity? *Int J Urol*. 2006;13(11):1398–404. doi:10.1111/j.1442-2042.2006.01589.x

55. Potts B, Belsante M, Peterson A, and Le N-B. Bladder outlet procedures are an effective treatment for patients with urodynamically-confirmed detrusor overactivity without bladder outlet obstruction. *J Urol*. 2016;195(4S). doi:10.1016/j.juro.2016.02.1712

56. Masumori N, Furuya R, Tanaka Y, Furuya S, Ogura H, and Tsukamoto T. The 12-year symptomatic outcome of transurethral resection of the prostate for patients with lower urinary tract symptoms suggestive of benign prostatic obstruction compared to the urodynamic findings before surgery. *BJU Int*. 2009;105(10):1429–33. doi:10.1111/j.1464-410X.2009.08978.x

57. Koyanagi T, Morita H, Takamatsu T, Taniguchi K, and Shinno Y. Radical transurethral resection of the prostate in male paraplegics revisited: Further clinical experience and urodynamic considerations for its effectiveness. *J Urol*. 1987;137(1):72–6. doi:10.1016/S0022-5347(17)43876-6

58. Pan D, Troy A, Rogerson J, Bolton D, Brown D, and Lawrentschuk N. Long-term outcomes of external sphincterotomy in a spinal injured population. *J Urol*. 2009;181(2):705–9. doi:10.1016/j.juro.2008.10.004

59. Vainrib M, Reyblat P, and Ginsberg DA. Long-term efficacy of repeat incisions of bladder neck/external sphincter in patients with spinal cord injury. *Urology*. 2014;84(4):940–5. doi:10.1016/j.urology.2014.06.009

60. Thorner DA, Blaivas JG, Tsui JF, Kashan MY, Weinberger JM, and Weiss JP. Outcomes of reduction cystoplasty in men with impaired detrusor contractility. *Urology*. 2014;83(4):882–7. doi:10.1016/j.urology.2013.10.068

61. Adot Zurbano JM, Salinas Casado J, Dambros M et al. Urodynamics of the bladder diverticulum in the adult male. *Arch Esp Urol*. 2005;58(7):641–9. http://www.ncbi.nlm.nih.gov/pubmed/16294786

62. Gepi-Attee S and Feneley RC. Bladder diverticulectomy revisited: Case reports of retention of urine caused by diverticula and discussion. *J Urol*. 1994;152(3):954–5. doi:10.1016/s0022-5347(17)32621-6

Chapter 4

PATHOPHYSIOLOGY OF THE LOW COMPLIANT BLADDER

W. Blair Townsend and Michael J. Kennelly

DEFINITION OF BLADDER COMPLIANCE

Bladder compliance (C) is defined as the change in bladder volume ($V_{bladder}$) relative to the corresponding change in detrusor pressure (P_{det}) and is measured in milliliters per centimeters of H_2O:

$$C = \Delta(V_{bladder})/\Delta(P_{det})$$

The International Continence Society (ICS) recommends two standard points of pressure to be measured. The first is P_{det} at initiation of bladder filling and is usually measured as zero with a bladder volume of zero. The second is P_{det} at cystometric capacity and is measured before any detrusor contractions occur.[1] Figure 4.1 represents a cystometric illustration of these points of measurement during bladder filling.

"Normal compliance" is difficult to define in terms of milliliters per centimeter (mL/cm) of H_2O as there is great variability in "normal" bladders. As such, there is not a clear, consistent definition of normal ranges; however, lower compliance values are generally thought to be unfavorable. Many have reported the low end of mean "healthy" compliance values to be 46 mL/cm H_2O, while others suggest compliance as low as 11 mL/cm H_2O could fall in the "normal" range.[2,3]

MECHANICAL PROPERTIES OF BLADDER COMPLIANCE

The behavior of the bladder during filling depends on both mechanical and neuromuscular properties. Mechanical properties depend on tissue composition and structure of the bladder wall. A normal human bladder has an estimated relative composition of smooth muscle, collagen, and elastin of 40%, 50%, and 2%, respectively. Collagen is a main component of the extracellular matrix of bladder tissues and contributes to the relative stiffness of the bladder wall during filling that can ultimately lead to higher intravesical pressures.

Type I and type III collagen are important to consider in the discussion of impaired bladder compliance and are present to varying degrees in bladder tissue.[4] Type I collagen is generally more nonelastic than type III collagen, and it contributes more resistance to tensile forces of bladder expansion. Type III collagen allows for more relative flexibility, in comparison.[5,6] When mixed type I/type III strands have been examined, the estimated elastic modulus of type III collagen is roughly one-half of type I collagen.[7]

Elastin fibers are sparse in the bladder compared with collagen but are found in all layers of the bladder wall.[8] During filling, smooth muscle bundles and collagen structures are rearranged providing for bladder expansion through thinning of the lamina propria at a faster rate than the muscle wall.[9] Additionally, the urothelium expands but also must preserve its barrier function while filling. It is suggested that numerous transducer proteins are activated during bladder filling and emptying due to mechanical inputs secondary to bladder wall and geometrical tension, bladder pressure and torsion, movement of adjacent visceral organs, and possibly even urine pH.[10] Studies using multiphoton imaging have revealed differences in collagen fiber structure and recruitment throughout the bladder wall during filling.[11]

In a highly compliant bladder, the bladder fills at a physiologic rate with little change in pressure. High compliance of the bladder during initial filling is due primarily to its elastic and viscoelastic properties. Elasticity allows the components of the bladder wall to stretch without increasing tension. Viscoelastic properties of the bladder, in slight contrast, are time dependent and can dissipate energy as a load is applied to the bladder wall during filling. This leads to transient tension after stretching followed by "stress relaxation" as the stimulus of bladder filling slows or ceases. The combination of these forces is secondary to the elastic and collagen fibers between smooth muscle cells, between muscle fibers, and in the bladder serosa.[12] There is also likely persistent smooth muscle contractile activity with dynamic adjustment of cellular length during filling.[13]

An intravesical pressure less than 10 cm H_2O should be maintained with normal filling of the

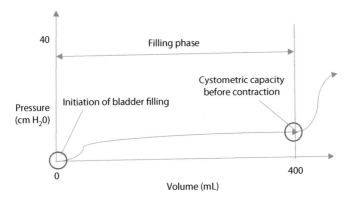

Figure 4.1   Cystometric points of pressure/volume measurements to calculate bladder compliance.

bladder at a slow physiologic rate.[14] In 559 women with stress incontinence, compliance and pressures were analyzed with a nonphysiologic fill rate of 50 mL/min. The mean maximum cystometric capacity (MCC) was 392 mL, and P_{det} rose from 2 cm H_2O at the beginning of fill to 6 cm H_2O at MCC.[15] With artificial filling such as that during urodynamics, compliance of the bladder may be dependent on the rate at which fluid is instilled into the bladder.[16] In patients with neurogenic bladder and severely impaired compliance on conventional cystometrogram (CMG), slowing of filling to natural rates led to normal compliance measurements.[17] Slowing or stopping the rate of filling alone can effectively reduce intravesical pressure.

NEUROMUSCULAR PROPERTIES OF BLADDER COMPLIANCE

Many have proposed that spinal sympathetic reflexes facilitate bladder filling and storage.[18–20] The inhibitory effect on bladder contraction is thought to be mediated by sympathetic regulation of cholinergic ganglionic transmission by a reflex mechanism. During bladder filling, inhibitory sympathetic transmission in the detrusor occurs, and neurotransmitters are released from sympathetic nerves to act directly on the smooth muscle of the bladder.[21,22] Moreover, these transmitters likely act on preganglionic parasympathetic nerves with cholinergic and purinergic inhibition.

Sympathetically mediated inhibition of α-adrenergic smooth muscle receptors ($\alpha 1$) at the bladder neck results in increased bladder outlet resistance, thereby promoting filling. Stimulation of β_3-adrenergic receptors in the bladder smooth musculature leads to increased bladder wall elasticity and decreased tension. Also, increased afferent pudendal nerve activity in the striated sphincter has been reported to directly inhibit detrusor motor neurons in the sacral

spinal cord. This action is regulated by inhibitory neurotransmitters such as γ-aminobutyric acid, glycine, opioids, purines, and noradrenergics.[23,24]

There may also be a nonneurogenic active component to the storage properties of the bladder. It has been proposed that a relaxing factor is released from urothelial cells during bladder filling.[25] Furthermore, it has been suggested that nitric oxide released from the urothelium of the bladder acts in an inhibitory manner on afferent pathways.[26] After a certain bladder capacity is reached, the urothelium of the distended bladder wall releases excitatory neurotransmitters such as acetylcholine, adenosine triphosphate, prostaglandins, and other peptides that result in bladder emptying.[27] It has been suggested that the bladder urothelium also responds to various other soluble factors released from nerves and blood vessels and some found in the urine to include epidermal growth factor (EGF), substance P, calcitonin gene-related peptide (CGRP), and corticotropin-releasing factor (CRF).[28,29]

INTRODUCTION TO THE LOW COMPLIANT BLADDER

Various definitions of impaired compliance have been described (e.g., between 10 and 20 mL/cm H_2O); however, no consistent definition exists. One group suggests impaired compliance is represented by a value less than 20 mL/cm H_2O.[30] When considering variables such as small cystometric capacity, defining low compliance becomes increasingly challenging. Therefore, utilization of absolute pressure measurements is arguably more helpful than compliance values to make clinical extrapolations. It has been commonly cited that storage pressures greater than 40 cm H_2O predicts harmful effects on the upper tract.[31,32] An example of a CMG with impaired compliance during bladder filling and P_{det} greater than 40 cm H_2O can be seen in Figure 4.2.

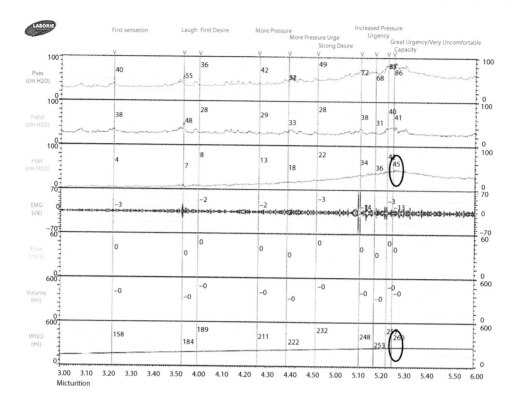

Figure 4.2 Example of impaired compliance in male patient after pelvic radiation therapy for cancer. Compliance is as follows: 260 mL/45 cm H_2O = 5.78 mL/cm H_2O.

MECHANISM OF THE LOW COMPLIANT BLADDER

Decreased compliance occurs due to several factors, including (Figure 4.3)

1. Fibrosis
2. Bladder muscle hypertrophy
3. Neurologic disease or injury affecting the lower urinary tract
4. Ischemia

FIBROSIS

Relative collagen content and subsequent fibrosis increase with tissue injury, chronic inflammation, persistent bladder outlet obstruction, or denervation.[9] As increases in collagen levels occur relative to elastin and healthy smooth muscle in the bladder wall, compliance decreases.

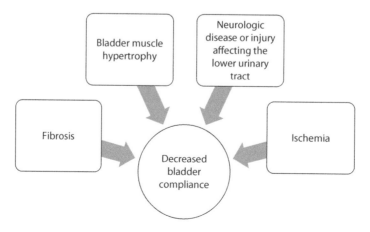

Figure 4.3 Factors leading to decreased bladder compliance.

Structural changes have been studied in patients with dysfunctional bladders, specifically those undergoing bladder augmentations.[33] Preoperatively, total bladder capacity, pressure-volume relationships, and bladder compliance were measured with urodynamic analysis. Intraoperatively, full-thickness bladder biopsy specimens were taken from the dome of the bladder. The ratio of connective tissue to smooth muscle was significantly increased in patients with poorly compliant bladders, and there was a change in the ratio of type III to type I collagen compared to healthier bladder tissue.

Conditions such as radiation cystitis and tuberculosis can lead to a low compliant bladder. When tuberculosis affects the bladder, an acute inflammatory process occurs with possible hyperemia, ulceration, and tubercle formation that can lead to fibrosis of the bladder wall.[34] Radiation cystitis is discussed later in the "Ischemia" section.

Collagen deposition can also occur with normal aging leading to bladder underactivity or underactive bladder (UAB) syndrome. The International Continence Society defines this as a "bladder contraction of reduced strength and/or duration, resulting in prolonged voiding and/or failure to achieve complete bladder emptying within a normal time span based on a urodynamic diagnosis." These patients often have low bladder compliance due to fibrosis.

BLADDER MUSCLE HYPERTROPHY

Bladder muscle hypertrophy is often secondary to chronic bladder outlet obstruction. Hypertrophic muscle is thought to be less elastic than normal detrusor, therefore leading to decreased compliance. This pathologic muscle tissue can also synthesize more collagen than normal bladder wall muscle.[35] After collagen has replaced normal components of the stroma, pharmacologic management and other more conservative management strategies to increase bladder compliance and capacity are often not effective.

NEUROLOGIC DISEASE OR INJURY AFFECTING THE LOWER URINARY TRACT

Impaired bladder compliance is seen in neurologic conditions that affect lower urinary tract function such as spinal cord injuries (SCIs) or lesions, spina bifida, and Parkinson's disease. Many of these patients can have increased outlet resistance secondary to detrusor external sphincter dyssynergia (DESD). In men, neurogenic causes of bladder outlet obstruction can be compounded with nonneurogenic phenomena such as benign prostatic obstruction that further exacerbate secondary bladder fibrosis and hypertrophy.[36]

Evidence has shown that bladder compliance is largely dependent upon central neural input.[37] During filling of a healthy bladder, afferent signals are conducted from the bladder wall to the spinal cord, which inhibits spontaneous detrusor contractility to allow compliance to remain high. Decreased compliance due to neurologic etiologies is usually caused by a process that injures the sacral cord or an infrasacral level to include sacral roots and pelvic nerves. With an autonomous neurogenic bladder, these patients have no communication between the motor and sensory components of the bladder and the sacral spinal cord. Loss of conscious awareness of bladder filling can result from this decentralizing of parasympathetic pathways to the detrusor muscle and loss of somatic innervation to the external sphincter.

Neurologic injury to the lower urinary tract also alters mechanical properties of the bladder. In spinal cord–injured rats, the elastin-to-collagen ratio was found to increase over the first 6 weeks from injury. During the same period, bladder compliance interestingly increased, cystometric capacity increased, and bladders became markedly overdistended. Ten weeks after the injury, the elastin-to-collagen ratio then decreased, bladder compliance decreased, and detrusor overactivity became evident.[38,39] Patients with neurogenic bladders can have chronic adrenergic activation of the detrusor muscle with transitioning of β-mediated adrenoreceptor relaxation to α-mediated bladder wall contraction.[40,41]

ISCHEMIA

In normal bladders, delivery of blood flow is able to increase to match the large increase in surface area during filling.[42] Increased intravesical pressure and intramural tension in low compliant bladders leads to a significant decrease in blood flow to the bladder wall.[43] When the detrusor muscle is chronically deprived of oxygen and undergoes ischemic damage, it loses its expansible and contractile ability.[44,45] Alterations and type I–to–type III collagen ratios and collagen-to-elastin ratios can be implicated as well. In addition to ischemia, reperfusion injury can occur after reduction in intramural tension and likely results in damage to intramural neurons with subsequent denervation and smooth muscle injury.[13]

Radiation cystitis is an example of an ischemic process that can ultimately lead to low bladder compliance. Radiation cystitis affects roughly 7% of those patients undergoing radiation treatment for prostate cancer and can develop as early as 6–12 months after treatment but often presents several years after.[46] The pathophysiology of decreased bladder compliance from late radiation damage to the bladder wall in these patients includes cellular depletion and obliterative endarteritis leading to fibrosis and increased collagen content.[47]

INVALID BLADDER COMPLIANCE MEASUREMENTS DURING URODYNAMICS

The measurement of compliance during urodynamic studies (UDS) can be affected by a number of factors. Inaccurate compliance measurements during UDS can occur due to technical factors (i.e., filling rate) and anatomic factors (i.e., vesicoureteral reflux, bladder diverticulum, and incontinence due to low outlet resistance). Optimal bladder compliance measurements are obtained with physiologic filling rates (body weight in kilograms divided by four, expressed as milliliters per minute [mL/min]). In some cases during nonphysiologic filling rates, the rapid filling causes a detrusor accommodation issue, and P_{det} arbitrarily increases. If this occurs, it is recommended to stop or reduce the filling rate to allow the detrusor to accommodate before determining the bladder compliance. One also needs to be cognizant that a sustained or lower amplitude involuntary detrusor contraction could be mistaken for low compliance.

Low outlet resistance (i.e., patients with spina bifida) can lead to invalid bladder compliance measurements during UDS. These patients often have persistent urinary leakage and an inability to fill the bladder. If the outlet pressure is increased to stop urinary leakage (i.e., a Foley catheter balloon at the bladder neck), the bladder is allowed to fill, and proper compliance can be obtained. Clinically, this becomes important when contemplating the placement of an artificial urinary sphincter in a patient with spina bifida, as poor bladder compliance could have adverse effects on the upper urinary tract.

Anatomic abnormalities of the lower urinary tract also can create compliance artifacts during urodynamic testing. Patients with significant vesicoureteral reflux (VUR) can transfer the pressure to the ipsilateral renal unit where reflux occurs. Ultimately, this could lead to recurrent pyelonephritis, renal scarring, and impaired kidney function, especially important to consider in the pediatric population. Similarly, a patient with a large bladder diverticulum could transfer pressure and urine volume from the true lumen of the bladder to the diverticulum. The addition of "video" or fluoroscopy to UDS is extremely useful in cases of VUR and bladder diverticulum (Figure 4.4).

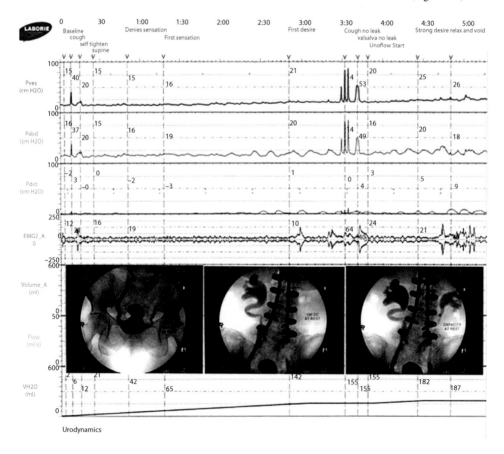

Figure 4.4 Example of video urodynamics demonstrating bilateral vesicoureteral reflux and "inaccurate" compliant bladder with "pop-off" mechanism.

Significant urinary incontinence due to a low-pressure urethra can also give false, misleading high-bladder compliance readings. If one treats the outlet (i.e., placement of an artificial urinary sphincter or sling), and increases the outlet resistance, the true bladder compliance can be measured. If there is a poorly compliant bladder after these interventions, there will be a "pop-off" mechanism where the transmission of bladder pressure is directed to the upper urinary tracts leading to hydronephrosis. This phenomenon is also depicted in Figure 4.4. Patients who are susceptible to poor bladder compliance (i.e., SCI, spina bifida, after radiation therapy, etc.) and who receive an artificial urinary sphincter should be monitored carefully for compliance changes.

REFERENCES

1. Abrams P Cardozo L, Fall M et al. The standardization of terminology in lower urinary tract function: Report from the standardization subcommittee of the International Continence Society. *Neurourol Urodyn.* 2002;21:167–78.
2. Sorensen S, Gregersen H, and Sorensen SM. Long term reproducibility of urodynamic investigations in healthy fertile females. *Scand J Urol Nephrol Suppl.* 1988;114:35–41.
3. van Waalwijk van Doorn ES, Remmers A, and Janknegt RA. Conventional and extramural ambulatory urodynamic testing of the lower urinary tract in female volunteers. *J Urol.* 1992;147:1319–26.
4. von der Mark K. Localization of collagen types in tissues. *Int Rev Connect Tissue Res.* 1981;9:265–324.
5. Liapis A, Bakas P, Pafiti A, Frangos-Plemenos M, Arnoyannaki N, and Creatsas G. Changes of collagen type III in female patients with genuine stress incontinence and pelvic floor prolapse. *Eur J Obstet Gynecol Reprod Biol.* 2001;97:76–9.
6. Kerkhof MH Hendriks L, and Brolmann HA. Changes in connective tissue in patients with pelvic organ prolapse—A review of the current literature. *Int Urogynecol J Pelvic Floor Dysfunct.* 2009;20:461–74.
7. Chao W Hao Z, Wen S, and Leng H. A quantitative study of the relationship between the distribution of different types of collagen and the mechanical behavior of rabbit medial collateral ligaments. *PLOS ONE.* 2014;9:e103363.
8. Murakumo M, Ushiki T, Abe K, Matsumura K, Shinno Y, and Koyanagi T. Three-dimensional arrangement of collagen and elastin fibers in the human urinary bladder: A scanning electron microscopic study. *J Urol.* 1995;154:251–6.
9. Macarak EJ, and Howard PS. The role of collagen in bladder filling. *Adv Exp Med Biol.* 1999;462:215–23, discussion 225–33.
10. Charrua A, Reguenga C, Cordeiro JM et al. Functional transient receptor potential vanilloid 1 is expressed in human urothelial cells. *J Urol.* 2009;182:2944–50.
11. Hornsby J, Cheng F, Kullmann A et al. Developing a mechanobiological model of the murine bladder: *In vivo, in vitro* and in silico modeling. *ECCOMAS.* 2016.
12. Andersson KE, and Anders A. Urinary bladder contraction and relaxation: Physiology and pathophysiology. *Physiol Rev.* 2004;84(3):935–86.
13. Brading AF. Alterations in the physiological properties of urinary bladder smooth muscle caused by bladder emptying against an obstruction. *Scand J Urol Nephrol Suppl.* 1997;184:51–8.
14. Klevmark B. Motility of the urinary bladder in cats during filling at physiological rates. Intravesical pressure patterns studied by a new method of cystometry. *Acta Physiol Scand.* 1974;90(3):565–77.
15. Nager CW, Albo ME, Fitzgerald MP et al. Reference urodynamic values for stress incontinent women. *Neurourol Urodyn.* 2007;26(3):333–40.
16. Coolsaet B. Bladder compliance and detrusor activity during the collection phase. *Neurourol Urodyn.* 1985;4(4):263–73.
17. Robertson AS. Behaviour of the human bladder during natural filling: The Newcastle experience of ambulatory monitoring and conventional artificial filling cystometry. *Scand J Urol Nephrol Suppl.* 1999;201:19–24.
18. Chancellor M, and Yoshimura N. Physiology and pharmacology of the bladder and urethra. In: Walsh PC, Retik AB, Vaughan ED, and Wein AJ, eds. *Campbell's Urology,* 8th ed. Philadelphia, PA: W.B. Saunders; 2002:831–86.
19. Yoshimura N, and Chancellor M. Physiology and pharmacology of the bladder and urethra. In: Wein AJ, Kavoussi LR, Novick AC, Partin AW, and Peters CA, eds. *Campbell-Walsh Urology,* 8th ed. Philadelphia, PA: W.B. Saunders; 2007:1922–72.
20. Zderic S Levin R, and Wein A. Voiding function: Relevant anatomy, physiology, pharmacology and molecular aspects. In: Gillenwater JY, Grayhack JT, Howards SS, and Mitchell ME, eds. *Adult and Pediatric Urology.* Philadelphia, PA: Lippincott, Williams & Wilkins; 2002:1061–113.
21. Labadia A, Rivera L, Costa G, and Garcia-Sacristan A. Influence of the autonomic nervous system in the horse urinary bladder. *Res Vet Sci.* 1988;44(3):282–5.
22. Maggi CA, Conte B, Furio M, Santicioli P, Giuliani S, and Meli A. Further studies on mechanisms regulating the voiding cycle of the rat urinary bladder. *Gen Pharmacol.* 1989;20(6):833–8.
23. Fuder H, and Muscholl E. Heteroreceptor-mediated modulation of noradrenaline and acetylcholine release from peripheral nerves. *Rev Physiol Biochem Pharmacol.* 1995;126:265–412.
24. Burnstock G. Purinergic signalling in the urinary tract in health and disease. *Purinergic Signal.* 2014;10(1):103–55.
25. Hawthorn MH, Chapple CR, Cock M et al. Urothelium-derived inhibitory factor(s) influences on detrusor muscle contractility *in vitro. Br J Pharmacol.* 2000;129:416–9.
26. Andersson KE. Relevant anatomy, physiology and pharmacology. In: Wein AJ, Andersson KE,and Drake MJ, eds. *Bladder Dysfunction in the Adult: The Basis for Clinical Management.* New York, NY: Humana Press; 2014:3–18.
27. McGuire EJ, Zhang S-C, and Horwinski E. Treatment for motor and sensory detrusor instability by electrical stimulation. *J Urol.* 1983;129:78–9.
28. Birder LA, and de Groat WC. Mechanisms of disease: Involvement of the urothelium in bladder dysfunction. *Nat Clin Pract.* 2007;4(1):46–54.
29. Hanna-Mitchell AT, Beckel, JM, Barbadora S, Kanai AJ, DeGroat WC, and Birder LA. Non-neuronal acetylcholine and urinary blader urothelium. *Life Sci.* 2007;80(24–25):2298–302.

30. Stöhrer M, Goepel M, Kondo A et al. The standardization of terminology in neurogenic lower urinary tract dysfunction with suggestions for diagnostic procedures. *Neurourol Urodyn.* 1999;18:139–58.

31. McGuire EJ. Urodynamic findings in patients after failure of stress incontinence operations. *Prog Clin Biol Res.* 1981;78:351–4.

32. McGuire EJ. Urodynamics of the neurogenic bladder. *Urol Clin North Am.* 2010;37(4):507–16.

33. Landau EH, Jayanthi VR, Churchill BM et al. Loss of elasticity in dysfunctional bladders: Urodynamic and histochemical correlation. *J Urol.* 1994; 152:702–5.

34. Gow J. Genitourinary tuberculosis. In: Walsh PC, Retik AB, Vaughan ED, and Wein AJ, eds. *Campbell's Urology*, 7th ed. Philadelphia, PA: W.B. Saunders; 1998.

35. Mostwin J. Clinical physiology of micturition. In: Cardozo L, and Staskin D, eds. *Textbook of Female Urology and Urogynecology*. Milton Park, UK: Informa Healthcare; 2006:141–55.

36. Leng WW, and McGuire EJ. Obstructive uropathy induced bladder dysfunction can be reversible: Bladder compliance measures before and after treatment. *J Urol.* 2003;169:563–6.

37. Smith PP, DeAngelis AM, and Kuchel GA. Evidence of central modulation of bladder compliance during filling phase. *Neurourol Urodyn.* 2012;31(1):30–5.

38. Nagatomi J, DeMiguel F, Torimoto K, Chancellor MB, Getzenberg RH, and Sacks MS. Early molecular-level changes in rat bladder wall tissue following spinal cord injury. *Biochem Biophys Res Commun.* 2005;334:1159–64.

39. Toosi KK, Nagatomi J, Chancellor MB, and Sacks MS. The effects of long-term spinal cord injury on mechanical properties of the rat urinary bladder. *Ann Biomed Eng.* 2008;36:1470–80.

40. Sundin T, Dahlström A, Norlen L, and Svedmyr N. The sympathetic innervation and adrenoreceptor function of the human lower urinary tract in the normal state and after parasympathetic denervation. *Invest Urol.* 1977;14(4):322–8.

41. Sundin T, and Dahlström A. The sympathetic innervation of the urinary bladder and urethra in the normal state and after parasympathetic denervation at the spinal root level. An experimental study in cats. *Scand J Urol Nephrol.* 1973;7(2):131–49.

42. Greenland JE, and Brading AF. Urinary bladder blood flow changes during the micturition cycle in a conscious pig model. *J Urol.* 1996;156(5):1858–61.

43. Ohnishi N, Kishima Y, Hashimoto K et al. A new method of measurement of the urinary bladder blood flow in patients with low compliant bladder. *Hinyokika Kiyo.* 1994;40(8):663–7.

44. Levin RM, Brendler K, Van Arsdalen KN, and Wein AJ. Functional response of the rabbit urinary bladder to anoxia and ischaemia. *Neurourol Urodyn.* 1983;42:54.

45. Pessina F, McMurray G, Wiggin A, and Brading AF. The effect of anoxia and glucose-free solutions on the contractile response of guinea-pig detrusor strips to intrinsic nerve stimulation and the application of excitatory agonists. *J Urol.* 1997;157:2375–80.

46. Smit SG, and Heyns CF. Management of radiation cystitis. *Nat Rev Urol.* 2013;10:713–22.

47. Manikandan R, Kumar S, and Dorairajan LN. Hemorrhagic cystitis: A challenge to the urologist. *Indian J Urol.* 2010;26(2):159–66.

Chapter 5

PATHOPHYSIOLOGY AND PREVALENCE OF DETRUSOR-SPHINCTER DYSSYNERGIA

Marcio Augusto Averbeck and Helmut Madersbacher

INTRODUCTION

According to the current terminology of the International Continence Society (ICS), detrusor sphincter dyssynergia (DSD) is defined by "a detrusor contraction concurrent with an involuntary contraction of the urethral and/or periurethral striated muscle."[1] Occasionally, flow may be prevented altogether. This is a common feature of neurogenic lower urinary tract dysfunction (NLUTD), especially among patients with spinal cord lesions (SCLs).

Neurologic lesions within the brainstem (pontine micturition center) and/or the sacral spinal cord are responsible for detrusor external sphincter dyssynergia. These include especially traumatic SCLs, and also multiple sclerosis (MS), myelodysplasia, and other forms of transverse myelitis. This chapter focuses on the pathophysiology and prevalence of DSD.

PATHOPHYSIOLOGY OF DETRUSOR EXTERNAL SPHINCTER DYSSYNERGIA

Bladder function relies on coordination between both central and peripheral nervous systems. In fact, the reciprocal innervation of bladder and external sphincter is essential to facilitate storage and emptying phases.[2] Normal micturition is controlled by neural circuits in the spinal cord and in the brain that coordinate the activity of visceral smooth muscle in the urinary bladder and urethra with activity of striated muscle in the urethral sphincter. Normal micturition is preceded by relaxation of the external urethral sphincter.[3]

In physiologic situations, a higher level of afferent activity results in inhibition of external sphincter activity via a spino-bulbo-spinal reflex, which is followed by inhibition of sympathetic outflow reflexes and activation of parasympathetic outflow to the bladder. Relaxation of the urethral smooth

muscle is mediated in animal models by activation of parasympathetic pathways to the urethra that trigger nitric oxide release, an inhibitory transmitter. Secondary reflexes elicited by urine flow through the urethra facilitate complete bladder emptying. These reflexes rely on the integrative action of neurons located at various levels of the neuroaxis.

Within the spinal cord, afferent neurons from the bladder synapse on interneurons, which send axons to the brain. These ascending neurons connect with structures in the brainstem, including the pons and the periaqueductal gray (PAG) of the midbrain. Afferent input from the spinal cord may pass through relay neurons in the PAG before reaching the pontine micturition center (PMC).[4] The PMC has a modulating effect on reflexes, such as those mediating excitatory outflow to the sphincter and sympathetic inhibitory outflow to the bladder, which are organized at the spinal level.

The dorsolateral pontine tegmentum is an essential control center for micturition and was first described by Barrington in the cat, being called "Barrington's nucleus," the "pontine micturition center," or the "M region."[5,6] Animal studies (cat model) also identified a region located laterally to the PMC, hence called the "L region," which provides input to the external urethral sphincter motoneurons in Onuf's nucleus, as well as projections to the thoracolumbar parasympathetic preganglionic neurons. Experimental findings let us assume that the M region is necessary to voiding and the L region is part of a larger, less specific area that probably relates to sphincter control in various circumstances, such as during increased abdominal pressure (coughing, sneezing, etc.).

Neurons in the PMC of the cat provide direct synaptic inputs to sacral parasympathetic preganglionic neurons, as well as to neurons in the sacral dorsal commissure.[7] The former neurons innervate the bladder (via the pelvic ganglia), while the latter are thought to have an important inhibitory influence on motoneurons that control the external urethral sphincter.[8] As a result of these connections, the PMC can promote coordinated reciprocal activity in the bladder and urethral sphincter.

De Groat et al. proposed that lower urinary tract function is controlled by complex pathways in the brain that act like switching circuits, which promote voluntary or reflex activity shifts resulting in either urine storage or micturition.[9] Later on, functional magnetic resonance imaging (fMRI) was used to visualize the brain switching circuits controlling reflex micturition in anesthetized rats.[10] The fMRI confirmed the hypothesis based on previous neuroanatomical and neurophysiological studies that the brainstem switch for reflex micturition control involves both the PAG and the PMC. During storage, the PAG is activated by afferent input from the urinary bladder, while the PMC is inactive. When bladder volume increases to the micturition threshold, the switch from storage to micturition is associated with PMC activation and enhanced PAG activity.[10]

In humans, Blok et al. carried out the first studies using positron emission tomography (PET) to assess the regulation of bladder function by brainstem activation during voiding. Increased blood flow in an area in the right dorsomedial pontine tegmentum close to the fourth ventricle has been demonstrated during voiding, and this was presumed to be the location of PMC in humans[11-13].

DSD causes *a functional bladder outlet obstruction, which is the primary driver for the high-pressure situation above the external urinary sphincter area* with all its consequences. Patients with suprasacral spinal cord lesions (SCL) are at risk for DSD secondary to the loss of coordination from pons that can lead to incomplete bladder emptying, high postvoid residual, and increased bladder pressure with resulting obstruction of kidneys leading to renal failure.[14] There is evidence that transurethral sphincterotomy abolishes the high-pressure situation and may prevent all the consequences of DSD on the lower and upper urinary tracts.[15]

As a consequence of an acute SCL, the normal connections between the sacral cord and the supraspinal circuits that control urine storage and release are disrupted. After the so-called "spinal shock phase," detrusor overactivity (DO) develops. DO is mediated by a spinal micturition reflex that emerges in response to a reorganization of synaptic connections in the spinal cord.[2] Bladder afferents that are normally unresponsive to low intravesical pressures become more mechanosensitive, leading to DO. A newly developed spinal reflex circuit, which is mediated by C fibers as a response to a reorganization of synaptic connections in the spinal cord, is thought to be responsible for the development of DO in response to low-volume filling after SCL. In normal micturition, the afferent reflex is carried by Aδ-nerve fibers to dorsal root ganglia. The unmyelinated C fibers are silent under normal conditions. In

neurogenic DO, this changes, and transmission is via unmyelinated C fibers, which leads to a shorter latency period.[16-18] C fiber–mediated reflexes may be relevant for future studies on new drugs. In complete suprasacral SCL (neurologically defined as ASIA A), there is no modulation of pelvic floor reflexes, such as the pudendo-anal (or urethral) reflex, whereas in incomplete injuries the reflex activity is variably facilitated. DO is therefore often accompanied by DSD.

ETIOLOGY AND PREVALENCE OF DSD

DSD has been reported in 70%–100% of patients with suprasacral SCL.[19] Autonomic dysreflexia (AD) is not an uncommon finding among these patients. Liu et al. carried out a retrospective study to assess AD among SCL patients with higher lesions (T6 and above). Individuals with cervical SCL, DSD, poor bladder compliance, or a time period of more than 2 years after SCL were associated with a higher possibility of developing AD during urodynamics. Furthermore, AD was more severe in individuals with complete suprasacral SCL (ASIA A) and was exacerbated with time after injury.[20]

Nontraumatic SCL may also be associated with DSD. Sakakibara et al. performed urodynamic studies and neurologic examinations on 128 patients with cervical myelopathies including 82 with spondylitic myelopathy and 46 with ossification of the posterior longitudinal ligament.[21] DO was detected in 61 (48%) and DSD in 22 (17%) patients. DSD was more frequent in patients with disturbed deep sensation and pyramidal signs ($P < 0.05$).

DSD has been reported as a frequent finding in patients with MS. A systematic review of contemporary MS urodynamic studies demonstrated that 53% of patients with MS have detrusor overactivity, and 43% have DSD.[22] However, DSD was not associated with high risk for upper urinary tract deterioration in this patient group.[23]

DSD has been described in various neurologic diseases, such as multiple system atrophy,[24] cerebral palsy,[25] and tuberculous meningitis.[26] Despite being uncommon in cerebrovascular disease, DSD was detected in up to 14% of patients with acute hemispheric stroke.[27]

CLASSIFICATION OF DSD

DSD has been classified not only as intermittent or continuous but also according to the consistency of sphincter contraction during the detrusor

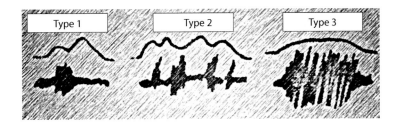

Figure 5.1 Different types of detrusor-sphincter dyssynergia (DSD). (Modified from Blaivas JG et al. *J Urol.* 1981; 125[4]:545–8.)

contraction.[28] Blaivas et al. described three types of DSD (Figure 5.1) based on the temporal relationship between urethral and sphincter contractions.[29] Type 1 is defined by a concomitant increase in both detrusor pressure and sphincter electromyography activity, but at the peak of the detrusor contraction the sphincter suddenly relaxes, and unobstructed voiding occurs. Type 2 DSD is characterized by sporadic contractions of the external urethral sphincter throughout the detrusor contraction (colonic sphincter contractions). In Type 3 DSD, there is a crescendo-decrescendo pattern of sphincter contraction that results in urethral obstruction throughout the entire detrusor contraction (sustained sphincter contraction).

TAKE-HOME MESSAGES

CURRENT TERMINOLOGY FROM THE INTERNATIONAL CONTINENCE SOCIETY (ICS)

The ICS defines DSD as "incoordination between detrusor and sphincter during voiding due to a neurological abnormality" (i.e., detrusor contraction synchronous with contraction of the urethral and/or periurethral striated muscle).[1]

PATHOPHYSIOLOGY

Suprasacral SCL may result in DSD due to the loss of the PMC coordinating function to the lower urinary tract, which may lead to incomplete bladder emptying, high postvoid residual, and increased bladder pressure.[14] DSD causes a *functional obstruction*, which is the primary driver for the high-pressure situation above the external sphincter area with all of its consequences.

ETIOLOGY

Neurological lesions within the brainstem (PMC) and/ or the sacral spinal cord cause DSD. These include especially traumatic spinal cord lesions, but also MS, myelodysplasia, and other neurologic diseases.

PREVALENCE

DSD is seen in 70%–100% of patients with suprasacral SCLs.[19] DSD is also a common finding in patients with MS (28%–82%).

REFERENCES

1. Gajewski JB, Schurch B, Hamid R et al. An International Continence Society (ICS) report on the terminology for adult neurogenic lower urinary tract dysfunction (ANLUTD). *Neurourol Urodyn.* 2018;37(3):1152–61.
2. Hamid R, Averbeck MA, Chiang H et al. Epidemiology and pathophysiology of neurogenic bladder after spinal cord injury. *World J Urol.* 2018;36(10):1517–27.
3. Vereecken RL and Verduyn H. The electrical activity of the paraurethral and perineal muscles in normal and pathological conditions. *Br J Urol.* 1970;42(4):457–63.
4. Blok BF. Central pathways controlling micturition and urinary continence. *Urology.* 2002;59(5 Suppl 1):13–7.
5. Morrison JF. The discovery of the pontine micturition centre by F. J. F. Barrington. *Exp Physiol.* 2008;93(6):742–5.
6. De Groat WC. Nervous control of the urinary bladder of the cat. *Brain Res.* 1975;87(2–3): 201–11.
7. Blok BF and Holstege G. Ultrastructural evidence for a direct pathway from the pontine micturition center to the parasympathetic preganglionic motoneurons of the bladder of the cat. *Neurosci Lett.* 1997;222(3):195–8.
8. Blok BF, van Maarseveen JT, and Holstege G. Electrical stimulation of the sacral dorsal gray commissure evokes relaxation of the external urethral sphincter in the cat. *Neurosci Lett.* 1998;249(1):68–70.
9. de Groat WC. Anatomy of the central neural pathways controlling the lower urinary tract. *Eur Urol.* 1998;34(Suppl 1):2–5.
10. Tai C, Wang J, Jin T et al. Brain switch for reflex micturition control detected by FMRI in rats. *J Neurophysiol.* 2009;102(5):2719–30.
11. Blok BF, Willemsen AT, and Holstege G. A PET study on brain control of micturition in humans. *Brain.* 1997;120 (Pt 1):111–21.
12. Blok BF, Sturms LM, and Holstege G. A PET study on cortical and subcortical control of pelvic floor musculature in women. *J Comp Neurol.* 1997;389(3):535–44.
13. Blok BF, Sturms LM, and Holstege G. Brain activation during micturition in women. *Brain.* 1998;121 (Pt 11):2033–42.
14. Kaplan SA, Chancellor MB, and Blaivas JG. Bladder and sphincter behavior in patients with spinal cord lesions. *J Urol.* 1991;146(1):113–7.

15. Ross JC, Gibbon NO, and Damanski M. Division of the external urethral sphincter in the treatment of the paraplegic bladder: A preliminary report on a new procedure. *Paraplegia*. 1987;25(3):185–95.

16. de Groat WC, Kawatani M, Hisamitsu T et al. Mechanisms underlying the recovery of urinary bladder function following spinal cord injury. *J Auton Nerv Syst*. 1990;30(Suppl):S71–7.

17. Kruse MN, Bray LA, and de Groat WC. Influence of spinal cord injury on the morphology of bladder afferent and efferent neurons. *J Auton Nerv Syst*. 1995;54(3):215–24.

18. Geirsson G, Fall M, and Sullivan L. Clinical and urodynamic effects of intravesical capsaicin treatment in patients with chronic traumatic spinal detrusor hyperreflexia. *J Urol*. 1995;154(5):1825–9.

19. Perkash I. Autonomic dysreflexia and detrusor-sphincter dyssynergia in spinal cord injury patients. *J Spinal Cord Med*. 1997;20(3):365–70.

20. Liu N, Zhou MW, Biering-Sørensen F, and Krassioukov AV. Cardiovascular response during urodynamics in individuals with spinal cord injury. *Spinal Cord*. 2017;55(3):279–84.

21. Sakakibara R, Hattori T, Tojo M, Yamanishi T, Yasuda K, and Hirayama K. The location of the paths subserving micturition: Studies in patients with cervical myelopathy. *J Auton Nerv Syst*. 1995;55(3):165–8.

22. Stoffel JT. Chronic urinary retention in multiple sclerosis patients: Physiology, systematic review of urodynamic data, and recommendations for care. *Urol Clin North Am*. 2017;44(3):429–39.

23. Lawrenson R, Wyndaele JJ, Vlachonikolis I, Farmer C, and Glickman S. Renal failure in patients with neurogenic lower urinary tract dysfunction. *Neuroepidemiology*. 2001;20(2):138–43.

24. Bloch F, Pichon B, Bonnet AM et al. Urodynamic analysis in multiple system atrophy: Characterisation of detrusor-sphincter dyssynergia. *J Neurol*. 2010;257(12):1986–91.

25. Gündoğdu G, Kömür M, Avlan D et al. Relationship of bladder dysfunction with upper urinary tract deterioration in cerebral palsy. *J Pediatr Urol*. 2013;9(5):659–64.

26. Gupta A, Garg RK, Singh MK et al. Bladder dysfunction and urodynamic study in tuberculous meningitis. *J Neurol Sci*. 2013;327(1–2):46–54.

27. Sakakibara R, Hattori T, Yasuda K, and Yamanishi T. Micturitional disturbance after acute hemispheric stroke: Analysis of the lesion site by CT and MRI. *J Neurol Sci*. 1996;137(1):47–56.

28. Weld KJ, Graney MJ, and Dmochowski RR. Clinical significance of detrusor sphincter dyssynergia type in patients with post-traumatic spinal cord injury. *Urology*. 2000;56(4):565–8.

29. Blaivas JG, Sinha HP, Zayed AA, and Labib KB. Detrusor-external sphincter dyssynergia: A detailed electromyographic study. *J Urol*. 1981;125(4):545–8.

Chapter 6

PATHOPHYSIOLOGY OF AUTONOMIC DYSREFLEXIA

Anne Cameron

ETIOLOGY

Autonomic dysreflexia (AD) occurs in approximately 60% of patients with cervical spinal cord injury (SCI) and 20% of patients with thoracic SCI.[1,2] The most common stimulus for AD is stimulation of the urethra/prostate/internal sphincter region or distention of the bladder or rectum, with the former being a much more potent stimulus.[3] This can be spontaneous or caused by manipulation or instrumentation during activities such as cystoscopy, urodynamic studies (UDS), or administration of an enema.[4] Other common causes include plugging of a catheter or clot retention. Less frequent causes include misplaced urethral catheters,[5] sexual activity or electroejaculation, upper or lower tract calculi, gastrointestinal pathology, long-bone fractures, and decubitus ulcers.[6,7] AD has also been reported during extracorporeal shock wave lithotripsy (ESWL) and during childbirth.[8] A more comprehensive list of etiologies for AD is presented in Table 6.1. Understanding and appreciating the pathophysiology of AD is important since it is preventable, and failure to recognize it may result in devastating consequences such as seizures, stroke, or even death.

SIGNS

AD is classically characterized by an increase in blood pressure (BP), which can occur suddenly, accompanied by bradycardia. Patients with T6 SCI and above usually have a normal baseline BP of 90–110 mm Hg. The International Standards to document remaining Autonomic Function After Spinal Cord Injury (ISAFSCI) recommends a threshold of a rise in systolic blood pressure (SBP) of greater than 20 mm Hg from baseline.[9] SBP has been reported to rise up to 300 mm Hg and diastolic up to 220 mm Hg.[10]

Although reflex bradycardia is traditionally thought to be part of the syndrome of AD, it is only seen in 10% of cases. Tachycardia or no significant change in heart rate is more commonly noted in most patients with AD.[2,4,11]

Other objective signs that may be associated with AD include the following:

- Tachycardia
- Cardiac arrhythmias including atrial fibrillation, premature ventricular contraction, and atrioventricular conduction abnormalities
- Cutaneous vasodilation or vasoconstriction
- Penile erection
- Changes in skin and rectal temperature
- Change in the level of consciousness

SYMPTOMS

Symptoms of AD usually start after the spinal shock period. However, AD can be seen at an early stage and should be considered in the differential diagnosis of patients immediately after an SCI.[12] Patients may experience a variety of symptoms.[10] SCI patients may present with one or more of the following signs or symptoms when experiencing an AD episode. These symptoms may be minimal or even absent, even with significant rises in BP.[13]

- Pounding headache, usually occipital, bitemporal, and bifrontal in greater than 50% of patients
- Flushing and sweating above the level of injury, especially, the face and neck with cold limbs
- Piloerection (goosebumps and shivering) above or below the lesion
- Blurred vision with or without the appearance of spots in the visual field
- Nasal congestion
- Anxiety
- Dyspnea
- Malaise
- Nausea

Table 6.1   Etiology of Autonomic Dysreflexia

Genitourinary	Bladder distention/urethral stimulation (catheter clogging, cystoscopy, urodynamic studies)
	Urethral/bladder neck stimulation (cystoscopy, catheter change, clean intermittent catheterization)
	Urinary tract infection, epididymitis, orchitis
	Detrusor-sphincter dyssynergia or detrusor overactivity (urodynamics)
	Sexual intercourse, penile vibration, ejaculation, electroejaculation
	Childbirth/pregnancy/menstruation
	Kidney stones
	Extracorporeal shock wave lithotripsy
	Testicular torsion
Gastrointestinal	Bowel/rectal distention/constipation
	Anal strictures
	Gastric ulcer
	Cholelithiasis or cholecystitis
	Gastroesophageal reflux
Cutaneous	Pressure ulcers
	Burns or sunburns
	Ingrown or infected toenails
	Insect bites
Musculoskeletal/extremities	Position changes
	Spasticity
	Long-bone fracture or trauma
	Tight clothing/leg strap/abdominal binder
	Deep venous thrombosis/severe lymphedema
	Heterotopic ossification
	Exercise

Source: Adapted from Courtois F et al., *Spinal Cord*, 50, 869–77, 2012.

Despite these classic symptoms of AD, some patients will be entirely asymptomatic. Linsenmeyer et al.[14] examined 45 men with SCI above T6 of which 35 had significant elevation of BP during voiding but 45% did not have any classic symptoms. Similarly, Giannantoni[4] showed that 35% of their patients only had an increase in BP during UDS without any symptoms. It is therefore extremely important to monitor these patients during any instrumentation, as a significant number of patients may be asymptomatic.

NEUROPHYSIOLOGY OF AUTONOMIC DYSREFLEXIA

AD in the patient with SCI generally occurs after the spinal shock phase of approximately 6–12 weeks. However, some patients may show evidence of AD before the end of spinal shock. About 90% of quadriplegic patients will have evidence of AD within 6 months of their injury.[15] Studies in rats have shown that soon after SCI, bulbospinal pathways are damaged, disrupting the control of sympathetic preganglionic neurons, and the neurons are less receptive to excitatory input.[16] This is followed by regeneration and reorganization of the preganglionic fibers via abnormal synapses within the spinal cord, which occurs approximately 30 days after SCI in the rat model. There may be upregulation of the normal receptors or formation of new receptors in the preganglionic neurons as a response to their deafferentation at the time of injury.[16,17] There is also growth of C-fibers, which is regulated by nerve growth factor.[18] This promotes the exaggerated excitatory response, thus leading to occurrence of AD. The occurrence and severity of AD are therefore time dependent.[19]

The spinal cord's sympathetic outflow lies from T5 to T12 and is inaccessible in patients with SCI T5–T6 and above, thus giving these patients no control of the splanchnic bed. The initial stimulus (usually distention of viscera) reflexively causes a large sympathetic response with the release of prostaglandins and norepinephrine (Figure 6.1a). This in turn leads to α-adrenergic smooth muscle stimulation, i.e., vasoconstriction. Vasoconstriction leads to increased venous return and a rise in BP. Studies have shown that the rise in norepinephrine is independent of renin levels, indicating that the

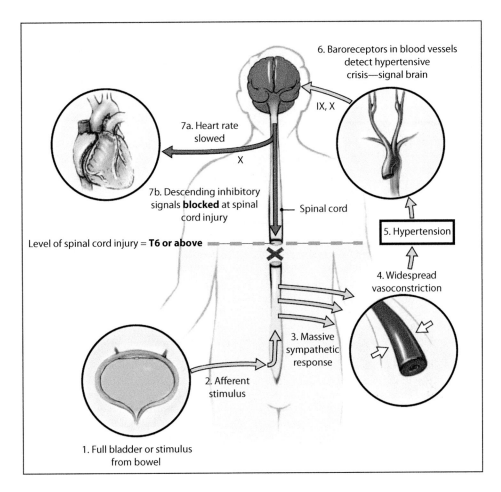

Figure 6.1 How autonomic dysreflexia occurs in spinal cord injury (SCI). An afferent stimulus (distended bladder) triggers unopposed peripheral sympathetic response causing vasoconstriction and hypertension. The usual descending inhibitory signals that normally counteract the rise in blood pressure are blocked at the level of the SCI. (Courtesy of Chelsey Sheppard.)

elevated BP is a primary sympathetic response as opposed to adrenal activity.[19,20]

PREVENTION AND TREATMENT

Urologists can play an important role in AD prevention since the primary driver of AD episodes is lower urinary tract stimulation. They can educate all patients on the importance of avoiding bladder overdistention either from infrequent catheterizations or from indwelling catheter kinking or clogging. They can also ensure that patients are not using their AD symptoms as a trigger for catheterizing, since bladder sensation is often diminished and onset of symptoms indicates that the bladder is overfilled. This results in hypertensive crisis from AD that can be prevented if the bladder is emptied sooner. Patients also need to have a rescue plan in place if they have AD episodes

from bladder distention and have difficulty with their catheter. Having a caregiver be able to assist with a Foley change should it get clogged or be able to perform clean intermittent catheterization (CIC) should the patient have acute difficulty is imperative, since there are reports of patients suffering fatal strokes after failure to perform CIC.[21] Good bladder management is key, since preventing detrusor overactivity can also prevent AD. Antimuscarinic agents, specifically fesoteridine,[22] are being investigated as a preventive treatment for AD. In one small prospective study, botulinum toxin bladder injections of 200 U decreased systolic and diastolic BP rise during urodynamics and during 24-hour ambulatory BP monitoring.[23] The frequency of AD events also decreased from a mean of four per day to one after the botulinum toxin injection. Alpha blockers such as prazosin are often used for the treatment of neurogenic bladder related incontinence and poor bladder compliance,[24] but these also have been shown to prevent AD episodes when used chronically by blocking α_1-adrenergic receptors in the peripheral vasculature without affecting resting BP or heart rate[25]; hence, if using alpha blockers consider these less-selective therapies over other alpha blockers in patients at risk for AD.

Urologists also frequently perform lower urinary tract procedures in the office on this patient population, and they can trigger AD episodes. Urodynamics (Figure 6.2), cystoscopy, cystoscopy with botulinum toxin injection, and catheter changes are all likely triggers. Urodynamics provokes AD so frequently that it is a proposed testing method for the presence of AD[14] and occurs between half and two-thirds[26–28] of patients with lesions above T6. There are certain patients who have been shown in studies to be at higher risk for AD during urodynamics, including those who have detrusor overactivity at higher pressure, are above 45 years old,[28] have a higher level of SCI, are more than 2 years postinjury, have the presence of DSD, and have poor bladder compliance[27,29]; older individuals are more likely to have asymptomatic AD,[1] and complete injuries are more likely to have more severe episodes.[27]

Unfortunately, local anesthetic of the bladder is not desirable since it will decrease the accuracy of the urodynamic test; hence, there is no clear method to prevent it, but the urologist can only recognize it early and intervene.

Cystoscopy is very stimulating to the urethra/bladder neck/prostate, which are potent drivers of AD,[3] and topical lidocaine 2% gel can be applied to the urethra several minutes ahead of the procedure and the cystoscopist should avoid bladder overdistention.

Cystoscopy with botulinum toxin is stimulating to the urethra and also the bladder through injections; hence, both the urethra and bladder require local anesthesia. Similar protocols as those used with able-bodied individuals should be applied, such as 30cc of 2% lidocaine left indwelling in the bladder for 20 minutes before the injection. It is a misconception that this analgesia can be skipped because of lack of pain perception; it is to prevent dysreflexia.

Most patients will not have dysreflexia during catheter changes and no special precautions need to be employed, but for those patients with a history of AD during catheter changes, premedicating with lidocaine 10–20 mL via the catheter and capping the tube for 10 minutes before the catheter change can be effective.[32] Also if a patient does get AD symptoms after a catheter change, the catheter placement should be verified. A catheter balloon inflated in the urethra is a potent stimulus for AD and needs to be remedied,[5] but if the catheter is confirmed to be in the correct location, lidocaine can be administered into the bladder and can be an effective treatment of an AD episode.[32]

Patients at risk for dysreflexia (SCI T6 and above), regardless of if they have AD episodes or not, should be monitored during all office procedures with a before-study baseline heart rate and BP, and at a minimum BP assessment every 3–5 minutes during the study. Also inquiring about previous episodes of AD and that patient's specific symptoms is also very helpful since the symptoms tend to be similar between episodes.

If a patient has a greater than 20 mm Hg BP rise during a urologic procedure, the procedure should be

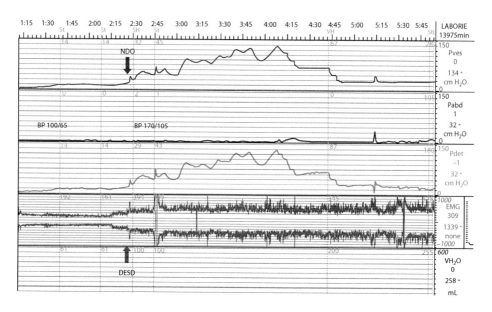

Figure 6.2   Elevation in blood pressure associated with a detrusor contraction and detrusor-sphincter dyssynergia during urodynamics in a quadriplegic patient. DESD, detrusor external sphincter dyssynergia; NDO, neurogenic detrusor overactivity.

stopped, the bladder should be drained quickly with a catheter, all urodynamics catheters including rectal should be removed, and the BP measurement should be repeated after 3–5 minutes. This is typically all that is needed for most events. If this is not effective, sit the patient upright and ensure the patient does not have any stimulus below the lesion by removing abdominal binders/compression socks, ensuring all limbs are padded and not compressed and that there are no impinging objects. Sitting the patient upright will reduce intracranial pressure during the episode, reducing the risk of complications. If this still does not resolve the episode, the patient may have impacted stool, and lidocaine gel can be instilled into the rectum and the patient gently de-impacted after waiting 2 minutes. If none of these measures are effective and SBP is greater than 150 mm Hg, 2.5 cm (1 inch) of nitropaste should be applied to the hairless portion of the chest. If BP is not improved after 10 minutes, then another 2.5 cm (1 inch) is placed. The advantage of nitropaste is that it can be wiped off as soon as SBP is less than 130 mm Hg, and it is less likely to cause reflex hypotension because of its quick

onset and clearance, unlike oral agents that take significant time. Nitropaste has an onset of action of typically 9–11 minutes and full clinical effectiveness in 14–20 minutes. In a study of 260 episodes of AD requiring nitroglycerin ointment with SBP greater than 160 mm Hg, 77% were controlled without requiring other pharmacotherapy.[34] If the two applications of nitropaste have not relieved the AD, then 10 mg of oral hydralazine can be given. In the past, beta blockers and calcium channel blockers were advocated, but these cause bradycardia and more severe hypotension once the episode is resolved. Any patient who received nitropaste or oral hydralazine should be monitored for several hours for recurrence of the hypertension and also for hypotension that occurs in approximately 4% of patients after nitropaste use[34]; hence, once these therapies are instituted, transfer to an emergency facility should be arranged since most clinics cannot accommodate this intensive monitoring (Figure 6.3).

All clinics that care for these patients should stock lidocaine gel, catheters, and at a minimum nitropaste

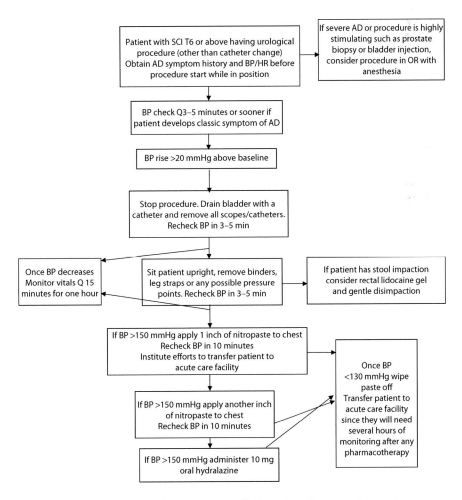

Figure 6.3   Monitoring and treatment of autonomic dysreflexia during office urologic procedures.

and should have a familiar protocol to all staff (urodynamics nurse, clinic medical assistants) so they can be familiar with these events.

An inpatient nursing-driven protocol of the treatment of AD was published by Solinski et al. that assessed its effectiveness in 445 AD episodes. When the protocol was followed, 97.6% achieved target BP, and the only adverse event was hypotension.[33]

ACKNOWLEDGMENT

The authors would like to acknowledge the editorial assistance of Gianna Rodriguez, MD, and the prior work by Dr. Inder Perkash, Teresa Danforth, and David Ginsberg, as this manuscript was modified from their chapters in the prior editions of this book.[30,31]

REFERENCES

1. Huang YH, Bih LI, Liao JM et al. Blood pressure and age associated with silent autonomic dysreflexia during urodynamic examinations in patients with spinal cord injury. *Spinal Cord.* 2013;51:401–5. http://dx.doi.org/10.1038/sc.2012.155

2. Huang YH, Bih LI, Chen GD et al. Autonomic dysreflexia during urodynamic examinations in patients with suprasacral spinal cord injury. *Arch Phys Med Rehabil.* 2011;92:1450–4.

3. Liu N, Fougere R, Zhou MW et al. Autonomic dysreflexia severity during urodynamics and cystoscopy in individuals with spinal cord injury. *Spinal Cord.* 2013;51:863–7. http://dx.doi.org/10.1038/sc.2013.113

4. Giannantoni A, Di Stasi SM, Scivoletto G et al. Autonomic dysreflexia during urodynamics. *Spinal Cord.* 1998;36:756–60.

5. Subramanian V, Soni BM, Hughes PL et al. The risk of intra-urethral Foley catheter balloon inflation in spinal cord-injured patients: Lessons learned from a retrospective case series. *Patient Saf Surg.* 2016;10:1–8. http://dx.doi.org/10.1186/s13037-016-0101-1

6. Wein AJ and Dmochowski RR. Neuromuscular dysfunction of the lower urinary tract. In: Partin A, Peters CA, Kavoussi LR, and Wein AJ, eds. *Campbell Walsh Wein Urology*, 12th ed. Amsterdam: Elsevier; 2020.

7. Arnold JMO, Feng QP, Delaney GA et al. Autonomic dysreflexia in tetraplegic patients: Evidence for α-adrenoceptor hyper-responsiveness. *Clin Auton Res.* 1995;5(5):267–70.

8. Wanner MB, Rageth CJ, and Zäch GA. Pregnancy and autonomic hyperreflexia in patients with spinal cord lesions. *Paraplegia.* 1987;25(6):482–90.

9. Krassioukov A, Biering-Sorensen F, Donovan W et al. International standards to document remaining autonomic function after spinal cord injury. *J Spinal Cord Med.* 2012;35:201–10.

10. Blackmer J. Rehabilitation medicine: 1. Autonomic dysreflexia. *CMAJ.* 2003;169:931–5.

11. Kewalramani LS. Autonomic dysreflexia in traumatic myelopathy. *Am J Phys Med.* 1980;59(1):1–21.

12. Silver JR. Early autonomic dysreflexia. *Spinal Cord.* 2000;38(4):229–33.

13. Calder KB, Estores IM, and Krassioukov A. Autonomic dysreflexia and associated acute neurogenic pulmonary edema in a patient with spinal cord injury: A case report and review of the literature. *Spinal Cord.* 2009;47:423–5.

14. Linsenmeyer TA, Campagnolo DI, and Chou IH. Silent autonomic dysreflexia during voiding in men with spinal cord injuries. *J Urol.* 1996;155:519–22.

15. Lindan R, Joiner E, Freehafer AA et al. Incidence and clinical features of autonomic dysreflexia in patients with spinal cord injury. *Paraplegia.* 1980;18:285–92.

16. Krassioukov AV and Weaver LC. Morphological changes in sympathetic preganglionic neurons after spinal cord injury in rats. *Neuroscience.* 1996;70:211–25.

17. Vaidyanathan S, Soni BM, Sett P et al. Pathophysiology of autonomic dysreflexia: Long-term treatment with terazosin in adult and paediatric spinal cord injury patients manifesting recurrent dysreflexic episodes. *Spinal Cord.* 1998; 36:761–70.

18. Elkelini MS, Bagli DJ, Fehlings M et al. Effects of intravesical onabotulinumtoxinA on bladder dysfunction and autonomic dysreflexia after spinal cord injury: Role of nerve growth factor. *BJU Int.* 2012;109:402–7.

19. Mathias CJ, Christensen NJ, Corbett JL et al. Plasma catecholamines during paroxysmal neurogenic hypertension in quadriplegic man. *Circ Res.* 1976;39(2):204–8.

20. Nanninga JB, Rosen JS, and Krumlovsky F. Effect of autonomic hyperreflexia on plasma renin. *Urology.* 1976;7:638–40.

21. Vaidyanathan S, Soni BM, Hughes PL et al. Fatal cerebral hemorrhage in a tetraplegic patient due to autonomic dysreflexia triggered by delay in emptying urinary bladder after unsuccessful intermittent catheterization by carer: Lessons learned. *Int Med Case Rep J.* 2018;11:53–8.

22. Walter M, Ramirez AL, Lee AH et al. Protocol for a phase II, open-label exploratory study investigating the efficacy of fesoterodine for treatment of adult patients with spinal cord injury suffering from neurogenic detrusor overactivity for amelioration of autonomic dysreflexia. *BMJ Open.* 2018;8:1–9.

23. Fougere RJ, Currie KD, Nigro MK et al. Reduction in bladder-related autonomic dysreflexia after onabotulinum toxin A treatment in spinal cord injury. *J Neurotrauma.* 2016;33:1651–7. http://www.liebertpub.com/10.1089/neu.2015.4278

24. Cameron AP, Clemens JQ, Latini JM et al. Combination drug therapy improves compliance of the neurogenic bladder. *J Urol.* 2009;182:1062–7.

25. Krum H, Louis WJ, Brown DJ et al. A study of the alpha-1 adrenoceptor blocker prazosin in the prophylactic management of autonomic dysreflexia in high spinal cord injury patients. *Clin Auton Res.* 1992;2:83–8.

26. Liu N, Zhou M, Biering-Sørensen F et al. Iatrogenic urological triggers of autonomic dysreflexia: A systematic review. *Spinal Cord.* 2015;53:500–9. http://www.ncbi.nlm.nih.gov/pubmed/25800696

27. Liu N, Zhou MW, Biering-Sørensen F et al. Cardiovascular response during urodynamics in individuals with spinal cord injury. *Spinal Cord.* 2017;55(3):279–84.

28. Vírseda-Chamorro M, Salinas-Casado J, Gutiérrez-Martín P et al. Risk factors to develop autonomic dysreflexia during urodynamic examinations in patients with spinal cord injury. *Neurourol Urodyn.* 2017;36(1):171–75.

29. Walter M, Knüpfer SC, Cragg JJ et al. Prediction of autonomic dysreflexia during urodynamics: A prospective cohort study. *BMC Med.* 2018;16:53.

30. Ginsberg D, and Danforth T. Pathophysiology of autonomic dysreflexia. In: *Corcos, Ginsberg, Karsenty Textbook of the Neurogenic Bladder.* Boca Raton, FL: CRC Press; 2016.

31. Perkash I. Pathophysiology of the autonomic dysreflexia. In: Corcos J, Schick E, eds. *Textbook of the Neurogenic Bladder,* 2nd ed. London, UK: CRC Press; 2008;207–11.

32. Solinsky R, and Linsenmeyer TA. Intravesical lidocaine decreases autonomic dysreflexia when administered prior to catheter change. *J Spinal Cord Med.* 2018;1–5. doi:10.1080/10790268.2018.1518764

33. Solinsky R, Svircev JN, James JJ et al. A retrospective review of safety using a nursing driven protocol for autonomic dysreflexia in patients with spinal cord injuries. *J Spinal Cord Med.* 2016;39(6):713–19.

34. Solinsky R, Bunnell AE, Linsenmeyer TA et al. Pharmacodynamics and effectiveness of topical nitroglycerin at lowering blood pressure during autonomic dysreflexia. *Spinal Cord.* 2017;55(10):911–14.

Chapter 7

PATHOPHYSIOLOGY OF SPINAL SHOCK

Siobhan M. Hartigan, Elizabeth A. Rourke, and Roger R. Dmochowski

INTRODUCTION

Spinal cord injury (SCI) results in interference with the autonomic nervous system which ultimately affects various systems including respiratory, cardiovascular, genitourinary, gastrointestinal, and sexual function. The severity of damage to the spinal cord determines the extent to which these systems are affected. SCI can be characterized by primary and secondary (modifiable) mechanisms of injury.

PRIMARY MECHANISM

Primary injury is the initial damage that occurs to the spinal cord as a result of various mechanisms. The initial trauma, damage to cord and/or cord vasculature, can be due to distraction (ligamentous tearing, dislocations), penetrating trauma (sporting accidents, gunshot wounds), and compression (spondylosis/stenosis, underlying spinal disease, etc.).[1-3] Distraction injury is the result of rapid acceleration and deceleration causing hyperextension of the spinal cord and/or shearing or stretching of the spinal cord in populations predisposed to ligament laxity, underdeveloped musculature, cord tethering, etc.[11] Compression injuries result from disk protrusions or vertebral encroachment on the spinal cord (often seen in cases of benign/malignant tumors). The goal in management of acute SCI is to prevent/minimize the cascade of secondary damage.

SECONDARY MECHANISM

Following initial injury to the spinal cord, a cascade of events occurs that results in complete/permanent injury. The initial clinical scenario in acute spinal shock, occurring within minutes of the primary injury, is due to compromise of motor, sensory, and autonomic systems resulting in flaccid paralysis, areflexia (absent somatic activity), and autonomic dysfunction driven by neurogenic shock.[4] Spinal cord shock can last days to weeks (typically 4–12 weeks) following the primary injury with studies demonstrating spinal cord edema at its peak around 3 days after injury.[5,6]

CARDIOVASCULAR AND HEMODYNAMIC INSTABILITY

In the acute phase, several physiologic derangements can occur within the autonomic nervous system, specifically, interference with the sympathetic nervous system resulting in a loss of innervation and signal transduction to the heart (bradycardia), hypotension, and hyperemia.[7] The splanchnic venous system, which mobilizes blood volume during times of stress or diminished circulating volume, is under sympathetic control. An injury to the cervical and thoracic spinal cord causes a disruption in this pathway resulting in pooling of venous blood, decreased cardiac return, and ultimately systematic hypotension.[8] In addition, parasympathetic (vagal) activity is unopposed when sympathetic nerve fibers are injured. The result is profound bradycardia that can be worsened with further stimulation of the vagal nerves and should be considered with managing a patient with an acute SCI.[9]

The secondary mechanisms of SCI include ischemia-driven edema and inflammation, hemorrhage, and hypoxia that can exacerbate cord damage and compression.[10] As discussed earlier, impaired perfusion due to sympathetic dysfunction can result in hypoxia of the spinal cord as well as direct trauma to microcirculation of the cord (arterioles, capillaries, venules, etc.). Traumatic ischemia has been demonstrated to cause intravascular thrombosis, vasospasm, and disruption of autoregulation of blood flow.[11-13] These periods of ischemia can also produce deleterious oxygen free radicals that contribute to secondary injury of the spinal cord.

CELL BIOLOGY

Vascular damage following spinal injury (both primary and secondarily mediated) is histologically demonstrated in endothelial cells and appears to be a prime mechanism of damage. Cyclooxygenase-1 (COX-1) expression is upregulated by endothelial cells following SCI as a result of an influx of intracellular messenger calcium. This causes a disruption in blood homeostasis that clinically manifests as decreases in blood flow, vasoconstriction, and platelet aggregation, as well as lipid peroxidation generating free radicals. COX-1 accumulation in macrophages, endothelial cells, and smooth muscle can persist for up to a month following initial injury and result in ischemia/necrosis at the site. In addition, COX-1 has been associated with site-specific edema secondary to vasogenic dysfunction and endothelial damage. COX-2 has also been demonstrated to undergo upregulation following SCI and is responsible for cell membrane damages and ultimately a neurotoxin causing neuronal death.[14]

Overall, COX-1 appears to be the primary source, over COX-2, driving damage at the cellular level following SCI.

ELECTROLYTE ABNORMALITIES

Secondary damage, through various mechanisms, results in a variety of electrolyte derangements including high intracellular calcium (Ca) and sodium (Na) concentrations, increased extracellular potassium (K), and depletion of intracellular magnesium (Mg).

Accumulation of intracellular Ca interferes with mitochondrial respiratory chain enzymes, which inhibits cellular respiration resulting in worsening of tissue hypoxia and ischemia. Select proteases and lipases (calpains, phospholipase A2 cyclooxygenase) are calcium mediated, and their activation can result in degradation of axon-myelin structural proteins, neurofilaments, and conversion of arachidonic acid into metabolites responsible for platelet aggregation (contributing to increased risk of thrombotic events in acute SCI patients) and vasoconstriction.[15,16] In addition, accumulation of Ca is magnified by Mg depletion. Mg serves as an important cofactor for several metabolic processes including glycolysis, phosphorylation, etc., as well as neuronal protection through the inhibition of N-methyl-D-aspartate (NMDA) receptors, and ultimately is depleted during spinal shock.[17]

Na-K ATPase inhibition occurs during the initial hours of injury and is responsible for the accumulation of intracellular Na and extracellular K. Elevated levels of extracellular K result in cellular depolarization, which decreases neuronal signal conduction and further perpetuates spinal shock.[18] Inhibition of the Na-K ATPase pump produces retention of sodium and water within the intracellular space, further contributing to deleterious edema.

APOPTOSIS

Programmed pathways of neuronal death have been implicated in the pathobiology of multiple neurologic disorders including SCI. Cellular apoptosis occurring in populations of neurons, oligodendrocytes, microglia, and possibly astrocytes plays an active role in central nervous system (CNS) injury.[19] Following SCI, the death of oligodendrocytes in white matter tracts continues for many weeks and may contribute to postinjury demyelination.[11]

There are two main pathways of apoptosis in SCI, extrinsic and intrinsic.[11] Extrinsic, or receptor-dependent, apoptosis is evoked by extracellular signals, the most significant of which is tumor necrosis factor. Tumor necrosis factor can rapidly accumulate in the injured spinal cord causing an activation of the Fas receptor of neurons, microglia, and oligodendrocytes, which subsequently induces a sequence of caspase activation involving caspase-8 and caspase-6.[20] Activation of these effector caspases results in the demise of the affected cell. Nitric oxide synthase also induces the extrinsic pathway, which brings caspace-3 activation to effect programmed cell death.[21]

The intrinsic, or receptor-independent, pathway for apoptosis after SCI is activated by intracellular signals such as high intraneuronal calcium concentrations. High calcium concentrations within neurons induce mitochondrial damage, cytochrome c release, and subsequent activation of an alternative programmed sequence of caspase activation.[11,20]

EXCITOTOXINS

The acidic amino acids glutamate and aspartate are widely distributed within the CNS and serve as excitatory neurotransmitters. When excitatory neurotransmitters are released and accumulate, there can be direct damage to the spinal cord and indirect damage from production of reactive oxygen species and nitrogen species and from alterations in microcirculatory function and secondary ischemia.[22-24] Microdialysis studies in humans with SCI[25] have shown that a massive release of glutamate and extensive and prolonged exposure of spinal neurons to glutamate is associated with excitotoxic signaling events such as an increase in intracellular Ca and dysfunction of the endoplasmic reticulum and mitochondria.[26] Consequently, release and activation of proapoptotic enzymes leads to DNA fragmentation and apoptosis.[27,28]

IMMUNOLOGIC

Historically, neuroinflammation was frequently viewed as deleterious to neurologic function and recovery following SCI, as it was previously thought that suppression of immune response would be neuroprotective; however, recent studies have revealed some beneficial aspects of inflammation that should not be inhibited.[29,30] Microglia and infiltrating macrophages in the CNS are heterogenous, with diverse functions that range from pro-inflammatory (M1-like) phenotypes to immunosuppressive (M2-like) phenotypes.[31] Microglia are the primary mediators of the innate immune response in the CNS and play a critical role in neuroinflammation and secondary injury following injury to the CNS, such as SCI. Inflammatory response following SCI for wound healing also includes leukocyte influx from the periphery, lesion debris clearance by neutrophils, tissue remodeling, axonal regrowth, and remyelination.[32] In order to develop therapeutic methods of modulating the immune system, further work needs to be conducted to better understand immune cell subtypes that are more detrimental than beneficial and those that are necessary in repair.

ENDOGENOUS OPIOIDS

Following primary SCI, there is a rise in endogenous opioids (endorphins) that activate opioid receptors and can contribute to the excitotoxic process described earlier.[33] The excitotoxic process can be prolonged by activation of μ and δ opioid receptors. Activation of κ receptors can exacerbate decreases in blood flow and promote the excitotoxic process.[34] With the release of endogenous opioids, levels of certain neurotransmitters, such as acetylcholine and 5-hydroytryptamine (5-HT, serotonin), also rise, which can contribute to secondary damage by causing vasoconstriction and promoting platelet activation and endothelial permeability.[11,35] Treatment with naloxone, an opiate antagonist, improves blood pressure and spinal cord blood flow and is associated with less prominent spinal cord changes and significantly improved neurologic recovery.[35]

EFFECT OF SPINAL CORD INJURY ON MICTURITION

The effect of SCI on lower urinary tract function is dependent on the level, duration, and completeness of the cord lesion. When damage to the spinal cord occurs rostral to the sacral cord, functional deficits give the picture of an upper motor neuron lesion. Alternatively, a lower motor neuron lesion clinical picture is seen when damage occurs to the sacral

cord and/or cauda equina that gives rise to the parasympathetic and somatic pathway to the bladder and urethral sphincter.[36] Upper motor neuron type SCI initially leads to a phase of spinal shock characterized by a flaccid paralysis and absence of reflex activity below the level of the lesion. Therefore, the detrusor becomes areflexic. However, activity of the internal and external sphincter persists or rapidly recovers after suprasacral injuries. Due to the presence of sphincter tone, urinary retention develops, and patients are treated with intermittent or continuous catheterization for bladder drainage until spinal shock subsides. Spinal shock usually lasts 6–12 weeks in complete suprasacral spinal cord lesions but may last up to 1–2 years.[36] In the case of incomplete suprasacral lesions, spinal shock may last for a shorter period of time or even just a few days.

REFERENCES

1. Winter B and Pattani H. Spinal cord injury. *Anaesth Intens Care Med.* 2011;12(9):403–5.
2. Devivo MJ. Epidemiology of traumatic spinal cord injury: Trends and future implications. *Spinal Cord.* 2012;50(5):365–72.
3. Sekhon LH and Fehlings MG. Epidemiology, demographics, and pathophysiology of acute spinal cord injury. *Spine (Phila Pa 1976).* 2001;26(24 Suppl):S2–12.
4. Ditunno JF, Little JW, Tessler A, and Burns AS. Spinal shock revisited: A four-phase model. *Spinal Cord.* 2004;42(7):383–95.
5. Yashon D, Bingham WG Jr, Faddoul EM, and Hunt WE. Edema of the spinal cord following experimental impact trauma. *J Neurosurg.* 1973; 38(6):693–7.
6. Biering-Sorensen F, Biering-Sorensen T, Liu N, Malmqvist L, Wecht JM, and Krassioukov A. Alterations in cardiac autonomic control in spinal cord injury. *Auton Neurosci.* 2018;209:4–18.
7. Atkinson PP and Atkinson JL. Spinal shock. *Mayo Clin Proc.* 1996;71(4):384–9.
8. Furlan JC, Fehlings MG, Shannon P, Norenberg MD, and Krassioukov AV. Descending vasomotor pathways in humans: Correlation between axonal preservation and cardiovascular dysfunction after spinal cord injury. *J Neurotrauma.* 2003;20(12):1351–63.
9. Lee J and Thumbikat P. Pathophysiology, presentation and management of spinal cord injury. *Surgery (Oxford).* 2015;33(6):238–47.
10. Rowland JW, Hawryluk GW, Kwon B, and Fehlings MG. Current status of acute spinal cord injury pathophysiology and emerging therapies: Promise on the horizon. *Neurosurg Focus.* 2008;25(5):E2.
11. Dumont RJ, Okonkwo DO, Verma S et al. Acute spinal cord injury, part I: Pathophysiologic mechanisms. *Clin Neuropharmacol.* 2001;24(5):254–64.
12. Tator CH and Fehlings MG. Review of the secondary injury theory of acute spinal cord trauma with emphasis on vascular mechanisms. *J Neurosurg.* 1991;75(1):15–26.

13. de la Torre JC. Spinal cord injury. Review of basic and applied research. *Spine (Phila Pa 1976)*. 1981;6(4):315–35.

14. Schwab JM, Brechtel K, Nguyen TD, and Schluesener HJ. Persistent accumulation of cyclooxygenase-1 (COX-1) expressing microglia/macrophages and upregulation by endothelium following spinal cord injury. *J Neuroimmunol*. 2000;111(1–2):122–30.

15. Fiskum G. Mitochondrial participation in ischemic and traumatic neural cell death. *J Neurotrauma*. 2000;17(10):843–55.

16. Schanne FA, Kane AB, Young EE, and Farber JL. Calcium dependence of toxic cell death: A final common pathway. *Science*. 1979;206(4419):700–2.

17. Rhoney DH, Luer MS, Hughes M, and Hatton J. New pharmacologic approaches to acute spinal cord injury. *Pharmacotherapy*. 1996;16(3):382–92.

18. Young W, and Koreh I. Potassium and calcium changes in injured spinal cords. *Brain Res*. 1986;365(1):42–53.

19. Beattie MS, Farooqui AA, and Bresnahan JC. Review of current evidence for apoptosis after spinal cord injury. *J Neurotrauma*. 2000;17(10):915–25.

20. Eldadah BA and Faden AI. Caspase pathways, neuronal apoptosis, and CNS injury. *J Neurotrauma*. 2000;17(10):811–29.

21. Satake K, Matsuyama Y, Kamiya M et al. Nitric oxide via macrophage iNOS induces apoptosis following traumatic spinal cord injury. *Brain Res Mol Brain Res*. 2000;85(1–2):114–22.

22. Panter SS, Yum SW, and Faden AI. Alteration in extracellular amino acids after traumatic spinal cord injury. *Ann Neurol*. 1990;27(1):96–9.

23. Faden AI, Lemke M, Simon RP, and Noble LJ. *N*-methyl-D-aspartate antagonist MK801 improves outcome following traumatic spinal cord injury in rats: Behavioral, anatomic, and neurochemical studies. *J Neurotrauma*. 1988;5(1):33–45.

24. Faden AI and Simon RP. A potential role for excitotoxins in the pathophysiology of spinal cord injury. *Ann Neurol*. 1988;23(6):623–6.

25. Chen S, Phang I, Zoumprouli A, Papadopoulos MC, and Saadoun S. Metabolic profile of injured human spinal cord determined using surface microdialysis. *J Neurochem*. 2016;139(5):700–5.

26. Schizas N, Perry S, Andersson B, Wahlby C, Kullander K, and Hailer NP. Differential neuroprotective effects of interleukin-1 receptor antagonist on spinal cord neurons after excitotoxic injury. *Neuroimmunomodulation*. 2017;24(4–5):220–30.

27. Nath R, Scott M, Nadimpalli R, Gupta R, and Wang KK. Activation of apoptosis-linked caspase(s) in NMDA-injured brains in neonatal rats. *Neurochem Int*. 2000;36(2):119–26.

28. Anguelova E, Boularand S, Nowicki JP, Benavides J, and Smirnova T. Up-regulation of genes involved in cellular stress and apoptosis in a rat model of hippocampal degeneration. *J Neurosci Res*. 2000;59(2):209–17.

29. Gaudet AD and Fonken LK. Glial cells shape pathology and repair after spinal cord injury. *Neurotherapeutics*. 2018;15(3):554–77.

30. Plemel JR, Wee Yong V, and Stirling DP. Immune modulatory therapies for spinal cord injury—Past, present and future. *Exp Neurol*. 2014;258:91–104.

31. Faden AI, Wu J, Stoica BA, and Loane DJ. Progressive inflammation-mediated neurodegeneration after traumatic brain or spinal cord injury. *Br J Pharmacol*. 2016;173(4):681–91.

32. Bowes AL and Yip PK. Modulating inflammatory cell responses to spinal cord injury: All in good time. *J Neurotrauma*. 2014;31(21):1753–66.

33. McIntosh TK, Hayes RL, DeWitt DS, Agura V, and Faden AI. Endogenous opioids may mediate secondary damage after experimental brain injury. *Am J Physiol*. 1987;253(5 Pt 1):E565–74.

34. Olsson Y, Sharma HS, Nyberg F, and Westman J. The opioid receptor antagonist naloxone influences the pathophysiology of spinal cord injury. *Prog Brain Res*. 1995;104:381–99.

35. Faden AI. Neuropeptides and central nervous system injury. Clinical implications. *Arch Neurol*. 1986;43(5):501–4.

36. Wein AJ and Dmochowski RR. Neuromuscular dysfunction of the lower urinary tract. In: Wein AJ, Kavoussi LR, Partin AW, and Peters CA, eds. *Campbell-Walsh Urology*, 11th ed. Philadelphia, PA: Elsevier; 2016:1761–95.

NEUROLOGIC PATHOLOGIES RESPONSIBLE FOR THE DEVELOPMENT OF THE NEUROGENIC BLADDER

Section A

PERIPHERAL NEUROPATHIES

Chapter 8

SYSTEMIC ILLNESSES (DIABETES MELLITUS, SARCOIDOSIS, ALCOHOLISM, AND PORPHYRIAS)

Stephanie Kielb and Jeremy Lai

INTRODUCTION

Neurogenic bladder can be a result of peripheral neuropathy due to various systemic illnesses. In this chapter, we discuss diabetes mellitus, sarcoidosis, alcoholism, and porphyria.

DIABETES MELLITUS

Diabetes can be divided into type 1 and type 2. Type 1 is characterized by insulin deficiency most commonly caused by an autoimmune destruction of the pancreatic Langerhans islet cells, and type 2 is characterized by a heterogenous group of genetic and environmental causes where insulin production cannot meet the body's demand.[1] In the past, type 1 was associated with people less than 30 years old, but it is now recognized that the autoimmune process can occur at any age. There is also an increase in the incidence of type 2 diabetes in adolescents and children.[2]

Almost one-third of all patients with diabetes have evidence of a peripheral neuropathy. It is estimated that 25.8 million cases or 8.3% of the U.S. population have diabetes, including an estimated 7 million cases that have been undiagnosed. Worldwide the prevalence is estimated to be 415 million people.[3] The prevalence is similar in men and women, although men may develop neuropathy earlier in their course.[4] Approximately 50% of all diabetics will have some form of nervous system damage.[5]

COMPLICATIONS
Chronic complications of diabetes affect many organ systems and can generally be divided into vascular and nonvascular complications. Vascular complications are more common and include retinopathy, neuropathy, nephropathy, coronary heart disease, peripheral artery disease, and cerebrovascular disease. It is thought that the high percentage of patients who present with complications on diagnosis of diabetes reflects delayed diagnosis, and neuropathy may be the presenting symptom in many of these patients.[6]

The most common neurologic complication of diabetes is diabetic peripheral neuropathy.[7] It is estimated that over 10% of patients present with diabetic neuropathy.[8] Diabetic neuropathy is heterogeneous and can be symmetric or multifocal. It can also be continuous or episodic and may manifest as polyneuropathy, mononeuropathy, and/or autonomic neuropathy. The cause of neurogenic bladder is autonomic neuropathy. The incidence of urinary tract complaints in patients with diabetes is estimated to be up to 1.5 times that of the general population and is associated with increased age, longer diabetes duration, and concomitant diabetes complications.[9]

The bladder is innervated by the autonomic nervous system, while the urethra is innervated by a combination of autonomic and somatic nerves. The mechanism for neurogenic bladder in diabetes can be a result of a sensory and/or a motor neuropathy. Sensory neuropathy affects the filling stage and can be a source of both overactive bladder (OAB) and impaired sensation of a full bladder. Motor neuropathy contributes to impaired detrusor contractility and affects the bladder's ability to empty completely. Diabetic cystopathy is classically thought of as an insidious onset of impaired bladder sensation due to impaired sensory afferent pathways accompanied by a decrease in voiding frequency. Eventually this can lead to unrecognized detrusor distension and then overdistension and decompensation. The end result is a hyposensitive, underactive neurogenic bladder (Figure 8.1).

PATHOGENESIS
Complications of diabetes arise from vascular and metabolic derangements, and it is likely that both contribute to peripheral neuropathies and voiding dysfunction.[10] Vascular hypoxia and ischemia have also been implicated in diabetic polyneuropathy via direct and indirect mechanisms such as structural changes to nerves.[11]

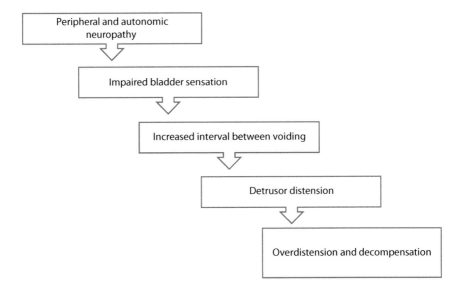

Figure 8.1   Classic diabetic cystopathy progression.

EVALUATION AND MANAGEMENT

The urodynamic findings associated with classic diabetic cystopathy include impaired bladder sensation, increased bladder capacity, decreased bladder contractility, impaired urinary flow, and, later, increased residual urine volume. The constellation of findings is often reported as a hyposensitive, underactive bladder. It is important to distinguish between outlet obstruction and decreased bladder contractility, especially in the case of impaired urinary flow. Pressure-flow urodynamics will distinguish between the two etiologies. It is uncommon to see sphincter dyssynergia in diabetic cystopathy, and one must be careful to identify abdominal straining on urodynamics (Figure 8.2) that can be associated with an interference electromyographic pattern (pseudodyssynergia).[12]

Management begins with behavioral modifications focused on general care of the diabetic patient. Weight loss, dietary changes, and medication adherence are important in addition to glycemic control for preventing neurogenic bladder. The strategy for bladder management specifically is to attempt to mimic normal capacity and emptying and to protect the upper tracts.

In the early phases of diabetic cystopathy, timed and double voiding may help to prevent some of the problems associated with overdistension. Some patients may require clean intermittent catheterization if they cannot generate an adequate contraction to empty their bladder. Oral medications (anticholinergics, β_3 agonists) may be useful for OAB symptoms, but these patients must be followed closely as they may not have adequate sensation or contractility to detect urinary retention. A postvoid residual should be obtained after initiation of therapy and periodically in follow-up. Sacral neuromodulation has also been studied as an option. Compared to non-diabetic patients, there are no significant differences in outcomes for the diabetic patients treated for incontinence, urgency/frequency, and retention with neuromodulation. There were however, more device explants secondary to infection for diabetic patients with sacral nerve stimulators.[13]

> **KEY POINTS**
>
> - Diabetes is an increasingly common condition with neurologic consequences on the bladder.
> - Autonomic neuropathy, both sensory and motor, is the foundation of diabetic cystopathy.
> - Diabetic cystopathy is characterized by impaired bladder sensation, increased capacity, decreased contractility, impaired flow, and increased postvoid residuals.
> - Initial management includes behavioral modification, timed voiding, and glucose control.

SARCOIDOSIS

PREVALENCE

Sarcoidosis is a relatively common disease that affects both males and females, and most races, ages, and regional locations. Females have been noted to have a slightly higher susceptibility than males.[14] Among adults worldwide, the prevalence of the disease varies between 10 and 60 per 100,000. In the United

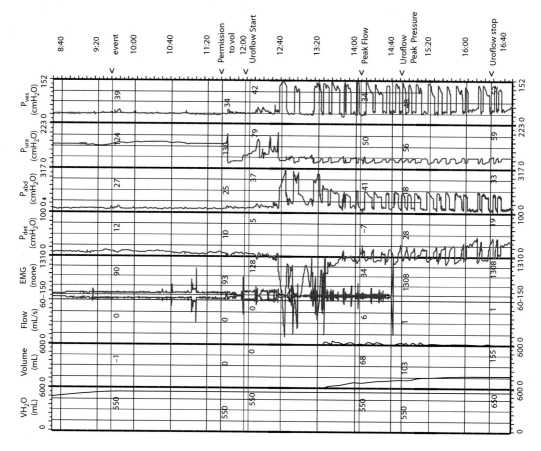

Figure 8.2   Classic urodynamic evidence of abdominal voiding: at initiation of flow, abdominal straining is noted.

States, African-Americans are three times more predisposed to it than whites. The highest prevalence is seen in the Netherlands, Great Britain, Ireland, and the Scandinavian countries.[15] Sarcoidosis usually develops before 50 years of age, and the peak of incidence in both sexes is around the ages of 25–29 years. Sarcoidosis is a chronic disease that can affect almost any organ in the body. The precise etiology remains unknown, though interplay between both environmental and recently identified immune-related genetic risk factors continues to be identified.[16] The main characteristic of sarcoidosis is noncaseating granulomas.[17] Because it can manifest variably in any organ, the disease can affect a variety of functions.[18]

NEUROSARCOIDOSIS

The prevalence of neurosarcoidosis is registered in 5% of patients with sarcoidosis.[19] Peripheral nervous system involvement ranges between 25% and 67%.[20] The central nervous system can also be affected; in the brain, patients can have leptomeningeal and intraparenchymal granulomatous infiltrates, but these lesions can be found anywhere along the spinal cord.[21] In a review of neurosarcoidosis literature, cranial neuropathy was the most common manifestation, with micturition abnormalities

reported in 23/206 (11%) patients. Spinal cord disease and peripheral neuropathies were identified in a larger portion of patients (185); however, it is not clear how many patients were evaluated for urinary tract symptoms.

If sarcoidosis affects the autonomic nerves innervating the lower urinary tract, it can cause neurogenic bladder dysfunction with manifestations dependent on the location of lesions. The exact incidence of patients with neurogenic bladder due to neurosarcoidosis is unknown because only a few cases have been urodynamically investigated and reported.[22–25] In 17 patients with known central nervous sarcoidosis, 35% were noted to have sphincter dysfunction with micturition difficulties.[26] According to their clinical symptoms, these patients likely experienced both upper and lower types of neurogenic bladder, making urodynamics a recommended part of the workup due to the unpredictability of neurosarcoidosis lesion location and impact when suspected.

TREATMENT

Overall, sarcoidosis is frequently a self-limiting disease, and prognosis is good as a whole. The therapeutic approach to the neurogenic bladder caused by neurosarcoidosis is directed by symptoms and urodynamics findings. If the disease is in remission or the patient is asymptomatic, no treatment is necessary. When indicated, the standard sarcoidosis therapy includes the use of corticosteroids, methotrexate, azathioprine, and hydroxychloroquine, an antimalarial drug. Cyclophosphamide is more specifically used to treat neurosarcoidosis.[27]

KEY POINTS

- Sarcoidosis is a common, chronic disease that can affect virtually any organ in the body.
- Neurosarcoidosis is present in roughly 5% of patients and occur more commonly cranially but can also affect the spinal cord or any peripheral nerve level.
- The exact incidence of neurogenic bladder is not clear, as few symptomatic or urodynamic studies have been reported in this patient population.
- Given the possible presence of cord and peripheral lesions, urodynamics studies should be undertaken in the patient with sarcoidosis with suspected urologic involvement.
- Management is symptom focused and may include cyclophosphamide for more specific neurosarcoidosis related symptoms.

ALCOHOLISM

DEFINITION AND PREVALENCE
In Western countries, about 80% of people have consumed alcohol (ethanol) at some point in their life. Although alcohol consumption is considered a universal behavior, repetitive alcohol usage and alcohol abuse can be seen in both men and women. Alcohol consumption can have adverse legal, occupational, social, psychological, and medical consequences. The *Diagnostic and Statistical Manual of Mental Disorders*, fifth edition (*DSM-5*) defines alcohol use disorder as meeting at least 2 of 11 specific criteria over a 12-month period.[28] Alcoholism is found in all races and ethnicities regardless of education or income, although it is difficult to determine the exact prevalence of alcoholism. In Western countries, the prevalence of alcohol dependence is about 10%–15% for men and 5%–8% for women.[29]

CLINICAL NEUROPATHOLOGY
Alcohol can affect the central nervous system in several ways. Polyneuropathy is the most common manifestation, affecting 5%–15% of alcoholics.[30] Ethanol can interfere with the absorption of both fat and water soluble vitamins, e.g., thiamine (B1), nicotinic

acid (B3), pyridoxine (B6), folate (B9), and vitamin A.[29] Polyneuropathy can be a result of nutritional deficiency (mainly thiamine deficiency) and/or direct toxic effect of ethanol and acetaldehyde.[31] Studies that propose direct toxicity of alcohol on the peripheral nervous system show cytochrome P450E1, an isozyme of cytochrome P450, to induce oxidative stress causing neurotoxicity[32] or a direct neurotoxic effect of ethanol or its metabolites.[33] Alcoholic neuropathy is uniformly shown to be slow progression of distal and symmetric sensory and motor disease. In some cases, damage can lead to loss of ganglionic neurons and sympathetic and parasympathetic nerve fibers.[40]

Patients with neurogenic bladder due to alcohol dependence show similar clinical neurourologic and urodynamic findings as a diabetic neurogenic bladder. Management of neurogenic bladder caused by this disease is thus in accordance with that suggested in the "Diabetes Mellitus" section.

KEY POINTS

- Alcoholism is found in all races and ethnicities regardless of education or income.
- Alcoholic neuropathy can affect both the central and peripheral nervous systems.
- Alcoholic neuropathy may be the result of nutritional deficiency (mainly thiamine) and direct toxic effect of alcohol on peripheral nerves.
- Alcoholic neuropathy has a slow progression of distal, symmetric, sensory, and motor disease.
- Neurogenic bladder due to alcohol use disorder is urodynamically similar to diabetic bladder.

PORPHYRIAS

DEFINITION AND BIOCHEMISTRY
Porphyrias consist of a group of eight metabolic hereditary disorders. They are further classified as either erythropoietic or hepatic depending on the main site of expression of the defective enzyme. The disease is caused by acquired or inherited partial deficiency of one of the enzymes in heme biosynthesis. Porphyrin precursor's overproduction is seen in acute hepatic porphyrias, whereas porphyrins are seen in the cutaneous types.[34] There are five hepatic porphyrias, four of which present with neurologic symptoms: acute intermittent porphyria (AIP), δ-aminolevulinic acid dehydratase-deficient porphyria (ADP), hereditary coproporphyria (HCP), and variegate porphyria (VP).[35] Acute attacks are usually precipitated by factors that fall into four categories: nutrition, endocrine factors, stress, and drugs. The consumption of various drugs includes,

but is not limited to, contraceptives, barbiturates, sulfonamides, griseofulvin, phenytoin, valproic acid, steroids, and succinimides.

NEUROPATHOLOGY

The most common manifestations of porphyric neuropathy are a product of involvement of small unmyelinated and myelinated nerve fibers throughout the nervous system along with destruction of the axis cylinders. By far the most affected seem to be the peripheral nerves and supporting cells, suffering from degenerated axons with secondary demyelination without inflammatory or vascular lesions.[36] Autonomic function studies have shown that during acute attacks both parasympathetic and sympathetic nerves are impaired.[37] The pathogenesis of neurologic symptoms is not certain but is thought to be due to a reduction in heme protein in neuronal cells or neurotoxic levels of δ-aminolevulinic acid.[38]

DIAGNOSIS AND TREATMENT

Clinical manifestations commonly present with abdominal pain, psychotic symptoms, and neuropathy ranging from peripheral acute or subacute distal or proximal mononeuritis or polyneuropathy. Other symptoms such as tachycardia, hypertension, postural hypotension, fever, excessive sweating, urinary retention, hesitancy, and dysuria are also due to autonomic failure.[39] Acute urinary retention has been reported in patients with porphyria, while cystoscopy was found to be normal.[40]

The treatment of porphyrias is mainly preventative. It is important to avoid precipitating factors, such as porphyrogenic drugs, excessive stress, and prolonged starvation. Intravenous heme is the most immediate and effective therapy in the acute setting. The mortality rate during acute attacks is less than 10%.[41] Motor neuropathy associated with acute attacks typically resolves within 1 year.[42] The same treatment as in the "Diabetes Mellitus" section is recommended. If bladder dysfunction is present, treatment is usually the same as noted for the diabetic neurogenic bladder. In addition, patients should be monitored for resolution of symptoms over time, though there is little published to provide additional guidance.

KEY POINTS

- Porphyria is caused by a hereditary defect in one of the eight steps in heme formation.
- They are grouped into hepatic and cutaneous forms, with manifestations of the overproduction of heme precursors and manifestations being due to nervous system effects.
- Acute presenting symptoms include abdominal pain, psychotic symptoms, and neuropathy.

- Neurogenic bladder has been reported in porphyria and should be managed similar to diabetic bladder.
- Treatment of porphyria includes heme and avoidance of precipitating factors.

CONCLUSION

The four systemic illnesses reviewed in this chapter—diabetes, sarcoidosis, alcoholism, and porphyrias—affect the bladder in diverse and heterogeneous ways. There is still much to be understood as far as the mechanisms of disease and prevention are concerned. A thorough evaluation of these patients, often involving urodynamics, is useful in personalizing clinical treatment plans.

REFERENCES

1. Diagnosis and classification of diabetes mellitus. *Diabetes Care*. 2010;34(Suppl 1):S62–9.
2. Powers A. Diabetes mellitus. In: Longo D, Fauci AS, Kasper DL, Hauser S, Jameson J, and Loscalzo J, eds. *Harrison's Principles of Internal Medicine*, 18th edn. New York, NY: McGraw-Hill; 2012.
3. Ogurtsova K, da Rocha Fernandes JD, Huang Y et al. IDF Diabetes atlas: Global estimates for the prevalence of diabetes for 2015 and 2040. *Diabetes Res Clin Pract*. 2017;128:40–50.
4. Aaberg ML, Burch DM, Hud ZR, and Zacharias MP. Gender differences in the onset of diabetic neuropathy. *J Diabetes Complications*. 2008;22(2):83–7.
5. Hicks CW, Selvin E. Epidemiology of peripheral neuropathy and lower extremity disease in diabetes. *Curr Diab Rep*. 2019;19(10):86.
6. Partanen J, Niskanen L, Lehtinen J, Mervaala E, Siitonen O, and Uusitupa M. Natural history of peripheral neuropathy in patients with non-insulin-dependent diabetes mellitus. *N Engl J Med*. 1995;333(2):89–94.
7. Tesfaye S, Boulton AJ, and Dickenson AH. Mechanisms and management of diabetic painful distal symmetrical polyneuropathy. *Diabetes Care*. 2013;36(9):2456–65.
8. Callaghan BC, Little AA, Feldman EL, and Hughes RAC. Enhanced glucose control for preventing and treating diabetic neuropathy. *Cochrane Database Syst Rev*. 2012;6:. CD007543, CD007543
9. Wiedemann AFl. The patient with diabetes in urologic practice: A special risk for lower urinary tract symptoms? Results of the Witten diabetes survey of 4071 type 2 diabetics. *Urol A*. 2010;49(2):238–44.
10. Stevens MJ, Feldman EL, and Greene DA. The aetiology of diabetic neuropathy: The combined roles of metabolic and vascular defects. *Diabet Med*. 1995;12(7):566–79.

11. Dyck PJ, and Giannini C. Pathologic alterations in the diabetic neuropathies of humans. *J Neuropathol Exp Neurol*. 1996;55(12):1181–93.

12. Wein AJ. Preface. In: Kavoussi LR, Partin AW, Peters CA, eds. *Campbell-Walsh Urology*. Elsevier; 2012:xxv.

13. Daniels DH, Powell CR, Braasch MR, and Kreder KJ. Sacral neuromodulation in diabetic patients: Success and complications in the treatment of voiding dysfunction. *Neurourol Urodynam*. 2010;29(4):578–81.

14. Baughman RP Lower EE. In: Longo D, Fauci AS, Kasper DL, Hauser S, Jameson J, and Loscalzo J, eds. *Harrison's Principles of Internal Medicine*, 18th edn. New York, NY: McGraw-Hill; 2012.

15. Nicholson TT, Plant BJ, Henry MT, and Bredin CP. Sarcoidosis in Ireland: Regional differences in prevalence and mortality from 1996–2005. *Sarcoidosis Vasc Diffuse Lung Dis*. 2010;27(2):111–20.

16. Fischer A, Ellinghaus D, Nutsua M et al. Identification of immune-relevant factors conferring sarcoidosis genetic risk. *Am J Respir Crit Care Med*. 2015;192(6):727–36.

17. Iannuzzi MC, Rybicki BA, and Teirstein AS. Sarcoidosis. *N Engl J Med*. 2007;357(21):2153–65.

18. Culver DA. Sarcoidosis. *Immunol Allergy Clin North Am*. 2012;32(4):487–511.

19. Titlic M, Bradic-Hammoud M, Miric L, and Punda A. Clinical manifestations of neurosarcoidosis. *Bratisl Lek Listy*. 2009;110(9):576–79.

20. Delaney P. Neurologic manifestations in sarcoidosis. *Ann Intern Med*. 1977;87(3):336.

21. Vargas D, and Stern B. Neurosarcoidosis: Diagnosis and management. *Semin Respir Crit Care Med*. 2010;31(04):419–27.

22. La Rochelle JC, and Coogan CL. Urological manifestations of sarcoidosis. *J Urol*. 2012;187(1):18–24.

23. Kim IY, Elliott DS, Husmann DA, and Boone TB. An unusual presenting symptom of sarcoidosis: Neurogenic bladder dysfunction. *J Urol*. 2001;165:903–4.

24. Sakakibara R, Hattori T, Uchiyama T, and Yamanishi T. Micturitional disturbance in a patient with neurosarcoidosis. *Neurourol Urodyn*. 2000;19(3):273–7.

25. Fitzpatrick KJ, Chancellor MB, Rivas DA, Kumon H, Mandel S, and Manon-Espaillat R. Urologic manifestation of spinal cord sarcoidosis. *J Spinal Cord Med*. 1996;19(3):201–3.

26. Koffman B, Junck L, Elias SB, Feit HW, and Levine SR. Polyradiculopathy in sarcoidosis. *Muscle Nerve*. 1999;22(5):608–13.

27. Judson MA. Sarcoidosis: Clinical presentation, diagnosis, and approach to treatment. *Am J Med Sci*. 2008;335(1):26–33.

28. *Diagnostic and Statistical Manual of Mental Disorders, Fifth edition (DSM-5)*. Washington, DC: American Psychiatric Publishing; 2013.

29. Schuckit MA. Alcohol and alcoholism. In: Longo D, Fauci AS, Kasper DL, Hauser S, Jameson J, and Loscalzo J, eds. *Harrison's Principles of Internal Medicine*, 18th edn. New York, NY: McGraw-Hill; 2012.

30. Albanese AP. Management of alcohol abuse. *Clin Liver Dis*. 2012;16(4):737–62.

31. Mellion M, Gilchrist JM, and De La Monte S. Alcohol-related peripheral neuropathy: Nutritional, toxic, or both? *Muscle Nerve*. 2011;43(3):309–16.

32. Ammendola A. Peripheral neuropathy in chronic alcoholism: A retrospective cross-sectional study in 76 subjects. *Alcohol Alcohol*. 2001;36(3):271–5.

33. Koike H, Iijima M, Sugiura M et al. Alcoholic neuropathy is clinicopathologically distinct from thiamine-deficiency neuropathy. *Ann Neurol*. 2003;54(1):19–29.

34. Desnick RJ, and Balwani M. The porphyrias. In: Longo D, Fauci AS, Kasper DL, Hauser S, Jameson J, and Loscalzo J, eds. *Harrison's Principles of Internal Medicine*, 18th edn. New York, NY: McGraw-Hill; 2012.

35. Schneider-Yin X, Harms J, and Minder EI. Porphyria in Switzerland, 15 years experience. *Swiss Med Wkly*. 2009;139(13–14):198–206.

36. Torpy JM. Peripheral neuropathy. *JAMA*. 2010;303(15):1556.

37. Tjandra BS, and Janknegt RA. Neurogenic impotence and lower urinary tract symptoms due to vitamin B1 deficiency in chronic alcoholism. *J Urol*. 1997;157:954–5.

38. Scott TS, Brillman J, and Gross JA. Sarcoidosis of the peripheral nervous system. *Neurol Res*. 1993;15(6):389–90.

39. Mumford CJ. Clinical neurology. *Brain*. 2003;126(5):1245–6.

40. Redeker AG. Atonic neurogenic bladder in porphyria. *J Urol*. 1956;75(3):465–9.

41. Phillips JD, Anderson KE. The porphyrias. In: Prchal JT, Kaushansky K, Lichtman MA, Kipps TJ, Seligsohn U, eds. *Williams Hematology*, 8th edn. New York, NY: McGraw-Hill, 2010.

42. Bissell DM, Anderson KE, and Bonkovsky HL. Porphyria. *N Engl J Med*. 2017;377(9):862–72.

Chapter 9

PERIPHERAL NEUROPATHIES OF THE LOWER URINARY TRACT FOLLOWING PELVIC SURGERY AND RADIATION THERAPY

David Ginsberg and Temitope Rude

INTRODUCTION

The peripheral nervous system is the end mediator for neuromuscular control of the lower urinary tract. As such, a thorough appreciation of this complex anatomy is required for the pelvic physician and surgeon. Such an understanding allows for optimized treatment approaches as well as expedient recognition of post-treatment injuries. In this chapter, we discuss the relevant anatomy and syndromes occurring after pelvic surgery and/or pelvic radiation therapy and their management.

PERIPHERAL NEUROANATOMY

Three main peripheral nerves innervate the pelvis, providing sensation and control to the bladder, urethra, pelvic floor, and external genitalia (Figure 9.1). Autonomic innervation is provided by the pelvic and hypogastric nerves.[1] The pelvic nerve provides parasympathetic inputs from its origin in the sacral spinal cord from the S2-S4 ventral rami. From there, presynaptic neurons course medially toward the inferior hypogastric plexus, located near the root of the middle rectal artery and covered by the endopelvic fascia where they join the sympathetic fibers.[2-4] The peripheral parasympathetic branches from this plexus then innervate the bladder, urethra, and internal urinary sphincter, as well as the prostate, seminal vesicles, rectum, and sexual organs.[5-7] Primarily via its neurotransmitter of acetylcholine (Ach), it causes detrusor excitation via the M3 receptor; it also causes relaxation of the internal urethral sphincter at level of the urethra and bladder neck via nitric oxide release.[8]

The opposing sympathetic innervation is from the hypogastric nerve. This nerve originates from the thoracolumbar segments T10-L2 after synapsing at the paravertebral sympathetic chains. The postsynaptic neurons then form the superior hypogastric plexus at the bifurcation of the aorta. The hypogastric nerves then travel 2 cm from the ureters and common iliac arteries,[3] to the inferior hypogastric plexus, then to its target organs. Sympathetic branches then release noradrenaline causing detrusor relaxation via β-adrenergic inhibition and internal urethral sphincter excitation via α-adrenergic receptors, in addition to rectal, prostatic, and sexual functions.

Somatic motor innervation to the external urethral sphincter occurs via the pudendal nerve. From its origin in Onuf's nucleus in the sacral spine at S2-S4, it travels from the sacrotuberous ligament and exits the pelvis through the grater sciatic foramen. The pudendal nerve then gives off inferior rectal and perineal branches which innervate the internal anal and striated urethral sphincters, respectively, mediated by Ach.[1]

Afferent signaling of bladder fullness is mediated by the autonomic nerves, while bladder neck and urethral sensations are carried by the pudendal and hypogastric nerves. These nerves are composed of A δ and C fibers, which are myelinated and unmyelinated, respectively. A δ fibers respond to bladder filling and are considered the primary source of signal in normal voiding, while C fibers relay nociceptive stimuli.[1]

HIGH-RISK PROCEDURES

Extirpative pelvic surgery is indicated for the treatment of multiple malignancies, most commonly colorectal, cervical, endometrial, and prostate cancers. The primary focus of these surgeries is complete resection of disease with adequate lymphadenectomy for diagnostic and therapeutic purposes. However, the autonomic nerves of the pelvis are intimately associated with the target organs. The superior hypogastric plexus is at or above the limits of most pelvic dissections, at the aortic bifurcation. The hypogastric nerves originate at the first sacral vertebra and travel in the presacral space toward

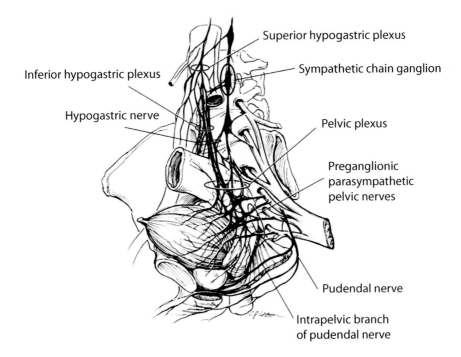

Superior hypogastric plexus

Sympathetic chain ganglion

Inferior hypogastric plexus

Hypogastric nerve

Pelvic plexus

Preganglionic
parasympathetic
pelvic nerves

Pudendal nerve

Intrapelvic branch
of pudendal nerve

Figure 9.1   Peripheral innervation of the lower urinary tract.

the lateral rectum. In a study of female cadavers, branches of hypogastric nerves were 0–0.5 mm from the midpoint of the uterosacral ligament.[6] The inferior hypogastric plexus is only 1–3 cm lateral to the rectum and upper third of the vagina.[6] The pelvic nerves enter the plexus posteriorly by traveling along the coccygeus muscle.[6] While many surgeries of the retroperitoneum and spine may risk peripheral nerve injury, here we focus on the procedures with the highest risk of causing lower urinary tract peripheral neuropathy.

COLORECTAL RESECTION

The rate of voiding dysfunction following rectal cancer surgeries, abdominoperineal resection, and low anterior resection, is estimated between 7% and 70%, depending on the breadth of dissection and extent of disease.[2,9,10] The lower aspect of the superior hypogastric plexus is at risk for injury during these surgeries due to its proximity to the rectal wall as the rectum is dissected off the sacrum. In addition, the inferior hypogastric plexus branches supplying the rectum must be transected to resect the rectum. Posterior to the rectum, the sacral sympathetic ganglia is exposed along with fragile terminal parasympathetic branches. Finally, during lymphadenectomy in advanced cancer, the middle rectal artery must be taken along with its lymphatic drainage and the inferior hypogastric plexus.[2] Beyond anatomic studies, Blavias and Barbalias performed urodynamic studies of patients following abdominoperineal resection of the rectum and

showed decreased proximal urethral closure pressures with an incompetent bladder neck, consistent with sympathetic denervation, in all patients. In addition, 38% of patients had evidence of parasympathetic denervation, and 52% had evidence of pudendal denervation.[11] Sympathetic nerve injury has been the predominant deficit seen in other post-operative cohorts as well.[12] However, as the S4 parasympathetic nerve enters the plexus distally, Hojo et al. developed a technique to spare this during the node dissection to avoid severe urinary dysfunction. In their series of 134 patients who underwent resection for rectal cancer, all but one patient regained the ability to volitionally void by 3–4 months after surgery; however, in patients without nerve sparing, their sensation of bladder fullness remained limited.[2] In a newer series (2003–2013), autonomic nerve sparing was associated with a decrease in urinary dysfunction from 22%–80% in non-nerve-sparing to 2%–24%, although the risk remained higher for patients with a pelvic lymph node dissection.[3]

RADICAL HYSTERECTOMY

Lower urinary tract dysfunction is the most common long-term side effect of radical hysterectomy for cervical and uterine malignancy, with rates of 8%–80% depending on the limits of dissection.[13-15] Urodynamic evaluation has shown rates of poor compliance, mixed urinary incontinence, and stress urinary incontinence to be present in 35%, 17%, and 38% percent of patients one year following surgery.[13] While patients may not develop complete retention, due to a decrease in midurethral closure pressure, patients may exhibit elevated residuals with decreased urinary flow 2–12 weeks following surgery due to parasympathetic injury to the pelvic splanchnic nerve as well as pudendal nerve injury.[16] The onset of post-operative stress urinary incontinence in some patients may be related to destruction of bladder neck support, but also to sympathetic nerve injury to the end branches as they leave the inferior hypogastric plexus.[13,15] The development of nerve sparing approaches has led to a reduction in post-operative urinary dysfunction; patients who undergo non-nerve sparing radical hysterectomy have an increased odds ratio of 3.4 for developing poor bladder compliance in one study by Oda et al, which is aligned with single center reports.[13] Minimally invasive approaches have also showed some promise in allowing greater magnification of pelvic nerves with improved nerve sparing and post-operative voiding function.[13]

RADICAL PROSTATECTOMY

Urinary dysfunction following prostatectomy is multifactorial, with neurologic injury as just one component among post-operative fibrosis, urethral length, and muscular changes, among others, contributing to risk of post-prostatectomy incontinence.[17] However, post-prostatectomy incontinence is quite prevalent; an average of 84% of patients require at least one pad following surgery.[18] The degree to which peripheral nerve injury contributes to post-prostatectomy incontinence is unclear, but there is evidence of its importance. In a prospective study of nerve density in the bladder trigone following prostatectomy, continent patients had a 44% decrease compared to a 20% decrease in incontinent patients.[19] In addition, anatomic studies show that the pudendal nerve supplies the external urinary sphincter and appears to have an intrapelvic component that may be injured during surgery.[20] The importance of the prostatic neurovascular bundle (NVB) in post-prostatectomy continence also remains controversial as the literature shows nerve-sparing prostatectomy both impacting long-term continence and having no impact. However, anatomic studies have shown direct afferents from the NVB to the membranous urethra, and clinically, preservation of the NVB appears to lead to earlier recovery of continence.[21]

RADICAL HYSTERECTOMY

Lower urinary tract dysfunction is the most common long-term side effect of radical hysterectomy for cervical and uterine malignancy, with rates of 8%–80% depending on the limits of dissection.[18–20] Urodynamic evaluation has shown rates of poor compliance, mixed urinary incontinence, and stress urinary incontinence to be present in 35%, 17%, and 38% of patients 1 year following surgery.[18] While

patients may not develop complete retention, due to a decrease in midurethral closure pressure, patients may exhibit elevated residuals with decreased urinary flow 2–12 weeks following surgery due to parasympathetic injury to the pelvic splanchnic nerve as well as pudendal nerve injury.[21] The onset of post-operative stress urinary incontinence in some patients may be related to destruction of bladder neck support, but also to sympathetic nerve injury to the end branches as they leave the inferior hypogastric plexus.[18,20] The development of nerve-sparing approaches has led to a reduction in post-operative urinary dysfunction; patients who undergo non-nerve-sparing radical hysterectomy have an increased odds ratio of 3.4 for developing poor bladder compliance in one study by Oda et al., which is aligned with single-center reports.[18] Minimally invasive approaches have also showed some promise in allowing greater magnification of pelvic nerves with improved nerve sparing and post-operative voiding function.[18]

URETERAL REIMPLANTATION

Ureteral reimplantation for pediatric vesicoureteral reflux was first described with an intravesical approach by Politano and Leadbetter with 97% resolution of reflux but significant morbidity.[22] Consequently, the extravesical technique was described by Lich and Gregoir. While better tolerated, bilateral reimplantation was associated with urinary retention in up to 22% of patients.[22–24] To mitigate this, staged reimplantations were performed if bilateral repair was needed.[25] Anatomic studies, such as that performed by Leissner et al., demonstrate the close proximity of the pelvic plexus, or inferior hypogastric plexus, to the ureterovesical junction (UVJ). Indeed, they found that the main body of the plexus was merely 1.5 cm dorsal and medial to the UVJ in adult cadavers with termination at the distal ureter, trigone, and rectum.[25] With modern modifications to the Lich-Gregoir repair to minimize ureteral dissection, Palmer reported bilateral ureteral reimplantation as an outpatient pediatric surgery with no post-operative voiding dysfunction.[26]

PELVIC RADIATION

Voiding dysfunction is commonly seen after radiation for pelvic malignancies.[27,28] This is attributed to the field defects to healthy tissue surrounding the target organ either by immediate cell death or as sequelae of free radicals.[29] Resultant atrophy and fibrosis of the bladder and urinary sphincter are typically cited as the main causes of post-treatment voiding dysfunction. However, it is unknown how much pathology is related to neurologic injury. The timing for the manifestation of these injuries is unclear; the symptoms would be delayed due to the slow reproductive cycles of neurons but may also be hastened by injury to neural blood supply.[30] In animal models, peripheral neuropathy was evident at 15–20 Gy, a low threshold that may be met even with modern techniques to minimize the radiated field.[31] In addition to injury to the nerves themselves, the radiated bladder has been shown to have decreased response to cholinergic signaling *in vitro*, which suggests a potential role for end organ–mediated neurologic deficits.[32]

PATIENT MANAGEMENT

EVALUATION

The evaluation of lower urinary tract dysfunction in a patient at risk from peripheral neuropathy begins with a heightened level of suspicion by the provider. The inferior hypogastric plexus, in particular, is a complex network of both sympathetic and parasympathetic nerves, leading to unpredictable outcomes following peripheral nerve injuries in this region. The examination of these patients begins with a careful history of preprocedural urinary symptoms to differentiate between new and old symptoms. Symptom questionnaires are useful in obtaining a clear picture of current symptoms but are also a reliable way to measure changes in patient symptoms over time. Postoperatively, patients may present with clear urinary retention.

The physical examination should include an examination of the urethra to ensure that there is no external etiology for incontinence, especially with prolonged catheterization, including meatal erosion or urinary-cutaneous fistula. A neurologic examination is indicated to assess sensation in the sacral distribution to isolate nerve roots that may be compromised. The bulbocavernosus reflex can be elicited by stimulating the clitoris and glans penis and should cause an anal wink. Absence of this response is indicative of pudendal nerve injury.[33]

Postvoid residual should be obtained with ultrasound or straight catheterization. For patients without volitional voiding, random bladder scans may be utilized. If the assumption is made that this patient has only urinary incontinence, and a postvoid residual is not obtained, there is a risk of delayed diagnosis and treatment of urinary retention. Laboratory analysis may include evaluation of renal function. Urinalysis and culture should also be obtained for symptomatic patients to exclude urinary tract infection as an etiology of new-onset urgency. Upper tract imaging with renal ultrasound may be indicated in the patient with urinary retention or elevated creatinine to evaluate for hydronephrosis and obstructive uropathy.

In the post-operative patient, evaluation typically occurs within the first week after the patient fails his or her first trial of void. These patients are quite early in their course and may recover nerve function rapidly if their symptoms are due to neuropraxia rather than more significant injuries. For these patients, repeat evaluation when they have returned to their functional baseline is most prudent. Even at this point, patients may continue to improve for several months. Out of the 2%–10% of patients requiring long-term catheterization following rectal cancer surgery, up to 40% had a successful trial of void in 6 months.[3] In a study of patients following radical hysterectomy, urinary symptoms appeared to stabilize approximately 12 months postoperatively.[34]

Urodynamic evaluation with fluoroscopic imaging (fluoroscopic urodynamic study [FUDS]) is the gold standard in assessing bladder contractility and urinary sphincter activity. FUDS is best employed after the patient demonstrates a plateau in urinary symptoms. For these studies, we prioritize an oblique view of the bladder neck during storage and voiding phases to best appreciate the activity of the internal and external sphincters.

TREATMENT OPTIONS

In the acute period, management of patients with lower urinary tract dysfunction due to peripheral neuropathy should focus on upper tract safety. That is, the bladder should be managed with catheterization until appropriate emptying is confirmed clinically or on urodynamic evaluation. Patients with storage predominant symptoms are typically managed according to American Urological Association treatment pathways for overactive bladder and bladder outlet obstruction (BOO).[14]

For patients with continued sphincter insufficiency and urinary incontinence 6–12 months following surgery, operative intervention with urethral sling, or artificial urinary sphincter in men, can be considered.[14] For impaired compliance refractory to medications and onabotulinumtoxinA injection, bladder augmentation is an option. Continued urinary retention due to poor detrusor contractility remains the most difficult to treat. Bladder outlet surgery may also be indicated in men with borderline BOO to decrease outlet resistance enough for adequate bladder emptying.[35] Some authors advocate for the use of sacral neurostimulation in these patients,[14] although its use has not been reported for patients with peripheral neuropathies in particular. There is also at least one current prospective trial of external electrical stimulation for bladder underactivity following radical hysterectomy,[14] which may provide an additional treatment option for these patients.

SUMMARY

Peripheral neuropathies are a significant complication following pelvic surgery and radiation, causing significant morbidity and distress to patients. While permanent injury is relatively rare, many patients who require wide resection for malignancy are at higher risk for these injuries despite ongoing improvements to treatment techniques. For this reason, the pelvic physician must remain attuned to the possibility that post-treatment urinary tract issues may reflect serious neurologic injury. Careful examination enables the physician to appropriately risk stratify patients, and tertiary studies of FUDS can provide additional prognostic information. Management options for patients remain relatively confined to catheterization with some promise being shown in nerve stimulation modalities.

REFERENCES

1. Clemens JQ. Basic bladder neurophysiology. *Urol Clin North Am.* 2010;37(4):487–94.
2. Hojo K, Vernava AM 3rd, Sugihara K, and Katumata K. Preservation of urine voiding and sexual function after rectal cancer surgery. *Dis Colon Rectum.* 1991;34(7):532–9.
3. Chew MH, Yeh YT, Lim E, and Seow-Choen F. Pelvic autonomic nerve preservation in radical rectal cancer surgery: Changes in the past 3 decades. *Gastroenterol Rep.* 2016;4(3):173–85.
4. deGroat WC and Booth AM. Physiology of the urinary bladder and urethra. *Ann Intern Med.* 1980;92(2 Pt 2):312–5.
5. Shah AP, Mevcha A, Wilby D et al. Continence and micturition: An anatomical basis. *Clin Anat (New York, NY).* 2014;27(8):1275–83.
6. Ripperda CM, Jackson LA, Phelan JN, Carrick KS, and Corton MM. Anatomic relationships of the pelvic autonomic nervous system in female cadavers: Clinical applications to pelvic surgery. *Am J Obstet Gynecol.* 2017;216(4):388.e1–e7.
7. Hollabaugh RS Jr, Steiner MS, Sellers KD, Samm BJ, and Dmochowski RR. Neuroanatomy of the pelvis: Implications for colonic and rectal resection. *Dis Colon Rectum.* 2000;43(10):1390–7.
8. Fowler CJ, Griffiths D, and de Groat WC. The neural control of micturition. *Nat Rev Neurosci.* 2008;9(6):453–66.
9. Burgos FJ, Romero J, Fernandez E, Perales L, and Tallada M. Risk factors for developing voiding dysfunction after abdominoperineal resection for adenocarcinoma of the rectum. *Dis Colon Rectum.* 1988;31(9):682–5.
10. Kirkegaard P, Hjortrup A, and Sanders S. Bladder dysfunction after low anterior resection for mid-rectal cancer. *Am J Surg.* 1981;141(2):266–8.
11. Blaivas JG and Barbalias GA. Characteristics of neural injury after abdominoperineal resection. *J Urol.* 1983;129(1):84–7.
12. Kinn AC and Ohman U. Bladder and sexual function after surgery for rectal cancer. *Dis Colon Rectum.* 1986;29(1):43–8.
13. Heesakkers J, Farag F, Bauer RM, Sandhu J, De Ridder D, and Stenzl A. Pathophysiology and contributing factors in postprostatectomy incontinence: A review. *Eur Urol.* 2017;71(6):936–44.
14. Ficarra V, Iannetti A, and Mottrie A. Urinary continence recovery after open and robot-assisted radical prostatectomy. *BJU Int.* 2013;112(7):875–6.
15. John H, Hauri D, Leuener M, Reinecke M, and Maake C. Evidence of trigonal denervation and reinnervation after radical retropubic prostatectomy. *J Urol.* 2001;165(1):111–3.
16. Hollabaugh RS, Steiner MS, and Dmochowski RR. Neuroanatomy of the female continence complex: Clinical implications. *Urology.* 2001;57(2):382–8.
17. Strasser H, Ninkovic M, Hess M, Bartsch G, and Stenzl A. Anatomic and functional studies of the male and female urethral sphincter. *World J Urol.* 2000;18(5):324–9.
18. Laterza RM, Sievert KD, de Ridder D et al. Bladder function after radical hysterectomy for cervical cancer. *Neurourol Urodynam.* 2015;34(4):309–15.
19. Cheung F and Sandhu JS. Voiding dysfunction after non-urologic pelvic surgery. *Curr Urol Rep.* 2018;19(9):75.
20. Forney JP. The effect of radical hysterectomy on bladder physiology. *Am J Obstet Gynecol.* 1980;138(4):374–82.
21. Chuang TY, Yu KJ, Penn IW, Chang YC, Lin PH, and Tsai YA. Neurourological changes before and after radical hysterectomy in patients with cervical cancer. *Acta Obstet Gynecol Scand.* 2003;82(10):954–9.
22. David S, Kelly C, and Poppas DP. Nerve sparing extravesical repair of bilateral vesicoureteral reflux: Description of technique and evaluation of urinary retention. *J Urol.* 2004;172(4 Pt 2):1617–20; discussion 20.
23. Barrieras D, Lapointe S, Reddy PP et al. Urinary retention after bilateral extravesical ureteral reimplantation: Does dissection distal to the ureteral orifice have a role? *J Urol.* 1999;162(3 Pt 2):1197–200.
24. Fung LC, McLorie GA, Jain U, Khoury AE, and Churchill BM. Voiding efficiency after ureteral reimplantation: A comparison of extravesical and intravesical techniques. *J Urol.* 1995;153(6):1972–5.
25. Leissner J, Allhoff EP, Wolff W et al. The pelvic plexus and antireflux surgery: Topographical findings and clinical consequences. *J Urol.* 2001;165(5):1652–5.
26. Palmer JS. Outpatient surgery for vesicoureteral reflux: Endoscopic injection vs extravesical ureteral reimplantation. *J Urol.* 2011;186(5):1765–7.
27. Parkin DE, Davis JA, and Symonds RP. Long-term bladder symptomatology following radiotherapy for cervical carcinoma. *Radiother Oncol: J Eur Soc Ther Radiol Oncol.* 1987;9(3):195–9.
28. Litwin MS, Pasta DJ, Yu J, Stoddard ML, and Flanders SC. Urinary function and bother after radical prostatectomy or radiation for prostate cancer: A longitudinal, multivariate quality of life analysis from the Cancer of the Prostate Strategic Urologic Research Endeavor. *J Urol.* 2000;164(6):1973–7.
29. Liberman D, Mehus B, and Elliott SP. Urinary adverse effects of pelvic radiotherapy. *Transl Androl Urol.* 2014;3(2):186–95.
30. Deangelis LM and Posner JB. *Side Effects of Radiation Therapy.* Oxford University Press; 2008.
31. Kinsella TJ, DeLuca AM, Barnes M, Anderson W, Terrill R, and Sindelar WF. Threshold dose for peripheral neuropathy following intraoperative

radiotherapy (IORT) in a large animal model. *Int J Radiat Oncol Biol Phys.* 1991;20(4):697–701.

32. Michailov MC, Neu E, Tempel K, Holzl H, and Breiter N. Influence of X-irradiation on the motor activity of rat urinary bladder *in vitro* and *in vivo*. *Strahlenther Onkol.* 1991;167(5):311–8.

33. Siroky MB, Sax DS, and Krane RJ. Sacral signal tracing: The electrophysiology of the bulbocavernosus reflex. *J Urol.* 1979;122(5):661–4.

34. Fishman IJ, Shabsigh R, and Kaplan AL. Lower urinary tract dysfunction after radical hysterectomy for carcinoma of cervix. *Urology.* 1986;28(6):462–8.

35. Gerstenberg TC, Nielsen ML, Clausen S, Blaabjerg J, and Lindenberg J. Bladder function after abdominoperineal resection of the rectum for anorectal cancer. Urodynamic investigation before and after operative in a consecutive series. *Ann Surg.* 1980;191(1):81–6.

HEREDITARY AND DEGENERATIVE DISEASES

Chapter 10

DEMENTIA AND LOWER URINARY TRACT DYSFUNCTION

Ryuji Sakakibara

INTRODUCTION

Urinary incontinence, dementia, and osteoporosis are major concerns in geriatric populations, which have grown rapidly in recent decades. Of the three, urinary incontinence is most often associated with dementia, since both conditions originate from the same underlying disorder, and urinary incontinence occurs secondarily from dementia. Urinary incontinence can result in medical morbidity, impaired self-esteem, early institutionalization, stress on caregivers, and considerable financial cost. Recently it has been acknowledged that many dementia patients have a stage of overactive bladder (OAB) before they develop urinary incontinence. OAB commonly occurs with brain diseases, since patients with brain diseases seldom have large postvoid residuals. This is particularly true in white matter disease (WMD), as discussed later. This chapter reviews prevalence, etiology, mechanism, and management of lower urinary tract (LUT) dysfunction associated with dementia.

PREVALENCE

PREVALENCE RATE OF URINARY INCONTINENCE

Of the LUT dysfunctions in patients with dementia, urinary incontinence and its prevalence have been the focus of most investigators. As expected, institutional samples had the highest prevalence (90%), with progressively lower rates reported for mixed institutional–community-dwelling samples (around 40%) and individuals attending outpatient clinics and living at home (lowest prevalence, 11%).[1-20] Regarding etiologies of dementia, Kotsoris et al.[20] found urinary incontinence in up to 50% of 84 outpatients with vascular dementia, which tends to appear earlier than in Alzheimer's disease. Of particular importance is that urinary incontinence in those patients was not always accompanied by dementia and was often preceded by urinary frequency and urgency.[21]

SEX DISTRIBUTION

Among adults older than 60 years, urinary incontinence is twice as common in women as in men, reflecting anatomic differences in the urethra and the pelvic floor muscles that lead to stress urinary incontinence.[17] Alzheimer's disease also occurs more commonly in women. However, it is also reported that men deteriorate more severely than women after admission to nursing homes.[18] The presence of prostatic hypertrophy predisposing to urinary overflow, combined with the male predominance of multi-infarct dementia, may explain these findings.[18,19]

ETIOLOGY

We now briefly discuss the underlying etiologies of both dementia and LUT dysfunction. It should be noted that in a clinical context, comorbidity of degenerative and vascular pathologies seems likely.

ALZHEIMER'S DISEASE

Alzheimer's disease is the most common cause of *severe* dementia in the elderly and accounts for more than 50% of dementia patients.[22] The pathologic hallmarks of this disease include senile plaques and neurofibrillary tangles, together with neuronal degeneration, which appears initially in the temporal and parietal cortices.[23] Neurofibrillary tangles are tau-positive, whereas senile plaques are amyloid-β 1–42 positive, both of which can increase the cerebrospinal fluid of patients with dementia. Positron emission tomography (PET) scans can visualize *in vivo* amyloid and tau deposits in the parietotemporal lobe of patients with Alzheimer's disease.[24] Coronal slices of magnetic resonance imaging (MRI) scans are feasible for showing atrophy of the cerebral cortex and hippocampus (Figure 10.1); the latter accounts for memory impairment.

In practice, dementia can be indicated by test scores, such as 23 or lower of 30 points on the Mini-Mental

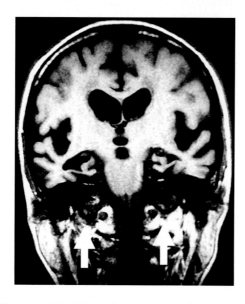

Figure 10.1 Magnetic resonance imaging of Alzheimer's disease. Atrophy in the hippocampus is the characteristic feature and is typically observed in coronal planes (arrows). (Courtesy of Dr. Shoichi Ito.)

State Examination (MMSE). Emotional disturbances include depression in about 25% patients, with agitation and restlessness also being common. Motor signs are particularly rare early in the course of the illness. Typically, patients with Alzheimer's disease have MMSE scores of less than 5 even though they can walk into the clinic without assistance. However, as the disease progresses, increased deep

tendon reflexes and parkinsonian syndrome may develop. Epilepsy and myoclonus are occasionally noted. Decreased motivation and initiative are also significant features. In most advanced cases, abulia (loss of psychomotor activity) or apallic syndrome (akinetic mutism, vegetative state) occurs, making the patient totally dependent. Urinary disturbances do occur in patients with Alzheimer's disease but are very uncommon at an early stage.

DEMENTIA WITH LEWY BODIES

Dementia with Lewy bodies (DLB) is the second most common degenerative cause of dementia.[25] Lewy bodies are cytoplasmic inclusion bodies, and they appear to be widespread in the cerebral cortex and basal ganglia in patients with this disorder.[26] Lewy bodies are α-synuclein-positive, presumably reflecting cytoskeletal alteration.[27] In DLB, fluorodopa PET imaging reveals decreased dopaminergic neurons,[28] while routine MRI scans are normal. In DLB, brain perfusion imaging by single-photon emission computed tomography (SPECT) shows diffuse decrease in perfusion including the occipital lobe (Figure 10.2), relevant to the visual hallucinations in this disorder. MIBG (metaiodo-benzylguanidine, a potent norepinephrine analog) myocardial scintigraphy shows decreased noradrenergic nerve terminals in the heart in patients with DLB. This is because DLB is a systemic disease affecting peripheral catecholaminergic autonomic fibers.

Del-Ser et al.[29] found that the onset of urinary incontinence was significantly earlier in patients

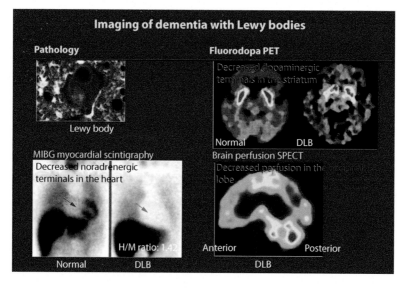

Figure 10.2 Imaging of dementia with Lewy bodies. Pathology shows a Lewy body in the cytoplasm. Fluorodopa positron emission tomography shows decreased dopaminergic nerve terminals in the striatum. Meta-iodobenzylguanidine (a potent norepinephrine analog) myocardial scintigraphy shows decreased noradrenergic nerve terminals in the heart. Brain perfusion single-photon emission computed tomography shows decreased brain perfusion including the occipital lobe.

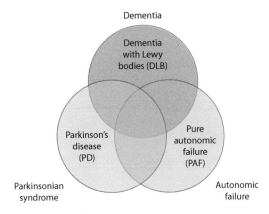

Figure 10.3 Spectrum of Lewy body diseases. When dementia is present, dementia with Lewy bodies is diagnosed (when motor disorder precedes dementia, it is also called Parkinson's disease with dementia). When motor disorder predominates, Parkinson's disease is diagnosed. When autonomic failure is the only manifestation, pure autonomic failure is diagnosed.

with DLB (3.2 years after dementia onset) than in patients with Alzheimer's disease (6.5 years after dementia onset). In patients with Alzheimer's disease, urinary incontinence is often associated with a severe cognitive decline, whereas in DLB it usually precedes severe mental failure. A significant though less common feature of DLB is widespread autonomic failure, which constitutes "pure autonomic failure" and "Lewy body constipation" (Figure 10.3).

WHITE MATTER DISEASE

WMD, also called multiple cerebral infarction, is regarded as the common cause of *mild* dementia in the elderly, and if dementia is the main problem, it is called a vascular dementia.[30] Clinically, a combination of degenerative cause (e.g., Alzheimer's disease, DLB) and vascular cause (WMD) is not uncommon. Kotsoris et al.[20] found that urinary disturbance, noted in 50% patients, frequently preceded the development of dementia by 5 years or more. Similarly, gait disturbance, noted in 24%, preceded the development of dementia by 2 years or more. MRI is the sensitive method for grading WMD. Sakakibara et al.[21] graded MRI-defined white matter multi-infarction on a scale of 1–4, and found that urinary disturbance was more common than cognitive or gait disorders, particularly in patients with mild (grade 1) lesions. In addition, nocturnal urinary frequency was a more common and earlier feature than urinary incontinence (Figures 10.4 and 10.5). Therefore, it is likely that urinary disturbance is the initial manifestation in WMD.[21]

There may be a cerebral vascular component in the etiology of elderly OAB and incontinence.[31] This is because MRI health surveys show that WMD occurs in around 10% of the general population, which is akin to that of OAB (10%–14%). In addition, WMD increases significantly with age and preferentially affects the prefrontal deep white matter.[32] The frequency of nocturia in patients with Alzheimer's disease (44%) was less than that in WMD (84%), and it was intermediate (60%) in patients with both Alzheimer's disease and WMD.[33] This suggests that WMD is a more significant burden of OAB in the geriatric population than Alzheimer's disease. In one study,[34] detrusor overactivity (DO) was independent of general cognitive status (the mean MMSE score or any of its subdomains). In contrast, the presence of DO was significantly associated with the inhibitory control subdomain in the frontal assessment battery (FAB) test ($p < 0.01$). This finding agrees with the fact that brain perfusion was most severely reduced in the frontal lobe of subjects with WMD.[32] The bladder is under general inhibitory control concerning decision-making and emotion by the prefrontal cortex. In patients with WMD, this neural network might be impaired, leading to both frontal cortex-related behavior changes and DO.[34]

OTHER CEREBRAL CAUSES

Less common but potentially treatable causes of urinary incontinence/dementia include normal pressure (communicating) hydrocephalus (NPH)[34–36] (Figure 10.6) and chronic subdural hematoma.

MECHANISM

There are several prerequisites for maintaining continence in the elderly:

1. Presence of a normal LUT with intact innervation for both urinary filling and voiding
2. Willingness to hold urine after having the first sensation and proper motivation to urinate in the toilet
3. Cognitive ability to know how to get to a toilet and how to adjust clothing
4. Physical ability to reach the toilet with hand dexterity sufficient to disrobe
5. Absence of medications that adversely affect the LUT innervation or alertness
6. Proper environment, including access to toilets and a lack of restraints

It is very likely that incontinence in elderly patients with dementia is multifactorial, and often one factor relates to another.

FUNCTIONAL INCONTINENCE

Functional incontinence is the major cause of urinary incontinence in dementia. It refers to incontinence that is not derived from an abnormality in the LUT or its innervation, but from immobility, cognitive disability, and decreased motivation (Figure 10.7).[36,37] In particular, a person who is unable to walk 5 m

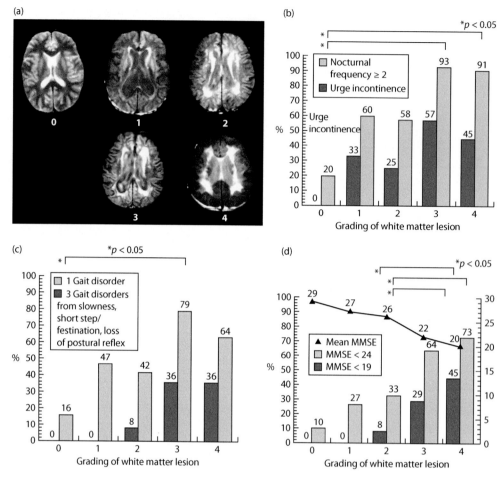

Figure 10.4 White matter disease and urinary dysfunction. (a) The grading of cerebral white matter lesions on MRI. Grade 1: punctate foci with high signal intensity in the white matter immediately at the top of the frontal horns of the lateral ventricles. Grade 2: white matter lesions were seen elsewhere but remained confined to the immediate subependymal region of the ventricles. Grade 3: periventricular as well as separate, discrete, deep white matter foci of signal abnormality. Grade 4: discrete white matter foci had become large and coalescent. (b) Urinary dysfunction and white matter lesions on MRI. (c) Gait disorder and white matter lesion on MRI. (d) Cognitive disorder and white matter lesion on MRI. MMSE, Mini-Mental State Examination; MRI, magnetic resonance imaging.

independently, or who has MMSE score less than 10, is prone to have functional incontinence.[38-46]

OVERACTIVE BLADDER

OAB is a major cause of urinary incontinence in dementia.[16] OAB is common in the general population, with its prevalence in individuals aged 18 years and older being estimated as 16.5%, and this prevalence significantly increases with age (20%–40%) (Figure 10.8).[47-50] Major etiologies for DO in elderly individuals are thought to be central and peripheral. Peripheral etiology includes detrusor muscle change, which may increase with age, as detected by electron microscopy.[51] *In vitro* muscle cells from patients with DO have greater spontaneous contractile activity than those from normal detrusor and greater sensitivity to electrical field stimulation and acetylcholine.[52] In men with outlet

obstruction, increased α-adrenergic receptors and morphological-biochemical changes of the detrusor muscles may lead to increased contractile activity and possible DO.[53] In such cases, surgical treatment of the obstruction may lessen DO. Central etiology is thought to be more significant. It is well known that cerebral diseases can lead to a loss of the brain's inhibitory influence on the spino-bulbo-spinal micturition reflex. The reflex that arises from the LUT reaches the pontine micturition center (PMC), which then activates the descending pathway to the sacral preganglionic neurons innervating the bladder.[54-57] Griffiths et al.[58] studied 128 geriatric incontinent patients, half of whom had dementia, and found that half of the 128 patients had DO by videourodynamic study. In addition, SPECT imaging showed that patients with DO had significant underperfusion in the right frontal lobe.[61,62] Similarly, cognitively intact,

(a)

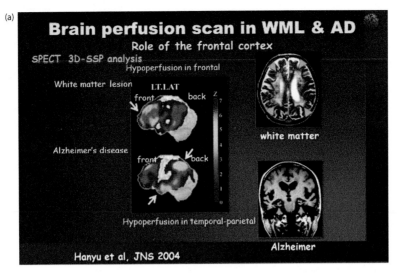

(b)

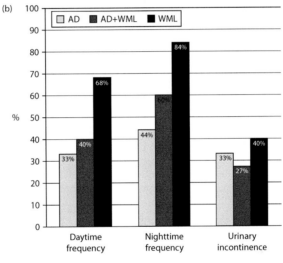

(c)

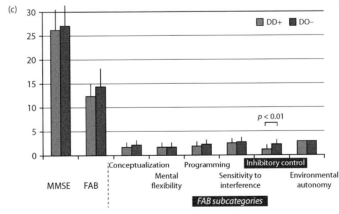

Figure 10.5 White matter disease (WMD) and urinary dysfunction (continued). (a) Brain perfusion single-photon emission computed tomography in Alzheimer's disease and WMD. (b) Incidence of daytime frequency, nighttime frequency, and urinary incontinence in Alzheimer's disease and WMD. (c) Cognitive task results in patients with WMD with/without detrusor overactivity (DO). FAB, frontal assessment battery (frontal function test); MMSE, Mini-Mental State Examination (general cognitive test). In total scores, MMSE and FAB did not differ between patients with and without DO. In contrast, looking at the six subcategories of FAB, inhibitory control task (also called go–no-go task, reflecting executive brain function) is decreased in those with DO (p < 0.05).

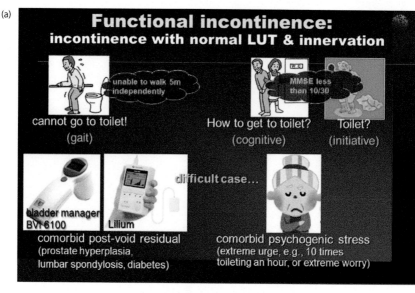

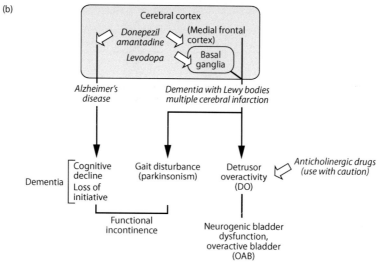

Figure 10.6   (a) Functional incontinence and (b) its relationship to brain function.

community-dwelling older individuals commonly show *silent* multiple cerebral infarction in MRI scans[20,36,59,60] (Figure 10.9).

Although not many studies have specified the types of dementia,[21,63–66] Mori et al.[63] examined 46 institutionalized dementia patients, 31 of whom had Alzheimer's disease, 11 of whom had vascular dementia, and 4 of whom had both; they found DO in 58%, 91%, and 50%, respectively. We examined LUT function in 11 DLB patients.[65] All patients had LUT symptoms: urinary incontinence in 10 (urgency type, 7; functional type due to dementia and immobility, 2; both urgency and stress type, 1) and OAB symptoms in 9. Sakakibara et al.[67] examined 19 patients with multi-infarct dementia. All of them had nocturnal frequency and urgency, and 70% had urinary incontinence of the urgency and stress types.

Urodynamic studies revealed DO in 70% and a low-compliance curve in 10%.

BLADDER UNDERACTIVITY

Bladder underactivity originates from various causes, including age-related bladder muscle change, and disturbed innervation such as diabetic neuropathy and cauda equina lesion by lumbar spondylosis. It is noteworthy that elderly individuals commonly have "detrusor hyperactivity with impaired contractile function (DHIC)," which is a combination of detrusor overactivity during bladder filling (due mostly to brain disease, and prostatic hypertrophy in elderly men) and bladder underactivity during voiding as described earlier.[68–72] However, the exact pathophysiology of DHIC is still uncertain. In brain diseases, one explanation is that two separate brain areas (the facilitatory and inhibitory brain sites for

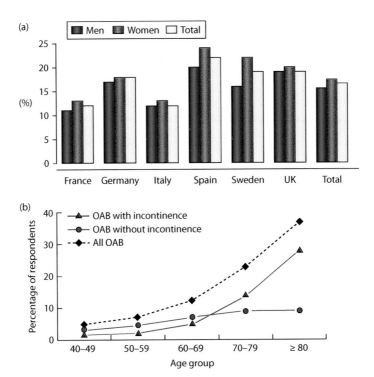

Figure 10.7 Frequency of overactive bladder (OAB) syndrome and its relation with age. (a) Frequency of OAB is around 12%–22% in many countries. (b) Frequency of OAB, particularly OAB-wet, increases with age. ([a] From Milsom I et al. *BJU Int.* 2001;87:760–6. [b] From Homma Y et al. *BJU Int.* 2005;96:1314–8.)

micturition) might be involved that lead to DHIC. In contrast, in spinal cord lesions, a single partial lesion in the spinal autonomic pathways could cause DHIC, since it disrupts the spino-bulbo-spinal micturition reflex arc, and could cause the emergence of a C-fiber-mediated novel sacral micturition reflex arc below the lesion.[54,55] These findings phenotypically mimic motor dysfunction caused by pyramidal tract lesion, i.e., in upper neuron–type spinal cord lesion, muscle weakness inevitably occurs. Concurrently, usually several times later, exaggerated reflexes may become obvious. In the LUT, detrusor-sphincter dyssynergia may further overlap during the voiding phase, which will lead to more severe voiding dysfunction and lower urinary tract symptom (LUTD). Also, concurrent bladder wall damages (age and/or obstruction related) may contribute to these dysfunctions.

STRESS URINARY INCONTINENCE

It is important to evaluate patients for comorbid stress incontinence since it is a very common condition due to pelvic floor weakness in older women and is potentially treatable.[60,73] Patients with MMSE scores of 9 or lower were still able to perform a stress maneuver.

NOCTURNAL POLYURIA

Cerebrovascular disease may also cause nocturnal polyuria, particularly when it involves the hypothalamic region that contains arginine

vasopressin (AVP) neurons. We had such patients; they lost the circadian rhythm of plasma AVP that normally rises at night. Diabetes is also a common cause of polyuria.

DRUG-INDUCED INCONTINENCE AND RETENTION

Drugs that may affect either the central nervous system (CNS) or the LUT are potential causes of transient incontinence.[74]

MANAGEMENT

In general, management for LUT dysfunction in patients with dementia needs to be individualized, and the risk/benefit ratio of these procedures, particularly invasive or irreversible treatments, needs to be carefully considered.

TREATMENT OF TRANSIENT CAUSES

The first step in management is to identify and treat transient acute causes of incontinence. Acute causes may be recalled from the mnemonic "DIAPPERS" (delirium, infection, atrophic vaginitis, pharmaceuticals, psychological factors, endocrine conditions, restricted mobility, stool impaction).[75]

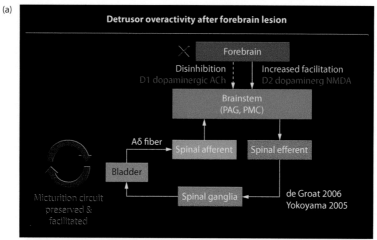

(a) Detrusor overactivity after forebrain lesion

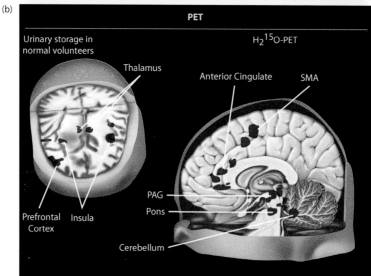

(b) PET

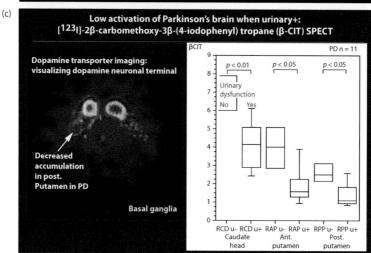

(c) Low activation of Parkinson's brain when urinary+:
[^{123}I]-2β-carbomethoxy-3β-(4-iodophenyl) tropane (β-CIT) SPECT

Figure 10.8   Neural mechanism of overactive bladder. (a) Micturitional reflex circuit is preserved in brain disease. Mainly disinhibition of this circuit by frontal/basal ganglia disease leads to facilitation of the reflex. (b) Brain areas activated by urinary storage in normal volunteers. (c) Marked depletion of basal ganglia activity in parkinsonian brain when urinary dysfunction was present. ([b] From Kavia RBC et al. *J Comp Neurol.* 2005;493:27–32.; [c] From Sakakibara R et al. *J Neurol Sci.* 2001;187:55–9.)

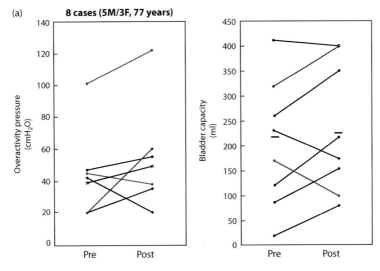

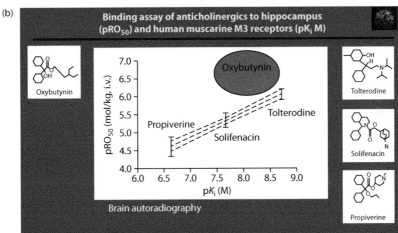

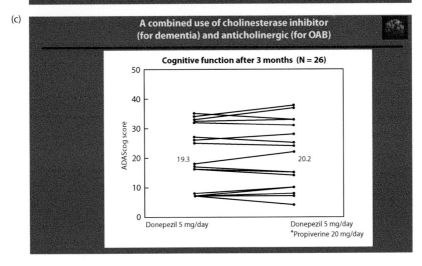

Figure 10.9 Cholinergic neural pathways, cognition and bladder. (a) Effect of donepezil (central cholinergic drug) on the micturition function in Alzheimer's disease. (b) Receptor binding of four cholinergics to hippocampus (pRO$_{50}$) and human muscarine M3 receptors (pKiM). Oxibutynin has more binding to hippocampus as compared with propiverine, solifenacin, and tolterodine. (c) Addition of propiverine (a peripheral anticholinergic) to donepezil (a central cholinesterase inhibitor) ameliorated OAB without worsening cognitive function in elderly patients with OAB with dementia.

TOILETING/BEHAVIORAL THERAPY

Toileting regimens (behavioral therapy) have been used to manage functional incontinence in elderly individuals.[76–80] Carefully selecting patients who can most benefit from toileting regimens is one possible way of reducing conflict between the cost and dryness. Environmental settings are also important for managing functional incontinence.[81]

MEDICATION
COGNITIVE IMPAIRMENT AND DECREASED MOTIVATION

The cognitive deficits in patients with Alzheimer's disease are thought to be due, at least in part, to a decrease in cholinergic innervation of the cerebral cortex and basal forebrain. The loss of cholinergic nerve terminals in patients with Alzheimer's disease is detected *in vivo* by PET using acetylcholinesterase (AChE) activities.[87] Central cholinergic agents are the mainstay in the treatment of cognitive decline. These agents inhibit AChE selectively in the brain.[82,83] Hashimoto et al.[84] reported that 7% of patients with Alzheimer's disease taking 5 mg/day of donepezil showed urinary incontinence as a potential initial adverse effect. However, we recently showed that donepezil ameliorated cognitive function without adverse effects on the LUT function in patients with Alzheimer's disease.[85] Experimental studies showed that lesions in the nucleus basalis of Meynert in the basal forebrain (central cholinergic nucleus) lessened bladder capacity.[27,86,88] In addition, improved cognitive status and alertness may give the patient sufficient initiative to hold urine (Figure 10.10a).

GAIT DISORDER

Gait disorder is a symptom of parkinsonian syndrome in multi-infarct dementia and DLB, but it also occurs mildly in Alzheimer's disease. Although levodopa seems less effective in Alzheimer's than in Parkinson's disease, 200–300 mg/day (usually coupled with peripheral dopa-decarboxylase inhibitor) ameliorates gait disorder in patients with dementia and may be of benefit in treating functional incontinence. Levodopa is better prescribed in conjunction with rehabilitation programs, since Jirovec[89] found that, in cognitively impaired nursing home residents, a daily exercise program designed to improve walking significantly reduced daytime incontinence. Physicians should also be aware of the potential adverse effects of levodopa, such as postural hypotension and hallucinations. Although levodopa seems to ameliorate urinary urgency in patients with early, untreated Parkinson's disease,[90,91] it may augment DO in a 1-hour time-window in patients with early[92] or advanced Parkinson's disease.[93]

OVERACTIVE BLADDER AND DETRUSOR OVERACTIVITY

Medications used to treat OAB and DO include anticholinergic agents and the newer adrenergic β_3-receptor-selective agonists.[63,94–96] The use of medications with anticholinergic side effects in older persons is a concern, particularly when there is a risk of exacerbating cognitive impairment. After they are ingested and absorbed from the intestine, anticholinergic drugs are systemically circulated. If they cross the blood-brain barrier (BBB), they reach the CNS and block cholinergic receptors, particularly M1-muscarinic receptors in the cerebral cortex, or M4 receptors in the basal ganglia. Although oxybutynin has been developed as a peripherally acting drug, research suggests that it has some adverse effects on cognitive function by penetrating the CNS with high lipophilicity.[97] To a much lesser extent, tolterodine[98] also affects cognitive function[99–101] (Figure 10.10b). Trospium, a quaternary amine, has a particularly high polarity. Other common anticholinergic side effects are dryness of the mouth (M3) and constipation (M2, M3). Extended-release formulations may lessen these adverse effects. It was recently shown that the addition of propiverine (a peripheral anticholinergic) to donepezil (a central cholinesterase inhibitor) ameliorated OAB without worsening cognitive function in elderly patients with OAB with dementia.[102]

STRESS INCONTINENCE

Tricyclic antidepressants are commonly used to treat both DO and stress incontinence, since they have both anticholinergic and α-adrenergic properties, the latter of which is expected to increase urethral tone. However, a randomized controlled study to examine the effect of a tricyclic on incontinence in an exclusively older group of patients did not find a statistically significant difference between imipramine hydrochloride (mean dose 54 mg) and placebo.[103] The α-adrenergic agonists, such as midodrine hydrochloride, have been shown to benefit some older women with stress incontinence.[97]

OUTLET OBSTRUCTION

The α_1-adrenergic antagonists such as prazosin, terazosin, doxazosin, alfuzosin, silodosin, etc., are effective in the symptomatic management of benign prostatic hypertrophy. The proximal urethra has an abundance of α_{1A-D}-adrenergic receptors. In contrast, the vascular wall has an abundance of α_{1B} receptors, particularly in the elderly.[104] Prazosin may block both α_{1B} receptors in the vascular wall and α_{1A-D} receptors in the proximal urethra. Selective α_{1A-D}-adrenergic blockers, such as tamsulosin hydrochloride and naftopidil, are the drugs of choice because they have fewer side effects such as orthostatic hypotension.

NOCTURNAL POLYURIA

Desmopressin, a potent analog of AVP, has been used to treat patients with nocturnal polyuria probably because of impaired circadian rhythm of the plasma AVP.[105] We prescribed 5 µg of intranasal desmopressin once a night in poststroke patients who had impaired circadian AVP rhythm, and noted improvement in nocturnal polyuria.[106]

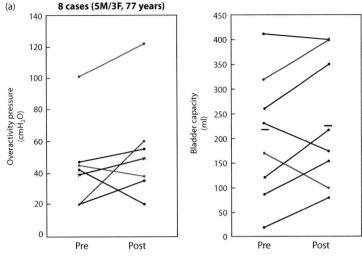

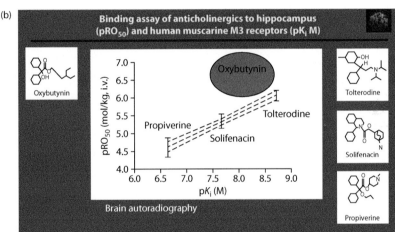

Figure 10.10 Cholinergic neural pathways, cognition and bladder. (a) Effect of donepezil (central cholinergic drug) on the micturition function in Alzheimer's disease. (b) Receptor binding of four cholinergics to hippocampus (pRO$_{50}$) and human muascarine M3 receptors (pKiM). Oxibutynin has more binding to hippocampus as compared with propiverine, solifenacin, and tolterodine.

PELVIC MUSCLE EXERCISES AND BIOFEEDBACK

Pelvic muscle exercises, sometimes combined with biofeedback, have been used successfully to treat stress incontinence in older women.[107] However, Tobin and Brocklehurst[89] note that, because most of their patients had severe cognitive and physical deterioration, they were unable to cooperate with treatment for stress incontinence.

ELECTRICAL STIMULATION

Although literature regarding dementia/nursing home residents is limited, in an uncontrolled trial, Lamhut et al.[108] studied the effectiveness of electrical stimulation in nine incontinent female nursing home patients with DO. Since tibial nerve stimulation (TNS) is a minimally invasive, safe, and easy method to treat OAB, TNS may have a role in treating OAB symptoms in patients with dementia

in the future, particularly when drug-based therapy is not favorable/contraindicated.

SURGERY

Surgery has been used to treat benign outlet obstruction and stress incontinence in older patients, when conservative methods and medications have failed or [were] not appropriate.[109] However, whether or not the repair of these outlet lesions reliably restores continence in frail, demented individuals remains to be established.

DEVICES, PADS, AND CATHETERS

Indwelling catheters are often used excessively and inappropriately in frail, demented patients, even for the relief of incontinence, and are associated with a high rate of morbidity. Clean intermittent catheterization (CIC) is used to treat an underactive detrusor and other causes of urinary retention.

However, it is often difficult to perform CIC in patients with dementia because of uncooperativeness, aggression, and agitation, and also because it increases demands on staff time. Indwelling catheterization might be chosen regarding situations.

CONCLUSION

Urinary incontinence is common in patients with dementia, and it is more prevalent in older individuals with dementia than in those without. Since the etiology of incontinence is multifactorial, factors within and outside the LUT must be assessed to maximize continence in these patients. A recent view has emerged that WMD is a significant burden in elderly patients with dementia with OAB. A person who is unable to walk 5 m independently, or who has a MMSE score less than 10, is likely to be functionally incontinent. A measurement of postvoid residuals and caring psychogenic factors are also important. Most research on the management of urinary incontinence in patients with dementia has focused on toileting programs for functional incontinence and on drug treatments for DO. To date, regarding cognitive adverse effects, the use of anticholinergic medications for DO is under debate, and the newer adrenergic β_3-receptor-selective agonists are becoming widely used. In the future, centrally acting drugs that can improve gait and cognitive function may also become an option for the treatment of urinary incontinence in patients with dementia.

REFERENCES

1. Teri L, Borson S, Kiyak A, and Yamagishi M. Behavioral disturbance, cognitive dysfunction, and functional skill; prevalence and relationship in Alzheimer's disease. *J Am Geriatr Soc.* 1989;37:109–16.
2. Teri L, Larson EB, and Reifler BV. Behavioral disturbance in dementia of the Alzheimer's type. *J Am Geriatr Soc.* 1988;36:1–6.
3. Teri L, Hughes JP, and Larson EB. Cognitive deterioration in Alzheimer's disease: Behavioral and health factors. *J Gerontol.* 1990;45:P58–P63.
4. Swearer JM, Drachman DA, O'Donnell BF, and Mitchell AL. Troublesome and disruptive behaviors in dementia. *J Am Geriatr Soc.* 1988;36:784–90.
5. Udaka F, Nishinaka K, Kameyama M et al. Urinary dysfunction in dementia; 1. Dementia of Alzheimer type. *Void Disord Dig.* 1994;2:271–5.
6. Berrios GE. Urinary incontinence and the psychopathology of the elderly with cognitive failure. *Gerontology.* 1986;32:119–24.
7. Ouslander JG, Zarit SH, Orr NK, and Muira SA. Incontinence among elderly community-dwelling dementia patients. *J Am Geriatr Soc.* 1990;38:440–5.
8. Rabins PV, Mace NL, and Lucas MJ. The impact of dementia on the family. *JAMA.* 1982;248:333–5.
9. Burns A, Jacoby R, and Levy R. Psychiatric phenomena in Alzheimer's disease. IV: Disorders of behaviour. *Br J Psychiatry.* 1990;157:S6–S94.
10. Campbell AJ, Reinken J, and McCosh L. Incontinence in the elderly: Prevalence and prognosis. *Age Ageing.* 1985;14:65–70.
11. Borrie MJ and Davidson HA. Incontinence in institutions: Costs and contributing factors. *Can Med Assoc J.* 1992;147:322–8.
12. Noto H. Urinary dysfunction in dementia; 2. Multi-infarct Dementia. *Void Disord Dig.* 1994;2:277–84.
13. Toba K, Ouchi Y, Orimo H et al. Urinary incontinence in elderly inpatients in Japan: A comparison between general and geriatric hospitals. *Aging Clin Exp Res.* 1996;8:47–54.
14. McLaren SM, McPherson FM, Sinclair F, and Ballinger BR. Prevalence and severity of incontinence among hospitalised, female psychogeriatric patients. *Health Bull.* 1981;39:157–61.
15. International Continence Society. Standardization of terminology of lower urinary tract function. *Scand J Urol Nephrol.* 1988;1(Suppl 14):5–19.
16. Abrams P, Cardozo L, Fall M et al. The standardization of terminology of lower urinary tract function: Report from the standardization sub-committee of the International Continence Society. *Neurourol Urodynam.* 2002;21:167–78.
17. Herzog AR and Fultz NH. Prevalence and incidence of urinary incontinence in community–dwelling populations. *J Am Geriatr Soc.* 1990;38:273–81.
18. Palmer MH, German PS, and Ouslander JG. Risk factors for urinary incontinence one year after nursing home admission. *Res Nurs Health.* 1991;14:405–12.
19. Ouslander JG, Palmer MH, Rovner BW, and German PS. Urinary incontinence in nursing homes: Incidence, remission and associated factors. *J Am Geriatr Soc.* 1993;41:1083–9.
20. Kotsoris H, Barclay LL, Kheyfets S et al. Urinary and gait disturbances as markers for early multi-infarct dementia. *Stroke.* 1987;18:138–41.
21. Sakakibara R, Hattori T, Uchiyama T, and Yamanishi T. Urinary function in elderly people with and without leukoaraiosis: Relation to cognitive and gait function. *J Neurol Neurosurg Psychiatry.* 1999;67(5):658–60.
22. American Psychiatric Association. *Diagnostic and Statistical Manual of Mental Disorders,* 4th ed. Washington, DC: American Psychiatric Association Press; 1994.
23. Braak H and Braak E. Diagnostic criteria for neuropathologic assessment of Alzheimer's disease. *Neurobiol Aging.* 1997;18(Suppl 1):S85–S88.
24. Kepe V, Huang SC, Small GW et al. Visualizing pathology deposits in the living brain of patients with Alzheimer's disease. *Methods Enzymol.* 2006;412:144–60.
25. McKieth IG, Galasko D, Kosaka K et al. Consensus guidelines for the clinical and pathologic diagnosis of dementia with Lewy bodies (DLB): Report of the consortium on DLB International Workshop. *Neurology.* 1996;47:1113–24.
26. Braak H, Del Tredici K, Rüb U et al. Staging of brain pathology related to sporadic Parkinson's disease. *Neurobiol Aging.* 2003;24:197–211.
27. Tateno F, Sakakibara R, Kawai T, Kishi M, and Murano T. Alpha-synuclein in the cerebrospinal fluid differentiates synucleinopathies (Parkinson Disease, dementia with Lewy bodies, multiple system atrophy) from Alzheimer disease. *Alzheimer Dis Assoc Disord.* 2012;26:213–6.
28. Hu XS, Okamura N, Arai H et al. 18F-fluorodopa PET study of striatal dopamine uptake in the diagnosis of dementia with Lewy bodies. *Neurology.* 2000;55:1575–7.

29. Del-Ser T, Munoz DG, and Hachinski V. Temporal pattern of cognitive decline and incontinence is different in Alzheimer's disease and diffuse Lewy body disease. *Neurology*. 1996;46:682–6.

30. Roman GC, Tatemichi TK, Erkinjuntti T et al. Vascular dementia, diagnostic criteria for research studies: Report of the NINDS-AIREN International Workshop. *Neurology*. 1993;43:250–60.

31. Sakakibara R, Panicker J, Fowler CJ et al. Vascular incontinence: Incontinence in the elderly due to ischemic white matter changes. *Neurol Int*. 2012;4:e13.

32. Hanyu H, Shimuzu S, Tanaka Y et al. Cerebral blood flow patterns in Binswanger's disease: A SPECT study using three-dimensional stereotactic surface projections. *J Neurol Sci*. 2004;220:79–84.

33. Takahashi O, Sakakibara R, Panicker J et al. White matter lesions or Alzheimer's disease: Which contributes more to overactive bladder and incontinence in elderly adults with dementia? *J Am Geriatr Soc*. 2012;60:2370–1.

34. Haruta H, Sakakibara R, Ogata T et al. Inhibitory control task is decreased in vascular incontinence patients. *Clin Auton Res*. 2013;23:85–9.

35. Sakakibara R, Panicker J, Fowler CJ et al. "Vascular incontinence" and normal-pressure hydrocephalus: Two common sources of elderly incontinence with brain etiologies. *Curr Drug Ther*. 2012;7:67–76.

36. Yu LC, Rohner TJ, Kaltreider DL et al. Profile of urinary incontinent elderly in long-term care institutions. *J Am Geriatr Soc*. 1990;38:433–9.

37. Della Sala S, Francescani A, and Spinnler H. Gait apraxia after bilateral supplementary motor area lesion. *J Neurol Neurosurg Psychiatry*. 2002;72:77–85.

38. Resnick NM, Baumann M, Scott M et al. Risk factors for incontinence in the nursing home: A multivariate study. *Neurourol Urodyn*. 1988;7:274–6.

39. Jirovec MM and Wells TJ. Urinary incontinence in nursing home residents with dementia: The mobility-cognition paradigm. *Appl Nurs Res*. 1990;3:112–7.

40. McGrother CW, Jagger C, Clarke M, and Castleden CM. Handicaps associated with incontinence: Implications for management. *J Epidemiol Commun Health*. 1990;44:246–8.

41. Luk JK, Cheung RT, Ho SL, and Li L. Does age predict outcome in stroke rehabilitation? A study of 878 Chinese subjects. *Cerebrovasc Dis*. 2006;21:229–34.

42. Singh R, Hunter J, Philip A, and Todd I. Predicting those who will walk after rehabilitation in a specialist stroke unit. *Clin Rehabil*. 2006;20:149–52.

43. Landi F, Onder G, Cesari M et al. Functional decline in frail community-dwelling stroke patients. *Eur J Neurol*. 2006;13:17.

44. Paolucci S, Antonucci G, Grasso MG, and Pizzamiglio L. The role of unilateral special neglect in rehabilitation of right brain-damaged ischemic stroke patients: A matched comparison. *Arch Phys Med Rehab*. 2001;82:743–9.

45. Himashree G, Banerjee PK, and Selvamurthy W. Sleep and performance—Recent trends. *Indian J Physiol Pharmacol*. 2002;46:6–24.

46. Shaw FE. Falls in cognitive impairment and dementia. *Clin Geriatr Med*. 2002;18:159–73.

47. Ouslander JG. Geriatric considerations in the diagnosis and management of overactive bladder. *Urology*. 2002;60(Suppl 1):50–5.

48. Wein AJ and Rackley RR. Overactive bladder: A better understanding of pathophysiology, diagnosis, and management. *J Urol*. 2006;175:S5–S10.

49. Milsom I, Abrams P, Cardozo L et al. How widespread are the symptoms of an overactive bladder and how are they managed? A population-based prevalence study. *BJU Int*. 2001;87:760–6.

50. Homma Y, Yamaguchi O, Hayashi K et al. An epidemiological survey of overactive bladder symptoms in Japan. *BJU Int*. 2005;96:1314–8.

51. Elbadawi A, Yalla SV, and Resnick NM. Structural basis of geriatric voiding dysfunction. 3. Detrusor overactivity. *J Urol*. 1993;150:1668–80.

52. Kinder RB and Mundy AR. Pathophysiology of idiopathic detrusor instability and detrusor hyper-reflexia: An *in vitro* study of human detrusor muscle. *Br J Urol*. 1987;60(6):509–15.

53. Elbadawi A, Yalla SV, and Resnick NM. Structural basis of geriatric voiding dysfunction. 4. Bladder outlet obstruction. *J Urol*. 1993;150:1681–95.

54. de Groat WC, Booth AM, and Yoshimura N. Neurophysiology of micturition and its modification in animal models of human disease. In: Maggi CA, ed. *The Autonomic Nervous System: Nervous Control of the Urogenital System*, Vol 3. London, United Kingdom: Horwood Academic; 1993:227–90.

55. Griffiths D. Basics of pressure-flow studies. *World J Urol*. 1995;13:30–3.

56. Aswal BS, Berkley KJ, Hussain I et al. Brain responses to changes in bladder volume and urge to void in healthy men. *Brain*. 2001;124:369–77.

57. Kavia RBC, Dasgupta R, and Fowler CJ. Functional imaging and the central control of the bladder. *J Comp Neurol*. 2005;493:27–32.

58. Griffiths DJ, McCracken PN, Harrison GM et al. Cerebral etiology of urinary urge incontinence in elderly people. *Age Ageing*. 1994;23:246–50.

59. Kitada S, Ikei Y, Hasui Y et al. Bladder function in elderly men with subclinical brain magnetic resonance imaging studies. *J Urol*. 1992;147:1507–9.

60. Resnick NM, Yalla SV, and Laurino E. The pathophysiology of urinary incontinence among institutionalized elderly persons. *N Engl J Med*. 1989;320:1–7.

61. Sakakibara R, Hattori T, Yasuda K, and Yamanishi T. Micturitional disturbance after acute hemispheric stroke: Analysis of the lesion site by CT and MRI. *J Neurol Sci*. 1996;137:47–56.

62. Sakakibara R, Shinotoh H, Uchiyama T et al. SPECT imaging of the dopamine transporter with [^{123}I]-β-CIT reveals marked decline of nigrostriatal dopaminergic function in Parkinson's disease with urinary dysfunction. *J Neurol Sci*. 2001;187: 55–9.

63. Mori S, Kojima M, Sakai Y, and Nakajima K. Bladder dysfunction in dementia patients showing urinary incontinence: Evaluation with cystometry and treatment with propiverine hydrochloride. *Jpn J Geriat*. 1999;36:489–94.

64. Sugiyama T, Hashimoto K, Kiwamoto H et al. Urinary incontinence in senile dementia of the Alzheimer type (SDAT). *Int J Urol*. 1994;1:337–40.

65. Sakakibara R, Ito T, Uchiyama T et al. Lower urinary tract function in dementia of Lewy body type (DLB). *J Neurol Neurosurg Psychiatry*. 2005;76:729–32.

66. Komatsu K, Yokoyama O, Otsuka N et al. Central muscarinic mechanism of bladder overactivity associated with Alzheimer type senile dementia. *Neurourol Urodyn*. 2000;4:539–40.

67. Sakakibara R, Hattori T, Tojo M et al. Micturitional disturbance in patients with cerebrovascular dementia. *Autonom Nerv Syst*. 1993;30:390–6.

68. Resnick NM and Yalla SV. Detrusor hyperactivity with impaired contractile function. *JAMA*. 1987;257:3076–81.

69. Eastwood H and Lord A. Are there two types of detrusor hyperreflexia? *Neurourol Urodyn*. 1990;9:415–6.

70. Elbadawi A, Yalla SV, and Resnick NM. Structural basis of geriatric voiding dysfunction. 2. Ageing detrusor: Normal versus impaired contractility. *J Urol.* 1993;150:1657–67.

71. Kuwabara S, Naramoto C, Suzuki N et al. Silent post-micturition residuals in elderly subjects with dementia: A study with ultrasound echography. *Senile Dementia.* 1997;11:417–21.

72. Yamamoto T, Sakakibara R, Uchiyama T et al. Neurological diseases that cause detrusor hyperactivity with impaired contractile function. *Neurourol Urodynam.* 2006;25(4):356–60.

73. Payne C. Epidemiology, pathophysiology and evaluation of urinary incontinence and overactive bladder. *Urology.* 1998;51(Suppl 2a):3–10.

74. Keister KJ and Creason NS. Medications of elderly institutionalized incontinent females. *J AdvNurs.* 1989;14:980–5.

75. Resnick NM and Yalla SV. Current concepts: Management of urinary incontinence in the elderly. *New Engl J Med.* 1985;313:800–15.

76. Skelly J and Flint AJ. Urinary incontinence associated with dementia. *J Austr Geriat Soc.* 1995; 43:286–94.

77. Ouslander JG, Blaustein J, Connor A, and Pitt A. Habit training and oxybutynin for incontinence in nursing home patients: A placebo controlled study. *J Am Geriatr Soc.* 1988;36:40–6.

78. Flint AJ and Skelly JM. The management of urinary incontinence in dementia. *Int J Geriatr Psychiatry.* 1994;9:245–6.

79. Jirovec MM. Effect of individualized prompted toileting on incontinence in nursing home residents. *Appl Nurs Res.* 1991;4:188–91.

80. Schnelle JF, Sowell VA, Hu TW, and Traughber B. Reduction of urinary incontinence in nursing homes: Does it reduce or increase costs? *J Am Geriatr Soc.* 1988;36:34–9.

81. Chanfreau-Rona D, Bellwood S, and Wylie B. Assessment of a behavioural programme to treat incontinent patients in psychogeriatric wards. *Br J Clin Psychol.* 1984;23:273–9.

82. Shinotoh H, Aotsuka A, Fukushi K et al. Effect of donepezil on brain acetylcholinesterase activity in patients with AD measured by PET. *Neurology.* 2001;56:408–10.

83. Burns A, Rossor M, Hecker J et al. The effects of donepezil in Alzheimer's disease: Results from a multinational trial. *Dement Geriatr Cogn Disord.* 1999;10:237–44.

84. Hashimoto M, Imamura T, Tanimukai S et al. Urinary incontinence: An unrecognised adverse effect with donepezil. *Lancet.* 2000;356:568.

85. Sakakibara R, Uchiyama T, Yoshiyama M et al. Preliminary communication: Urodynamic assessment of donepezil hydrochloride in patients with Alzheimer's disease. *Neurourol Urodyn.* 2005;24:273–5.

86. Gillon G and Stanton SL. Long-term follow-up of surgery for urinary incontinence in elderly women. *Br J Urol.* 1984;56:478–81.

87. Nieuwenhuys R. *Chemoarchitecture of the Brain.* Berlin, Germany: Springer-Verlag; 1985:8.

88. Kumon Y, Sakaki S, Takeda S et al. Effect of aneracetam on psychiatric symptoms after stroke. *J New Remedies Clin.* 1997;46:231–43.

89. Jirovec MM. The impact of daily exercise on the mobility, balance and urine control of cognitively impaired nursing home residents. *Int J Nurs Stud.* 1991;28:145–51.

90. Aranda B and Cramer P. Effects of apomorphine and L-dopa on the parkinsonian bladder. *Neurourol Urodyn.* 1993;12:203–9.

91. Sakakibara R, Uchiyama T, Hattori T, and Yamanishi T. Urodynamic evaluation in Parkinson's disease before and after levodopa treatment. *9th International Catechecholamine Symposium,* Kyoto, Japan, 2001.

92. Brusa L, Petta F, Pisani A et al. Central acute D2 stimulation worsens bladder function in patients with mild Parkinson's disease. *J Urol.* 2006;175:202–6.

93. Uchiyama T, Sakakibara R, Hattori T et al. Short-term effect of a single levodopa dose on micturition disturbance in Parkinson's disease patients with the wearing-off phenomenon. *Mov Disord.* 2003;18:573–8.

94. Tobin GW and Brocklehurst JC. The management of urinary incontinence in local authority residential homes for the elderly. *Age Ageing.* 1986;15:292–8.

95. Burgio KL, Locher JL, Goode PS et al. Behavioural vs drug treatment for urge urinary incontinence in older women: A randomized controlled trial. *JAMA.* 1998;280:1995–2000.

96. Zorzitto ML, Jewett MS, and Fernie GR. Effectiveness of propantheline bromide in the treatment of geriatric patients with detrusor instability. *Neurourol Urodyn.* 1986;5:133–40.

97. Donnellan CA, Fook L, McDonald P, and Playfer JR. Oxybutynin and cognitive dysfunction. *BMJ.* 1997;315:1363–4.

98. Womack KB and Heilman KM. Tolterodine and memory: Dry but forgetful. *Arch Neurol.* 2003;60:771–3.

99. Maruyama S, Tsukada H, Nishiyama S et al. *In vivo* quantitative autoradiographic analysis of brain muscarinic receptor occupancy by antimuscarinic agents for overactive bladder treatment. *JPET.* 2008;25:774–81.

100. Sakakibara R, Uchiyama T, Yamanishi T, and Kishi M. Dementia and lower urinary dysfunction: With a reference to anticholinergic use in elderly population. *Int J Urol.* 2008;15:778–88.

101. Scheife R and Takeda M. Central nervous system safety of anticholinergic drugs for the treatment of overactive bladder in the elderly. *Clin Ther.* 2005;27:144–53.

102. Sakakibara R, Ogata T, Uchiyama T et al. How to manage overactive bladder in elderly individuals with dementia? A combined use of donepezil, a central acetylcholinestrase inhibitor, and propiverine, a peripheral muscarine receptor antagonist. *J Am Geriatr Soc.* 2009;57:1515–7.

103. Castleden CM, Duffin HM, and Gulati RS. Double-blind study of imipramine and placebo for incontinence due to bladder instability. *Age Ageing.* 1986;15:299–303.

104. Schwinn DA. Novel role for $\alpha 1$ adrenergic receptor subtypes in lower urinary tract symptoms. *BJU Int.* 2000;86(Suppl 2):11–22.

105. Cannon A, Carter PG, McConnell PG, and Abrams P. Desmopressin in the treatment of nocturnal polyuria in the male. *BJU Int.* 1999;84:20–4.

106. Sakakibara R, Uchiyama T, Liu Z et al. Nocturnal polyuria with abnormal circadian rhythm of plasma arginine vasopressin in poststroke patients. *Intern Med.* 2005;44:281–4.

107. Wells TJ, Brink CA, Diokno AC et al. Pelvic muscle exercise for stress urinary incontinence in elderly women. *J Am Geriatr Soc.* 1991;39:785–91.

108. Lamhut P, Jackson TW, and Wall LL. The treatment of urinary incontinence with electrical stimulation in nursing home patients: A pilot study. *J Am Geriatr Soc.* 1992;40:48–52.

109. Booth J, Connelly L, Dickson S, Duncan F, and Lawrence M. The effectiveness of transcutaneous tibial nerve stimulation (TTNS) for adults with overactive bladder syndrome: A systematic review. *Neurourol Urodyn.* 2018;37:528–41.

Chapter 11

PATHOLOGIES OF THE BASAL GANGLIA, SUCH AS PARKINSON'S AND HUNTINGTON'S DISEASES

Teruyuki Ogawa and Naoki Yoshimura

INTRODUCTION

The basal ganglia in the brain are a group of anatomically closely related subcortical nuclei. They have been implicated in a wide range of behavioral functions including motor, cognitive, and emotional.[1-3] Damage to these nuclei such as in Parkinson's disease (PD) and Huntington's disease (HD) usually causes dramatic motor abnormalities without weakness, as well as lower urinary tract dysfunction.[4,5] In this chapter we provide an overview of the current concept of the contribution of the basal ganglia to lower urinary tract function and review the lower urinary tract dysfunction in patients with disorders of the basal ganglia, such as PD and HD.

FUNCTIONAL ANATOMY OF THE BASAL GANGLIA

The basal ganglia consist of several subcortical nuclei including the striatum, the globus pallidus (GP), the subthalamic nucleus (STN), and the substantia nigra (SN) (Figure 11.1a).

The striatum receives various inputs from other regions in the brain such as glutamatergic inputs from the cerebral cortex and thalamus,[6] dopaminergic inputs from the SN,[7] and serotonergic inputs from the raphe nuclei.[8] The outputs from the striatum use γ-aminobutyric acid (GABA) as its principal transmitter[9] colocalized with the neuropeptides enkephalin or substance P/dynorphin.[10-13]

The SN is a dopaminergic nucleus, which is divided into two parts: the substantia nigra pars compacta (SNpc) and the substantia nigra pars reticulata (SNpr). The SNpc receives inputs from the striatum and sends information right back. The SNpr also receives inputs from the striatum but sends information outside the basal ganglia. Dopamine is important for the micturition reflex as well as normal movement.[14]

The GP consists of the globus pallidus externa (GPe) and the globus pallidus interna (GPi). Both receive inputs from the striatum and communicate with the STN. GPi and SNpr are considered as the output structure that modulates the activity of motor control centers in the thalamus and brainstem.

PHYSIOLOGY OF THE BASAL GANGLIA

Cortical information that reaches the striatum is conveyed to the basal ganglia output structure (GPi-SNpr complex) via two pathways (Figure 11a). One is a direct pathway in which the striatum project directly to the GPi-SNpr complex by GABAergic neurons. Another is an indirect pathway, which includes (1) a projection from the striatum to the GPe, (2) a projection from GPe to STN, and (3) an excitatory projection from the STN to the GPi-SNpr complex. These two inhibitory pathways (striato-GPe and GPe-STN) use GABA as a neurotransmitter, and the excitatory pathway (the STN to the GPi-SNpr complex) uses glutamate.[15]

The information is then transmitted back to the cerebral cortex via the thalamus. The activity of spiny striatal neurons, which are the origins of the direct and indirect pathways, is modulated by dopamine released from nerve terminals of dopaminergic neurons in the SNpc. Dopamine D2 receptors are expressed in striatopallidal neurons in the indirect pathway, while dopamine D1 receptors are located on neurons in the direct pathway (striatonigral/striatoentopeduncular neurons)[16] (Figure 11.1a). Increased activity of the direct pathway is associated with facilitation of movement, while activation of the indirect pathway is associated with inhibition of movement. Dopamine is thought to inhibit neuronal activity through dopamine D2 receptors in the indirect pathway and to excite neurons via dopamine D1 receptors in the direct pathway (Figure 11.1a). In conclusion, activation of dopamine D1/D2 receptors in the striatum provides excessive facilitation of motor systems by exerting the dual effects on the direct and indirect pathways.

PHYSIOLOGY AND PATHOPHYSIOLOGY OF LOWER URINARY TRACT DYSFUNCTION IN PARKINSON'S DISEASE

DOPAMINERGIC SYSTEMS RELATED TO THE MICTURITION REFLEX

The GP has been reported to suppress spontaneous detrusor contractions, and the subthalamus and the SN inhibit the micturition reflex in early studies.[17,18] Electrical stimulation of the basal ganglia including the SNpc[19,20] and STN[21] inhibits the micturition reflex in the cat. The inhibitory effect is activated by the dopamine D1 receptor in the brain.[19] In other words, dopaminergic neurons originating in the SN tonically inhibit the micturition reflex through dopamine D1 receptors under the normal condition (Figure 11.1a).[22] Interestingly, in the normal condition, stimulation of dopamine D1 receptors did not affect the micturition reflex, whereas in an animal model of PD,[23-25] detrusor overactivity was suppressed by stimulation of dopamine D1 receptors (Figure 11.1b).[24,25] In addition, the striatal dopamine level is significantly increased during bladder filling as compared with that during voiding in normal cats.[26] Taken together, it is assumed that detrusor overactivity in patients with PD is due to activation failure of inhibitory mechanisms via dopamine D1 receptors (Figure 11.1b). Stimulation of dopamine D2 receptors facilitates the micturition reflex.[14,19,22,24,25,27,28] The precise mechanism is unclear; however, it is possible that D2 receptor-mediated effects on bladder function might be mediated by dopaminergic mechanisms in systems other than the nigrostriatal dopaminergic pathways.[29,30] In addition, stimulation of D3 receptors seems to have no influence on the micturition reflex.[14]

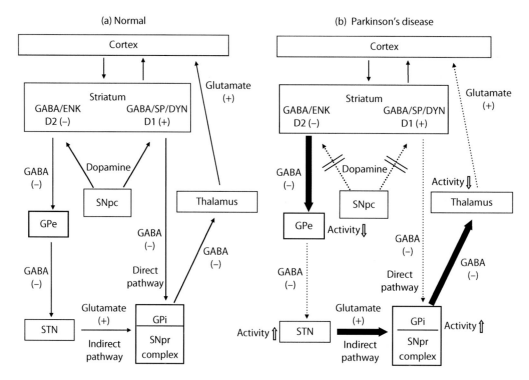

Figure 11.1 Simplified scheme of neural organization in the basal ganglia under (a) the normal condition and (b) in Parkinson's disease. (a) The striatum receives multiple afferent inputs from the cerebral cortex. The GPi-SNpr complex exerts a tonic GABAergic inhibitory output upon excitatory premotor neurons located in the thalamus. The direct pathway arises from striatal neurons that contain GABA plus peptides substance P (SP) or dynorphin (DYN) and project monosynaptically to the GPi-SNpr complex. The indirect pathway originates from striatal neurons that contain GABA and enkephalin (ENK). Its output is conveyed polysynaptically to the GPi-SNpr complex via GPe and STN. Dopamine increases neuronal activity in the direct pathway via D1 receptor and inhibits neurons in the indirect pathway via D2 receptor. Bradykinesia or akinesia observed in Parkinson's disease is thought to result from increased GABAergic inhibition of thalamic premotor neurons. (Thick and broken arrows indicate increased and decreased activity, respectively) GABA, gamma-aminobutyric acid; GPe, globus pallidus externa; GPi, globus pallidus interna; SNpc, substantia nigra pars compacta; SNpr, substantia nigra pars reticulata; STN, subthalamic nucleus.

The interaction between dopamine and other neurotransmitters in the periaqueductal gray (PAG) is involved in the urinary symptoms in patients with PD.[31] Dopamine and glutamate levels are increased during micturition, while GABA levels are decreased in the normal condition. The blockade of D1 receptors in the PAG increased GABA levels, whereas dopamine and glutamate levels were not affected. In 6-OHDA lesioned rats, mimicking the urinary symptoms in patients with PD, GABA levels are increased during micturition. In summary, changes in extracellular GABA levels in the PAG during micturition are modulated by D1 receptor activation, and the loss of dopamine did not affect the GABA levels. Therefore, it is assumed that the dopamine depletion loses control of GABA levels, leading to bladder dysfunction in patients with PD.[31]

In human positron emission tomography, it has been revealed that brain activation sites in response to bladder filling were altered in patients with PD,[32] and another imaging study using single-photon emission computed tomography also suggested that a reduction in the nigrostriatal dopaminergic neurons is related to the urinary disturbance in patients with PD.[33,34]

The ventral tegmentum area (VTA) that lies close to the SN and is abundant in dopaminergic and serotonergic neurons seems to be functionally heterogeneous. Both inhibitory and facilitatory responses were reported.[20,35] We do not know the exact mechanism regarding how VTA neurons exert their effects. However, the inhibitory and facilitatory effects might be mediated via the dopamine D1 and D2 receptors, respectively[35] (Figure 11.1a).

CLINICAL FEATURES OF LOWER URINARY TRACT DYSFUNCTION IN PATIENTS WITH PARKINSON'S DISEASE
SYMPTOMS

Most patients are diagnosed as having PD for about 5–6 years before the onset of urinary symptoms.[36–38] Storage symptoms, such as increased daytime frequency, nocturia, urgency, and urgency urinary incontinence, are most commonly found in PD,[36,37,39–42] whereas voiding symptoms alone or a combination is thought to be infrequent and moderate.[37] It should be noted that voiding function may be influenced by other conditions such as bladder outlet obstruction, diabetes, and so on.

Several studies have also shown that the severity of urinary symptoms is related to the neurologic disability or disease severity.[33,37,38,43–45] In any case, we should pay attention to various aspects of lower urinary tract function since results of self-report measurements such as questionnaires are unlikely to reflect its real problems.[43]

BLADDER FUNCTION
It is widely accepted that neurogenic detrusor overactivity during bladder filling[46] is most commonly found in urodynamic observations in patients with PD, ranging from 36% to 93%,[37,39,40,42,43,47–52] while bladder sensation is preserved. In the voiding phase, acontractile or underactive detrusor is also found (0%–48%).[33,37,39,40,43,49,51] However, previous studies have shown that patients with multiple system atrophy (MSA) have larger residual volumes of urine (>100 mL) than those with PD.[48,53]

URETHRAL FUNCTION
Previous studies have shown that patients with PD have impaired urethral function, although there are some controversies it has been unclear. Detrusor-sphincter dyssynergia (DSD) in patients with PD has been reported in some studies[43,49] but not in others.[39,40,48,50] At present it seems likely that impaired relaxation or delay in striated sphincter relaxation might exist in patients with PD.[39,51] In other words, sphincter bradykinesia is a characteristic of PD and represents a manifestation of skeletal muscle hypertonicity involving pelvic floor muscles. DSD might be mimicked by and misdiagnosed as MSA,[48] with misinterpretation of electromyography[54] and intake of dopamine D2 receptor agonists.[55] Smooth muscle urethral sphincter dysfunction has not been reported in patients with PD. More recently, dopamine depletion has been shown to impair the urethral closure pressure in 6-OHDA rats, and activation of dopamine D1 receptor partially compensates for the impaired urethral function.[56]

TREATMENT
Previous reports showed a high incidence of urinary incontinence after prostatic surgery in patients with PD[57]; however, the urethra was not impaired in patients with PD, as mentioned previously.[36,58,59] Therefore, various therapeutic options are available for voiding dysfunction in patients with PD as well as other diseases such as benign prostatic hyperplasia (BPH), which is common in the elderly.[41] Alpha-blockers are also preferred as the first-line treatment, especially for male patients with voiding and even storage symptoms, although patients may have orthostatic hypotension due to PD and/or its medication. Although multiple factors may contribute to postprostatectomy incontinence, it is essential to consider detrusor overactivity. It is unlikely that prostatic surgery for voiding dysfunction due to PD is a contraindication, since detrusor overactivity can be controlled by antimuscarinics.

Based on the results of the basic research, nonselective dopamine receptor agonists such as levodopa and apomorphine facilitates micturition reflex via dopamine D2 receptors, resulting in worsening of detrusor overactivity. However, clinical studies have shown conflicting results.[40,47,51,60–63] It is well known that dopamine replacement therapy is the most effective for motor dysfunction in patients with PD, but the treatment is less effective with time. Therefore, there is a demand for developing an alternative therapy that would allow the possibility of giving equal efficacy with fewer side effects. In this regard, adenosine A2A receptor antagonists might be a therapeutic option in the future[64–66] (Figure 11.2b). Recently, deep brain stimulation of the subthalamic nucleus (STN-DBS) has been established as a surgical treatment of motor symptoms in PD patients. In a similar fashion, several clinical studies have demonstrated that STN-DBS improved voiding

dysfunction in PD patients,[67–69] although it is still uncertain whether suppression of neuronal activities in the subthalamic nucleus by STN-DBS directly or indirectly suppresses the pontine micturition center or whether similar inhibitory effects were also observed in animal studies.[21,70]

Various antimuscarinic drugs are currently available for the treatment of overactive bladder. Clinical and urodynamic data provide significant improvements in patients with PD.[5,71] However, it should be noted that these patients might have bowel dysfunction such as constipation secondary to PD.[72] If medical treatment fails and patients

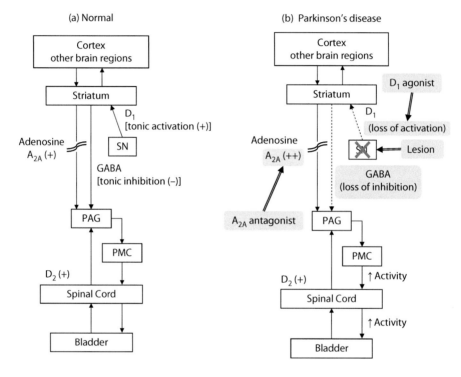

Figure 11.2 Hypothetical diagram showing dopaminergic and adenosinergic mechanisms inducing bladder dysfunction in PD. The micturition reflex is controlled by the spino-bulbo-spinal pathway passing through the PAG in the midbrain and the PMC in the brainstem. This neural circuit is under the control of higher centers including the striatum and the cortex region. (a) Under normal conditions (intact), tonic activation (+) of dopaminergic neurons in the SN activates dopamine D1 receptors expressed on GABAergic inhibitory neurons (GABA [tonic inhibition] [−]) in the striatum in order to inhibit the micturition reflex. At the same time, D1 receptor stimulation suppresses the activity of adenosinergic neurons, which exert an excitatory effect on micturition via adenosine A_{2A} receptors (Adenosine A_{2A} [+]). (b) In PD, dopaminergic neurons in the SN are lost (lesion), leading to the loss of dopamine D1 receptor activation (D1 [loss of activation]), which results in reduced activation of inhibitory GABAergic neurons in the striatum (GABA [loss of inhibition]). At the same time, reduced D1 receptor stimulation enhances the adenosinergic mechanism to stimulate adenosine A_{2A} receptors (Adenosine A_{2A} [++]), leading to facilitation of the spino-bulbo-spinal pathway controlling the micturition reflex (activity↑). Administration of dopamine D1 receptor agonists (D1 agonist) could restore the GABAergic nerve activity and suppress A_{2A} receptor-mediated activation to reduce bladder overactivity in PD. Also, administration of adenosine A_{2A} receptor antagonists (A_{2A} antagonist) could suppress A_{2A} receptor-mediated activation of the micturition reflex to reduce bladder overactivity in PD. Dopamine D2 receptors (D2 [+]) expressed in the spinal cord enhance the micturition reflex. D1, dopamine D1 receptor; D2, dopamine D2 receptor; GABA, gamma-aminobutyric acid; PAG, periaqueductal gray matter; PMC, pontine micturition center; SN, substantia nigra pars compacta.

have large residual volumes, the introduction of clean intermittent catheterization is an option. For the refractory overactive bladder, intradetrusor injection of botulinumtoxinA is available for patients with PD.[73,74] Stem cell implantation therapy is also investigated for the treatment of motor dysfunction and lower urinary tract symptoms in patients with PD, although it is not available in clinical settings.[75-78]

HUNTINGTON'S DISEASE

HD is a degenerative disease characterized by progressive neuronal loss in the basal ganglia, especially in the caudate nucleus, and cerebral cortex.[79,80] The exact mechanisms underlying neuronal death in HD are still unknown. Although the disease may begin at any time from childhood to old age (average age of onset is approximately 40 years), adult-onset HD is characterized by a triad of progressive motor, cognitive, and emotional symptoms.

There has been little investigation regarding urinary tract dysfunction in patients with HD. Wheeler et al. reviewed the neuro-urologic findings in six patients with HD who complained of lower urinary tract symptoms, and found that four out of six patients had detrusor overactivity with a normal sphincter, while the remaining two patients exhibited no abnormal findings. Symptoms include urinary frequency, urgency, nocturia, and incontinence, and the onset of these symptoms was 6.1 years after the onset of HD.[81] A previous survey of 1283 symptomatic individuals with HD found that lower urinary tract symptoms occurred in the late stage of HD, typically more than 10 years after onset.[82]

Anticholinergic agents could be useful to alleviate urologic symptoms. However, in patients with severe neurologic disability, a permanent indwelling catheter may be required.

REFERENCES

1. Flowers KA. Visual "closed-loop" and "open-loop" characteristics of voluntary movement in patients with Parkinsonism and intention tremor. *Brain.* 1976;99(2):269–310.
2. Evarts EV, Teravainen H, and Calne DB. Reaction time in Parkinson's disease. *Brain.* 1981;104(Pt 1):167–86.
3. Sakakibara R, Tateno F, Kishi M, Tsuyuzaki Y, Uchiyama T, and Yamamoto T. Pathophysiology of bladder dysfunction in Parkinson's disease. *Neurobiol Dis.* 2012;46(3):565–71.
4. Fowler CJ. Update on the neurology of Parkinson's disease. *Neurourol Urodyn.* 2007;26(1):103–9.
5. Winge K and Fowler CJ. Bladder dysfunction in Parkinsonism: Mechanisms, prevalence, symptoms, and management. *Mov Disord.* 2006;21(6):737–45.
6. Bolam JP, Hanley JJ, Booth PA, and Bevan MD. Synaptic organisation of the basal ganglia. *J Anat.* 2000;196(Pt 4):527–42.
7. Tritsch NX, Ding JB, and Sabatini BL. Dopaminergic neurons inhibit striatal output through non-canonical release of GABA. *Nature.* 2012;490(7419):262–66.
8. Mathur BN and Lovinger DM. Serotonergic action on dorsal striatal function. *Parkinsonism Relat Disord.* 2012;18(Suppl 1):S129–31.
9. Kita H and Kitai ST. Glutamate decarboxylase immunoreactive neurons in rat neostriatum: Their morphological types and populations. *Brain Res.* 1988;447(2):346–52.
10. Vincent SR, Hokfelt T, Christensson I, and Terenius L. Dynorphin-immunoreactive neurons in the central nervous system of the rat. *Neurosci Lett.* 1982;33(2):185–90.
11. Vincent S, Hokfelt T, Christensson I, and Terenius L. Immunohistochemical evidence for a dynorphin immunoreactive striato-nigral pathway. *Eur J Pharmacol.* 1982;85(2):251–52.
12. Beckstead RM. Complementary mosaic distributions of thalamic and nigral axons in the caudate nucleus of the cat: Double anterograde labeling combining autoradiography and wheat germ-HRP histochemistry. *Brain Res.* 1985;335(1):153–59.
13. Kanazawa I, Emson PC, and Cuello AC. Evidence for the existence of substance P-containing fibres in striato-nigral and pallido-nigral pathways in rat brain. *Brain Res.* 1977;119(2):447–53.
14. Yoshimura N, Kuno S, Chancellor MB, de Groat WC, and Seki S. Dopaminergic mechanisms underlying bladder hyperactivity in rats with a unilateral 6-hydroxydopamine (6-OHDA) lesion of the nigrostriatal pathway. *Br J Pharmacol.* 2003;139(8):1425–32.
15. Levy R, Hazrati LN, Herrero MT et al. Re-evaluation of the functional anatomy of the basal ganglia in normal and Parkinsonian states. *Neuroscience.* 1997;76(2):335–43.
16. Le Moine C and Bloch B. D1 and D2 dopamine receptor gene expression in the rat striatum: Sensitive cRNA probes demonstrate prominent segregation of D1 and D2 mRNAs in distinct neuronal populations of the dorsal and ventral striatum. *J Comp Neurol.* 1995;355(3):418–26.
17. Lewin RJ, Dillard GV, and Porter RW. Extrapyramidal inhibition of the urinary bladder. *Brain Res.* 1967;4:301–7.
18. Raz S. Parkinsonism and neurogenic bladder. Experimental and clinical observations. *Urol Res.* 1976;4(3):133–8.
19. Yoshimura N, Sasa M, Yoshida O, and Takaori S. Dopamine D1 receptor-mediated inhibition of micturition reflex by central dopamine from the substantia nigra. *Neurourol Urodyn.* 1992;11:535–45.
20. Sakakibara R, Nakazawa K, Uchiyama T, Yoshiyama M, Yamanishi T, and Hattori T. Micturition-related electrophysiological properties in the substantia nigra pars compacta and the ventral tegmental area in cats. *Auton Neurosci.* 2002;102(1–2):30–8.
21. Sakakibara R, Nakazawa K, Uchiyama T, Yoshiyama M, Yamanishi T, and Hattori T. Effects of subthalamic nucleus stimulation on the micturation reflex in cats. *Neuroscience.* 2003;120(3):871–5.

22. Seki S, Igawa Y, Kaidoh K, Ishizuka O, Nishizawa O, and Andersson KE. Role of dopamine D1 and D2 receptors in the micturition reflex in conscious rats. *Neurourol Urodyn.* 2001;20(1):105–13.

23. Albanese A, Jenner P, Marsden CD, and Stephenson JD. Bladder hyperreflexia induced in marmosets by 1-methyl-4-phenyl-1,2,3,6-tetrahydropyridine. *Neurosci Lett.* 1988;87(1–2):46–50.

24. Yoshimura N, Mizuta E, Kuno S, Sasa M, and Yoshida O. The dopamine D_1 receptor agonist SKF 38393 suppresses detrusor hyperreflexia in the monkey with parkinsonism induced by 1-methyl-4-phenyl-1,2,3,6-tetrahydropyridine (MPTP). *Neuropharmacology.* 1993;32:315–21.

25. Yoshimura N, Mizuta E, Yoshida O, and Kuno S. Therapeutic effects of dopamine D1/D2 receptor agonists on detrusor hyperreflexia in 1-methyl-4-phenyl-1,2,3,6-tetrahydropyridine-lesioned parkinsonian cynomolgus monkeys. *J Pharmacol Exp Ther.* 1998;286(1):228–33.

26. Yamamoto T, Sakakibara R, Hashimoto K et al. Striatal dopamine level increases in the urinary storage phase in cats: An in vivo microdialysis study. *Neuroscience.* 2005;135(1):299–303.

27. Kontani H, Inoue T, and Sakai T. Dopamine receptor subtypes that induce hyperactive urinary bladder response in anesthetized rats. *Jpn J Pharmacol.* 1990;54:482–86.

28. Kuno S, Mizuta E, and Yoshimura N. Different effects of D1 and D2 agonists on neurogenic bladder in Parkinson's disease and MPTP-induced parkinsonian monkeys. *Mov Disord.* 1997;12(S1).

29. de Groat WC, Booth AM, and Yoshimura N. Neurophysiology of micturition and its modification in animal models of human disease. In: Maggi CA, ed. *The Autonomic Nervous System, Nervous Control of the Urogenital System.* Vol 3. London: Harwood Academic; 1993:227–90.

30. Roppolo JR, Noto H, Mallory BS, and de Groat WC. Dopaminergic and cholinergic modulation of bladder reflexes at the level of the pontine micturition center in the cat. *Soc Neurosci Abstr.* 1987;13:733.

31. Kitta T, Matsumoto M, Tanaka H, Mitsui T, Yoshioka M, and Nonomura K. GABAergic mechanism mediated via D receptors in the rat periaqueductal gray participates in the micturition reflex: An in vivo microdialysis study. *Eur J Neurosci.* 2008;27(12):3216–25.

32. Kitta T, Kakizaki H, Furuno T et al. Brain activation during detrusor overactivity in patients with Parkinson's disease: A positron emission tomography study. *J Urol.* 2006;175(3 Pt 1):994–98.

33. Sakakibara R, Shinotoh H, Uchiyama T, Yoshiyama M, Hattori T, and Yamanishi T. SPECT imaging of the dopamine transporter with [(123)I]-beta-CIT reveals marked decline of nigrostriatal dopaminergic function in Parkinson's disease with urinary dysfunction. *J Neurol Sci.* 2001;187(1–2):55–9.

34. Winge K, Friberg L, Werdelin L, Nielsen KK, and Stimpel H. Relationship between nigrostriatal dopaminergic degeneration, urinary symptoms, and bladder control in Parkinson's disease. *Eur J Neurol.* 2005;12(11):842–50.

35. Hashimoto K, Oyama T, Sugiyama T, Park YC, and Kurita T. Neuronal excitation in the ventral tegmental area modulates the micturition reflex mediated via the dopamine D1 and D2 receptors in rats. *J Pharmacol Sci.* 2003;92(2):143–48.

36. Chandiramani VA, Palace J, and Fowler CJ. How to recognize patients with parkinsonism who should not have urological surgery. *Br J Urol.* 1997;80(1):100–4.

37. Bonnet AM, Pichon J, Vidailhet M et al. Urinary disturbances in striatonigral degeneration and Parkinson's disease: Clinical and urodynamic aspects. *Mov Disord.* 1997;12(4):509–13.

38. Winge K, Skau AM, Stimpel H, Nielsen KK, and Werdelin L. Prevalence of bladder dysfunction in Parkinson's disease. *Neurourol Urodyn.* 2006;25(2):116–22.

39. Pavlakis AJ, Siroky MB, Goldstein I, and Krane RJ. Neurologic findings in Parkinson's disease. *J Urol.* 1983;129:80–3.

40. Fitzmaurice H, Fowler CJ, Rickards D et al. Micturition disturbance in Parkinson's disease. *Br J Urol.* 1985;57(6):652–6.

41. Lemack GE, Dewey RB Jr., Roehrborn CG, O'Suilleabhain PE, and Zimmern PE. Questionnaire-based assessment of bladder dysfunction in patients with mild to moderate Parkinson's disease. *Urology.* 2000;56(2):250–4.

42. Defreitas GA, Lemack GE, Zimmern PE, Dewey RB, Roehrborn CG, and O'Suilleabhain PE. Distinguishing neurogenic from non-neurogenic detrusor overactivity: A urodynamic assessment of lower urinary tract symptoms in patients with and without Parkinson's disease. *Urology.* 2003;62(4):651–5.

43. Araki I and Kuno S. Assessment of voiding dysfunction in Parkinson's disease by the International Prostate Symptom Score. *J Neurol Neurosurg Psychiatry.* 2000;68(4):429–33.

44. Hattori T, Yasuda K, Kita K, and Hirayama K. Voiding dysfunction in Parkinson's disease. *Jpn J Psychiatry Neurol.* 1992;46(1):181–6.

45. Winge K, Werdelin LM, Nielsen KK, and Stimpel H. Effects of dopaminergic treatment on bladder function in Parkinson's disease. *Neurourol Urodyn.* 2004;23(7):689–96.

46. Abrams P, Cardozo L, Fall M et al. The standardisation of terminology of lower urinary tract function: Report from the Standardisation Sub-committee of the International Continence Society. *Neurourol Urodyn.* 2002;21(2):167–78.

47. Christmas TJ, Kempster PA, Chapple CR et al. Role of subcutaneous apomorphine in parkinsonian voiding dysfunction. *Lancet.* 1988;2(8626–8627):1451–3.

48. Sakakibara R, Hattori T, Uchiyama T, and Yamanishi T. Videourodynamic and sphincter motor unit potential analyses in Parkinson's disease and multiple system atrophy. *J Neurol Neurosurg Psychiatry.* 2001;71(5):600–6.

49. Khan Z, Starer P, and Bhola A. Urinary incontinence in female Parkinson disease patients. Pitfalls of diagnosis. *Urology.* 1989;33(6):486–9.

50. Gray R, Stern G, and Malone-Lee J. Lower urinary tract dysfunction in Parkinson's disease: Changes relate to age and not disease. *Age Ageing.* 1995;24(6):499–504.

51. Stocchi F, Carbone A, Inghilleri M et al. Urodynamic and neurophysiological evaluation in Parkinson's disease and multiple system atrophy. *J Neurol Neurosurg Psychiatry.* 1997;62(5):507–11.

52. Myers DL, Arya LA, and Friedman JH. Is urinary incontinence different in women with Parkinson's disease? *Int Urogynecol J Pelvic Floor Dysfunct.* 1999;10(3):188–91.

53. Hahn K and Ebersbach G. Sonographic assessment of urinary retention in multiple system atrophy and idiopathic Parkinson's disease. *Mov Disord.* 2005;20(11):1499–502.

54. Uchiyama T, Sakakibara R, Yamamoto T et al. Urinary dysfunction in early and untreated Parkinson's disease. *J Neurol Neurosurg Psychiatry.* 2011;82(12):1382–6.

55. Ogawa T, Seki S, Masuda H et al. Dopaminergic mechanisms controlling urethral function in rats. *Neurourol Urodyn.* 2006;25(5):480–9.

56. Ouchi M, Kitta T, Kanno Y et al. Dopaminergic urethral closure mechanisms in a rat model of Parkinson's disease. *Neurourol Urodyn.* 2019;38(5):1203–11.

57. Staskin DS, Vardi Y, and Siroky MB. Post-prostatectomy continence in the parkinsonian patient: The significance of poor voluntary sphincter control. *J Urol.* 1988;140(1):117–18.

58. Fowler CJ. Urinary disorders in Parkinson's disease and multiple system atrophy. *Funct Neurol.* 2001;16(3):277–82.

59. Quinn N. Parkinsonism—Recognition and differential diagnosis. *BMJ.* 1995;310(6977):447–52.

60. Benson GS, Raezer DM, Anderson JR, Saunders CD, and Corriere JN Jr. Effect of levodopa on urinary bladder. *Urology.* 1976;7(1):24–8.

61. Aranda B and Cramer P. Effects of apomorphine and L-dopa on the parkinsonian bladder. *Neurourol Urodyn.* 1993;12(3):203–9.

62. Uchiyama T, Sakakibara R, Hattori T, and Yamanishi T. Short-term effect of a single levodopa dose on micturition disturbance in Parkinson's disease patients with the wearing-off phenomenon. *Mov Disord.* 2003;18(5):573–8.

63. Brusa L, Petta F, Pisani A et al. Central acute D2 stimulation worsens bladder function in patients with mild Parkinson's disease. *J Urol.* 2006;175(1):202–6; discussion 6–7.

64. Pinna A, Wardas J, Simola N, and Morelli M. New therapies for the treatment of Parkinson's disease: Adenosine A2A receptor antagonists. *Life Sci.* 2005;77(26):3259–67.

65. Schwarzschild MA, Agnati L, Fuxe K, Chen JF, and Morelli M. Targeting adenosine A2A receptors in Parkinson's disease. *Trends Neurosci.* 2006;29(11):647–54.

66. Kitta T, Chancellor MB, de Groat WC, Kuno S, Nonomura K, and Yoshimura N. Suppression of bladder overactivity by adenosine A2A receptor antagonist in a rat model of Parkinson disease. *J Urol.* 2012;187(5):1890–7.

67. Finazzi-Agro E, Peppe A, D'Amico A et al. Effects of subthalamic nucleus stimulation on urodynamic findings in patients with Parkinson's disease. *J Urol.* 2003;169(4):1388–91.

68. Seif C, Herzog J, van der Horst C et al. Effect of subthalamic deep brain stimulation on the function of the urinary bladder. *Ann Neurol.* 2004;55(1):118–20.

69. Herzog J, Weiss PH, Assmus A et al. Subthalamic stimulation modulates cortical control of urinary bladder in Parkinson's disease. *Brain.* 2006;129(Pt 12):3366–75.

70. Dalmose AL, Bjarkam CR, Sorensen JC, Djurhuus JC, and Jorgensen TM. Effects of high frequency deep brain stimulation on urine storage and voiding function in conscious minipigs. *Neurourol Urodyn.* 2004;23(3):265–72.

71. Palleschi G, Pastore AL, Stocchi F et al. Correlation between the Overactive Bladder questionnaire (OAB-q) and urodynamic data of Parkinson disease patients affected by neurogenic detrusor overactivity during antimuscarinic treatment. *Clin Neuropharmacol.* 2006;29(4):220–9.

72. Sakakibara R, Shinotoh H, Uchiyama T et al. Questionnaire-based assessment of pelvic organ dysfunction in Parkinson's disease. *Auton Neurosci.* 2001;92(1–2):76–85.

73. Kulaksizoglu H and Parman Y. Use of botulinum toxin-A for the treatment of overactive bladder symptoms in patients with Parkinsons's disease. *Parkinsonism Relat Disord.* 2010;16(8):531–4.

74. Giannantoni A, Rossi A, Mearini E, Del Zingaro M, Porena M, and Berardelli A. Botulinum toxin A for overactive bladder and detrusor muscle overactivity in patients with Parkinson's disease and multiple system atrophy. *J Urol.* 2009;182(4):1453–7.

75. Hegarty SV, Sullivan AM, and O'Keeffe GW. Midbrain dopaminergic neurons: A review of the molecular circuitry that regulates their development. *Dev Biol.* 2013;379(2):123–38.

76. Lindvall O. Developing dopaminergic cell therapy for Parkinson's disease—Give up or move forward? *Mov Disord.* 2013;28(3):268–73.

77. Nishimura K and Takahashi J. Therapeutic application of stem cell technology toward the treatment of Parkinson's disease. *Biol Pharm Bull.* 2013;36(2):171–5.

78. Soler R, Fullhase C, Hanson A, Campeau L, Santos C, and Andersson KE. Stem cell therapy ameliorates bladder dysfunction in an animal model of Parkinson disease. *J Urol.* 2012;187(4):1491–7.

79. Feigin A and Zgaljardic D. Recent advances in Huntington's disease: Implications for experimental therapeutics. *Curr Opin Neurol.* 2002;15(4):483–9.

80. Walker FO. Huntington's disease. *Lancet.* 2007;369(9557):218–28.

81. Wheeler JS, Sax DS, Krane RJ, and Siroky MB. Vesico-urethral function in Huntington's chorea. *Br J Urol.* 1985;57(1):63–6.

82. Kirkwood SC, Su JL, Conneally P, and Foroud T. Progression of symptoms in the early and middle stages of Huntington disease. *Arch Neurol.* 2001;58(2):273–8.

DEMYELINATING NEUROPATHIES

Chapter 12

MULTIPLE SCLEROSIS, TRANSVERSE MYELITIS, TROPICAL SPASTIC PARAPARESIS, PROGRESSIVE MULTIFOCAL LEUKOENCEPHALOPATHY, LYME DISEASE

Michele Fascelli and Howard B. Goldman

MULTIPLE SCLEROSIS

Multiple sclerosis (MS) is an autoimmune disorder of the central nervous system (CNS) causing disabling neurologic deficits. Disease manifestations result from axon demyelination and differ depending on the location of the CNS involvement (Figure 12.1). Cerebral lesions cause cognitive, sensory, and motor impairment, with or without epilepsy and focal cortical deficits.[1–3] Optic nerve lesions lead to painful loss of vision, whereas cerebellum and brainstem lesions present with tremor, ataxia, vertigo, and impaired speech and swallowing. Spinal cord involvement alters motor, sensory, and autonomic function, often including bowel, bladder, and erectile dysfunction.[1,2,4] Diagnosis is based on clinical presentation, cerebrospinal fluid (CSF) analysis (oligoclonal bands), visually evoked potentials, and magnetic resonance imaging (MRI).[5]

UROLOGIC SYMPTOMS ASSOCIATED WITH MULTIPLE SCLEROSIS

Urologic symptoms occur in over 50% of patients with MS and most commonly involve frequency and urgency (incidence: 31%–86%).[6] Incontinence and obstructive symptoms with or without urinary retention are reported in 34%–72% and 2%–49%, respectively.[7–9] Seven percent will develop serious renal or bladder problems. While symptoms may occur in early stages, most experience urologic symptoms within 6–10 years of their neurologic disease.[7,10–12] MRI findings do not correlate with the presence of urologic symptoms, and urodynamic evaluation does not correlate with the extent of vesical dysfunction.[13–15] Thus, the physician must attribute urologic symptoms to underlying neurologic disease with thoughtful caution, as common urologic disorders may coexist with, mimic, or aggravate MS.

NEUROLOGIC EFFECT OF MULTIPLE SCLEROSIS ON THE URINARY TRACT

Bladder and sphincter function require autonomic, somatic, and CNS coordination to facilitate efficient, low-pressure storage and expulsion of urine. Demyelination of suprasacral, sacral, and intracranial tracts alters detrusor and external urethral sphincter innervation, resulting in varying forms of lower urinary tract dysfunction (LUTD).[9] Interruption of the reticulospinal pathways between the pontine and sacral micturition centers causes loss of synergism between the detrusor and urethral sphincter, leading to detrusor external sphincter dyssynergia (DESD).[16] Lesions in the corticospinal tract negate supraspinal suppression of autonomous bladder contractions to cause detrusor overactivity (DO).

Autopsy studies reported 20% incidence of sacral cord involvement.[17,18] Detrusor hypocontractility was observed in 66% and acontractility in 5%.[19] Plaques located in the spinal afferents and efferents of the sacral reflex arc may inhibit bladder contraction, impairing emptying.

Intracranial plaques develop in the periventricular zone of approximately 60%–80% of cases, resulting in loss of voluntary control of initiation or prevention of voiding, as the perception of fullness and ability to inhibit bladder contraction depend on alert and normally functioning sensorium.[9] Micturition reflex and the bladder-urethral sphincter synergy remain intact.

Site	Symptoms	Signs	Treatment		
			Established efficacy	Equivocal efficacy	Speculative
Cerebrum	Cognitive impairment	Deficits in attention, reasoning, and executive function (early); dementia (late)	–	–	–
	Hemisensory and motor	Upper motor neuron signs	–	–	–
	Affective (mainly depression)		Antidepressants	–	–
	Epilepsy (rare)		Anticonvulsants	–	–
	Focal cortical deficits (rare)		–	–	–
Optic nerve	Unilateral painful loss of vision	Scotoma, reduced visual acuity, color vision, and relative afferent papillary defect	Low vision aids	–	–
Cerebellum and cerebellar pathways	Tremor	Postural and action tremor, dysarthria	–	–	Wrist weights, carbamazepine, isoniazid, beta-blockers, clonazepam, thalamotomy, and thalamic stimulation
	Clumsiness and poor balance	Limb incoordination and gait ataxia	–	–	–
Brainstem	Diplopia	Nystagms, internuclear, and other complex opthamoplegias	–	–	Baclofen, gabapentin, isoniazid
	Vertigo		–	Prochlorpherazine, cinnarizine	–

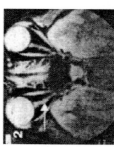
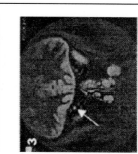

Figure 12.1 Lesion sites, syndromes, and symptomatic treatments in multiple sclerosis. T2-weighted magnetic resonance imaging (MRI) abnormalities (arrows) in the cerebrum (1), right optic nerve, longitudinal section, (2), transverse section (3). (Continued)

Lesion site	Symptom	Syndrome			
Spinal cord	Impaired speech and swallowing	Dysarthria and pseudobulbar palsy	Tricyclic antidepressants	—	Speech therapy
	Paroxysmal symptoms		Carbamazepine, gabapentin	—	—
	Weakness	Upper motor neuron signs	—	—	—
	Stiffness and painful spasms	Spasticity	Tizanidine, baclofen, dantrolene, benzodiazepines intrathecal baclofen	Botulinum toxin, IV corticosteroids	Cannabinoids
	Bladder dysfunction		Anticholinergics and intermittents self-catheterization, suprapubic catheterization	Desmopressin, intravescial capsaicin	Abdominal vibration, cranberry juice
	Erectile impotence		Sidenafil	—	—
	Constipation	Bulk laxatives, enemas	—	—	—
Other	Pain		Carbamazepine, gabapentin	Tricyclic antidepressants, TENS	—
	Fatigue		Amantadine	Modafanil	4-aminopyridine, pemoline fluoxetine
	Temperature sensitivity and exercise intolerance	—	—	—	Cooling suit, 4-aminopyridine

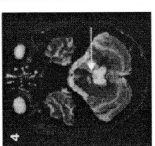

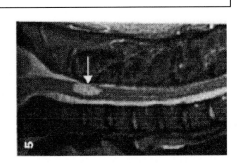

Figure 12.1 (Continued) Lesion sites, syndromes, and symptomatic treatments in multiple sclerosis. Brainstem and cerebellar peduncle (4), and cervical spinal cord (5). TENS, transcutaneous electric nerve stimulation. (Reproduced from *The Lancet*, 347, Sadovnick A, Eberg G, Dyment D, Rish N, Canadian Collaborative Study Group. Evidence for genetic basis of multiple sclerosis, 1728–30, Copyright 1996, with permission from Elsevier.)

EVALUATION OF URINARY TRACT DYSFUNCTION IN PATIENTS WITH MULTIPLE SCLEROSIS

HISTORY

Initial assessment should characterize urologic symptoms and voiding dysfunction. Insight into temporal and spatial details, protective absorbent pad use, fluid intake, and quality of life (QOL) should be solicited.[9] One should identify the presence or absence of urologic complications: upper or lower urinary tract infection, hematuria, and stones. Past medical and surgical history are mandatory; urologic pathologies like BPH or stress incontinence are common in older populations and may confound the neuro-urologic profile. Note current medications, as many drugs may affect bladder function. It is critical to recognize the presentation of a young patient with unexplained urologic symptoms. Every effort should be made to elicit neurologic symptoms suggestive of MS, and prompt referral is mandatory.[20,21]

PHYSICAL EXAMINATION

Thorough genitourinary evaluation includes abdominal examination to ensure no overt evidence of bladder distention. A complete pelvic examination should evaluate sensory and motor pelvic floor function and sacral dermatomes; it is also important to determine concomitant urethral hypermobility or vaginal prolapse. A directed neurologic examination may not only help understand the disease extent but can also help predict urologic dysfunction.

The incidence of upper tract abnormalities was reported in 7% of 2076 MS patients, suggesting that upper tract deterioration is the exception rather than the rule.[22,23] The presence of an indwelling catheter, DESD, and poor bladder compliance have been previously linked to upper tract deterioration.[13,24–26] Patient disability scores are associated with unfavorable urodynamic findings and increased risk for upper tract damage.[24,27] Although baseline radiographic assessment remains part of initial evaluation, the low incidence of upper tract deterioration has led many urologists to abandon routine yearly upper tract imaging unless baseline studies are abnormal or there is a change in clinical status.[28]

URODYNAMIC EVALUATION

The purpose of urodynamic testing is to determine and classify the voiding dysfunction and to identify risk factors such as DESD, decreased bladder compliance, and high detrusor filling pressures. Predisposing factors to upper tract problems include vesicoureteral reflux, bladder and kidney stones, hydronephrosis, pyelonephritis, and renal insufficiency. A retrospective analysis of 66 MS patients revealed no predictive urodynamic parameters for upper tract deterioration as identified by ultrasound.[29,30]

The incidence of abnormal urodynamic findings in MS patients with voiding dysfunction approaches 100%. The incidence of normal urodynamic findings in symptomatic patients is approximately 10%, as revealed by a meta-analysis of 1900 patients.[9,29–31] MS patients without urinary complaints demonstrated 52% incidence of clinically silent urodynamic abnormalities.[17] Even MS patients who deny urologic symptoms can exhibit significant underlying urodynamic pathology.

Three major patterns of urodynamic dysfunction have been described.

DETRUSOR OVERACTIVITY WITHOUT BLADDER OUTLET OBSTRUCTION

The most common urodynamic abnormality in MS is DO, which manifests as urinary frequency, urgency, nocturia, and incontinence.[32] These findings correlate with the high incidence of intracranial and cervical spinal plaques.[33] Systematic reviews and meta-analyses report 53%–62% of patients had DO on urodynamics.[9,34,35]

DETRUSOR OVERACTIVITY WITH BLADDER OUTLET OBSTRUCTION

Second most common is DO with DESD and is reported in 25%–43% of patients.[9,35] Detrusor overactivity occurs without proper relaxation of the external urethral sphincter, presenting with obstructive symptoms and incomplete emptying, the latter likely related to sphincteric dysfunction or incomplete bladder contraction.[36] Compared to DESD in spinal cord patients, DESD is rarely associated with upper tract dysfunction, suggesting that detrusor overactivity and extent of external sphincter spasms may be less severe than in patients with spinal cord injury (SCI).[14,37,38]

HYPOCONTRACTILE DETRUSOR

Finally, hypocontractile detrusor is reported in approximately 10%–20% of patients, and symptoms include straining, incapacity to void, or overflow incontinence.[9,35] Changes in urodynamic patterns have also been observed given fluctuating disease course and in response to treatments. Generalizations concerning patterns cannot be drawn, but a significant proportion of patients (15%–55%) will develop urodynamic changes, emphasizing periodically repeating the studies.[28,39]

MANAGEMENT OF URINARY MANIFESTATIONS OF MULTIPLE SCLEROSIS

The aim of treatment of the neurogenic patient is management of lower urinary tract symptoms, prevention of UTIs, preservation of the upper urinary tract, and improvement of QOL. Treatment should be based on understanding the pathology and on objective parameters, as well as on the patient's disability, autonomy, manual dexterity, and motivation. Since symptoms can change, treatment modalities should preferably be reversible, deferring permanent surgical procedures as much as possible. Table 12.1 summarizes different therapeutic options.

BEHAVIORAL MODIFICATIONS AND PELVIC FLOOR REHABILITATION

Voiding symptoms can improve with behavioral manipulations, but the success relies on patient motivation. Regular voiding reduces hyperreflexic contraction by emptying the bladder before a critical state of filling. Pelvic floor rehabilitation (PFR) has been reported of some value in the treatment of detrusor instability and urgency by influencing the sacral micturition reflex arc, thus inhibiting DO. In 77% of PFR patients, improvement in functional bladder capacity, frequency, incontinence, and QOL were reported.[40,41]

Patients with high PVRs can practice double-voiding and often Valsalva to assist with bladder emptying. Timed voiding helps by avoiding bladder overdistention. Pelvic floor stimulation in the hyporeflexic bladder plays a very limited role.[42]

CLEAN INTERMITTENT CATHETERIZATION AND CATHETER DRAINAGE

Clean intermittent catheterization (CIC) is a simple, very effective treatment for neurogenic voiding dysfunction in patients with primary emptying difficulties or after pharmacologic therapy for DO.[7,43–46] For patients with advanced disease, poor hand dexterity, or pain with catheterization, CIC is problematic.[45,46] These patients may require an indwelling catheter or suprapubic cystostomy. The latter is attractive as it has several advantages over a conventional indwelling catheter: urethral erosion and traumatic hypospadias in males and bladder neck and urethral damage in females are avoided, and personal hygiene/catheter care are simplified because of the catheter's accessibility and its position remote from perineal or vaginal soilage.[41] The external genitalia can be free of foreign bodies and may render sexual activity possible.[42,47]

BOTULINUM TOXIN

Botulinum toxin, the neurotoxin produced by *Clostridium botulinum*, inhibits calcium-mediated release of acetylcholine vesicles at the neuromuscular junction, reducing muscle contractility.[48] Injections into the detrusor muscle are a safe conservative treatment for DO in MS patients. In 2011, onabotulinumtoxinA was approved by the U.S. Food and Drug Administration for the treatment of neurogenic DO. After therapy, 19 of 21 patients experienced complete continence at 6 weeks and 11 out of 22 at 36 weeks.[49,50] In 16 patients with

Table 12.1 Management Options of Patients with Multiple Sclerosis Based on Urologic Dysfunction

Detrusor overactivity without bladder outlet obstruction:
- Behavioral modification and pelvic floor rehabilitation
- Clean intermittent catheterization/catheter drainage
- Pharmacologic therapy
- Surgical management
  - Denervation procedures
  - Augmentation cystoplasty
- Neuromodulation
- Botulinum toxin

Detrusor overactivity with bladder outlet obstruction:
- Clean intermittent catheterization/catheter drainage
- Augmentation cystoplasty
- Ileal conduit
- Cutaneous ileovesicostomy
- Neuromodulation
- Botulinum toxin

Hypocontractile detrusor:
- Clean intermittent catheterization/catheter drainage
- Urinary diversion

MS evaluated for refractory DO to anticholinergics, injection therapy increased PVR, decreased frequency, and improved incontinence.[51] Urodynamic parameters measured increased reflex volume, mean cystometric capacity, and decreased mean detrusor pressure. Patient satisfaction and QOL were rated highly, and all patients indicated a willingness to undergo repeated injections.[51]

The risks of bladder calculi, infection, hematuria, and squamous cell carcinoma should be weighed against the advantages for the patient.[42,52]

NEUROMODULATION

Neuromodulation has proven efficacy in relieving neurogenic overactivity symptoms secondary to MS, especially in DO with or without DESD. Commonly used approaches include sacral neuromodulation (SNM), pudendal nerve stimulation, and posterior tibial nerve stimulation.[34,53–55] In patients with DO, an SNM was associated with overall patient satisfaction of 75%–85% with improvement in frequency, volume voided, and urinary incontinence.[56–59] Current SNM devices are not MRI compatible except for 1.5 T head imaging. This limitation, however, will be obviated with upcoming newer device generations.[60]

SURGICAL MANAGEMENT

Surgical intervention in the management of neurogenic dysfunction secondary to MS has dramatically reduced with increased adoption of CIC. As a general principle, nonoperative treatments should be utilized. Permanent procedures are deferred due to progressive disease course and performed only after neurologic status stabilizes and after conservative options have been exhausted. Evaluation of manual dexterity, disability, life expectancy, and social support should be undertaken. Patients with DESD are at higher risk of upper tract damage.[16] In those males who cannot be treated with conservative measures, outlet reducing procedures may be necessary.

Augmentation cystoplasty with or without a catheterizable limb (using the ileocecal valve or intussuscepted portion of the small bowel) is usually reserved for refractory DO. Bladder augmentation will allow large urine volumes stored in the bladder at low-filling pressures.[61] Excellent results can be expected.[61,62] Most will require CIC; thus, the ability to perform CIC is mandatory if considering this procedure.[62,63] Evaluation of sphincteric competence may obviate the need for a concomitant outlet procedure such as pubovaginal sling or sphincter prosthesis.

CONCLUSION

The majority of patients with MS with advancing disease suffer from LUTD. Poor correlation between subjective symptoms and objective parameters requires thorough urinary tract evaluation in individuals with and without symptoms. Although treatment options exist, a stepwise approach with conservative and initially reversible therapy is important.[36] Follow-up aims to preserve renal function while minimizing symptoms and enhancing QOL.

TRANSVERSE MYELITIS

Transverse myelitis (TM) is a clinical syndrome following an immune-mediated process causing neural injury to the spinal cord, and manifests varying degrees of weakness, sensory alterations, and autonomic dysfunction. Acute transverse myelitis (ATM) has an incidence of one to four cases per million people per year with bimodal prevalence between the ages of 10–19 and 30–39 years. ATM is commonly parainfectious. Classification is based on speed of symptom progression (acute, subacute, or chronic) or etiology (viral, bacterial, idiopathic, etc.).[2,64–66]

DIAGNOSIS

ATM is characterized by onset of symptoms and signs of neurologic dysfunction with clearly defined upper borders of sensory dysfunction; spinal MRI and lumbar puncture show acute inflammation. Upon reaching maximal deficit level, approximately 50% of patients experience paraplegia, virtually all patients have LUTD, and 80%–94% have numbness, paresthesias, or band-like dysesthesias. Autonomic symptoms consist variably of increased urinary urgency, bowel or bladder incontinence, difficulty or inability to void, incomplete evacuation, or constipation.[67]

LOWER URINARY TRACT DYSFUNCTION IN TRANSVERSE MYELITIS

Lower urinary tract abnormalities in ATM correlate with evoked potentials, MRI, and urodynamic findings.[68] Complaints of increased urgency, frequency, and urge incontinence predominanted in 84% of patients with ATM in a prospective study from a neurorehabiliation unit of a tertiary university.[69] Early abnormal urodynamic findings commonly persisted at the 6- and 12-month examinations, with persistent abnormalities including DO, dyssynergia, and acontractile bladder.[68,70] No patient characteristics were predictive of urodynamic findings.[69,70]

A retrospective review of 21 children reported that bladder sphincter dysfunction occurred on the first days of disease in 85% of cases.[71] Abnormal perception of micturition was one of the most constant and specific symptoms. Regression occured in 40% of patients, and no upper tract deterioration was noted after 3 years. Favorable prognostic factors were early motor function recovery and early management of bladder dysfunction.

Abnormal detrusor function persisted in six patients with TM and lower urinary tract symptoms, despite motor recovery.[72] Computed tomography scans and myelograms were inconclusive. Of those neuro-urologically evaluated, four were neurologically intact, while the remainder had residual deficits. Urodynamic studies revealed persistent DESD and DO; urodynamic study findings should determine bladder management with ongoing urologic surveillance.[69,70,72]

PROGNOSIS

Longitudinal case series reveal approximately one-third of patients recovered with little to no sequelae, one-third experience moderate degree of permanent disability, and one-third have severe disabilities. Rapid symptom progression, back pain, and spinal shock predict poor recovery. Paraclinical findings (absent central conduction on evoked potential testing, the presence of 14-3-3 protein in the CSF, a marker of neuronal injury) predict a poor outcome. Some authors reported that the recovery rate is generally complete.[73]

TROPICAL SPASTIC PARAPARESIS

Tropical spastic paraparesis (TSP) is associated with and probably caused by the retrovirus human T-cell lymphotropic virus type 1 (HTLV-1).[74-76] HTLV-1 has an affinity for CD4 cells. It remains a common cause of paraparesis in the West Indies, in the Japanese southern islands, where it is called HTLV-1-associated myelopathy (HAM), but it is also widely found in the tropics and subtropics.[74-76]

Transmission is through sexual contact, blood, and breastfeeding. HTLV-1 is associated with adult T-cell leukemia/lymphoma (ATL), HAM/TSP, and HTLV-associated uveitis as well an infectious dermatitis of children.

Meningomyelitis with demyelination and axonal loss affecting the corticospinal tracts is usually present. These findings are most prominent in lower thoracic and upper lumbar regions.[77,78]

HAM/TSP is a progressive, chronic myelopathy characterized by spasticity, hyperreflexia, muscle weakness, and sphincter disorders. Pathologic changes within the CNS result in a variety of urodynamic and neurophysiologic features. Gait disturbance is a main symptom; however,

bladder dysfunction is one of the major symptoms characteristic of HAM.[79]

URODYNAMIC FINDINGS

Progressive paraparesis associated with back pain and voiding disturbances are classically described. Despite reports concerning the clinical and immunologic features of this condition, little attention has been paid to the bladder dysfunction that commonly accompanies it.

Most patients had urodynamic evidence of DO and DESD.[52,80,81] Supranuclear voiding dysfunction seems to be in accordance with the known pathologic lesions of this disease. In 31 untreated patients with HAM undergoing urodynamic evaluation, two cases (11%) had no urinary symptoms; 19 (89%) had dysuria, frequency, incontinence, or urgency.[82] The combination of irritative and obstructive urinary disturbance was a characteristic symptom.[79] Urodynamics revealed DO in 14 cases (66%), although 3 (15%) showed underactive or acontractile bladder with decrease in urinary sensation.[82]

Patients with untreated HAM demonstate coexistence of both irritative and obstructive symptoms, and DESD was the main cause of symptoms identified.[83] As the activities of daily living deteriorated, the mean PVR, incidence of DO, and DESD all increased. Medical treatment relieved subjective symptoms, but urodynamics did not necessarily confirm improvement.[52,80,81]

PROGNOSIS AND TREATMENT

Approximately one-third of patients recover with little to no sequelae, one-third suffer a moderate degree of permanent disability, and one-third have severe disabilities. Rapid progression of symptoms, back pain, and spinal shock predict poor recovery. Long-term urological follow-up in patients with TM is recommended, as an increased risk of conversion to MS exists when associated with oligoclonal bands in CSF and brain MRI findings.[73] In some cases, symptoms are persistent, progressive, and do not correlate with the severity of other neurologic symptoms of the lower spinal cord.[81,84]

PROGRESSIVE MULTIFOCAL LEUKOENCEPHALOPATHY

Progressive multifocal leukoencephalopathy (PML) is an infectious demyelinating brain disease caused by JC virus (JCV), which is associated with significant morbidity and mortality in the immunosuppressed (IS) host. Considered a rare opportunistic infection of the CNS, PML has recently been associated with select IS patients with MS, particularly those treated with natalizumab.[85]

Approximately 400 CSF samples from IS individuals with neurologic symptoms investigated by polymerase chain reaction (PCR) for the presence of polyomaviruses demonstrated two widespread human polyomaviruses, BK virus (BKV) and JCV.[86] Both were found to establish latency in the urinary tract and can be reactivated in AIDS. Although reports of BKV in CNS are rare, there is now evidence for its occurrence in IS patients; the diagnosis should be considered in patients with neurologic symptoms and signs of renal disease.[86]

Prophylactic and therapeutic interventions for these viruses are limited by our current understanding of pathogenesis. Clinical trials are limited by the few numbers of patients with clinically significant disease, no defined risk factors and disease definitions, no existing proven effective treatment, and overall significant morbidity and mortality.[87]

LYME DISEASE

Lyme disease (LD) is a multisystemic, tick-borne illness caused by Borrelia burgdorferi, a spirochete. Infected deer ticks transmit the spirochete to humans and animals via bites. Untreated, the bacterium travels through the bloodstream, enters various body tissues, and causes a number of symptoms. Lyme borreliosis is a multiorgan infection caused by spirochete infection.

The erythema migrans (EM) rash, occuring in 90% of reported cases, is a specific feature of LD, and treatment should begin immediately. In the absence of an EM rash, diagnosis of early LD should be made solely on symptoms and evidence of a tick bite, and not blood tests, which can often give false results if performed in the first month after initial innoculation.[88]

A major clinical and epidemiologic study reporting Lyme borreliosis cases delineated the common clinical manifestations: EM, diagnosed in 70% of the patients, followed by voiding disorders (20%), lyme arthritis (8%), and cardiac (1.1%) and ocular manifestations (0.9%).[89]

LOWER URINARY TRACT DYSFUNCTION IN LYME DISEASE

Micturition disorders in LD can occur by two mechanisms. First, cystitis occurs because the spirochete directly invades the urinary bladder. The second mechanism is related to neuroborreliosis, such as meningoencephalopathy, TM, myeloradiculitis, and demyelinating lesions of the spinal cord.

Micturition disorders can appear in diverse forms such as DO, DSD, and detrusor acontractility. Lower urinary tract dysfunction can appear as an initial or a later-stage symptom, though this generally develops after other neurologic symptoms have appeared.[90,91]

TREATMENT

Conservative bladder management including CIC guided by urodynamic evaluation is recommended. Chancellor et al. published the first report of urinary retention as the initial presentation of LD.[92] Paralysis and urinary retention resolved with antibiotic treatment. Olivares et al. reported a case of ATM related to Lyme neuroborreliosis, isolated acute urinary retention, and no lower extremity impairment.[93] This case, confirmed by urodynamic and electrophysiologic investigations, partially resolved after 6 weeks of antibiosis, affording the removal of the indwelling catheter. Alpha-blocker therapy was needed for 3 months until complete normalization of urodynamic and electrophysiologic findings. This case study indicates that whenever urinary retention is encountered associated with ATM or alone, the patient should be investigated for LD.[93]

Relapses of active LD and residual neurologic deficits are common. Urologists practicing in areas endemic for LD need to be aware of B burgdorferi infection in the differential diagnosis of neurogenic bladder dysfunction.

REFERENCES

1. Compston A and Coles A. Multiple sclerosis. *Lancet (London, England)*. 2002;359(9313):1221–31. doi:10.1016/S0140-6736(02)08220-X
2. Sakakibara R. Neurogenic lower urinary tract dysfunction in multiple sclerosis, neuromyelitis optica, and related disorders. *Clin Auton Res*. 2019;29(3):313–20. doi:10.1007/s10286-018-0551-x
3. Dobson R and Giovannoni G. Multiple sclerosis—A review. *Eur J Neurol*. 2019;26(1):27–40. doi:10.1111/ene.13819
4. Keegan BM and Noseworthy JH. Multiple sclerosis. *Annu Rev Med*. 2002;53(1):285–302. doi:10.1146/annurev.med.53.082901.103909
5. McDonald WI, Compston A, Edan G et al. Recommended diagnostic criteria for multiple sclerosis: Guidelines from the International Panel on the diagnosis of multiple sclerosis. *Ann Neurol*. 2001;50(1):121–7.
6. Tubaro A, Puccini F, De Nunzio C et al. The treatment of lower urinary tract symptoms in patients with multiple sclerosis: A systematic review. *Curr Urol Rep*. 2012;13(5):335–42. doi:10.1007/s11934-012-0266-9
7. Schneider MP, Tornic J, Sýkora R et al. Alpha-blockers for treating neurogenic lower urinary tract dysfunction in patients with multiple sclerosis: A systematic review and meta-analysis.

A report from the Neuro-Urology Promotion Committee of the International Continence Society (ICS). *Neurourol Urodyn.* 2019;38(6):1482–91. doi:10.1002/nau.24039

8. Fernández O. Mechanisms and current treatments of urogenital dysfunction in multiple sclerosis. *J Neurol.* 2002;249(1):1–8.

9. Litwiller SE, Frohman EM, and Zimmern PE. Multiple sclerosis and the urologist. *J Urol.* 1999;161(3):743–57.

10. Phé V, Schneider MP, Peyronnet B et al. Desmopressin for treating nocturia in patients with multiple sclerosis: A systematic review: A report from the Neuro-Urology Promotion Committee of the International Continence Society (ICS). *Neurourol Urodyn.* 2019;38(2):563–71. doi:10.1002/nau.23921

11. Nortvedt MW, Riise T, Frugård J et al. Prevalence of bladder, bowel and sexual problems among multiple sclerosis patients two to five years after diagnosis. *Mult Scler.* 2007;13(1):106–12. doi:10.1177/1352458506071210

12. Panicker JN, Fowler CJ, and Kessler TM. Lower urinary tract dysfunction in the neurological patient: Clinical assessment and management. *Lancet Neurol.* 2015;14(7):720–32. doi:10.1016/S1474-4422(15)00070-8

13. Wiedemann A, Kaeder M, Greulich W et al. Which clinical risk factors determine a pathological urodynamic evaluation in patients with multiple sclerosis? An analysis of 100 prospective cases. *World J Urol.* 2013;31(1):229–33. doi:10.1007/s00345-011-0820-y

14. Koldewijn EL, Hommes OR, Lemmens WA, Debruyne FM, and van Kerrebroeck PE. Relationship between lower urinary tract abnormalities and disease-related parameters in multiple sclerosis. *J Urol.* 1995;154(1):169–73.

15. Sirls LT, Zimmern PE, and Leach GE. Role of limited evaluation and aggressive medical management in multiple sclerosis: A review of 113 patients. *J Urol.* 1994;151(4):946–50. doi:10.1016/S0022-5347(17)35131-5

16. Blaivas JG and Barbalias GA. Detrusor-external sphincter dyssynergia in men with multiple sclerosis: An Omjnous urologic condition. *J Urol.* 1984;131(1):91–4. doi:10.1016/S0022-5347(17)50216-5

17. Bemelmans BLH, Hommes OR, Van Kerrebroeck PEV, Lemmens WAJG, Doesburg WH, and Debruyne FMJ. Evidence for early lower urinary tract dysfunction in clinically silent multiple sclerosis. *J Urol.* 1991;145(6):1219–24. doi:10.1016/S0022-5347(17)38581-6

18. Philp T, Read DJ, and Higson RH. The urodynamic characteristics of multiple sclerosis. *Br J Urol.* 1981;53(6):672–5.

19. Mayo ME and Chetner MP. Lower urinary tract dysfunction in multiple sclerosis. *Urology.* 1992;39(1):67–70.

20. De Ridder D, Van Der Aa F, Debruyne J et al. Consensus guidelines on the neurologist's role in the management of neurogenic lower urinary tract dysfunction in multiple sclerosis. *Clin Neurol Neurosurg.* 2013;115(10):2033–40. doi:10.1016/j.clineuro.2013.06.018

21. Brucker BM, Nitti VW, Kalra S et al. Barriers experienced by patients with multiple sclerosis in seeking care for lower urinary tract symptoms. *Neurourol Urodyn.* 2017;36(4):1208–13. doi:10.1002/nau.23101

22. Musco S, Padilla-Fernández B, Del Popolo G et al. Value of urodynamic findings in predicting upper urinary tract damage in neuro-urological patients: A systematic review. *Neurourol Urodyn.* 2018;37(5):1522–40. doi:10.1002/nau.23501

23. Nseyo U and Santiago-Lastra Y. Long-term complications of the neurogenic bladder. *Urol Clin North Am.* 2017;44(3):355–66. doi:10.1016/j.ucl.2017.04.003

24. Ineichen B V, Schneider MP, Hlavica M, Hagenbuch N, Linnebank M, and Kessler TM. High EDSS can predict risk for upper urinary tract damage in patients with multiple sclerosis. *Mult Scler.* 2018;24(4):529–34. doi:10.1177/1352458517703801

25. Dray E, Cameron AP, Clemens JQ, Qin Y, Covalschi D, and Stoffel J. Does post-void residual volume predict worsening urological symptoms in patients with multiple sclerosis? *J Urol.* 2018;200(4):868–74. doi:10.1016/j.juro.2018.04.068

26. Shakir NA, Satyanarayan A, Eastman J, Greenberg BM, and Lemack GE. Assessment of renal deterioration and associated risk factors in patients with multiple sclerosis. *Urology.* 2019;123:76–80. doi:10.1016/j.urology.2018.09.014

27. Tornic J and Panicker JN. The management of lower urinary tract dysfunction in multiple sclerosis. *Curr Neurol Neurosci Rep.* 2017;18(8). doi:10.1007/s11910-018-0857-z

28. Averbeck MA and Madersbacher H. Follow-up of the neuro-urological patient: A systematic review. *BJU Int.* 2015;115(Suppl 6):39–46. doi:10.1111/bju.13084

29. Lemack GE, Hawker K, and Frohman E. Incidence of upper tract abnormalities in patients with neurovesical dysfunction secondary to multiple sclerosis: Analysis of risk factors at initial urologic evaluation. *Urology.* 2005;65(5):854–7. doi:10.1016/j.urology.2004.11.038

30. Fletcher SG, Dillon BE, Gilchrist AS et al. Renal deterioration in multiple sclerosis patients with neurovesical dysfunction. *Mult Scler J.* 2013;19(9):1169–74. doi:10.1177/1352458512474089

31. Ukkonen M, Elovaara I, Dastidar P, and Tammela TLJ. Urodynamic findings in primary progressive multiple sclerosis are associated with increased volumes of plaques and atrophy in the central nervous system. *Acta Neurol Scand.* 2004;109(2):100–5.

32. Phé V, Chartier-Kastler E, and Panicker JN. Management of neurogenic bladder in patients with multiple sclerosis. *Nat Rev Urol.* 2016;13(5):275–88. doi:10.1038/nrurol.2016.53

33. Oppenheimer DR. The cervical cord in multiple sclerosis. *Neuropathol Appl Neurobiol.* 4(2):151–62.

34. Tracey JM and Stoffel JT. Secondary and tertiary treatments for multiple sclerosis patients with urinary symptoms. *Investig Clin Urol.* 2016;57(6):377–83. doi:10.4111/icu.2016.57.6.377

35. Stoffel JT. Chronic urinary retention in multiple sclerosis patients: Physiology, systematic review of urodynamic data, and recommendations for care. *Urol Clin North Am.* 2017;44(3):429–39. doi:10.1016/j.ucl.2017.04.009

36. Jaggi A, Drake M, Siddiqui E, and Fatoye F. A comparison of the treatment recommendations for neurogenic lower urinary tract dysfunction in the National Institute for Health and Care Excellence, European Association of Urology and international consultations on incontinence guidelines. *Neurourol Urodyn.* 2018;37(7):2273–80. doi:10.1002/nau.23581

37. Tsang B, Stothers L, Macnab A, Lazare D, and Nigro M. A systematic review and comparison of questionnaires in the management of spinal cord injury, multiple sclerosis and the neurogenic bladder. *Neurourol Urodyn.* 2016;35(3):354–64. doi:10.1002/nau.22720

38. Drake MJ, Apostolidis A, Cocci A et al. Neurogenic lower urinary tract dysfunction: Clinical management recommendations of the Neurologic Incontinence committee of the fifth International Consultation on Incontinence 2013. *Neurourol Urodyn.* 2016;35(6):657–65. doi:10.1002/nau.23027

39. Ciancio SJ, Mutchnik SE, Rivera VM, and Boone TB. Urodynamic pattern changes in multiple sclerosis. *Urology.* 2001;57(2):239–45.

40. De Ridder D, Vermeulen C, Ketelaer P, Van Poppel H, and Baert L. Pelvic floor rehabilitation in multiple sclerosis. *Acta Neurol Belg.* 1999;99(1):61–4.

41. De Ridder D, Ost D, Van der Aa F et al. Conservative bladder management in advanced multiple sclerosis. *Mult Scler.* 2005;11(6):694–9. doi:10.1191/1352458505ms1237oa

42. Rashid TM and Hollander JB. Multiple sclerosis and the neurogenic bladder. *Phys Med Rehabil Clin N Am.* 1998;9(3):615–29.

43. Lapides J, Diokno AC, Silber SJ, and Lowe BS. Clean, intermittent self-catheterization in the treatment of urinary tract disease. *J Urol.* 2017;197(2):S122–4. doi:10.1016/j.juro.2016.10.097

44. Barbosa CD, Balp M-M, Kulich K, Germain N, and Rofail D. A literature review to explore the link between treatment satisfaction and adherence, compliance, and persistence. *Patient Prefer Adherence.* 2012;6:39–48. doi:10.2147/PPA.S24752

45. Kessler TM, Ryu G, and Burkhard FC. Clean intermittent self-catheterization: A burden for the patient? *Neurourol Urodyn.* 2009;28(1):18–21. doi:10.1002/nau.20610

46. Castel-Lacanal E, Gamé X, De Boissezon X et al. Impact of intermittent catheterization on the quality of life of multiple sclerosis patients. *World J Urol.* 2013;31(6):1445–50. doi:10.1007/s00345-012-1017-8

47. Chancellor MB and Blaivas JG. Urological and sexual problems in multiple sclerosis. *Clin Neurosci.* 1994;2(3–4):189–95.

48. Phelan MW, Franks M, Somogyi GT et al. Botulinum toxin urethral sphincter injection to restore bladder emptying in men and women with voiding dysfunction. *J Urol.* 2001;165(4):1107–10.

49. Schurch B, Stöhrer M, Kramer G, Schmid DM, Gaul G, and Hauri D. Botulinum-A toxin for treating detrusor hyperreflexia in spinal cord injured patients: A new alternative to anticholinergic drugs? Preliminary results. *J Urol.* 2000;164(3 Pt 1):692–7.

50. Schurch B, Deseze M, Denys P et al. Botulinum toxin type A is a safe and effective treatment for neurogenic urinary incontinence: Results of a single treatment, randomized, placebo controlled 6-month study. *J Urol.* 2005;174(1):196–200. doi:10.1097/01.ju.0000162035.73977.1c

51. Schulte-Baukloh H, Schobert J, Stolze T, Stürzebecher B, Weiss C, and Knispel HH. Efficacy of botulinum-A toxin bladder injections for the treatment of neurogenic detrusor overactivity in multiple sclerosis patients: An objective and subjective analysis. *Neurourol Urodyn.* 2006;25(2):110–5. doi:10.1002/nau.20153

52. Carneiro Neto JA, Santos SB, Orge GO et al. Onabotulinumtoxin type A improves lower urinary tract symptoms and quality of life in patients with human T cell lymphotropic virus type 1 associated overactive bladder. *Braz J Infect Dis.* 22(2):79–84. doi:10.1016/j.bjid.2017.10.009

53. Le N-B, and Kim J-H. Expanding the role of neuromodulation for overactive bladder: New indications and alternatives to delivery. *Curr Bladder Dysfunct Rep.* 2011;6(1):25–30. doi:10.1007/s11884-010-0074-3

54. Zecca C, Panicari L, Disanto G et al. Posterior tibial nerve stimulation in the management of lower urinary tract symptoms in patients with multiple sclerosis. *Int Urogynecol J.* 2016;27(4):521–7. doi:10.1007/s00192-015-2814-6

55. Gross T, Schneider MP, Bachmann LM et al. Transcutaneous electrical nerve stimulation for treating neurogenic lower urinary tract dysfunction: A systematic review. *Eur Urol.* 2016;69(6):1102–11. doi:10.1016/j.eururo.2016.01.010

56. Chartier-Kastler EJ, Ruud Bosch JL, Perrigot M, Chancellor MB, Richard F, and Denys P. Long-term results of sacral nerve stimulation (S3) for the treatment of neurogenic refractory urge incontinence related to detrusor hyperreflexia. *J Urol.* 2000;164(5):1476–80.

57. Puccini F, Bhide A, Elneil S, and Digesu GA. Sacral neuromodulation: An effective treatment for lower urinary tract symptoms in multiple sclerosis. *Int Urogynecol J.* 2016;27(3):347–54. doi:10.1007/s00192-015-2771-0

58. Engeler DS, Meyer D, Abt D, Müller S, and Schmid H-P. Sacral neuromodulation for the treatment of neurogenic lower urinary tract dysfunction caused by multiple sclerosis: A single-centre prospective series. *BMC Urol.* 2015;15:105. doi:10.1186/s12894-015-0102-x

59. Andretta E, Simeone C, Ostardo E, Pastorello M, and Zuliani C. Usefulness of sacral nerve modulation in a series of multiple sclerosis patients with bladder dysfunction. *J Neurol Sci.* 2014;347(1-2):257–61. doi:10.1016/j.jns.2014.10.010

60. Guzman-Negron JM, Pizarro-Berdichevsky J, Gill BC, and Goldman HB. Can lumbosacral magnetic resonance imaging be performed safely in patients with a sacral neuromodulation device? An in vivo prospective study. *J Urol.* 2018;200(5):1088–92. doi:10.1016/j.juro.2018.05.095

61. Hoen L, Ecclestone H, Blok BFM et al. Long-term effectiveness and complication rates of bladder augmentation in patients with neurogenic bladder dysfunction: A systematic review. *Neurourol Urodyn.* 2017;36(7):1685–702. doi:10.1002/nau.23205

62. Kalkan S, Jaffe WI, Simma-Chiang V, Li ESW, and Blaivas JG. Long term results of augmentation cystoplasty and urinary diversion in multiple sclerosis. *Can J Urol.* 2019;26(3):9774–80.

63. Luangkhot R, Peng BCH, and Blaivas JG. Ileocecocystoplasty for the management of refractory neurogenic bladder: Surgical technique and urodynamic findings. *J Urol.* 1991;146(5):1340–4. doi:10.1016/S0022-5347(17)38086-2

64. Transverse Myelitis Consortium Working Group. Proposed diagnostic criteria and nosology of acute transverse myelitis. *Neurology.* 2002;59(4):499–505. doi:10.1212/wnl.59.4.499

65. Flanagan EP. Autoimmune myelopathies. In: *Handbook of Clinical Neurology.* Eds. Pittock SJ and Vincent A. Vol 133. Elsevier B.V.; 2016:327–51. doi:10.1016/B978-0-444-63432-0.00019-0

66. Wingerchuk DM. Immune-mediated myelopathies. *Contin Lifelong Learn Neurol.* 2018;24(2, Spinal Cord Disorders):497–522. doi:10.1212/CON.0000000000000582

67. Hiraga A, Sakakibara R, Mori M, Yamanaka Y, Ito S, and Hattori T. Urinary retention can be the sole initial manifestation of acute myelitis. *J Neurol Sci.* 2006;251(1–2):110–2. doi:10.1016/j.jns.2006.09.010

68. Kalita J. Bladder dysfunction in acute transverse myelitis: Magnetic resonance imaging and neurophysiological and urodynamic correlations. *J Neurol Neurosurg Psychiatry.* 2002;73(2):154–9. doi:10.1136/jnnp.73.2.154

69. Gupta A, Kumar SN, and Taly AB. Urodynamic profile in acute transverse myelitis patients: Its correlation with neurological outcome. *J Neurosci Rural Pract.* 8(1):44–8. doi:10.4103/0976-3147.193547

70. Gliga LA, Lavelle RS, Christie AL et al. Urodynamics findings in transverse myelitis patients with lower urinary tract symptoms: Results from a tertiary referral urodynamic center. *Neurourol Urodyn.* 2017;36(2):360–3. doi:10.1002/nau.22930

71. Leroy-Malherbe V, Sébire G, Hollenberg H, Tardieu M, and Landrieu P. [Neurogenic bladder in children with acute transverse myelopathy]. *Arch Pediatr.* 1998;5(5):497–502. doi:10.1016/S0929-693X(99)80313-3

72. Berger Y, Blaivas JG, and Oliver L. Urinary dysfunction in transverse myelitis. *J Urol.* 1990;144(1):103–5. doi:10.1016/S0022-5347(17)39381-3

73. Bourre B. Prognostic factors of acute partial transverse myelitis-reply. *Arch Neurol.* 2012;69(11):1523–4. doi:10.1001/archneurol.2012.2593

74. Bangham CRM, Araujo A, Yamano Y, and Taylor GP. HTLV-1-associated myelopathy/tropical spastic paraparesis. *Nat Rev Dis Prim.* 2015;1(1):15012. doi:10.1038/nrdp.2015.12

75. Nozuma S and Jacobson S. Neuroimmunology of human T-lymphotropic virus type 1-associated myelopathy/tropical spastic paraparesis. *Front Microbiol.* 2019;10:885. doi:10.3389/fmicb.2019.00885

76. Tamiya S, Matsuoka M, Takemoto S et al. Adult T cell leukemia following HTLV-I-associated myelopathy/tropical spastic paraparesis: Case reports and implication to the natural course of ATL. *Leukemia.* 1995;9(10):1768–70.

77. Cruickshank JK, Rudge P, Dalgleish AG et al. Tropical spastic paraparesis and human T cell lymphotropic virus type 1 in the United Kingdom. *Brain.* 1989;112(4, Pt 4):1057–90. doi:10.1093/brain/112.4.1057

78. Iwasaki Y. Pathology of chronic myelopathy associated with HTLV-I infection (HAM/TSP). *J Neurol Sci.* 1990;96(1):103–23.

79. Coler-Reilly ALG, Yagishita N, Suzuki H et al. Nation-wide epidemiological study of Japanese patients with rare viral myelopathy using novel registration system (HAM-net). *Orphanet J Rare Dis.* 2016;11(1):69. doi:10.1186/s13023-016-0451-x

80. de Castro NM, Freitas DM, Rodrigues W, Muniz A, Oliveira P, and Carvalho EM. Urodynamic features of the voiding dysfunction in HTLV-1 infected individuals. *Int Braz J Urol.* 2007;33(2):238–44. doi:10.1590/s1677-55382007000200016

81. Troisgros O, Barnay J-L, Darbon-Naghibzadeh F, Olive P, and René-Corail P. Retrospective clinic and urodynamic study in the neurogenic bladder dysfunction caused by human T cell lymphotrophic virus type 1 associated myelopathy/tropical spastic paraparesis (HAM/TSP). *Neurourol Urodyn.* 2017;36(2):449–52. doi:10.1002/nau.22952

82. Sakiyama H, Nishi K, Kikukawa H, and Ueda S. [Urinary disturbance due to HTLV-1 associated myelopathy]. *Nihon Hinyokika Gakkai Zasshi.* 1992;83(12):2058–61.

83. Imamura A. [Studies on neurogenic bladder due to human T-lymphotropic virus type-I associated myelopathy (HAM)]. *Nihon Hinyokika Gakkai Zasshi.* 1994;85(7):1106–15.

84. Nomata K, Nakamura T, Suzu H et al. Novel complications with HTLV-1-associated myelopathy/tropical spastic paraparesis: Interstitial cystitis and persistent prostatitis. *Jpn J Cancer Res.* 1992;83(6):601–8. doi:10.1111/j.1349-7006.1992.tb00132.x

85. Baldwin KJ and Hogg JP. Progressive multifocal leukoencephalopathy in patients with multiple sclerosis. *Curr Opin Neurol.* 2013;26(3):318–23. doi:10.1097/WCO.0b013e328360279f

86. Bratt G, Hammarin AL, Grandien M et al. BK virus as the cause of meningoencephalitis, retinitis and nephritis in a patient with AIDS. *AIDS.* 1999;13(9):1071–5.

87. Roskopf J, Trofe J, Stratta RJ, and Ahsan N. Pharmacotherapeutic options for the management of human polyomaviruses. *Adv Exp Med Biol.* 2006;577:228–54. doi:10.1007/0-387-32957-9_17

88. Lipsker D, Hansmann Y, Limbach F et al. Disease expression of Lyme borreliosis in northeastern France. *Eur J Clin Microbiol Infect Dis.* 2001; 20(4):225–30.

89. Christova I and Komitova R. Clinical and epidemiological features of Lyme borreliosis in Bulgaria. *Wien Klin Wochenschr.* 2004;116(1–2):42–6.

90. Puri BK, Shah M, Julu PO, Kingston MC, and Monro JA. Urinary bladder detrusor dysfunction symptoms in lyme disease. *Int Neurourol J.* 2013;17(3):127–9. doi:10.5213/inj.2013.17.3.127

91. Kim M, Kim WC, and Park D-S. Neurogenic bladder in Lyme disease. *Int Neurourol J.* 2012;16(4):201. doi:10.5213/inj.2012.16.4.201

92. Chancellor MB, Dato VM, and Yang JY. Lyme disease presenting as urinary retention. *J Urol.* 1990;143(6):1223–4. doi:10.1016/S0022-5347(17)40231-X

93. Olivares JP, Pallas F, Ceccaldi M et al.. Lyme disease presenting as isolated acute urinary retention caused by transverse myelitis: An electrophysiological and urodynamical study. *Arch Phys Med Rehabil.* 1995;76(12):1171–2.

VASCULAR PATHOLOGIES AND TUMORS OF THE BRAIN PRESENTS

Chapter 13

CEREBROVASCULAR ACCIDENTS, INTRACRANIAL TUMORS, AND VOIDING DYSFUNCTION

Ahmed Ibrahim and Roger R. Dmochowski

INTRODUCTION

Intact cerebral cortical and pontine function is required for normal voiding and urinary continence. Cerebrovascular accidents (CVAs) and intracranial tumors are common pathologic processes that alter higher cortical function and normal urologic function. Therefore, these disease entities and their subsequent urologic consequences are clinically important to urologists. Voiding dysfunction is the most common urologic consequence of CVAs and intracranial tumors; however, patients may also have sexual problems related to these two disease processes. Voiding dysfunction is usually characterized by urinary incontinence, frequency, and urgency.[1] Incontinence is the most common and disruptive chronic concern; however, in the acute phase of disease, patients may present with urinary retention.

EPIDEMIOLOGY

Approximately 1 million CVAs occur in the United States each year and 15 million worldwide.[2,3] Fifty-seven percent are initial episodes, and the remainder are recurrent strokes.[4] Additionally, following heart disease, cancer, and pulmonary disease, CVAs are the fourth leading cause of death in the United States.[5] A rising incidence of strokes and a declining mortality rate greatly increase the number of individuals needing poststroke care.[6] Intracranial tumors are far less common than CVAs with a worldwide incidence rate of 26.8 per 100,000 adults (17.9 benign, 8.9 malignant) (Table 13.1).[7,8]

Ueki found a 12.6% incidence of incomplete emptying, 5.4% of urinary incontinence, and 2% of urinary retention in patients with brain tumors.[9] Epidemiology, type, and frequency of urologic symptoms for CVA and brain tumors are summarized in Table 13.1.[10–12]

PATHOPHYSIOLOGY

CEREBROVASCULAR ACCIDENTS (STROKES)

There are two broad categories of CVAs: (1) occlusive lesions and (2) hemorrhagic lesions from trauma or vascular malformation.

The pathophysiology of micturition disturbance after CVA involves two separate mechanisms. First, there is often decreased sensation and awareness of bladder filling (postponed desire to urinate). Second, there is damage to higher cortical centers, especially in the frontal lobe, that leads to an inability to suppress a bladder contraction. Therefore, incomplete emptying, bladder overflow, or detrusor overactivity may produce voiding dysfunction after cortical events.[12]

The pathophysiology of CVAs may also be related to *underperfusion* of brain areas involved in micturition. Single-photon emission computed tomography (SPECT) studies in elderly incontinent patients revealed that, compared to normal subjects, there was significantly decreased perfusion to the right superior and left cortical areas of their frontal lobes and reduced awareness of bladder sensations.[13]

BRAIN TUMORS

Brain tumors produce clinical symptoms by three mechanisms: (1) infiltration along nerve fiber tracts, (2) displacement of brain tissue with resulting increased intracranial pressure from vasogenic edema, and (3) destruction of brain tissue by a rapidly growing tumor.[14,15]

The frontal cortex is where *cognitive control* of voiding is located, whereas the pontine micturition center is where regulation and coordination of voiding occur.[16] During normal storage, there is a net inhibitory effect by the central nervous system (CNS) on the detrusor muscle, and the external sphincter is closed. When the need to void is sensed, the CNS "allows" the urethral sphincter to relax and the detrusor to contract reflexively, and voiding is initiated.[17]

Table 13.1 Epidemiology, Type, and Frequency of Urologic Symptoms for Cerebrovascular Accidents and Brain Tumors

	Incidence Rate	Type and Frequency of Urologic Symptoms	Urodynamic Finding
Cerebrovascular accident (strokes)	450 cases/100,000/ year (Europe), 10% of cardiovascular mortality	• Nocturia-overactive bladder-urgency incontinence • 57%–83% of neuro-urological symptoms at 1-month poststroke • 71%–80% spontaneous recovery at 6 months • Persistence of urinary incontinence correlates with poor prognosis	• Detrusor overactivity (DO)± • Impaired voluntary control • Normal compliance • Synergic sphincter • Possible decreased sensation of LUT
Brain tumors	26.8/100,000/year (17.9 benign, 8.9 malignant)	Incontinence occurs mainly in frontal location (part of frontal syndrome or isolated in frontal location)	• DO • Normal compliance • Synergic sphincter • Possible decreased sensation of LUT

A CVA or brain tumor causes disruption of this normal control results in losing the main inhibitory input from the CNS and subsequently detrusor overactivity, and urge incontinence.[18] It was reported that stimulation of the dorsal pontine tegmentum in animal study causes relaxation of the urinary sphincter and leads to a coordinated detrusor contraction, thus initiating voiding.[19] Additionally, ablation of this area disables sphincter relaxation and detrusor contraction and causes *urinary retention*.[20] This explains why retention is commonly found in patients with tumors or CVAs that affect the pons.[21]

UROLOGIC PRESENTATION

Acute Stage Cerebrovascular Accident

Urinary retention may be the first urologic event to occur after a CVA. The exact mechanism is unclear, but this phenomenon has been termed *cerebral shock*. The retention may not be a direct result of the neurologic lesion itself but rather may be a result of impaired consciousness, immobility, and an inability to communicate, with resultant overdistention of the bladder and failure to void.[22] This lack of appreciation of bladder events appears to be more commonly associated with cortical insults in the *frontal lobe*. Interestingly, Burney et al. showed an 85% incidence of *urinary retention and areflexia* in patients with hemorrhagic CVAs of the frontal lobe.[12] Premorbid detrusor dysfunction or concomitant medications may also contribute to retention in the acute setting.[23] In addition, retention cohort was associated with a higher rate of diabetes, cognitive impairment, aphasia, and decreased functional status in another study.[24]

Although urinary retention is common in the acute phase, Patel et al. also found a high (39%) rate of

incontinence in 511 subjects 7 days after a CVA.[25] This early incontinence was found to be a *negative prognostic factor* for the patients, portending a much higher mortality rate. Additionally, they found *detrusor overactivity and incomplete emptying* in the acute period after cortical events. These findings were partially dependent on the premorbid urinary function of the patient, overall size of the stroke, and affected area of the brain.[25]

CHRONIC STAGE CEREBROVASCULAR ACCIDENT

The vast majority of patients (96%) with acute urinary retention from a CVA usually have resolution within 6 months; however, not all patients return to normal voiding. There appears to be an evolution from retention to a more fixed dysfunction, usually manifested by *urinary urgency, frequency,* and *urinary incontinence*. In fact, incontinence is one of the most prevalent and bothersome urologic symptoms of a CVA. It was found that approximately 29%–79% of stroke survivors experience *urinary incontinence*.[26–28] Additionally, studies show that incontinence is an important prognostic indicator for both mortality and quality of life in stroke patients, whereas patients who are able to regain continence typically have a better functional status and a lower institutionalization rate than those who remain incontinent.[10] The presence of incontinence after a CVA can also predict impaired functional recovery in these patients.[30,31]

QUALITY OF LIFE AND SEXUAL FUNCTION

Urinary symptoms also play a major role in the *quality of life* and overall well-being of patients after stroke. In a population-based study by Brittain et al., 10,000 community members underwent evaluation for the incidence of stroke and urinary symptoms.[32] Overall, they found a significant relationship between severity of urinary symptoms and both decreased quality of life and difficulty with activities of daily living. Also, patients who remained continent or regained continence after their stroke had better quality-of-life outcomes than those who did not. It has also been suggested that recovery of continence expedites recovery and improves morale and self-esteem.[33,34]

It is also clear that CVA has a negative impact on the *sexual function* of patients and their spouses.[35] In a prospective study of 192 patients with stroke and their spouses, Korpelainen et al. found that the most important factors contributing to changes in sexual function after a stroke were a worsened attitude toward sexuality, fear of impotence, and inability to discuss sexuality.[35] In addition, multiple studies have shown that incontinence has a significant negative impact on sexual function in both men and women.[36,37]

BRAIN TUMORS

Unlike a CVA, the early symptoms of a brain tumor are nonspecific, and urinary complaints are not generally thought of as part of the initial presentation.[38] Raised intracranial pressure resulting from space-occupying lesions (primary or metastatic) is the cause of the majority of early symptoms. Although headache and seizure are the most common presenting symptoms

of a brain tumor, disturbance of bladder functions has been associated with both primary and metastatic brain tumors.[38] Lower urinary tract dysfunction is usually related to the localized area involved in the brain. It has been reported that 14% of patients with frontal lobe tumors have *overactive bladder with or without urinary incontinence* (Table 13.1). Additionally, 3.4% of patients may have *urinary retention* in the acute phase in the absence of other associated neurologic deficits.[9] Moreover, patients with pontine lesions are more likely to present with urinary retention.[9,39] This urinary retention is most likely the result of inflammation and edema in the pons and may resolve after treatment with corticosteroids.[40]

LOCATION AND CLINICAL PRESENTATION

Location of a tumor or CVA has a direct effect on the clinical presentation. It appears that patients with frontal cerebral lesions are more likely to have incontinence and other urinary storage symptoms than patients with lesions elsewhere in the cerebrum. Patients with brainstem lesions are more likely to have urinary retention and obstructive symptoms. Sakakibara et al. found a urinary symptom rate of 53% after CVA, and patients with urinary symptoms were significantly more likely to have frontal lobe and fronto-parietal-temporal and fronto-parietal-occipital lesions than temporal, parietal, and occipital lesions (Figure 13.1).

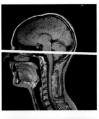

A. Suprapontine lesion

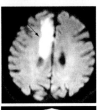

B. Acute ischemic frontal lobe stroke

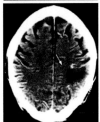

C. Fronto-parietal-temporal lobe ischemic stroke

Figure 13.1   Different locations of cerebrovascular accident lesions and clinical presentation.

The authors also demonstrated frequent uninhibited sphincter relaxation in patients with frontal lobe lesions and *detrusor external sphincter dyssynergia (DESD)* in patients with basal ganglia lesions.[41]

The cerebellum has a role in normal bladder storage and emptying.[18] It was found that patients with cerebellar infarctions had *detrusor areflexia with synergistic sphincter activity*.[42] In another study using functional magnetic resonance imaging (fMRI) to study activation of brain regions, the cerebellum was found to be involved in the inhibition of the micturition reflex as well.[43] So, while the cerebellum's normal function is inhibitory on the detrusor, its role after a CVA is not well understood.

It is unclear whether the sidedness of the brain lesion matters. One study reported that urgency, frequency, and incontinence were more common in right-sided lesions.[44] However, other studies found no difference among patients with respect to continence and the side of the lesion.[12,23]

Besides CVAs, location of a brain tumor and the corresponding symptoms has also been examined in several studies. While Ueki et al.[9] found a higher rate of *incontinence* in patients with cerebral hemisphere tumors compared to patients with posterior fossa tumors (7.2 versus 1.9%), other studies have shown that patients with *pontine tumors* are more likely to have problems with *urinary retention*, ranging from 71% to 77%.[9,39] Additionally, Andrew and Nathan confirmed that patients with frontal lobe tumors are more likely to have voiding difficulties than patients with tumors elsewhere in the cerebrum.[45]

URODYNAMICS

When incontinence occurs after a CVA or brain tumor, the main urodynamic finding is usually *detrusor overactivity*. Cystometrogram tracings representative of detrusor dysfunction found after a CVA can be seen in Figures 13.2 and 13.3. Figure 13.2 shows *multiple phasic* episodes of detrusor overactivity that culminate in a large sustained contraction. Although this finding is related to incontinence in this patient, there is also evidence of suppression of the contractions, which may be a good prognostic indicator for future continence. In Figure 13.3, the detrusor overactivity is more pronounced, and there is a much higher amplitude contraction that is not suppressed. This is the pattern of loss of inhibitory control normally found in patients with frontal cortex lesions. *Detrusor areflexia* can also be seen in patients with cerebellar lesions or in the acute phase related to *cerebral shock*.

Another common urodynamic finding in patients with frontal lobe lesions is *uninhibited sphincter relaxation with detrusor overactivity*.[29,41,42] The external sphincter is under higher cortical control; therefore, when uninhibited relaxation occurs, it is often associated with more profound urine loss and reduced awareness.[42] The other sphincter finding that

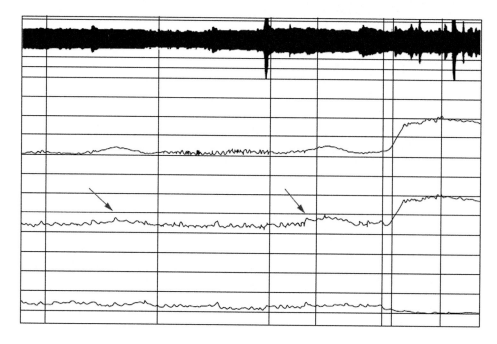

Figure 13.2   Cystometrogram tracing demonstrating phasic detrusor contractions. Note that contractions (marked with arrows) are initially suppressed, a good prognostic indicator.

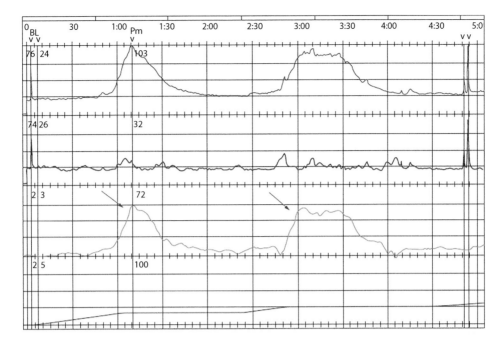

Figure 13.3 Cystometrogram demonstrating large-amplitude detrusor contractions. Note how the contractions (marked with arrows) are not suppressed, indicating loss of frontal lobe input.

is of concern is that of DESD. Fortunately, *DESD is a rare finding* after a CVA and is usually confused with *pseudodyssynergia*.[46] True DESD usually implies a contemporaneous cord lesion occurring with the cortical lesion. In multiple clinical studies, the presence of sphincteric dysfunction ranges from 8.3% to 17%.[41,42] Last, DESD and other forms of sphincteric dysfunction are frequently seen when there is involvement of the basal ganglia.[41]

TREATMENT

There is a relative paucity of information on the treatment of incontinence in patients who have experienced a CVA or tumor. Different scenarios could be encountered throughout the course of CVA. The proposed treatment algorithm for postcerebrovascular accident incontinence is illustrated in Figure 13.4.

In the acute phase, when there may be retention and loss of consciousness, *indwelling or intermittent catheterization* is an acceptable strategy. Indwelling catheterization should be discontinued as early as reasonably possible. Behavioral therapies such as timed voids (especially in aphasic patients) and fluid restriction can be of assistance.[12] *Pelvic floor muscle training* in women has been shown to be effective in reducing incontinence episodes in the poststroke time frame.[47]

Medical management of symptoms can be difficult in this patient population, and surgical management can be fraught with complications. Alpha-blockers have the unfortunate side effects of dizziness and hypotension, which are especially detrimental to functioning and rehabilitation of these patients. Additionally, when there is baseline impairment, anticholinergic medications have negative effects on cognitive functioning.[48]

For patients with persistent urge incontinence, intravesical botulinum type A toxin (*Botox*) injections may be successful. Botox was found to be 50% effective in increasing bladder volume and decreasing incontinence episodes in patients with incontinence after CVA.[49] In addition, it was associated with significant improvement in quality of life in other multicenter study.[50] *Sacral neuromodulation* is another possible form of treatment. It is approved for idiopathic detrusor overactivity; however, it is not approved for patients with neurologic disease and may not be as effective.[51]

Augmentation cystoplasty or urinary diversion should be considered in patients with refractory incontinence with poor urodynamic findings considering the medical fitness and life expectancy of the patient. Suburethral bulking agents may also be a valid option for a patient with primarily stress incontinence. Patients with brain tumors will often show improvement in urinary symptoms after surgical excision or radiotherapy. Ueki found that five out of ten patients treated with radiotherapy for pontine tumors showed remarkable

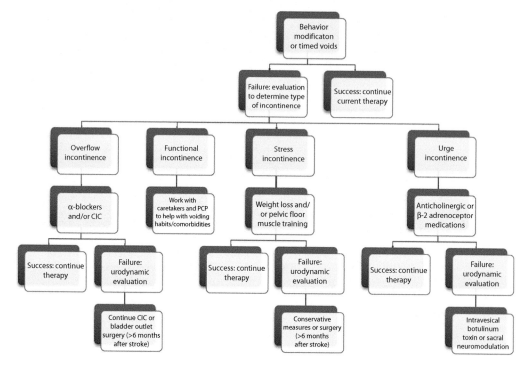

Figure 13.4   Proposed treatment algorithm for postcerebrovascular accident incontinence.

improvement in voiding complaints after therapy.[9] In addition, the majority of patients with urinary symptoms who underwent surgical resection also saw improvement. Overall, patients with brain tumors can be treated in a similar fashion to stroke patients.

FUTURE PERSPECTIVES

The mechanisms of bladder overactivity after CVA remain vague. Experimental models revealed that there are neural signaling changes involving glutaminergic, dopaminergic, γ-aminobutyric acid (GABA), and neuronal nitric oxide synthase gene mechanisms. Such results open the door for theoretical possibilities for central pharmacologic management. However, these findings are still not yet optimized and further basic and clinical research are needed.

CONCLUSIONS

Patients with CVAs and brain tumors often develop a disturbance in their voiding and sexual habits. Incontinence usually occurs in the early periods after an acute event. Subsequently, the typical presentation is an overactive detrusor that results in urgency and urge incontinence. Incontinence after a CVA is a very important prognostic factor for the mortality, severity of stroke, and recovery of the patient. Though management can be challenging in these patients, social continence should be the ultimate goal, as this can affect their overall sense of well-being and quality of life.

REFERENCES

1. Calabro RS and Bramanti P. Post-stroke sexual dysfunction: An overlooked and under-addressed problem. *Disabil Rehabil.* 2014;36(3):263–4.
2. Ovbiagele B, Goldstein LB, Higashida RT et al. Forecasting the future of stroke in the United States: A policy statement from the American Heart Association and American Stroke Association. *Stroke.* 2013;44(8):2361–75.
3. Townsend N, Wilson L, Bhatnagar P et al. Cardiovascular disease in Europe—Epidemiological update 2016. *Eur Heart J.* 2016 7;37(42):3232–45.
4. Rosamond W, Flegal K, Friday G et al. Heart disease and stroke statistics—2007 update: A report from the American Heart Association Statistics Committee and Stroke Statistics Subcommittee. *Circulation.* 2007;115:e69–171.
5. Towfighi A and Saver JL. Stroke declines from third to fourth leading cause of death in the United States: Historical perspective and challenges ahead. *Stroke.* 2011;42:2351–5.
6. May DS and Kittner SJ. Use of Medicare claims data to estimate national trends in stroke incidence, 1985–1991. *Stroke.* 1994;25:2343–7.

7. Dolecek T, Propp J, Stroup N et al. CBTRUS statistical report: Primary brain and central nervous system tumors diagnosed in the United States in 2005–2009. *Neuro Oncol.* 2012;14(Suppl 5):v1.
8. Siegel R, Naishadham D, and Jemal A. Cancer statistics, 2012. *CA Cancer J Clin.* 2012;62:10–29.
9. Ueki K. Disturbances of micturition observed in some patients with brain tumor. *Neurologia Medico-Chirurgica.* 1960;2:25–33.
10. Rotar M, Blagus R, Jeromel M et al. Stroke patients who regain urinary continence in the first week after acute first-ever stroke have better prognosis than patients with persistent lower urinary tract dysfunction. *Neurourol Urodyn.* 2011;30:1315–8.
11. Maurice-Williams RS. Micturition symptoms in frontal tumours. *J Neurol Neurosurg Psychiatry.* 1974;37:431.
12. Burney TL, Senapati M, Desai S et al. Effects of cerebrovascular accident on micturition. *Urol Clin North Am.* 1996;23:483–90.
13. Griffiths D. Clinical studies of cerebral and urinary tract function in elderly people with urinary incontinence. *Behav Brain Res.* 1998;92:151–5.
14. Abeloff DMD, Armitage JO, and Niederhuber JE. *Abeloff's Clinical Oncology.* New York, NY: Churchill Livingstone; 2008.
15. Plum F and Posner JB. *The Diagnosis of Stupor and Coma.* New York, NY: Oxford University Press; 1982.
16. Carlsson CA. The supraspinal control of the urinary bladder. *Acta Pharmacol Toxicol (Copenh)* 1978;43(Suppl 2):8–12.
17. Siracusa G, Sparacino A, and Lentini V. Neurogenic bladder and disc disease: A brief review. *Curr Med Res Opin.* 2013;29(8):1025–31.
18. Bradley WE and Sundin T. The physiology and pharmacology of urinary tract dysfunction. *Clin Neuropharmacol.* 1982;5:131–58.
19. De Groat WC. Nervous control of the urinary bladder of the cat. *Brain Res.* 1975;87:201–11.
20. Sacco RL. Risk factors, outcomes, and stroke subtypes for ischemic stroke. *Neurology.* 1997;49: S39–44.
21. Sakakibara R, Hattori T, Yasuda K et al. Micturitional disturbance and the pontine tegmental lesion: Urodynamic and MRI analyses of vascular cases. *J Neurol Sci.* 1996;141:105–10.
22. Borrie MJ, Campbell AJ, Caradoc-Davies TH et al. Urinary incontinence after stroke: A prospective study. *Age Ageing.* 1986;15:177–81.
23. Gelber DA, Good DC, Laven LJ et al. Causes of urinary incontinence after acute hemispheric stroke. *Stroke.* 1993;24:378–82.
24. Kong KH and Young S. Incidence and outcome of poststroke urinary retention: A prospective study. *Arch Phys Med Rehabil.* 2000;81:1464–7.
25. Patel M, Coshall C, Lawrence E et al. Recovery from poststroke urinary incontinence: Associated factors and impact on outcome. *J Am Geriatr Soc.* 2001;49:1229–33.
26. Tsuchida S, Noto H, Yamaguchi O et al. Urodynamic studies on hemiplegic patients after cerebrovascular accident. *Urology.* 1983;21:315–8.
27. Kalra L, Smith DH, and Crome P. Stroke in patients aged over 75 years: Outcome and predictors. *Postgrad Med J.* 1993;69:33–6.
28. Brocklehurst JC, Andrews K, Richards B et al. Incidence and correlates of incontinence in stroke patients. *J Am Geriatr Soc.* 1985;33:540–2.
29. Amundsen CL, Romero AA, Jamison MG et al. Sacral neuromodulation for intractable urge incontinence: Are there factors associated with cure? *Urology.* 2005;66:746–50.
30. Thommessen B, Bautz-Holter E, and Laake K. Predictors of outcome of rehabilitation of elderly stroke patients in a geriatric ward. *Clin Rehabil.* 1999;13:123–8.
31. Samanci N, Dora B, Kizilay F et al. Factors affecting one year mortality and functional outcome after first ever ischemic stroke in the region of Antalya, Turkey (a hospital-based study). *Acta Neurol Belg.* 2004;104:154–60.
32. Brittain KR, Perry SI, Peet SM et al. Prevalence and impact of urinary symptoms among community-dwelling stroke survivors. *Stroke.* 2000;31:886–91.
33. Barer DH. Continence after stroke: Useful predictor or goal of therapy? *Age Ageing.* 1989;18:183–91.
34. Sims J, Browning C, Lundgren-Lindquist B et al. Urinary incontinence in a community sample of older adults: Prevalence and impact on quality of life. *Disabil Rehabil.* 2011;33:1389–98.
35. Korpelainen JT, Nieminen P, and Myllyla VV. Sexual functioning among stroke patients and their spouses. *Stroke.* 1999;30:715–9.
36. Hayder D. The effects of urinary incontinence on sexuality: Seeking an intimate partnership. *J Wound Ostomy Continence Nurs.* 2012;39:539–44.
37. Coyne KS, Sexton CC, Thompson C et al. The impact of OAB on sexual health in men and women: Results from EpiLUTS. *J Sex Med.* 2011;8:1603–15.
38. Grant R. Overview: Brain tumour diagnosis and management/Royal College of Physicians guidelines. *J Neurol Neurosurg Psychiatr.* 2004;75(Suppl 2):ii18–23.
39. Renier WO and Gabreels FJ. Evaluation of diagnosis and non-surgical therapy in 24 children with a pontine tumour. *Neuropediatrics.* 1980;11:262–73.
40. Yaguchi H, Soma H, Miyazaki Y et al. A case of acute urinary retention caused by periaqueductal grey lesion. *J Neurol Neurosurg Psychiatr.* 2004; 75:1202–3.
41. Sakakibara R, Hattori T, Yasuda K et al. Micturitional disturbance after acute hemispheric stroke: Analysis of the lesion site by CT and MRI. *J Neurol Sci.* 1996;137:47–56.
42. Burney TL, Senapati M, Desai S et al. Acute cerebrovascular accident and lower urinary tract dysfunction: A prospective correlation of the site of brain injury with urodynamic findings. *J Urol.* 1996;156:1748–50.
43. Zhang H, Reitz A, Kollias S et al. An fMRI study of the role of supra-pontine brain structures in the voluntary voiding control induced by pelvic floor contraction. *Neuroimage.* 2005;24:174–80.
44. Kuroiwa Y, Tohgi H, Ono S et al. Frequency and urgency of micturition in hemiplegic patients: Relationship to hemisphere laterality of lesions. *J Neurol.* 1987;234:100–2.
45. Andrew J and Nathan PW. Lesions on the anterior frontal lobes and disturbances of micturition and defaecation. *Brain.* 1964;87:233–62.
46. Wein A and Barrett DM. Etiologic possibilities for increased pelvic floor electromyography activity during cystometry. *J Urol.* 1982;127:949–52.
47. Tibaek S, Gard G, and Jensen R. Pelvic floor muscle training is effective in women with urinary incontinence after stroke: A randomised, controlled and blinded study. *Neurourol Urodyn.* 2005;24:348–57.
48. Bottiggi KA, Salazar JC, Yu L et al. Long-term cognitive impact of anticholinergic medications in older adults. *Am J Geriatr Psychiatry.* 2006;14:980–4.
49. Kuo H-C. Therapeutic effects of suburothelial injection of botulinum a toxin for neurogenic detrusor overactivity due to chronic cerebrovascular accident and spinal cord lesions. *Urology.* 2006;67:232–6.
50. Kennelly M, Dmochowski R, Ethans K et al. Long-term efficacy and safety of onabotulinumtoxinA in patients with urinary incontinence due to neurogenic detrusor overactivity: An interim analysis. *Urology.* 2013;81:491–7.

DISK PROLAPSE AND TUMORS OF THE SPINAL CORD

Chapter 14

TUMORS OF THE SPINE, INTERVERTEBRAL DISK PROLAPSE, THE CAUDA EQUINA SYNDROME

Patrick J. Shenot and M. Louis Moy

INTRODUCTION

Spinal pathology may result in neurogenic bladder dysfunction by impact on nerve function in both the central and peripheral nervous systems. Spinal tumors and intervertebral disk prolapse are relatively uncommon causes of neurogenic bladder dysfunction. Cauda equina syndrome (CES) occurs when the nerve roots of the cauda equina are compromised, resulting in disruption of motor and sensory function to the pelvic floor, bladder, and lower extremities.

TUMORS OF THE SPINE

Primary tumors of the spinal cord, spinal nerve roots, and dura are relatively rare, while the bony spinal column is a common site of metastases in patients with visceral cancers. Delayed diagnosis of primary spinal tumors is common, and neurogenic lower urinary tract dysfunction is dependent upon the neural tracts involved. Spinal tumors are anatomically characterized into extradural, intradural but extramedullary, and intradural intramedullary[1] (Figure 14.1). Extradural spinal tumors are most common and are usually of metastatic origin. Intramedullary and extramedullary components may coexist, with communication through the intervertebral foramina or at the conus-filum terminale transition.[2] Magnetic resonance imaging (MRI) allows for anatomic localization and staging of primary and metastatic neoplasms and understanding of normal tracts involved.[3,4]

INTRADURAL EXTRAMEDULLARY TUMORS

About two-thirds of primary spinal tumors are benign extramedullary lesions (Table 14.1) with schwannomas, meningiomas, and ependymomas comprising 95% of these tumors. Nerve sheath tumors typically present as a single lesion in the vertebral canal. Approximately two-thirds of nerve sheath tumors are schwannomas with most of the remaining tumors neurofibromas. Malignant neural sheath tumors are rare, have a poor prognosis, and are often associated with neurofibromatosis.

Meningiomas are extra-axial lesions originating from arachnoid cap cells embedded in dura near the spinal nerve root sleeve. About 90% of spinal meningiomas are intradural with 80% in the thoracic segment (Figure 14.2).

Ependymomas are primary central nervous system (CNS) tumors arising from ependymal cells. Ependymomas are usually intramedullary and may arise anywhere in the CNS; intradural, extramedullary filum terminale ependymomas represent 40% of spinal ependymomas. Less common intradural, extramedullary tumors include dermoid cysts, lipomas, teratomas, and neuroenteric cysts, typically occurring in the lumbar and thoracolumbar areas.

INTRAMEDULLARY TUMORS

Intramedullary spinal cord tumors are the least common spinal neoplasm but can severely impair neurologic function and result in poor quality of life, or death.[5] Intramedullary astrocytomas tend to be associated with neurofibromatosis type 1. Malignant tumors are more frequent in the pediatric population. In adults, approximately 25% of primary intramedullary spinal tumors are malignant, while less than 5% of intramedullary spinal tumors are metastatic lesions.[6]

EXTRADURAL METASTATIC SPINAL LESIONS

The spinal muscular and bone structures are the third most common place for metastasis, after the lungs and liver. Extradural compression represents 97% of spinal cord metastatic lesions.[7] Metastasis usually arises in the posterior aspect of the vertebral body, with later invasion of the epidural space (Figure 14.3). Pathophysiologically, vascular insult is more important than direct spinal cord compression.[8] Bone metastases are found in approximately 70% of patients with advanced breast or prostate cancer, and approximately 15%–30% of patients with lung, colon, kidney, or bladder cancer develop bone metastasis.[9]

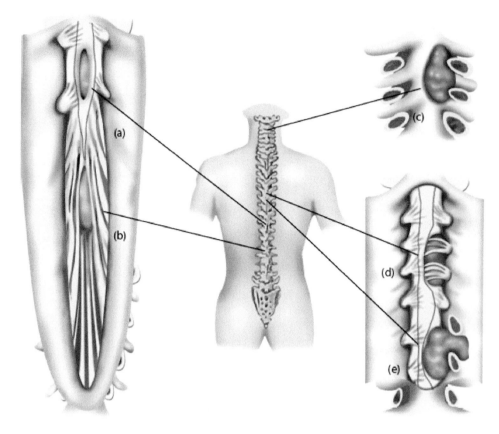

Figure 14.1 Anatomic relationship of spinal tumors with other spine structures: (a) intramedullary tumor, (b) filum terminale ependymoma, (c) extradural neurofibroma, (d) intradural extramedullary meningioma, and (e) schwannoma growing through the vertebral foramina.

Extracranial metatstatic spread of intracranial glioblastoma multiforme to the spine has been reported but appears to be very rare. [10]

CLINICAL FINDINGS

Intradural extramedullary tumors, which are typically benign, often grow slowly, causing pain and neurologic dysfunction at the area of innervation. Bladder and sphincter dysfunction is unusual and may present only as a late symptom. Malignant neoplasms have a shorter evolutionary course. Progressive pain

Table 14.1 Incidence of Tumors in Adults

Extramedullary (Two-Thirds of Cases)	%	Intramedullary (One-Third of Cases)	%
Nerve sheath tumors	40	Ependymoma	45
Meningioma	40	Astrocytoma	40
Filum ependymoma	15	Hemangioblastoma	5
Miscellaneous	5	Miscellaneous	10

Source: Schwartz H, McCormick PC. Spinal cord tumors in adults. In: Winn HR, ed. *Neurological Surgery*, vol 4, 5th ed. Philadelphia, PA: WB Saunders; 2004:4817–34.

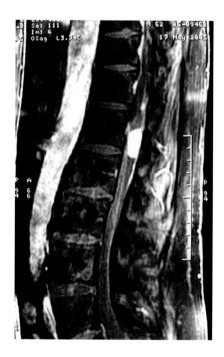

Figure 14.2 Magnetic resonance imaging of an extramedullary intradural thoracic meningioma.

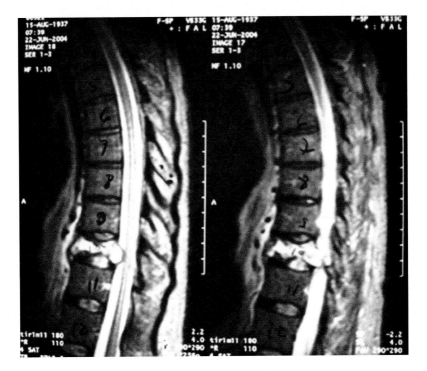

Figure 14.3   Breast neoplasia causing bone metastasis to T10 and invading the medullary space.

is the first complaint in vertebral metastasis in 90% of patients, followed by weakness, paresthesia, and loss of voluntary control of sphincters.[11]

Urologic management must take into account the general condition of the patient, life expectancy, and the origin of the primary tumor.[12] Bladder and sphincter dysfunction is related to the neurologic area involved rather than to the tumor type. Underlying disease and life expectancy should inform the type of bladder management in these patients.[13]

INTERVERTEBRAL DISK PROLAPSE

Symptoms of disk prolapse may vary depending on the location and severity of the herniation. The frequency of lumbar disk prolapse is highest at L4-L5 and L5-S1 levels, representing approximately 90% of symptomatic cases. The association of intervertebral disk prolapse with voiding dysfunction has long been recognized and typically results from the impact of spinal nerve root compression causing axonal dysfunction, ischemia, inflammation, and biochemical sensitization by the protruding disk.[14]

ANATOMY OF THE INTERVERTEBRAL DISK
The intervertebral disk in the adult is a complex avascular structure (Figure 14.4). The nucleus pulposus is restrained by dense collagenous annulus fibrosis. Herniated disks in the lower lumbar spine

most often result from avulsion of the vertebral endplate junction with unilateral posterolateral herniations impinging on the anterolateral aspect of the traversing nerve root being most common.[15,16] Central zone posterior disk herniation may affect nerve roots bilaterally.

Lumbar disk protrusion is highly prevalent in the adult population with 27% of asymptomatic adults having a protrusion (focal extension of the disk beyond the interspace) and 1% an extrusion (more extreme extension of the disk beyond the interspace).[17]

Asymptomatic thoracic and cervical disk herniation is also common and increases with age. Posterior cervical and thoracic disk prolapse may lead to radiculopathy and myelopathy, but mild cord compression does not necessarily result in clinical symptoms or myelopathy.

CLINICAL FINDINGS
Compression of nerve roots will typically result in lower back pain and pain that radiates along the dermatomes of the affected nerve roots. Most patients with symptomatic lumbar disk prolapse are initially managed medically, and only a minority will have clinical signs and symptoms of bladder dysfunction. Patients with urologic symptoms will usually complain of urinary hesitancy and intermittency, straining to urinate, and sometimes a sensation of incomplete bladder emptying. Incontinence is much less common and implies a more severe insult

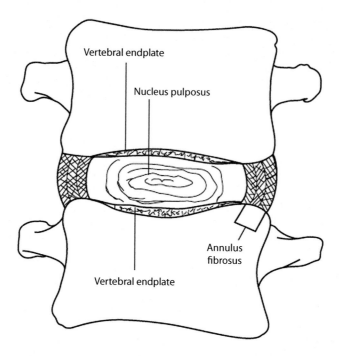

Figure 14.4   Anatomy of the intervertebral disk.

resulting in overflow incontinence, sphincteric dysfunction from pelvic floor denervation, or a combination of both processes.

Changes in perineal and lower extremity motor function, sensation, and reflexes may be appreciated on physical examination (Table 14.2).

The increase in anal sphincter tone with compression of the glans penis or clitoris, known as the bulbocavernous reflex (BCR), may be used to surmise sacral nerve involvement and sphincter function Although this reflex is expected to be absent in all patients with complete lower motor neuron lesions of the sacral cord, nearly 20% of healthy female subjects do not have a detectable BCR on physical examination. There is, however, a significant correlation between a compromised BCR and neuropathic pelvic floor dysfunction.[18,19]

Many neurologic insults from intervertebral disk prolapse are incomplete and slowly progressive, resulting in nerve irritation and detrusor overactivity that progress to detrusor areflexia as the degree of compression increases.[20] Acute compression of nerve roots, as may occur with acute traumatic disk rupture and herniation, may acutely interrupt nerve transmission resulting not only in a neurogenic acontractile detrusor but also in sphincteric dysfunction from the effect on the somatic nerve roots supplying the pudendal nerve.

DIAGNOSTIC STUDIES

Lumbar spine MRI with gadolinium contrast should be obtained in patients with lower urinary tract dysfunction presumed secondary to spinal disease (Figure 14.5). Because of the high rate of disk degeneration noted in asymptomatic individuals, MRI findings are nonspecific and must always be correlated with clinical findings.

Urodynamic testing with simultaneous pelvic floor electromyography will provide the urodynamic

Table 14.2   Clinical Features of Lumbar Nerve Root Compression

Disk	Nerve Root	Pain	Sensory	Motor	Reflex
L3-L4	L4	Anterior thigh	Anterior thigh to medial ankle	Knee extension	Patellar
L4-L5	L5	Posterolateral leg	Dorsum of foot	Dorsiflexion, foot drop	Medial hamstring
L5-S1	S1	Posterior calf and plantar surface of foot	Lateral and plantar foot	Plantar flexion and eversion	Achilles

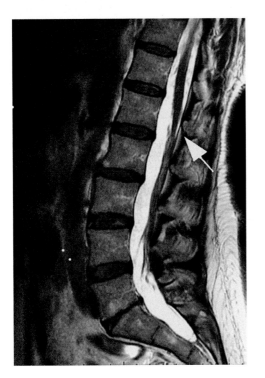

Figure 14.5 Sagittal T2-weighted image of the lumbar spine. The conus medullaris (indicated by the arrow) ends at the L1-L2 interspace. The nerve roots forming the cauda equina are visible traveling from the cauda to the conus.

diagnosis. Pressure flow studies are helpful in cases where obstruction may be present, such as in middle-aged males who may have coexisting bladder outlet obstruction from benign prostatic hyperplasia.

In symptomatic patients, detrusor function correlates with location of disk prolapse. A study of patients with cervical, thoracic, and lumbar disk prolapse not only confirmed the finding of diminished detrusor contractility in lumbar disease but also showed, as expected, detrusor overactivity with or without sphincter dyssynergia in thoracic and cervical lesions.[21]

CAUDA EQUINA SYNDROME

INTRODUCTION
CES is characterized by a constellation of symptoms including low back pain, unilateral or bilateral lower extremity pain and weakness, bowel disturbance, bladder and sexual dysfunction, and saddle or perineal paresthesia. It results from the simultaneous compression of multiple lumbosacral nerve roots below the level of the conus medullaris. Numerous

causes of CES have been reported, including traumatic injury, disk herniation, spinal tumors, spinal stenosis, inflammatory conditions, infectious conditions, and iatrogenic causes by medical intervention.[22,33] Intervertebral disk protrusion causing CES is usually in the L4–L5 or L5–S1 disk space.[22,24,32]

ETIOLOGY OF CAUDA EQUINA SYNDROME
Disk herniations usually occur in a dorsolateral direction, thereby leading to compression of individual spinal nerve roots. Central disk herniations result in a disproportionate number of cases that result in severe lower urinary tract dysfunction. The signs and symptoms resulting from central disk prolapse vary depending on the rate and extent of the herniation, the size of the spinal canal, and the number of nerve roots involved. Sacral roots travel closest to the midline in the cauda equina and, consequently, the nerve roots are most likely to be damaged by central disk herniations.

CLINICAL FINDINGS
The physical examination may reveal a distended bladder or a positive cough test for incontinence. Examination usually shows weakness in muscles innervated by S1 and S2 (gastrocnemius, hamstrings, gluteal muscles) and sensory loss extending from the soles of the feet to the perianal region that may be variable and patchy. There may be laxity of the anal sphincter and loss of the BCR. The pattern of sensory loss restricted to the medial buttocks and perianal area is termed *saddle anesthesia*.

Patients with voiding symptoms may present with obstructive voiding symptoms including urinary hesitancy, intermittency, diminished urinary flow rate, straining to void, elevated residual urine volume, and incontinence. These symptoms are primarily due to the diminished detrusor contractility. Incontinence may result from either overflow due to poor or absent detrusor contractility or due to diminished lack of resistance at the level of the external sphincter.

DIAGNOSTIC STUDIES
The predominant urodynamic pattern found in cauda equina syndrome is a neurogenic acontractile detrusor associated with neuropathic sphincter dysfunction.[22,33] Bladder scanning may be useful in the diagnosis of CES. A PVR less than 200 mL has a negative predictive value for CES of 97%.[26] Some patients have preserved bladder sensation because of the presence of numerous exteroceptive sensory nerves in the bladder trigone and vesical neck that bypass the sacral spinal cord by entering thoracolumbar spinal segments.[27,28]

MRI precisely shows the spinal cord, nerve roots, and surrounding areas and should be performed in cases where spinal pathology is the suspected cause of voiding dysfunction (Figure 14.6).

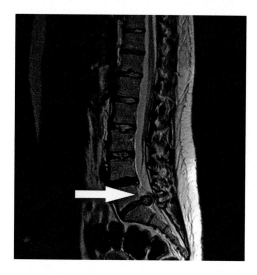

Figure 14.6 T2-weighted sagittal magnetic resonance imaging of the lumbar spine showing a large central disk prolapse with extrusion at L5-S1 resulting in acute cauda equina syndrome in a 23-year-old female.

UROLOGIC MANAGEMENT

Urologic management of a patient with neurogenic voiding dysfunction due to spinal pathology should be guided by the patient's symptoms and in accordance with sound urologic principles. In patients with significant urinary retention, intermittent catheterization is generally preferred since most of these patients do not have compromised upper extremity function. Management of incontinence should be guided by clinical and urodynamic findings. Detrusor overactivity can be managed with regular bladder emptying combined with antimuscarinic medications or intradetrusor botulinum toxin.

Surgical options for sphincteric incontinence may require major reconstructive urologic surgery. Bladder neck slings have been used to increase outlet resistance in patients with neurogenic lower urinary tract dysfunction with mixed results.[29,30] Implantation of an artificial sphincter has achieved excellent results in a small series of men with neurogenic sphincteric incontinence.[23,31,32] In women, a pubovaginal sling procedure will generally afford excellent continence and may be combined with intermittent catheterization to completely empty the bladder.

CONCLUSION

Bladder and sphincter dysfunction secondary to spinal pathology can result in devastating urologic

impairment including the loss of volitional voiding and marked urinary incontinence. MRI is critical to evaluation of spinal pathology, and urodynamics evaluation is invaluable in guiding management. Conservative management, particularly intermittent catheterization, should be the initial intervention. Surgical intervention should be deferred until such a time that a reasonable chance of functional recovery is unlikely.

REFERENCES

1. Schwartz H and McCormick PC. Spinal cord tumors in adults. In: Winn HR, ed. *Neurological Surgery*, vol 4, 5th ed. Philadelphia, PA: WB Saunders; 2004:4817–34.
2. Duong LM, McCarthy BJ, McLendon RE et al. Descriptive epidemiology of malignant and nonmalignant primary spinal cord, spinal meninges, and cauda equina tumors. *Cancer.* 2012;118:4220–7.
3. Bloomer CW, Ackerman A, and Bhatia RG. Imaging for spine tumors and new applications. *Top Magn Reson Imaging.* 2006;17(2):69–87.
4. Mechtler L and Nandingam K. Spinal cord tumors—New views and future directions. *Neuro Clin.* 2013;31:241–68.
5. Fisher CG, Goldschlager T, Boriani S et al. A novel scientific model for rare and often neglected neoplastic conditions. *Evid Based Spine Care J.* 2013;4(2):160–2.
6. Grimm S and Chamberlain MC. Adult primary spinal cord tumors. *Expert Rev Neurother.* 2009;9(10):1487–95.
7. Spinazze S, Careceni A, and Schrijvers D. Epidural spinal cord compression. *Crit Rev Oncol Hematol.* 2005;56(3):397–406.
8. Mut M, Schiff D, and Shaffrey ME. Metastasis to nervous system: Spinal epidural and intramedullary metastases. *J Neurooncol.* 2005;75(1):43–56.
9. Roodman GD. Mechanisms of bone metastasis. *N Engl J Med.* 2004;350(16):1655–98.
10. Slowik F and Balogh I. Extracranial spreading of glioblastoma multiforme. *Zentralbl Neurochir.* 1980;41(1):57–68.
11. Helweg-Larsen S and Sorensen PS. Symptoms and signs in metastatic spinal cord compression: A study of progression from first symptom until diagnosis in 153 patients. *Eur J Cancer.* 1994;30(3):39–8.
12. Byrne TN, Borges LF, and Loeffler JS. Metastatic epidural spinal cord compression: Update on management. *Semin Oncol.* 2006;33(3):307–11.
13. Reitz A, Haferkamp A, Wagener N, Gerner HJ, and Hohenfellner M. Neurogenic bladder dysfunction in patients with neoplastic spinal cord compression: Adaptation of the bladder management strategy to the underlying disease. *NeuroRehabilitation.* 2006;21(1):65–9.
14. Shephard RH. Diagnosis and prognosis of cauda equina syndrome produced by protrusion of lumbar disc. *Br Med J.* 1959;2:1434–9.
15. Rajasekaran S, Bajaj N, Tubaki V et al. ISSLS Prize winner: The anatomy of failure in lumbar disc herniation: An *in vivo,* multimodal, prospective study of 181 subjects. *Spine.* 2013;38:1491–500.
16. O'Flynn KJ, Murphy R, and Thomas DG. Neurogenic bladder dysfunction in lumbar intervertebral disc prolapse. *Br J Urol.* 1992;69:38–40.

17. Jensen MC, Brant-Zawadzki MN, Obuchowski N et al. Magnetic resonance imaging of the lumbar spine in people without back pain. *N Engl J Med.* 1994;331:69–73.

18. Blaivas JG, Zayed AAH, and Labib KB. The bulbocavernosus reflex in urology: A prospective study of 299 patients. *J Urol.* 1981;126:197–9.

19. Pavlakis AJ, Siroky MB, Goldstein I, and Krane RJ. Neurourologic findings in conus medullaris and cauda equina injury. *Arch Neurol.* 1983;40:570–3.

20. Jones D and Moore T. The types of neuropathic bladder dysfunction associated with prolapsed lumbar intervertebral discs. *Br J Urol.* 1973;45: 39–43.

21. Dong D, Xu Z, Shi B, Chen J et al. Clinical significance of urodynamic studies in neurogenic bladder dysfunction caused by intervertebral disk hernia. *Neurourol Urodyn.* 2006;25:446–50.

22. Andersen JT and Bradley WE. Neurogenic bladder dysfunction in protruded lumbar disc and after laminectomy. *Urology.* 1976;8:94–6.

23. Yates DR, Phé V, Rouprêt M et al. Robot-assisted laparoscopic artificial urinary sphincter insertion in men with neurogenic stress urinary incontinence. *BJU Int.* 2013;111:1175–9.

24. Scott PJ. Bladder paralysis in cauda equina lesions from disc prolapse. *J Bone Joint Surg.* 1965;47:224–7.

25. Chartier Kastler E, Genevois S, Gamé X et al. Treatment of neurogenic male urinary incontinence related to intrinsic sphincter insufficiency with an artificial urinary sphincter: A French retrospective multicentre study. *BJU Int.* 2011;107:426–32.

26. Venkatesan M, Nasto M, Tsegaye L, Magnum MD, and Grevitt, M. Bladder scans and postvoid residual volume measurement improve diagnostic accuracy of cauda equina syndrome. *Spine.* 2019;44:1303–8.

27. Reitz A. Afferent pathways arising from the lower urinary tract after complete spinal cord injury or cauda equina lesion: Clinical observations with neurophysiological implications. *Urol Int.* 2012;89:462–7.

28. Bradley WE, Timm GW, Scott FB, and Cystometry V. Bladder sensation. *Urology.* 1975;6:654–8.

29. Castellan M, Gosalbez R, Labbie A et al. Bladder neck sling for treatment of neurogenic incontinence in children with augmentation cystoplasty: Long-term follow-up. *J Urol.* 2005;173:2128–31.

30. Barthold JS, Rodriguez E, Freedman AL et al. Results of the rectus fascial sling and wrap procedures for the treatment of neurogenic sphincteric incontinence. *J Urol.* 1999;16:272–4.

31. Bersch U, Göcking K, and Pannek J. The artificial urinary sphincter in patients with spinal cord lesion: Description of a modified technique and clinical results. *Eur Urol.* 2009;55:687–93.

32. Chartier Kastler E, Genevois S, Gamé X et al. Treatment of neurogenic male urinary incontinence related to intrinsic sphincter insufficiency with an artificial urinary sphincter: A French retrospective multicentre study. *BJU Int.* 2011;107:426–32.

33. Yates DR, Phé V, Rouprêt M et al. Robot-assisted laparoscopic artificial urinary sphincter insertion in men with neurogenic stress urinary incontinence. *BJU Int.* 2013;111:1175–9.

Chapter 15

TETHERED CORD SYNDROME

Nishant Garg and Yahir Santiago-Lastra

INTRODUCTION

Tethered cord syndrome (TCS) is a functional disorder of the spinal cord caused by pathologic anchoring of its caudal end, causing neurologic dysfunction.[1] While there was originally disagreement within the neurosurgical community regarding the existence of TCS as a separate entity from other neurologic conditions, it is now recognized as a distinct disorder. Despite being a distinct pathologic condition with its own clinical manifestations, TCS has been observed to need subsequent treatment in 20%–50% of children with spina bifida, highlighting the interrelated nature of lumbar cord disorders.[2]

Current understanding of TCS describes its pathogenesis as stretching provoked by an inelastic structure anchored to the caudal portion of the cord.[1] This anchoring has progressively severe manifestations as children continue their growth into adults with the inelastic structure causing disruption of the nervous pathways and the blood flow to the spinal cord, eventually resulting in the sequelae of TCS.

The purpose of this chapter is to provide an overview of the workup and symptomatology of TCS, with a focus on the urologic complications and the ensuing management options for the clinician. The clinical urologist should be aware of the nonurologic complications of TCS, and these are briefly discussed here.

CATEGORIZATION OF TETHERED CORD SYNDROME

The terms *tethered cord* and *cord tethering* were subcategorized into three distinct entities by Yamada and Won[2] and are summarized by Düz[1]:

Category One: Lumbosacral cord anchored by an inelastic filum.

Category Two: Caudal myelomeningoceles (MCCs) and many sacral MCC.

Category Three (two subgroups):

1. Paraplegia and lipomyelomeningocele (LMMC) and MCC. These patients do not have any functional lumbosacral neurons; therefore, there is no beneficial role for surgery in these patients.

2. Asymptomatic patients with an elongated cord and a thick filum. These patients require close monitoring for subtle signs, especially urinary incontinence, as this indicates progressive irreversible worsening of the disorder.

For the purposes of this chapter and per the original categorization by Yamada and Won,[1] only those patients in category one meet the definition of true TCS.

INCIDENCE

The true incidence of occult spinal defects (OSDs) and more specifically, TCS, is unknown.[3] When looking only at MMCs and other midline dorsal anomalies, the literature reports 1 in every 1000 live births, and this rate is lower among African Americans than Caucasians.[4] In contrast to open neural tube defects (spina bifida, MMCs), TCS is difficult to diagnose unless there are active clinical manifestations. TCS is often diagnosed on workup for unrelated or possibly related disorders, such as imperforate anus.[5] With an increased utilization of MRI over time, the incidence of diagnosed TCS has also risen. Although not a perfect surrogate for TCS, OSD tends to have a 2:1 predominance among females relative to males,[6] but it is not known if that is true for TCS. Ultimately, greater clinical awareness, continued screening for the sequelae of TCS, and expanding use of MR and other imaging modalities will help elicit the true incidence of TCS.

ETIOLOGY (PATHOLOGIC CONSIDERATIONS AND NEUROLOGIC DYSFUNCTION)

Understanding of TCS is broken down into an appreciation of embryological development and the neurulation process as well as the local cellular and anatomic anomalies present from the postnatal period to the time of eventual diagnosis. These two contributing processes to TCS are briefly discussed separately in this section.

EMBRYOLOGY

The central nervous system is formed through three major processes over the first 2 months postconception, with the most critical portion for TCS occurring during the first 2–4 weeks and then during weeks 9–11.[7] These stages are broken down into the following: *neurulation* (neural tube formation), *canalization* of the tail bud, and *regression*.[8] Neurulation results in folding of the neural plate on itself to form the neural tube. Any

errors during this process are likely to result in disorders associated with TCS such as LMMCs, MMCs, and other spinal dysraphisms. The second major process, canalization of the tail bud, occurs when the caudal cell mass is stimulated through an unknown mechanism to undergo canalization and eventual regression.[9] This process continues until the only remaining components are the medulla spinalis below T12 and a distal filum terminale, and any anomalies in this process are thought to result in the increased risk and eventual development of TCS.

PATHOPHYSIOLOGY

The decreased elasticity transferred upon the spinal cord as a result of an abnormal filum impacts the oxidative metabolism capacity of the cord.[10] This impaired metabolism mimics the mechanisms seen in hypoxemia.[11] The range of these hypoxemic effects is directly concordant with the degree of the stretch induced on the cord[12]; minor stretching results in milder hypoxemia,[13] whereas marked stretching results in more pronounced hypoxemic and ischemic effects.[12,14] Ultimately these hypoxemic effects parallel diminished glucose metabolism within the cord as well as decreases in overall blood flow due to the pathologic stretch mechanisms.[15]

One other important consideration is that associated spinal dysraphisms, such as LMMCs, MMCs, lipomas, and meningocele manqué, when located at the lumbosacral cord, can have mass effect that result in symptoms similar to TCS despite not having the typical TCS pathophysiology.[11] When symptoms are so pronounced so as to result in total paraplegia, this no longer is considered to represent TCS.

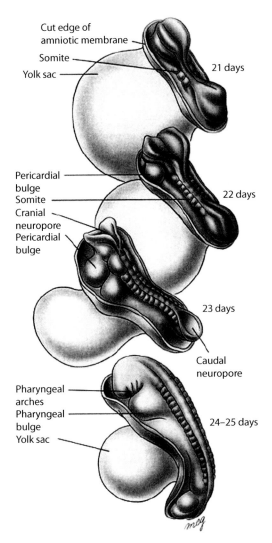

Figure 15.1 Primary neurulation. The lateral edges of the neural folds meet in the midline and fuse. (Reproduced with permission from Larsen WJ. *Human Embryology*, 3rd ed. Elsevier Science, 2001; Hertzler DA et al. *Neurosurg Focus*. 2010;29(1):E1.)

Cut edge of amniotic membrane
Somite
Yolk sac
21 days

Pericardial bulge
Somite
Cranial neuropore
Pericardial bulge
22 days

23 days

Caudal neuropore

Pharyngeal arches
Pharyngeal bulge
Yolk sac
24–25 days

PATIENT PRESENTATION

The presentation of TCS should be separated into the two categories of pediatric presentation and adult presentation in order to more accurately identify the symptomatology of which the clinician should be aware.

PEDIATRIC

Infants are typically asymptomatic[16,17] but may have suspicious lesions such as a sacral midline hair tuft (known as a "faun's tail"), a sacral lipomatous mass, or musculoskeletal deformities including limb atrophy, shortening, or possibly club foot. The predominant symptoms of urinary leakage and continuous dribbling are difficult to elucidate in a child prior to toilet training.

Young children, once ambulatory, may have historical features of gait abnormalities despite prior

Table 15.1 Common Features Pediatric-Onset Tethered Cord Syndrome

1. Gait anomalies after having had a normal gait during their childhood
2. Eventual development of urinary incontinence or dribbling despite successful toilet training
3. Development of lower extremity motor neuropathies such as foot drop
4. Presence of suspicious lesions in the lumbosacral region
5. Spinal deformities including scoliosis or lumbosacral lordosis

Table 15.2 Common Features of Adult-Onset Tethered Cord Syndrome

1. Back and leg pain that is frequently affected by postural changes
2. Difficulty with bowel or bladder control, with possible increases in postvoid residual urine volume
3. Challenges with performing day-to-day activities (exercise, sitting for prolonged periods of time)
4. Weakness and/or hyporeflexia in lower limbs
5. Sensory deficits in distal lower limbs and perianal area
6. Diminished sphincter tone

normal gait.[18] Pain and sensory loss are typically rare features, and their presence may indicate severe mass effect or other underlying pathology.[18] During the adolescent period, rapid growth of the child may result in scoliosis, and if concurrent with lumbosacral lordosis and lower extremity deformities, TCS is more likely.[18] The primary anomalies that should be noted in pediatric patients are summarized in Table 15.1.[18,19]

ADULT

Studies have shown that oftentimes adults presenting with symptoms of TCS have had these symptoms for 8–9 years prior to the initial office visit.[20] Patients present after progressive or precipitating events that, in line with the pathophysiology of TCS, induce severe and prolonged ischemia and reduced oxidative metabolism to the cord[21]; precipitating events can include obesity, sudden stressors on the back including exaggerated bending, trauma, and for women, pregnancy. In contrast to children, who typically have more neurologic dysfunction, adults will generally present complaining of pain.[21–23]

Adults with TCS have generally been classified into two categories[18]:

1. Patients with prior history of spinal dysraphisms that were diagnosed and subsequently repaired
2. Patients with a slow onset of symptoms that could be exacerbated by a sudden event

Patients in the first group, with a known history of TCS, are easier to monitor given their prior experiences and should be followed given that they have a 15% chance of developing TCS despite prior repair.[24] It is typically more challenging to diagnose group 2 TCS patients, and they should be monitored for the key symptoms summarized in Table 15.2.[25]

One key point to consider is that lumbar disk herniation may act as a confounding factor; however, it can be ruled out in the absence of lower limb pain with coughing or straight leg raise, and subsequent imaging may further delineate the correct diagnosis.[18]

IMAGING

The primary imaging modality for TCS is MRI, but clinicians may rely on adjunct information from computed tomography (CT) and ultrasound. Some key findings include:

1. An elongated cord or thickened filum (greater than 2 mm)[37]
2. Posterior displacement of conus and filum[18]
3. Spinal dysraphisms, MMC, LMMC, and lipomas

UROLOGIC CONSIDERATIONS

The normal physiology and function of the bladder, as well as the neurologic control mechanisms, were covered earlier in this book (see Part I chapter by Rose Khavari) and will not be discussed here.

Bladder dysfunction is noted as a complaint in 40% of TCS patients and is the sole complaint in 4% of these patients.[26–28] The earliest and most common issue is exacerbated or *de novo* incontinence in adults, and regression of toilet training in children. The pathophysiology of TCS is based on a lesion in the spinal cord gray matter rather than in the long tracts,[26,29,30] resulting in the loss of spinal synaptic reflex arcs. These arcs, composed of synapses between pelvic and pudendal afferent neurons to efferent neurons on the intermediolateral cell column as well as the anterior horn, disrupt the normal micturition reflex. The key disruption is due to afferent fiber entry into the conus, which as a result of TCS is under significant stretch. This stretch disrupts parasympathetic motor outflow but has no disruption on sympathetic pathways since they pass at higher cord levels.

TCS combined with bladder dysfunction is seen either as an acontractile detrusor or neurogenic detrusor overactivity, and detrusor sphincter dyssynergia (DSD) may or may not be present.[31,32] Prior studies have demonstrated that patients with TCS have an acontractile detrusor in 55% of cases (up to 71% in other studies),[33] neurogenic detrusor overactivity in 18%, mixed lesions in 12% (these are lesions with both decreased compliance and overactivity), as well as two less commonly found pathologies.[34] With an acontractile detrusor, the predominant pathology is urine leakage from overflow incontinence, specifically due to the synergistic effects of both bladder filling exceeding compliance as well as urethral sphincter capacity. By contrast, patients may experience urgency and urge incontinence with neurogenic detrusor overactivity causing involuntary bladder contraction.[26]

Ultimately, a thorough history can elucidate urinary symptoms, especially incontinence, suspicious of TCS. However, many of these symptoms are nonspecific; therefore, a high index of suspicion is required, particularly in cases of patients with neural tube defects with newly exacerbated symptoms who had previously had a stable period of symptom control. These symptoms can include the following[27]:

1. Urgency
2. Dysuria
3. Hesitation
4. Sensations of fullness
5. Incontinence
6. Straining to void
7. Erection, emission, and ejaculation

URODYNAMICS AND IMAGING STUDIES

The role of urodynamics is to gain an understanding of voiding function but should not be the primary mode of understanding TCS-related voiding dysfunction, as it will not identify TCS as the cause. Generally, an evaluation will begin with urinary flow rate (uroflow) and postvoid residual volumes to understand voiding function. This is followed by a cystometrogram to look at storage function.[26] Understanding both TCS and urinary dysfunction involves both a lumbosacral x-ray as well as a voiding cystourethrogram (VCUG).[35] The purpose of the x-ray is to examine spinal pathologies, while the VCUG examines the presence of vesicoureteral reflux, bladder atony or overactivity, and possible bladder outlet obstruction. The use of any of these studies is reliant on clinical suspicion for urinary dysfunction.

MANAGEMENT

Treatment of TCS is primarily indicated in cases of progressive neurologic decline, including motor signs, orthopedic deformities, and incontinence.

Although subtle, progression of incontinence has the potential to become irreversible if not monitored and treated appropriately.[36,37]

Generally, the treatment of TCS is based on surgical untethering of the cord.[16,38] Some surgeons advocate LMMC repair for cord untethering at 4 years old, even if the patient is asymptomatic.[39]

With regard to management of urologic symptoms, case series[33] have demonstrated that despite untethering of the cord, many patients continue to exhibit voiding dysfunction requiring continued intervention. Some estimates show that up to 40% of patients continue to have voiding dysfunction despite surgery, with the three most important prognostic features being[40]:

1. Symptoms for longer than 3 years
2. Loss of bladder sensation
3. Severe tethering with the conus fixed to the bottom of the dural sac

For an acontractile detrusor, clean intermittent catheterization remains a mainstay of treatment, and in those patients unable to carry this out, urinary diversion, augmentation with catheterizable stoma, or indwelling catheters are options.[26] By contrast, detrusor overactivity is best addressed with anticholinergic, antispasmodic agents and chemodenervation, such as onabotulinumtoxinA injections.[26]

CASE PRESENTATIONS

The following case reports are adapted from Yamada et al.[41] and were found in the previous edition of this book.

CASE 1

A 4-year-old girl began to have urinary dribbling after successful toilet training, starting 4 months before admission. Episodes of dribbling continued to increase. No other neurologic signs and symptoms were noted. Spina bifida was demonstrated at S5 and the sacral spine on plain x-ray films. A large soft swelling of the left gluteal area corresponded to cerebrospinal fluid accumulation underneath the skin on myelography. Surgical repair of a caudal LMMC was performed, and the caudal end of the spinal cord was disconnected from fat tissue in the wall of the anomaly. The patient regained continence in 2 weeks.

CASE 2

A 14-year-old girl was known as an infrequent voider in early infancy. At 3 years of age, toilet training was successful except for occasional enuresis. At the age of 7 years, enuresis became frequent and progressed to total incontinence, associated with a lack of urgency or sensation of a full bladder. Urinary loss was related to overflow and to stress or Valsalva maneuvers, requiring continuous pad protection. On examination, minimal suprapubic pressure would express urine. Two small dimples in the sacral area and pes cavus were noted. She had notable neurologic anomalies including perianal anesthesia. Postvoid urinary residual was greater than 200 mL. Plain films revealed spina bifida at S1 through S5. VCUG showed bilateral promptly functioning kidneys, a cellule and diverticula formation in the bladder, right vesicoureteral reflux, and a large postvoid residual. A myelogram showed LMMC in the sacral level with a cord tip at the S2 level. Surgical repair of a large transitional LMMC consisted of removal of the entire fibroadipose mass, with dissection from the caudal end of the spinal cord. Within 1 week after the operation, the patient began to regain bladder control without evidence of stress incontinence. VCUG clarified resolution of the reflux and a normal residual urine. This patient underwent 18 urologic procedures from the age of 7–14 years to manage her neurogenic bladder and vesicoureteral reflux.

CONCLUSIONS

TCS remains a rare but critical disorder among children and adults that is characterized by a stretch-induced functional disorder of the lumbar spinal cord due to anchoring by an inelastic structure. Patients have motor deficits in the lower limbs, incontinence, and musculoskeletal deformities. The physiology of TCS is due to impaired oxidative metabolism within the lumbosacral cord. Urinary incontinence may be the sole complaint in some patients and should be suspected by the clinical urologist in cases of sudden incontinence or regression of toilet training in a child. Incontinence in particular must be carefully monitored as its progression indicates the possibly irreversible nature of TCS. Surgery remains a mainstay of treatment with good results, but the urologist must be prepared to manage continued urologic dysfunction despite surgery. Management of the neurogenic bladder is based on the presence of either bladder atony or detrusor overactivity. Ultimately, the goal of managing TCS is to improve the quality of life for patients while also protecting the upper tracts.

REFERENCES

1. Düz B, Gocmen S, Ibrahim Secer H, Basal S, and Gönül E. Tethered cord syndrome in adulthood. *J Spinal Cord Med.* 2008;31(3):272–8.
2. Zalatimo O. Tethered Spinal Cord Syndrome, 2019. American Association of Neurological Surgeons. https://www.aans.org/Patients/Neurosurgical-Conditions-and-Treatments/Tethered-Spinal-Cord-Syndrome
3. Bui CJ, Tubbs RS, and Oakes WJ. Tethered cord syndrome in children: A review. *Neurosurg Focus.* 2007;23(2):1–9.
4. Dias MS. Neurosurgical management of myelomeningocele (spina bifida). *Pediatr Rev.* 2005; 26(2):50–60.
5. Golonka NR, Haga LJ, Keating RP et al. Routine MRI evaluation of low imperforate anus reveals unexpected high incidence of tethered spinal cord. *J Pediatr Surg.* 2002;37(7):966–9.
6. Carter CO, Evans KA, and Till, K. Spinal dysraphism: Genetic relation to neural tube malformations. *J Med Genet.* 1976;13(5):343–50.
7. Hertzler DA, DePowell JJ, Stevenson CB, and Mangano FT. Tethered cord syndrome: A review of the literature from embryology to adult presentation. *Neurosurg Focus.* 2010;29(1):E1.
8. Warder DE. Tethered cord syndrome and occult spinal dysraphism. *Neurosurg Focus.* 2001;10(1):1–9.
9. Tu A, and Steinbok P. Occult tethered cord syndrome: A review. *Childs Nerv Syst.* 2013;29(9):1635–40.
10. Yamada S, Won DJ, Pezeshkpour G et al. Pathophysiology of tethered cord syndrome and similar complex disorders. *Neurosurg Focus.* 2007;23 (2):1–10.
11. Filippidis AS, Kalani MY, Theodore N, and Rekate HL. Spinal cord traction, vascular compromise, hypoxia, and metabolic derangements in the pathophysiology of tethered cord syndrome. *Neurosurg Focus.* 2010;29(1):E9.
12. Yamada, S, Won DJ, and Yamada SM. Pathophysiology of tethered cord syndrome: Correlation with symptomatology. *Neurosurg Focus.* 2004;16(2):1–5.
13. Yamada S, Sanders D, and Haugen G. Functional and metabolic responses of the spinal cord to anoxia and asphyxia. In: Austin GM, ed. *Contemporary Aspects of Cerebrovascular Disease*; 1976:239.
14. Yamada S, Zinke DE, and Sanders D. Pathophysiology of "tethered cord syndrome." *J Neurosurg.* 1981;54(4):494–503.
15. Yamada S et al. Pathophysiology of tethered cord syndrome. In: Yamada S, ed., 2nd edition. *Tethered Cord Syndrome in Children and Adults.* New York, NY: Thieme; 2010:19–40.
16. Hoffman HJ, Hendrick B, and Humphreys RP. The tethered spinal cord: Its protean manifestations, diagnosis and surgical correction. *Pediatr Neurosurg.* 1976;2(3):145–55.
17. Schneider, Sanford. Neurological assessment of tethered spinal cord. In: Yamada S, ed., 2nd edition. *Tethered Cord Syndrome in Children and Adults.* New York, NY: Thieme; 2010:43–9.
18. Yamada S, Won D, and Kido DK. Adult tethered cord syndrome: New classification correlated with symptomatology, imaging and pathophysiology. *Neurosurg Q.* 2001;11(4):260–75.
19. Drake JM. Occult tethered cord syndrome: Not an indication for surgery. *J Neurosurg Pediatr.* 2006;104(5):305–8.
20. Klekamp J. Tethered cord syndrome in adults. *J Neurosurg Spine.* 2011;15(3):258–70.
21. Aufschnaiter K, Fellner F, and Wurm G. Surgery in adult onset tethered cord syndrome (ATCS): Review of literature on occasion of an exceptional case. *Neurosurg Rev.* 2008;31(4):371.

22. Hüttmann S, Krauss J, Collmann H, Sörensen N, and Roosen K. Surgical management of tethered spinal cord in adults: Report of 54 cases. *J Neurosurg Spine*. 2001;95(2):173–8.

23. Rajpal S, Tubbs RS, George T et al. Tethered cord due to spina bifida occulta presenting in adulthood: A tricenter review of 61 patients. *J Neurosurg Spine*. 2007;6(3):210–5.

24. Pang D and Wilberger JE. Tethered cord syndrome in adults. *J Neurosurg*. 1982;57(1):32–47.

25. Yamada S, Siddiqi J, Won DJ et al. Symptomatic protocols for adult tethered cord syndrome. *Neurol Res*. 2004;26(7):741–4.

26. Hadley R, Ruckle H, Yamada B, and Richards G. Urological aspect of tethered cord syndrome I: Lower urinary tract dysfunction in tethered cord syndrome. In: Yamada S, ed., 2nd edition. *Tethered Cord Syndrome in Children and Adults*. New York, NY: Thieme, 2010:74–84.

27. Hadley R and Holevas RE. Lower urinary tract dysfunction in tethered cord syndrome. In: 2nd edition, *Tethered Cord Syndrome*. Park Ridge, IL: American Association of Neurological Surgeons; 1996:79–88.

28. French BN. Midline fusion defects and defects of formation. In: Youmans JR, ed. *Neurological Surgery*. Philadelphia, PA: WB Saunders; 1990;2:1081–235.

29. Yamada S, Zinke DE, and Sanders, D. Pathophysiology of "tethered cord syndrome." *J Neurosurg*. 1981;54(4):494–503.

30. Fuse T, Patrickson JW, and Yamada S. Axonal transport of horseradish peroxidase in the experimental tethered spinal cord. *Pediatr Neurosurg*. 1989;15(6):296–301.

31. Kuru M. Nervous control of micturition. *Physiol Rev*. 1965;45:425–94.

32. Holtzman RN and Stein BM. *The Tethered Spinal Cord*. New York, NY: Thieme Medical; 1985.

33. Giddens JL, Radomski SB, Hirshberg ED, Hassouna M, and Fehlings M. Urodynamic findings in adults with the tethered cord syndrome. *J Urol*. 1999;161(4):1249–54.

34. Hellstrom WJ, Edwards MS, and Kogan BA. Urological aspects of the tethered cord syndrome. *J Urol*. 1986;135(2):317–9.

35. Khoury AE, Balcom A, McLorie GA, and Churchill BM. Clinical experience in urological involvement with tethered cord syndrome. In: Yamada S, 2nd edition. *Tethered Cord Syndrome*. Park Ridge, IL: American Association of Neurological Surgeons; 1996:89–98.

36. McLaurin RL. *Pediatric Neurosurgery: Surgery of the Developing Nervous System*. Philadelphia, PA: WB Saunders; 1989.

37. Pang D. Tethered cord syndrome. In: Hoffman HJ, ed. *Advances in Neurosurgery*. Vol 1, No 1. Philadelphia, PA: Hanley & Belfus; 1986:45–79.

38. Drake J, Hoffman H. Indication and treatment of tethered spinal cord. In: Yamada S, ed. *Tethered Cord Syndrome in Children and Adults*. New York, NY: Thieme; 2010:110–7.

39. Hoffman HJ, Taecholarn C, Hendrick EB, and Humphreys RP. Management of lipomyelomeningoceles: Experience at the Hospital for Sick Children, Toronto. *J Neurosurg*. 1985;62(1):1–8.

40. Kondo A, Kato K, Kanai S, and Sakakibara T. Bladder dysfunction secondary to tethered cord syndrome in adults: Is it curable? *J Urol*. 1986;135(2):313–6.

41. Corcos J, Ginsberg DD, and Karsenty G, eds. *Textbook of the Neurogenic Bladder*. Boca Raton, FL: CRC Press; 2015.

TRAUMATIC INJURIES OF THE CENTRAL NERVOUS SYSTEM

Chapter 16

SPINAL CORD INJURY AND CEREBRAL TRAUMA

Thomas M. Kessler

INTRODUCTION

Neurogenic lower urinary tract dysfunction (NLUTD) is very common after spinal cord injury (SCI) and cerebral trauma. The site and nature of the lesion in the neurological axis determine the type of lower urinary tract dysfunction that is reflected in the patient's symptoms (Figure 16.1).[1,2]

SPINAL CORD INJURY

BACKGROUND
SCI is a devastating event with far-reaching consequences for the individual's health and the family's economic and social future. It affects each year 15–53 new individuals per million in Western countries.[3] In the past, renal disease was responsible for more than 40% of deaths following SCI.[4] The introduction of intermittent self-catheterization, the use of regular urodynamic investigation, and modern management have since revolutionized the prognosis of patients with SCI.[5] Hence, urinary disease now accounts for only about 13% of deaths in patients with SCI, and the most common cause of death is related to pneumonia.[6] It follows that adequate function of the urinary tract is essential to prevent morbidity and mortality in patients with SCI.

CLASSIFICATION
The most comprehensive classification is that developed by the American Spinal Injury Association (ASIA), the International Standards for Neurological Classification of SCI (ISNCSCI) Worksheet, including the ASIA Impairment Scale (AIS) (Figure 16.2). It uses the examination of dermatomes and myotomes to determine the level and completeness of the sensory and motor functions and distinguishes five grades ranging from A to E (with A being the most severe injury) and five clinical syndromes:

- *Central cord syndrome* is a result of hemorrhagic necrosis of the central gray matter and some of the medial white matter and is most commonly due to hyperextension injury. More caudal fibers of the corticospinal and spinothalamic tract are localized in the spine more lateral (from the center) and hence are better protected from the central necrosis; consequently, arms are more affected than legs. NLUTD is also less common.
- *Brown-Séquard syndrome* is a rare unilateral cord condition that can result from penetrating injury or asymmetric disk herniation. It presents as ipsilateral motor weakness and sense impairment of fine touch and position and contralateral sensory impairment of pain and temperature. NLUTD in the pure condition is uncommon.
- *Anterior cord syndrome* is characterized by injury to the anterior aspects of the cord, with preservation of the posterior columns and dorsal horns. There is a motor deficit and loss of pain and temperature sensation below the level of the injury.
- *Posterior cord syndrome* is characterized by injury to the posterior aspects of the cord. It causes loss of light touch sensation below the level of injury, but it preserves movement, pain, and temperature sensation.
- *Conus medullaris and cauda equina syndrome* result from damage to the conus and spinal nerve roots, leading to flaccid paraplegia and sensory loss. Sacral reflexes can be partially or totally lost.

THE BLADDER IN "SPINAL SHOCK"
The initial phase following acute SCI is that of spinal shock.[7] This is related to the loss or the depression of most spinal reflex activity below the level of injury.[8] Spinal shock is thought to result from the sudden withdrawal of facilitatory descending input from the supraspinal tracts, which disrupts transmission at synapses and stops interneuronal conduction in the distal cord.[8] The loss of skeletal reflexes leads to flaccid paralysis and the loss of deep tendon reflexes. The duration of spinal shock varies widely, from several days to several months. It is not an "all or nothing" entity but depends on the extension and completeness of the spinal lesion. However, there is no generally accepted definition of spinal shock, since there are no high-level evidence studies on this issue. Nevertheless, Ditunno et al.[9] have proposed a spinal shock model, which is very helpful in understanding this phenomenon. It includes an initial phase of loss

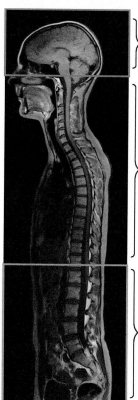

Suprapontine lesion
• History: predominantly storage symptoms
• Ultrasound: insignificant PVR urine volume
• Urodynamics: detrusor overactivity

Normoactive

Spinal (infrapontine-suprasacral) lesion
• History: both storage and voiding symptoms
• Ultrasound: PVR urine volume usually raised
• Urodynamics: detrusor overactivity, detrusor-sphincter dyssynergia

Overactive

Sacral/infrasacral lesion
• History: predominantly voiding symptoms
• Ultrasound: PVR urine volume raised
• Urodynamics: hypocontractile or acontractile detrusor

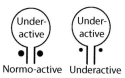

Normo-active   Underactive

Figure 16.1 Patterns of lower urinary tract dysfunction following different lesion levels in the neurologic axis. (Adapted from Panicker JN, Fowler CJ, and Kessler TM. *Lancet Neurol.* 2015;14[7]:720–32).

of reflexes and three subsequent recovery phases.[9] In addition to the effects on skeletal muscle, spinal shock may result in NLUTD. Indeed, it was generally assumed that patients with SCI have an acontractile detrusor during the spinal shock, but very recently detrusor overactivity was found in about 6 of 10 patients within the first 40 days after SCI.[10] Overall, almost two-thirds of the patients showed unfavorable urodynamic parameters that jeopardized the lower and upper urinary tracts.[10]

SUPRASACRAL TO INFRAPONTINE LESION (FORMER UPPER MOTOR NEURON LESION)
NEUROGENIC DETRUSOR OVERACTIVITY
This follows the stage of spinal shock resulting from a cord injury above the S2 level. Reflex bladder function eventually occurs after suprasacral SCI. This function is different from normal in that:

- It involves different afferent fibers (C-fibers in the cat)[11]
- Bladder contractions are poorly sustained
- The urethra and bladder become discoordinated

Consciousness of bladder sensation may not be totally absent, but voluntary inhibition of the micturition

reflex arc is lost. The bladder empties incompletely because of the dyssynergic contraction of the external urethral sphincter, reflex inhibition from the dyssynergic sphincter, and primary detrusor failure (discoordinated contraction). Overall, this alteration in central organization results in a high voiding pressure, postvoid residual, and urinary incontinence. These subsequently lead to recurrent infection, hydronephrosis, and finally to renal failure.

AFFERENT FIBERS
Normal micturition reflex involves Aδ-fiber afferents. Only in inflammatory states are C-fiber afferents involved (chemosensitivity). After SCI, C-fiber afferents mediate (mechanosensitivity) the abnormal sacral segmental bladder reflex.[11] The mechanism of this change from chemosensitivity to mechanosensitivity of C-fibers is unclear.

DETRUSOR UNDERACTIVITY
It has been assumed that poor detrusor function in patients with suprasacral SCI is primarily due to reflex inhibition from the dyssynergic sphincter, but primary detrusor failure might also be of significance. In some instances of cervical and high thoracic SCI, detrusor acontractility and external sphincter

ASIA IMPAIRMENT SCALE

☐ A = Complete: No motor or sensory function is preserved in the sacral segments S4–S5.

☐ B = Incomplete: Sensory but not motor function is preserved below the neurological level and includes the sacral segments S4–S5.

☐ C = Incomplete: Motor function is preserved below the neurological level, and more than half of key muscles below the neurological level have a muscle grade less than 3.

☐ D = Incomplete: Motor function is preserved below the neurological level, and at least half of key muscles below the neurological level have a muscle grade of 3 of more.

☐ E = Normal: Motor and sensory function are normal.

CLINICAL SYNDROMES

☐ Central cord
☐ Brown-Séquard
☐ Anterior cord
☐ Conus medullaris
☐ Cauda equina

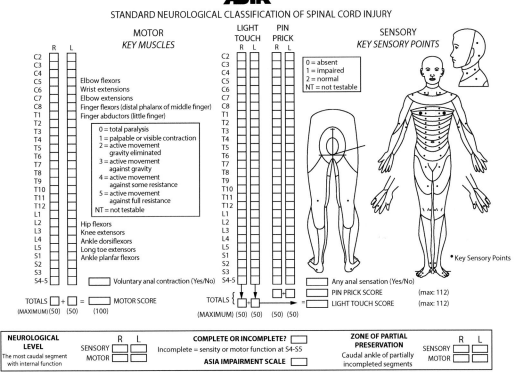

ASIA

STANDARD NEUROLOGICAL CLASSIFICATION OF SPINAL CORD INJURY

Figure 16.2 International standards for neurological classification of spinal cord injury (ISNCSCI) worksheet. (American Spinal Injury Association).

denervation are present, indicating a distinct and separate lesion in the sacral area.[12,13]

DETRUSOR SPHINCTER DYSSYNERGIA (INTERNAL AND EXTERNAL)

The pons coordinates the micturition reflex. Any lesion between the sacral and pontine level may produce discoordinated voiding, which results in increased external sphincter activity during detrusor contraction, i.e., detrusor external sphincter dyssynergia, which is responsible for the bladder outlet obstruction and, in combination with neurogenic detrusor overactivity, for high, sustained intravesical pressure, which is the most common cause of upper tract complications in SCI.[1,2] Combined pelvic floor electromyography (EMG) and videocystourethrography during urodynamic investigation are the most acceptable and widely agreed methods for diagnosing detrusor sphincter dyssynergia.[14]

The sympathetic system controls the bladder neck and proximal urethra from the T10 to L2 spinal cord segments. A spinal cord lesion above T10 removes supraspinal inhibitory control of the sympathetic vesicourethral neurons, resulting in bladder neck functional obstruction, i.e., detrusor internal sphincter dyssynergia (bladder neck dyssynergia).

Urologic manifestations of detrusor internal and external dyssynergia are the same.

AUTONOMIC DYSREFLEXIA

Autonomic dysreflexia (AD) is a sudden and exaggerated autonomic response to various stimuli in patients with SCI or spinal dysfunction. It generally manifests in patients with SCI at or above T6 (but a relevant percentage of patients may have a lesion level below T6 since the sympathetic outflow originates from T1 to L2)[15] and is defined by an increase in systolic blood pressure greater than 20 mm Hg from baseline.[16] Furthermore, AD can have life-threatening consequences if not properly managed. AD is caused by spinal reflex mechanisms that are initiated when a noxious stimulus enters the spinal cord below the level of injury. This afferent stimulus generates sympathetic overactivity leading to vasoconstriction below the neurologic lesion, along with involvement of splanchnic circulation causing vasoconstriction and hypertension. The excessive compensatory parasympathetic activity (and lack of sympathetic tone) leads to vasodilation above the level of the lesion and is thought to be responsible for headache, flushing, sweating, and nasal congestion. The reflex bradycardia is secondary to vagal stimulation. Bladder distension is the most common triggering factor for AD. The distension that can result from urinary retention or catheter blockage accounts for up to 85% of cases.[17] The second most common triggering factor for AD is bowel distension due to fecal impaction. Other potential factors include hemorrhoids and anal fissures, gastrointestinal precipitants (appendicitis, cholecystitis, etc.), pressure ulcers, ingrown toenails, fractures, heterotopic ossification, menstruation, pregnancy or labor, deep vein thrombosis, pulmonary embolism, and sexual activity. Medications, especially nasal decongestants and misoprostol, may also induce AD. Education of patients, caregivers, and family members regarding AD is vital to prevent it and to recognize its occurrence without delay.

If AD occurs, it is essential to find and eliminate the triggering stimulus (e.g., bladder distension or bowel impaction). Initial management also involves placing the patient in an upright position to take advantage of any orthostatic reduction in blood pressure, and loosening tight clothing and/or constrictive devices.

Blood pressure should be monitored until the patient is stable. These steps will resolve the problem in most patients, but in some, pharmacotherapy (in general, antihypertensive agents that have a rapid onset and short duration of action [nitrates]) may become necessary.

SACRAL/INFRASACRAL LESION (FORMER LOWER MOTOR NEURON LESION)

SCI to the sacral paths at S2 through S5 results in parasympathetic decentralization of the detrusor and somatic denervation of the external urethral sphincter, and loss of some afferent pathways. In a complete lesion, conscious awareness of bladder fullness will be lost, and the micturition reflex is absent. Some pain sensation can be preserved because the hypogastric (sympathetic) nerve is intact.

CEREBRAL TRAUMA

BACKGROUND

Cerebral trauma is a major health and socioeconomic problem throughout the world affecting people of all ages.[18] An estimated 69 million individuals sustain cerebral trauma from all causes each year, with the Southeast Asian and Western Pacific regions experiencing the greatest overall burden of disease.[19]

COMA

Cerebral trauma can cause temporary dysfunction (coma) or permanent lesion. Unconsciousness after cerebral trauma relates to compression, hemorrhage, or ischemia. The brainstem can be displaced downward or the temporal lobe herniates through the tentorial opening. Classification of the different coma stages is best described by the Glasgow Coma Scale.[20] In most cases of coma, spontaneous voiding is possible. Because only the suprapontine area is affected, coordination between the detrusor and sphincter remains generally intact, i.e., voiding is synergistic, without postvoid residual. Some patients, however, show decreased detrusor compliance (ability of the bladder to accommodate a larger volume with low pressure), which depends on both neural and nonneural factors. An indwelling catheter, which is placed in most coma patients, may cause detrusor irritation resulting in an increased stiffness of the bladder. Lack of sympathetic inhibition of bladder activity by the brain, as in progressive autonomic and multiple system failure, can be another explanation. In some comatose patients, there is temporary bladder retention that may be caused by bladder overdistention immediately after the accident or by an active cerebral bladder inhibition (i.e., pontine shock similar to spinal shock).

SUPRAPONTINE NEUROGENIC DETRUSOR OVERACTIVITY

If the amount of cortical inhibition running in descending pathways is reduced by a suprapontine injury, there will be diminished ability to inhibit the micturition reflex. This results in an uninhibited detrusor contraction, with synergistic relaxation of the internal and external urethral sphincter. During the filling phase, when the bladder contains a comparatively small volume of urine, inhibition of the suprapontine reflex arc will fail, and the detrusor will contract. There is no resistance from the urethra because of adequate relaxation of the sphincters due to the preserved sacropontine reflex arc. Patients with suprapontine detrusor overactivity will complain of frequency, urgency, and urgency incontinence and, in severe cases of complete lesion, lack of sensory or motor control of the micturition reflex. They have generally no postvoid residual and thus are not prone to bladder infections. Urodynamic studies may show early (small-volume) detrusor contractions, no detrusor sphincter dyssynergia (the sphincter relaxes during detrusor contraction), and voiding without postvoid residual.

REFERENCES

1. Panicker JN, Fowler CJ, and Kessler TM. Lower urinary tract dysfunction in the neurological patient: Clinical assessment and management. *Lancet Neurol.* 2015;14(7):720–32.
2. Groen J, Pannek J, Castro Diaz D et al. Summary of European Association of Urology (EAU) Guidelines on Neuro-Urology. *Eur Urol.* 2016;69(2):324–33.
3. Pavese C, Schneider MP, Schubert M et al. Prediction of bladder outcomes after traumatic spinal cord injury: A longitudinal cohort study. *PLOS Med.* 2016;13(6):e1002041.
4. Hackler RH. A 25-year prospective mortality study in the spinal cord injured patient: Comparison with the long-term living paraplegic. *J Urol.* 1977;117(4):486–8.
5. Schops TF, Schneider MP, Steffen F, Ineichen BV, Mehnert U, and Kessler TM. Neurogenic lower urinary tract dysfunction (NLUTD) in patients with spinal cord injury: Long-term urodynamic findings. *BJU Int.* 2015;115(Suppl 6):33–8.
6. Lidal IB, Snekkevik H, Aamodt G, Hjeltnes N, Biering-Sorensen F, and Stanghelle JK. Mortality after spinal cord injury in Norway. *J Rehabil Med.* 2007;39(2):145–51.
7. Hiersemenzel LP, Curt A, and Dietz V. From spinal shock to spasticity: Neuronal adaptations to a spinal cord injury. *Neurology.* 2000;54(8):1574–82.
8. Atkinson PP and Atkinson JL. Spinal shock. *Mayo Clin Proc.* 1996;71(4):384–9.
9. Ditunno JF, Little JW, Tessler A, and Burns AS. Spinal shock revisited: A four-phase model. *Spinal Cord.* 2004;42(7):383–95.
10. Bywater M, Tornic J, Mehnert U, and Kessler TM. Detrusor acontractility after acute spinal cord injury—Myth or reality? *J Urol.* 2018;199(6):1565–70.
11. de Groat WC, Kawatani M, Hisamitsu T et al. Mechanisms underlying the recovery of urinary bladder function following spinal cord injury. *J Auton Nerv Syst.* 1990;30(Suppl):S71–7.
12. Beric A, Dimitrijevic MR, and Light JK. A clinical syndrome of rostral and caudal spinal injury: Neurological, neurophysiological and urodynamic evidence for occult sacral lesion. *J Neurol Neurosurg Psychiatry.* 1987;50(5):600–6.
13. Light JK and Beric A. Detrusor function in suprasacral spinal cord injuries. *J Urol.* 1992;148(2 Pt 1):355–8.
14. Suzuki Bellucci CH, Wollner J, Gregorini F et al. External urethral sphincter pressure measurement: An accurate method for the diagnosis of detrusor external sphincter dyssynergia? *PLOS ONE.* 2012;7(5):e37996.
15. Walter M, Knupfer SC, Cragg JJ et al. Prediction of autonomic dysreflexia during urodynamics: A prospective cohort study. *BMC Med.* 2018;16(1):53.
16. Krassioukov A, Biering-Sorensen F, Donovan W et al. International standards to document remaining autonomic function after spinal cord injury. *J Spinal Cord Med.* 2012;35(4):201–10.
17. Shergill IS, Arya M, Hamid R, Khastgir J, Patel HR, and Shah PJ. The importance of autonomic dysreflexia to the urologist. *BJU Int.* 2004;93(7):923–6.
18. Peeters W, van den Brande R, Polinder S et al. Epidemiology of traumatic brain injury in Europe. *Acta Neurochir (Wien).* 2015;157(10):1683–96.
19. Dewan MC, Rattani A, Gupta S et al. Estimating the global incidence of traumatic brain injury. *J Neurosurg.* 2018:1–18. doi:10.3171/2017.10.JNS17352
20. Born JD. The Glasgow-Liege Scale. Prognostic value and evolution of motor response and brain stem reflexes after severe head injury. *Acta Neurochir (Wien).* 1988;91(1–2):1–11.

OTHER NEUROLOGIC PATHOLOGIES RESPONSIBLE FOR NEUROGENIC BLADDER DYSFUNCTION

CEREBRAL PALSY, CEREBELLAR ATAXIA, AIDS, PHACOMATOSIS, NEUROMUSCULAR DISORDERS, AND EPILEPSY

Ali Alsulihem and Jacques Corcos

INTRODUCTION

In comparison to most neurologic diseases, some infrequent neurologic conditions are rarely associated with urologic symptoms. Although urinary disturbance is well recognized in some of these conditions, in others, such as neuromuscular disorders, cases are rare and reports are anecdotal.

CEREBRAL PALSY

Cerebral palsy is becoming increasingly common as more premature, low birth weight infants are surviving. The combination of mental, neurologic, and physical handicap results in urinary symptoms and incontinence and are relatively common in patients with cerebral palsy.

Roijen et al.[1] reported a prevalence for primary urinary incontinence (UI) of 23.5%. In this study, 96% of all children with cerebral palsy who had normal intelligence (intelligence quotient [IQ] greater than 65) were continent; children with spastic tetraplegia and low intelligence (IQ less than 65) were the least likely to become continent. Other lower urinary tract symptoms (LUTS) are not exceptional mainly in spastic patients[2–6] (Table 17.1).

As shown in Table 17.2, overactive detrusor consistent with an upper motor neuron injury was the most common urodynamic finding in symptomatic patients with cerebral palsy.[2–5,8,9]

Given the risk of upper tract damage in neurogenic voiding dysfunction, Brodak et al.[10] used ultrasound to prospectively screen 90 patients (aged 1–25 years old), with or without urologic symptoms. The authors concluded that routine urinary tract screening was not justified because urinary tract abnormalities were only detected in 2% of the patients studied. Reliability of usual questionnaires in this population is good enough to recommend their use.[11] Urodynamic study remains the best test to characterize the type of voiding dysfunction in this population.[12]

Treatment for patients with overactive bladders (OABs) and symptoms of urge and frequency consists primarily of anticholinergic drugs. Postmicturition bladder residuals should then be closely monitored, as clean intermittent catheterization (CIC) may be necessary with increasing residuals. Using a combination of medication and behavioral modification (e.g., frequent voiding schedule), Decter et al.[4] were able to improve incontinence in 21 of the 27 patients with cerebral palsy (78%). Murphy et al.[8] instigated a functional toileting review in 35 patients with neurogenic bladder, 26 of whom also required oxybutynin therapy, with the addition of desmopressin and pseudoephedrine hydrochloride in 3. Positive continence outcomes were seen in 32 (91%), with no apparent relationship to motor severity or mobility status. Karaman et al.[6] advocated early intermittent catheterization with or without anticholinergics for increased residual urine and voiding. Several authors have demonstrated an increase in bladder capacity by carrying out pre- and postsacral rhizotomy urodynamic studies.[10,11]

CEREBELLAR AND SPINOCEREBELLAR DISORDERS

In cerebellar ataxia, the cerebellum and/or the pathways connecting the cerebellum with other parts of the nervous system undergo progressive, premature neuronal death and atrophy. The result is a heterogeneous spectrum of motor abnormalities that manifests as an abnormal broad-based gait, incoordination, tremor, dysarthria, and motor and autonomic dysfunction. The etiology in many

Table 17.1   Distribution of the Common Lower Urinary Tract Symptoms in Patients with Cerebral Palsy Undergoing Urologic Assessment

	McNeal et al.[5]	Decter et al.[4]	Mayo[3]	Reid and Borzyskowski[2]
Number of patients Symptoms	50	57	33	27
Incontinence[a]	54%	86%	48%	74%
Urgency	18%			37%
Frequency		51%		56%
Dribbling	6%			
Hesitancy/voiding difficulties		3.5%	46%	11%
Retention		2%	6%	7%

Note: Some patients had multiple symptoms.
[a] Incontinence includes urge/stress/day and/or enuresis.

Table 17.2   Urodynamic Findings in Patients with Cerebral Palsy

	Reid et al.[2]	Mayo[3]	Decter et al.[4]	McNeal et al.[5]	Drigo et al.[9]	Karaman et al.[6]
Number of patients	27	33	57	13	9	36
Detrusor overactivity	21 (78%)	22 (67%)	35 (61%)	4 (31%)	9 (100%)	17 (47%)
End-fill instability				2 (15%)		
Detrusor sphincter dyssynergia	5 (19%)	1 (3%)	7 (17%)		2 (22%)	4 (11%)
Acontractile bladder	2		1			

cases is an underlying genetic abnormality, of which Friedreich's ataxia is the most common and accounts for at least 50% of hereditary ataxias. In isolated cerebellar disorders, urinary disturbance is generally absent.[19] More frequently, the degenerative neuropathologic process affects multiple systems including the brainstem, cerebrum, and spinal cord, in which case urinary symptoms are more likely.

Chami et al.[15] found 23% had urgency and 6% had UI in a cohort of 195 patients. Detrusor-sphincter dyssynergia and acontractility are less common and correlate with the extent of neuronal damage in the spinal cord. In Chami's work, 23 (64%) patients had normal urodynamic studies, but detrusor overactivity was found in 6 and detrusor acontractility in 2, even though the majority of patients were asymptomatic. This has been confirmed by many authors (Table 17.33).[16–18]

More recent studies have found that urinary dysfunction in patients with genetically defined causes of spinocerebellar ataxia (SCA) was very rare.[21–24]

Treatment for urgency and urge incontinence in patients with ataxia ideally should be specific to the urodynamic findings. However, the likelihood is an underlying OAB, and these patients could be treated empirically with anticholinergics if they

do not carry large residual volumes. Patients with underactive detrusor can be treated with intermittent catheterization. Leach et al.[14] successfully treated their three patients with sphincter dyssynergia with a combination of α-sympathetic blockade (phenoxybenzamine), diazepam, and baclofen.

Nonhereditary ataxias with a multitude of etiologies, e.g., alcohol intoxication, neurosarcoidosis, central nervous system (CNS) infection, and superficial siderosis, can present acutely or subacutely, with UI as a common symptom.

HUMAN IMMUNODEFICIENCY VIRUS INFECTION AND ACQUIRED IMMUNODEFICIENCY SYNDROME

LUTS in the well HIV-positive patient is uncommon. Impaired micturition becomes more common with disease progression, due to global neurologic dysfunction or infection.[25,26] Urodynamic abnormality, either an overactive, underactive detrusor, or DSD, was identified in 87% of patients, and 61% of them had AIDS-related neurologic problems (cerebral toxoplasmosis, HIV demyelination disorders, AIDS-related dementia).

Table 17.3 Urodynamic Findings in Patients with Cerebellospinal Ataxia

	Leach et al.[14]	Vezina et al.[16]	Chami et al.[15]	Sakakibara et al.[17]
Number of patients	15	17	55	11
Hyperreflexia	8 (53%)	7 (41%)	14 (25%)	5 (45%)
Detrusor-sphincter dyssynergia	3 (6%)	6 (37%)		2 (18%)
Detrusor acontractility	4 (27%)		9 (16%)	3 (27%)

This has a poor prognosis, as 43% in this group died after 2–24 months.[27]

Urinary sphincter abnormalities leading to UI or retention occur secondary to spinal cord compression (metastatic lymphoma, tuberculoma) or infection of the spinal cord or nerve roots by opportunistic infections.[28]

Detrusor failure due to lower motor lesions is uncommon and caused by malignancy or infection. Patients should do CIC. Indwelling catheters should be avoided to reduce risks of infections.

NEUROCUTANEOUS SYNDROMES (PHACOMATOSIS)

Neurocutaneous syndromes encompass a number of hereditary conditions involving nervous system, eyeball, retina, and skin. They present in childhood and slowly progress through adolescence.[29,30]

NEUROFIBROMATOSIS TYPES 1 AND 2
Various NF1-associated tumors affect the urinary system and particularly the bladder. They are derived from nerves of the pelvic, vesical, and prostatic plexuses,[31] and include benign and, less commonly, malignant tumors. Plexiform neurofibromas can involve the perineal region leading to local urinary tract involvement. These should be suspected when patients develop symptoms (LUTS, enuresis, flank pain, incontinence, or symptoms related to urinary tract obstruction, localized pain, low back pain, and lower limb dysesthesia).[32] These symptoms may result from tumor size and/or neurogenic involvement.[33–36] Conservative management is suggested, as it is likely to damage adjacent organs if removed. Careful follow-up is necessary to detect signs of upper tract obstruction, a sign of tumor progression or malignant transformation.[33]

NF2 is characterized by the presence of schwannomas.[37] Spinal schwannomas may lead to upper motor neuron syndromes due to spinal cord compression.[38–39] Other tumors can involve the spinal cord, including ependymomas, meningiomas, or hamartomas.[39–45] Those may involve the conus or cauda equina and may present with mixed upper and/or lower motor neuron bladder symptoms.[45–47]

KLIPPEL-TRENAUNAY-WEBER SYNDROME
Klippel-Trenaunay-Weber syndrome (KTWS) is characterized by cutaneous port wine stains, complex vascular anomalies (angiomas) that combine capillary, venous and lymphatic components, and soft tissue and/or bony hypertrophy of an extremity. Genitourinary (GU) manifestations are present in up to 30% of patients, and intermittent gross hematuria from vascular anomalies in the GU tract is the most common symptom (65%).[48] LUTS would be expected if symptomatic spinal cord pathology occurred due to pressure or bleeding from large spinal angiomas.[49–51] In a case report, a patient with KTWS with extensive spinal arteriovenous malformation presented with progressive paraparesis and urinary retention. After surgical treatment, bladder dysfunction disappeared after 6 months.[52]

NEUROMUSCULAR DISORDERS

NEUROMUSCULAR JUNCTION DISORDERS
MYASTHENIA GRAVIS
Bladder disturbance attributable to myasthenia gravis (MG) is unusual.[53–58] The bladder dysfunction in most reported cases resembles lower motor neuron patterns (incomplete bladder emptying, hypotonic bladder, etc.).

Varying degrees of voiding dysfunction have been reported.[53–58] It can be complete and prolonged.[57] Urinary symptoms may respond to medications directed to treat MG.[54,56] Voiding dysfunction may be the initial presenting symptom[53,55] and may be associated with an exacerbation of generalized MG.[55,57] The fluctuation in severity related to drug treatment of MG suggests a causal relationship in some cases.

Few studies reported MG patients with OAB and urodynamic detrusor overactivity.[59–60] Anticholinergics are contraindicated in MG patients, and β_3-agonists is usually the first treatment option.[59–60] Successful posterior tibial nerve stimulation in a MG patient with OAB was reported.[60] Intradetrusor onabotulinumtoxinA (Botox-100 units) has been used without exacerbations of MG.[59]

LUTS in MG is reported in patients who had prostatic surgery. Patients with bladder outlet obstruction who underwent complete transurethral resection of the prostate (TURP) have developed UI, caused probably by injuring external sphincters compromised by MG.[61] In incomplete TURP, a patient initially remained dry but developed urgency urinary incontinence (UUI) 3 months later.[61] It was found that incontinence after TURP was associated with the use of blended current. Patients treated with high-frequency unblended current, partial proximal resection, or open prostatectomy, have remained dry.[62]

LAMBERT-EATON MYASTHENIC SYNDROME
Bladder involvement is rare in Lambert-Eaton myasthenic syndrome (LEMS). Bladder dysfunction has been reported in five cases,[63–65] and urodynamic findings were reported in a woman with LEMS[65] who had urinary frequency, reduced maximal urinary flow rate, and elevated PVR (underactive detrusor). After treatment with 3,4-diaminopyridine, urinary frequency improved. Posttreatment anal sphincter EMG and detrusor and abdominal pressures also increased markedly during voiding, suggesting that neurogenic lower urinary tract dysfunction (NLUTD) was caused by defective neurotransmission in autonomic detrusor muscle and skeletal abdominal muscle due to LEMS.

MUSCULAR DYSTROPHIES

MYOTONIC DYSTROPHY
Urinary tract dysfunction is less common in this disease.[66] Urinary retention[67–69] and symptomatic bladder dysfunction were found in a few patients.[70–71] Symptoms included urinary urgency, frequency, and stress urinary incontinence (SUI). Urodynamic investigation revealed reduced urethral pressures and abnormal motor units in the external sphincter. Pelvic floor muscle involvement could cause SUI, particularly in females.[72]

DUCHENNE MUSCULAR DYSTROPHY
NLUTD in Duchenne muscular dystrophy (DMD) is unusual.[73–78] Several reports[73–75] showed various presentations, including UI or retention. The mechanism of NLUTD is unclear. Myopathic changes within the detrusor muscle would be expected to cause a flaccid bladder, while pathology in skeletal pelvic floor muscles could account for SUI.[75] The upper motor neuron lesions are likely due to scoliosis, or complications of its surgical treatment, or due to altered expression of dystrophin on the CNS.[74–75] NLUTD might be associated with fatty infiltration of the filum terminale. Sectioning of the filum terminale has resulted in recovery of urinary continence in a reported case.[78]

EPILEPSY

CORTICAL BLADDER CONTROL AND SEIZURE LOCALIZATION
Several brain regions are implicated in cortical control of urinary function. Functional studies suggest lateralization to the right hemisphere for cortical bladder control,[79–81] which explains the urinary symptoms during partial seizures arising from the right hemisphere.

UI can occur following resection of a seizure focus in the supracallosal portion of the left medial frontal gyrus, with urodynamic features of reduced bladder sensation, increased bladder capacity, and involuntary detrusor contraction.[82]

INCONTINENCE IN SEIZURES
Incontinence is the most reported LUTS in epilepsy, followed by urgency, frequency, retention, and hesitancy.[83]

During absence seizures, detrusor overactivity has been recorded.[84] Enuresis following generalized tonic-clonic seizures is due to relaxation of the external sphincter.[85] During absence status, UI occurs as a result of micturitional automatism or neglect. The prevalence of incontinence in seizure subtypes is unknown.

MICTURITION IN LOCALIZATION RELATED EPILEPSY (PARTIAL SEIZURES)
Seizures involving the autonomic nervous system are associated with LUTS. Autonomic seizures arise from mediobasal limbic, frontal, orbital, or opercular regions.[86–88] Autonomic phenomena comprise one-third of all simple partial seizures.[87–89]

EARLY ONSET BENIGN CHILDHOOD SEIZURES WITH OCCIPITAL SPIKES (PANAYIOTOPOULOS SYNDROME)
Autonomic symptoms are prominent in Panayiotopoulos syndrome (PS).[90] UI occurs in 10%. It is benign with good prognosis. Half of patients have a single attack, and in the majority of the remainder, spontaneous remission occurs within a few years.

ICTAL URINARY URGE IN PARTIAL SEIZURES (AURAS)
This is a well-recognized feature of temporal lobe seizures, and it presents in up to 8%.[87,91–95] Electroencephalogram (EEG) and imaging suggested its onset in the nondominant temporal lobe.[93,95]

MICTURITION-INDUCED REFLEX EPILEPSY
Micturition-induced reflex epilepsy (MIRE) was reported in a few children.[96–103] Some had learning difficulties[97–98] or structural pathology.[99] EEG recordings, semiology,

video-EEG, and ictal single-photon emission computed tomography (SPECT) studies were used to determine the location of onset. Areas reported include central anterior or right frontal lobe, deep midline structures, supplementary sensorimotor region, central midline region, anterior cingulate gyrus and anterolateral right frontal lobe, and supplementary sensorimotor area of the right frontal lobe.[96-103]

URINARY SYMPTOMS RELATED TO ANTIEPILEPTIC DRUGS

Frequency and UI have been reported as adverse reactions to antiepileptic medications. They are unusual side effects of carbamazepine and valproate.[104] UI was reported with gabapentin, which persisted with taking the drug and disappeared after it was discontinued or reduced.[105]

Retigabine may cause urinary hesitancy and retention. It should be used with caution in patients at risk of urinary retention.[106-107]

TREATMENT OF BLADDER SYMPTOMS IN EPILEPSY

Treatment of incontinence related to epilepsy should be aimed toward treating seizures by antiepileptic drugs. Oxybutynin might be beneficial in selected patients.[7] However, anticholinergics may not be effective, particularly if incontinence is related to autonomic seizures.

REFERENCES

1. Roijen LE, Postema K, Limbeek VJ, and Kuppevelt VH. Development of bladder control in children and adolescents with cerebral palsy. *Dev Med Child Neurol.* 2001;43:103–7.
2. Reid CJ and Borzyskowski M. Lower urinary tract dysfunction in cerebral palsy. *Arch Dis Child.* 1993;68:739–42.
3. Mayo ME. Lower urinary tract dysfunction in cerebral palsy. *J Urol.* 1992;147:419–20.
4. Decter RM, Bauer SB, Khoshbin S et al. Urodynamic assessment of children with cerebral palsy. *J Urol.* 1987;138:1110–2.
5. McNeal DM, Hawtrey CE, Wolraich ML, and Mapel JR. Symptomatic neurogenic bladder in a cerebral-palsied population. *Dev Med Child Neurol.* 1983;25:612–6.
6. Karaman MI, Kaya C, Caskurlu T, Guney S, and Ergenekon E. Urodynamic findings in children with cerebral palsy. *Int J Urol.* 2005;12:717–20.
7. Harari D and Malone-Lee JG. Oxybutynin and incontinence during grand mal seizures. *Br J Urol.* 1991;68:658.
8. Murphy KP, Boutin SA, and Ide KR. Cerebral palsy, neurogenic bladder, and outcomes of lifetime care. *Dev Med Child Neurol.* 2012;54:945–50.
9. Drigo P, Seren F, Artibani W, Laverda AM, Battistella PA, and Zacchello G. Neurogenic vesico-urethral dysfunction in children with cerebral palsy. *Ital J Neurol Sci.* 1988;9:151–4.
10. Brodak PP, Scherz HC, Packer MG, and Kaplan GW. Is urinary tract screening necessary for patients with cerebral palsy? *J Urol.* 1994;152:1586–7.
11. Pariser JJ, Welk B, Kennelly M, and Elliott SP. Reliability and validity of the neurogenic bladder symptom score in adults with cerebral palsy. *Urology.* 2019;128:107–11.
12. Cotter KJ, Levy ME, Goldfarb RA et al. Urodynamic findings in adults with moderate to severe cerebral palsy. *Urology.* 2016;95:216–21.
13. Moulin F, Quintart A, Sauvestre C, Mensah K, Bergeret M, and Raymond J. [Nosocomial urinary tract infections: Retrospective study in a pediatric hospital]. *Arch Pediatr.* 1998;5(Suppl 3):274S–8S.
14. Leach GE, Farsaii A, Kark P, and Raz S. Urodynamic manifestations of cerebellar ataxia. *J Urol.* 1982;128:348–50.
15. Chami I, Miladi N, Ben Hamida M, and Zmerli S. [Continence disorders in hereditary spinocerebellar degeneration. Comparison of clinical and urodynamic findings in 55 cases]. *Acta Neurol Belg.* 1984;84:194–203.
16. Vezina JG, Bouchard JP, and Bouchard R. Urodynamic evaluation of patients with hereditary ataxias. *Can J Neurol Sci.* 1982;9:127–9.
17. Sakakibara R, Uchiyama T, Arai K, Yamanishi T, and Hattori T. Lower urinary tract dysfunction in Machado-Joseph disease: A study of 11 clinical-urodynamic observations. *J Neurol Sci.* 2004;218:67–72.
18. Sugiyama M, Sakakibara R, Tateno F et al. Voiding dysfunction in spinocerebellar ataxia type 31. *Low Urin Tract Symptoms.* 2014;6(1):64–7.
19. Yamamoto T, Yamanaka Y, Sugiyama A et al. The severity of motor dysfunctions and urinary dysfunction is not correlated in multiple system atrophy. *J Neurol Sci.* 2019;400:25–9.
20. Coon EA, Sletten DM, Suarez MD et al. Clinical features and autonomic testing predict survival in multiple system atrophy. *Brain.* 2015;138(Pt 12):3623–31.
21. Schols L, Amoiridis G, Epplen JT, Langkafel M, Przuntek H, and Riess O. Relations between genotype and phenotype in German patients with the Machado-Joseph disease mutation. *J Neurol Neurosurg Psychiatry.* 1996;61:466–70.
22. Watanabe M, Abe K, Aoki M et al. Analysis of CAG trinucleotide expansion associated with Machado-Joseph disease. *J Neurol Sci.* 1996;136:101–7.
23. Yeh TH, Lu CS, Chou YH et al. Autonomic dysfunction in Machado-Joseph disease. *Arch Neurol.* 2005;62:630–6.
24. Schmitz-Hubsch T, Coudert M, Bauer P et al. Spinocerebellar ataxia types 1, 2, 3, and 6: Disease severity and nonataxia symptoms. *Neurology.* 2008;71:982–9.
25. Gyrtrup HJ, Kristiansen VB, Zachariae CO, Krogsgaard K, Colstrup H, and Jensen KM. Voiding problems in patients with HIV infection and AIDS. *Scand J Urol Nephrol.* 1995;29:295–8.
26. Zeman A and Donaghy M. Acute infection with human immunodeficiency virus presenting with neurogenic urinary retention. *Genitourin Med.* 1991;67:345–7.
27. Hermieu JF, Delmas V, and Boccon-Gibod L. Micturition disturbances and human immunodeficiency virus infection. *J Urol.* 1996;156:157–9.
28. Thurnher MM, Post MJ, and Jinkins JR. MRI of infections and neoplasms of the spine and spinal cord in 55 patients with AIDS. *Neuroradiology.* 2000;42:551–63.

29. Baraister M. Neurocutaneous disorders. In: Baraister M, ed. *The Genetics of Neurological Disorders*, 3rd ed. Oxford, United Kingdom: Oxford University Press; 1997:85–101.

30. Dahan D, Fenichel GM, and El-Said R. Neurocutaneous syndromes. *Adolesc Med*. 2002;13:495–509.

31. Hintsa A, Lindell O, and Heikkila P. Neurofibromatosis of the bladder. *Scand J Urol Nephrol*. 1996;30:497–9.

32. Dominguez J, Lobato RD, Ramos A, Rivas JJ, Gomez PA, and Castro S. Giant intrasacral schwannomas: Report of six cases. *Acta Neurochir (Wien)*. 1997;139:954–9; discussion 959–60.

33. Chakravarti A, Jones MA, and Simon J. Neurofibromatosis involving the urinary bladder. *Int J Urol*. 2001;8:645–7.

34. Clark SS, Marlett MM, Prudencio RF, and Dasgupta TK. Neurofibromatosis of the bladder in children: Case report and literature review. *J Urol*. 1977;118:654–6.

35. Daneman A and Grattan-Smith P. Neurofibromatosis involving the lower urinary tract in children. A report of three cases and a review of the literature. *Pediatr Urol*. 1976;4:161–6.

36. Cheng L, Scheithauer BW, Leibovich BC, Ramnani DM, Cheville JC, and Bostwick DG. Neurofibroma of the urinary bladder. *Cancer*. 1999;86:505–13.

37. Evans DGR. Neurofibromatosis 2. In: Ferner RE, Huson SM, and Evans DGR, eds. *Neurofibromatoses in Clinical Practice*. London, United Kingdom: Springer-Verlag; 2011:46–71.

38. Huson SM. The neurofibromatoses: Differential diagnosis and rare subtypes. In: Ferner RE, Huson SM, and Evans DGR, eds. *Neurofibromatoses in Clinical Practice*. London, United Kingdom: Springer-Verlag; 2011:71–122.

39. Evans DG, Mason S, Huson SM, Ponder M, Harding AE, and Strachan T. Spinal and cutaneous schwannomatosis is a variant form of type 2 neurofibromatosis: A clinical and molecular study. *J Neurol Neurosurg Psychiatry*. 1997;62:361–6.

40. Brownlee RD, Clark AW, Sevick RJ, and Myles ST. Symptomatic hamartoma of the spinal cord associated with neurofibromatosis type 1. Case report. *J Neurosurg*. 1998;88:1099–103.

41. Chaparro MJ, Young RF, Smith M, Shen V, and Choi BH. Multiple spinal meningiomas: A case of 47 distinct lesions in the absence of neurofibromatosis or identified chromosomal abnormality. *Neurosurgery*. 1993;32:298–301; discussion 301–2.

42. Babjakova L, Jurkovic I, Krajcar R, and Kocan P. [Multiple intracranial and intraspinal meningiomas in the neurocristopathy (phacomatosis) type of neurofibromatosis]. *Cesk Patol*. 2000;36:150–5.

43. Kawsar M and Goh BT. Spinal schwannoma as a cause of erectile dysfunction with urinary incontinence and groin and testicular pain. *Int J STD AIDS*. 2002;13:584–5.

44. Honda E, Hayashi T, Goto S et al. [Two different spinal tumors (meningioma and schwannoma) with von Recklinghausen's disease in a case]. *No Shinkei Geka*. 1990;18:463–8.

45. Mizuo T, Ando M, Azima J, Ohshima H, and Yamauchi A. [Manifestation of mictional disturbance in four cases of von Recklinghausen's disease]. *Hinyokika Kiyo*. 1987;33:125–32.

46. Caputo LA and Cusimano MD. Schwannoma of the cauda equina. *J Manipulative Physiol Ther*. 1997;20:124–9.

47. Acharya R, Bhalla S, and Sehgal AD. Malignant peripheral nerve sheath tumor of the cauda equina. *Neurol Sci*. 2001;22:267–70.

48. Husmann DA, Rathburn SR, and Driscoll DJ. Klippel-Trenaunay syndrome: Incidence and treatment of genitourinary sequelae. *J Urol*. 2007;177(4):1244–9.

49. Klippel M and Trenaunay P. Du naevus variquex osteo-hypertropique. *Arch Genet Med*. 1900;3:641–72.

50. Weber FP Angioma formation in connection with hypertrophy of limbs and hemihypertrophy. *Br J Dermatol*. 1907;19:231–5.

51. Weber FP. Hemiangioectatic hypertrophy of limbs. Congenital phlebarteriectasia and so-called congenital varicose veins. *Br J Child Dis*. 1918;15:13–7.

52. Kojima Y, Kuwana N, Sato M, and Ikeda Y. Klippel-Trenaunay-Weber syndrome with spinal arteriovenous malformation—Case report. *Neurol Med Chir (Tokyo)*. 1989;29:235–40.

53. Berger AR, Swerdlow M, and Herskovitz S. Myasthenia gravis presenting as uncontrollable flatus and urinary/fecal incontinence. *Muscle Nerve*. 1996;19:113–4.

54. Christmas TJ, Dixon PJ, and Milroy EJ. Detrusor failure in myasthenia gravis. *Br J Urol*. 1990;65:422.

55. Howard JFJ, Donovan MK, and Tucker MS. Urinary incontinence in myasthenia gravis: A single fibre electromyographic study. *Ann Neurol*. 1992;32:254.

56. Matsui M, Enoki M, Matsui Y et al. Seronegative myasthenia gravis associated with atonic urinary bladder and accommodative insufficiency. *J Neurol Sci*. 1995;133:197–9.

57. Sandler PM, Avillo C, and Kaplan SA. Detrusor areflexia in a patient with myasthenia gravis. *Int J Urol*. 1998;5:188–90.

58. Kaya C and Karaman MI. Case report: A case of bladder dysfunction due to myasthenia gravis. *Int Urol Nephrol*. 2005;37:253–5.

59. Wright I, Civitarese A, and Baverstock R. The use of intra-detrusor onabotulinumtoxinA in patients with myasthenia gravis. *Can Urol Assoc J*. 2016;10(5–6):E184–5.

60. Antoniou A, Mendez Rodrigues J, and Comi N. Successful treatment of urodynamic detrusor over-activity in a young patient with Myasthenia gravis using pretibial nerve stimulation with follow-up to two years. *JRSM Open*. 2016;7(8). doi:10.1177/2054270416653684

61. Greene LF, Ghosh MK, and Howard FM. Transurethral prostatic resection in patients with myasthenia gravis. *J Urol*. 1974;112:226–7.

62. Wise GJ, Gerstenfeld JN, Brunner N, and Grob D. Urinary incontinence following prostatectomy in patients with myasthenia gravis. *Br J Urol*. 1982;54:369–71.

63. Khurana RK, Koski CL, and Mayer RF. Autonomic dysfunction in Lambert-Eaton myasthenic syndrome. *J Neurol Sci*. 1988;85:77–86.

64. Henriksson KG, Nilsson O, Rosen I, and Schiller HH. Clinical, neurophysiological and morphological findings in Eaton Lambert syndrome. *Acta Neurol Scand*. 1977;56:117–40.

65. Satoh K, Motomura M, Suzu H et al. Neurogenic bladder in Lambert-Eaton myasthenic syndrome and its response to 3,4-diaminopyridine. *J Neurol Sci*. 2001;183:1–4.

66. Harper PS. Smooth muscle in myotonic dystrophy. In: Harper PS, ed. *Major Problems in Neurology: Myotonic Dystrophy*, 3rd ed, No 37. London, United Kingdom: WB Saunders; 2001:91–108.

67. Harvey JC, Sherbourne DH, and Siegel CI. Smooth muscle involvement in myotonic dystrophy. *Am J Med.* 1965;39:81–90.

68. Kohn NN, Faires JS, and Rodman T. Unusual manifestations due to involvement of involuntary muscle in dystrophia myotonica. *N Engl J Med.* 1964;271:1179–83.

69. Pruzanski W. Myotonic dystrophy. A multisystem disease. Report of 67 cases and a review of the literature. *Psychiatr Neurol (Basel).* 1965;149:302–22.

70. Bernstein IT, Andersen BB, Andersen JT, and Arlien-Oborg P. Bladder function in patients with myotonic dystrophy. *Neurol Urody.* 1992;11:219–23.

71. Sakakibara R, Hattori T, Tojo M, Yamanishi T, Yasuda K, and Hirayama K. Micturitional disturbance in myotonic dystrophy. *J Auton Nerv Syst.* 1995;52:17–21.

72. Dickson MJ, Massiah N, and Church E. Urinary stress incontinence as the presenting feature of myotonic dystrophy. *J Obstet Gynaecol.* 2012;32:102.

73. Boland BJ, Silbert PL, Groover RV, Wollan PC, and Silverstein MD. Skeletal, cardiac, and smooth muscle failure in Duchenne muscular dystrophy. *Pediatr Neurol.* 1996;14:7–12.

74. Caress JB, Kothari MJ, Bauer SB, and Shefner JM. Urinary dysfunction in Duchenne muscular dystrophy. *Muscle Nerve.* 1996;19:819–22.

75. MacLeod M, Kelly R, Robb SA, and Borzyskowski M. Bladder dysfunction in Duchenne muscular dystrophy. *Arch Dis Child.* 2003;88:347–9.

76. van Wijk E, Messelink BJ, Heijnen L, and de Groot IJ. Prevalence and psychosocial impact of lower urinary tract symptoms in patients with Duchenne muscular dystrophy. *Neuromuscul Disord.* 2009;19:754–8.

77. Smith MD, Seth JH, Hanna MG, and Panicker JN. Detrusor overactivity in Becker muscular dystrophy. *Muscle Nerve.* 2013;47:464–5.

78. Tubbs RS, and Oakes WJ. Urinary incontinence in a patient with Duchenne muscular dystrophy and cord in the normal position with fatty filum terminale. *Childs Nerv Syst.* 2004;20:717–9.

79. Blok BF and Holstege G. The central control of micturition and continence: Implications for urology. *BJU Int.* 1999;83(Suppl 2):1–6.

80. Blok BF, Sturms LM, and Holstege G. Brain activation during micturition in women. *Brain.* 1998;121(Pt 11):2033–42.

81. Blok BF, Willemsen AT, and Holstege G. A PET study on brain control of micturition in humans. *Brain.* 1997;120(Pt 1):111–21.

82. Sekido N and Akaza H. Neurogenic bladder may be a side effect of focus resection in an epileptic patient. *Int J Urol.* 1997;4:101–3.

83. Jang HJ, Kwon MJ, and Cho KO. Central regulation of micturition and its association with epilepsy. *Int Neurourol J.* 2018;22(1):2–8.

84. Gastaut H, Batini C, Broughton R, Lob H, and Roger J. Polygraphic study of enuresis during petit mal seizures. *Electroencephalogr Clin Neurophysiol.* 1964;16(6)616–26.

85. Gastaut H, Broughton R, Roger J, and Tassinari C. Generalized nonconvulsive seizures without local onset. In: Vinken PJ, and Bruyn GW, eds. *Handbook of Clinical Neurology.* New York, NY; 1974:130–44.

86. Liporace JD and Sperling MR. Simple autonomic seizures. In: Engel JJ, and Pedley TA, eds. *Epilepsy: The Comprehensive CD-ROM.* Philadelphia, PA: Lippincott Williams and Wilkins; 1999.

87. Gupta AK, Jeavons PM, Hughes RC, and Covanis A. Aura in temporal lobe epilepsy: Clinical and electroencephalographic correlation. *J Neurol Neurosurg Psychiatry.* 1983;46:1079–83.

88. Palmini A and Gloor P. The localizing value of auras in partial seizures: A prospective and retrospective study. *Neurology.* 1992;42:801–8.

89. Devinsky O, Kelley K, Porter RJ, and Theodore WH. Clinical and electroencephalographic features of simple partial seizures. *Neurology.* 1988;38:1347–52.

90. Panayiotopoulos CP. Autonomic seizures and autonomic status epilepticus specific to childhood. *Arch Pediatr Adolesc Med.* 2002;156:945.

91. Feindel W and Penfield W. Localization of discharge in temporal lobe automatism. *AMA Arch Neurol Psychiatry.* 1954;72:603–30.

92. Inthaler S, Donati F, Pavlincova E, Vassella F, and Staldemann C. Partial complex epileptic seizures with ictal urogenital manifestation in a child. *Eur Neurol.* 1991;31:212–5.

93. Baumgartner C, Groppel G, Leutmezer F et al. Ictal urinary urge indicates seizure onset in the nondominant temporal lobe. *Neurology.* 2000;55:432–4.

94. O'Donovan C, Burgess R, and Luders H. *Aura in Temporal Lobe Epilepsy.* New York, NY: Churchill Livingstone; 2000.

95. Loddenkemper T, Foldvary N, Raja S, Neme S, and Luders HO. Ictal urinary urge: Further evidence for lateralization to the nondominant hemisphere. *Epilepsia.* 2003;44:124–6.

96. Glass HC, Prieur B, Molnar C, Hamiwka L, and Wirrell E. Micturition and emotion-induced reflex epilepsy: Case report and review of the literature. *Epilepsia.* 2006;47:2180–2.

97. Bourgeois BF. A retarded boy with seizures precipitated by stepping into the bath water. *Semin Pediatr Neurol.* 1999;6:151–6; discussion 156–7.

98. Spinnler H and Valli G. [Micturition "reflex" epilepsy. Presentation of a clinical case]. *Riv Patol Nerv Ment.* 1969;90:212–20.

99. Pradhan S and Kalita J. Micturition-induced reflex epilepsy. *Neurol Ind* 1993;41:221–3.

100. Okumura A, Kondo Y, Tsuji T et al. Micturition induced seizures: Ictal EEG and subtraction ictal SPECT findings. *Epilepsy Res.* 2007;73:119–21.

101. Ikeno T, Morikawa A, and Kimura I. A case of epileptic seizure evoked by micturition. *Rinsho Nouha* 1998;40:205–8.

102. Yamatani M, Murakami M, Konda M et al. [An 8-year-old girl with micturition-induced epilepsy]. *No To Hattatsu.* 1987;19:58–62.

103. Zivin I and Rowley W. Psychomotor epilepsy with micturition. *Arch Intern Med.* 1964;113:8–13.

104. *Physicians' Desk Reference,* 50th ed. Montvale, NJ: Medical Economics; 1996:2350.

105. Gil-Nagel A, Gapany S, Blesi K, Villanueva N, and Bergen D. Incontinence during treatment with gabapentin. *Neurology.* 1997;48:1467–8.

106. Brickel N, Gandhi P, VanLandingham K, Hammond J, and DeRossett S. The urinary safety profile and secondary renal effects of retigabine (ezogabine): A first-in-class antiepileptic drug that targets KCNQ ($K(v)7$) potassium channels. *Epilepsia.* 2012;53:606–12.

107. Ciliberto MA, Weisenberg JL, and Wong M. Clinical utility, safety, and tolerability of ezogabine (retigabine) in the treatment of epilepsy. *Drug Healthc Patient Saf.* 2012;4:81–6.

Chapter 18

SYRINGOMYELIA AND LOWER URINARY TRACT DYSFUNCTION

Jairam R. Eswara

INTRODUCTION

Syringomyelia is a condition that presents within the spinal cord. While there are many methods of formation, each method results in a fluid-filled cavity known as a "syrinx." The cavity that forms fills with cerebrospinal fluid and can cause a variety of symptoms. If the syrinx is left untreated, it may continue to grow. Generally, the larger the syrinx is, the more symptomatic a patient will be. Syringomyelia develops over long periods of time and can have very devastating effects on the body. A major problem that can arise in patients with syringomyelia is the development of lower urinary tract disorder. *Syringomyelia can be diagnosed using magnetic resonance imaging* and can be detected through neurologic, urologic, and clinical signs. The major forms of syringomyelia are split into primary cases with unknown causes and secondary cases with known causes.

PRIMARY SYRINGOMYELIA

ETIOPATHOGENY

There are a handful of theories that explain why syringomyelia occurs. The dysraphic theory was one of the first theories attempting to correctly identify syringomyelia's cause of formation. The theory states that *a closing defect prevents the neural tube from sealing between the 21st and 28th days of embryonal life. This embryopathy would arise from abnormal constitution of the posterior raphe. Bony anomalies associated with cervico-occipital transition and Chiari malformation would have no physiopathologic link.* A more recent theory was formed by Gardner in the 1950s. In his theory, Gardner stated that cerebrospinal fluid (CSF) plays a pathogenic role in the formation of syringomyelia. *This primitive embryologic disorder comprises a lack or late opening of the roof orifices of the fourth ventricle that links the great cistern with the perimedullary and pericerebral subarachnoid spaces. Thus, a CSF hyperpressure is responsible*

for downward dilation of the spinal central canal. Individuals with Chiari malformations experience a similar hyperpressure, as the cerebellar tonsils extend into the foramen magnum, which restricts the flow of CSF. This hyperpressure can cause physical pain and neurologic damage over time as the resulting syrinx extends down the canal.

Aboulker's theory insists on the transition effect. Any effort generating venous hyperpressure creates growth of CSF pressure in the perimedullary spaces. This hyperpressure is normally transmitted upward to the cranious spaces. In the case of cervico-occipital bony abnormalities, CSF passage to the great cistern is held up, and the consequent hyperpressure furthers CSF entry into the medullary spaces, about the level of the posterior rootlets. Coalescence of the liquid lakes forms the syringomyelic cavity.

CLINICAL AND NEUROLOGICAL SIGNS

Although syringomyelia is difficult to diagnose, it often presents a number of identifiable signs that can be found when working with a patient. The most common signs are paresthesia, *walking incapacity, cervical or cephalic pain, vertigo, motor deficiency of a limb, trophic signs (painless burn), and rapidly progressing thoracic scoliosis of adolescence.* The pressure that the syrinx and CSF exert in patients with syringomyelia has the potential to cause neurologic deterioration, which visibly presents as one or more of the symptoms described earlier. This neurologic deterioration, however, does not always occur, and a patient with syringomyelia may not show any of the related symptoms until late in the condition's development. It can also be difficult to determine the difference between syringomyelia and other spinal cord pathologies. Magnetic resonance imaging (MRI) should be performed if a patient presents any of the previously mentioned symptoms as they often relate to spinal cord pathologies, including syringomyelia.

When performing an MRI on a patient with syringomyelia, a few things are clearly seen. The *syrinx is tube shaped and extends beyond the spinal cord injury (SCI) site to at least two vertebral levels. The signal is homogeneous and clearly delimits the upper and lower limits of the syringomyelia. The extension is always much more significant than the clinics suppose.*

UROLOGIC SIGNS

While they often present late in the development of syringomyelia, there are a handful of neuro-urologic disorders that may potentially hint at the development of syringomyelia in a patient. As pressure builds within and the syrinx grows within the spinal cord, there is the potential for neurologic damage to occur, which may result in a variety of urologic disorders. A patient with this deterioration may experience difficulty voiding, nocturia, urge incontinence, hesitancy, or many other disorders not discussed.

SECONDARY SYRINGOMYELIA

ETIOPATHOGENY

A secondary syringomyelia has the potential to form due to a few known causes: *arachnoiditis, tumors, or overall post-traumatic condition* (Figure 18.1). The two main steps in the development of secondary syringomyelia involve the formation of a cavity and the resulting cavity's extension. When a syringomyelic cavity forms, there are often two reasons for its occurrence. Many patients with SCIs will experience varying levels of necrosis within the affected area. It is for this reason that a cavity may form, as the tissue within the spinal cord deteriorates. The other main reason for a cavity's occurrence in patients is arachnoiditis. The inflammation of the arachnoid creates a tightness within the spinal cord and may irreversibly stretch as a patient bends and moves during the day (Figure 18.2).

CLINICAL AND NEUROLOGIC SIGNS

Pain is the most common symptom associated with syringomyelia. The pain often localized to the affected area of the spinal cord; however, the pain may also radiate from its origin due to strain and pressure on the spinal cord. Other symptoms include paresthesia and numbness. Similar to primary syringomyelias, secondary syringomyelias can easily be seen using an MRI. On average, the spinal cavity tends to extend *3.5 vertebral segments in asymptomatic patients and 10 vertebral segments in symptomatic cases.*

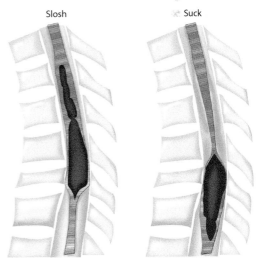

Figure 18.2   According to Williams' theory, secondary extension from the initial necrosis zone is a consequence of increased epidural venous pressure at the origin of intrachordal fluid movements due to thoracic and/or abdominal pressure increase. "Slush" leads to rostral extension and breaks down the zones of structural weakness; "suck" is the consequence of a pressure gradient at the origin of the caudal extension and filling of the cavity. These two phenomena are increased in the case of blockage in the subarachnoid space, notably in the case of arachnoiditis after a traumatic spinal cord injury. (Reproduced with permission from Macmillan Publishers Ltd. *Paraplegia*, Williams B, Posttraumatic syringomyelia, an update, June 1990;28(5), 296–313, copyright 1990.)

Figure 18.1   Post-traumatic syringomyelia.

UROLOGIC SIGNS

When spinal injuries occur, secondary syringomyelia can form in the affected area. As the secondary syringomyelia progresses, the resulting syrinx that forms within the damaged area of the spinal cord, along with other forms of deterioration, can result in urologic symptoms. Syringomyelia has been found to cause urologic problems when a spinal injury is located near the sacrum. The pressure within the spinal cord and the developing syrinx can deteriorate the surrounding nervous tissue. This deterioration of nervous tissue at the sacrum can result in a variety of neuro-urologic disorders. For patients with syringomyelia, a major part of their recovery is focused on preventing the formation of a syrinx. *Follow-up must be regular during the first 2 years and then it should become annual with clinical, urodynamic, and morphologic studies. Less frequent follow-up can be discussed in case there is no significant risk factor.*

CONCLUSION

Lower urinary tract dysfunction can result from the neurologic deterioration that is caused by syringomyelia. Both primary and secondary syringomyelia develop slowly over time and result in a variety of symptoms, many of which are urologic. A patient with either primary or secondary syringomyelia may experience incontinence, nocturia, as well as other nonurologic symptoms. As knowledge of syringomyelia's occurrence continues to grow, many theories are beginning to form that provide plausible reasons for its occurrence. When it comes to treating the disease, there are a few procedures that can be performed in order to stabilize a patient with syringomyelia. *Treatment indications have not yet been perfectly determined, but surgery is decided on the basis of the patient's clinical status and MRI findings.* Surgeries for patients with syringomyelia aim to alleviate symptoms. *The most suited surgical technique combines spinal laminectomy, a drainage of the cavity, an arachnoid liberation, and a dural plasty enlargement.* Removal of the syrinx and decreasing pressure within the spine are common procedures that help to improve a patient's symptoms and stabilize the patient's overall condition.

BIBLIOGRAPHY

1. Sichez JP, and Capelle L. Syringomyélie. Editions techniques. *EMCNeurologie*, 1997;17077A10:4.
2. Gardner WJ, and Angel J. The mechanism of syringomyelia and its surgical correction. *Clin Neurosurg.* 1959;6:131–40.
3. Aboulker J. La syringomyélie et les liquides intra-rachidiens. *Neurochirurgie (Paris)* 1979;25(Suppl 1):9–22.
4. Xenos C, Sgouros S, Walsh R, and Hockley A. Spinal lipomas in children. *Pediatr Neurosurg.* 2000;32:295–307.
5. Anderson NE, Frith RW, and Synek VM. Somatosensory evoked potentials in syringomyelia. *J Neurol Neurosurg Psychiatr.* 1986;49:1407–10.
6. Wilberger JE, Maroon JC, Prostko ER et al. Magnetic resonance imaging and intraoperative neurosonography in syringomyelia. *Neurosurg.* 1987;20:599–606.
7. Aubin ML, Baleriaux D, Cosnard G et al. IRM dans les syringomyélies d'origine congénitale, infectieuse, traumatique ou idiopathique. A propos de 142 cas. *J Neuroradiol (Paris).* 1987;14:313–36.
8. La Marca F, Herman M, Grant JA, and MacLone DG. Presentation and management of hydromyelia in children with Chiari type II malformation. *Pediatr Neurosurg.* 1997;26:57–67.
9. Sakakibara R, Hattori T, Yasuda K, and Yamanishi T. Micturitional disturbance in syringomyelia. *J Neurol Sci.* 1996;143:100–6.
10. Taskinen S, Valanne L, and Rintala R. The effect of spinal cord abnormalities on the function of the lower urinary tract in patients with anorectal abnormalities. *J Urol.* 2002;168:1147–9.
11. Amoiridis G, Meves S, Schöls L, and Przuntek H. Reversible urinary retention as the main symptom in the first manifestation of a syringomyelia. *J Neurol Neurosurg Psychiatry.* 1996;61:407–8.
12. Houang M, Leroy B, Forin V et al. Rétention aiguë d'urines: Un mode de révélation rare d'une syringomyélie cervicodorsale à l'occasion de la prise de cyproheptadine. *Arch Pédiatre (Paris).* 1994;1:260–3.
13. Holly LT, and Batzdorf U. Syringomyelia associated with intradural arachnoid cysts. *J Neurosurg Spine.* 2006;5:111–6.
14. Ozerdemoglu RA, Transfeldt EE, and Denis F. Value of treating primary causes of syrinx in scoliosis associated with syringomyelia. *Spine* 2003;28(8):806–14.
15. Umbach I, and Heilporn A. Post spinal-cord injury syringomyelia. Review. *Paraplegia.* 1991;29:219–21.
16. Williams B. Post-traumatic syringomyelia, an update. *Paraplegia.* 1990;28(5):296–313.
17. MacLean DR, Miller JDR, Allen PBR, and Ezzedin SA. Post traumatic syringomyelia. *J Neurosurg.* 1973;39:485–92.
18. Ball MJ, and Dayan AD. Pathogenesis of syringomyelia. *Lancet.* 1972;2:799–800.
19. Perrouin-Verbe B, Lenne-Aurier K, Robert R et al. Post-traumatic syringomyelia and post-traumatic spinal canal stenosis: A direct relationship: Review of 75 patients with a spinal cord injury. *Spinal Cord.* 1998;36:137–43.
20. Rossier AB, Foo D, Shillito J, and Dyro FM. Post traumatic cervical syringomyelia: Incidence, clinical presentation, electrological studies, syrinx protein and results of conservative and operative treatment. *Brain* 1985;108:439–61.
21. Vernon JD, Silver JR, and Ohry A. Post traumatic syringomyelia. *Paraplegia.* 1982;20:339–64.
22. Perrouin-Verbe B, Robert R, Le Fort M et al. Syringomyélie posttraumatique. *Neurochirurgie (Paris).* 1999;45(Suppl 1):58–66.
23. Schurch B, Wichmann W, and Rossier AB. Post-traumatic syringomyelia (cystic myelopathy): A prospective study of 449 patients with spinal cord injury. *J Neurol Neurosurg Psychiatr.* 1996;60:61–7.

24. Jaksche H, Schaan M, Schulz J, and Bosczcyk B. Post-traumatic syringomyelia a serious complication in tetra-and paraplegic patients. *Acta Neurochir Suppl.* 2005;93:165–7.

25. Lee TT, Almeda GJ, Camilo E, and Green BA. Surgical treatment of posttraumatic myelopathy associated with syringomyelia. *Spine.* 2001;26(24 Suppl):S119–27.

26. Caremel R, Hamel O, and Gerardin E et al. Post-traumatic syringomyelia: What should know the urologist? *Prog Urol.* 2013;23(1):8–14.

27. Taskinen S, Valanne L, Rintala R Effect of spinal cord abnormalities on the function of the lower urinary tract in patients with anorectal abnormalities. *J Urol.* 2002;168(3):1147–9. https://www.ncbi.nlm.nih.gov/pubmed/12187257

28. Levine DN. The pathogenesis of syringomyelia associated with lesions at the foramen magnum: A critical review of existing theories and proposal of a new hypothesis. *J Neurol Sci.* 2004;220:3–21. https://www.ncbi.nlm.nih.gov/pubmed/15140600

Part III

EVALUATION OF NEUROGENIC BLADDER DYSFUNCTION

Chapter 19

CONSIDERATIONS FOR THE FOCUSED NEURO-UROLOGIC HISTORY AND PHYSICAL EXAM

Laura L. Giusto, Patricia M. Zahner, and Howard B. Goldman

INTRODUCTION

We present a framework of a basic history that centers on the patient's bladder, bowel, and sexual function. Other key portions of the history include the etiology of the patient's neurologic disease (if known), current medications, functional status, past medical, surgical, and social history, as well as allergies.[1,2]

Essential elements of the focused neuro-urologic physical exam include an evaluation of the patient's gross motor function, an abdominal exam, and a genitourinary exam that consists of a rectal examination, sacral sensitivity, and reflex testing.[3] The order of this exam is meant to go from less to more invasive and flows so it is both a logical and convenient progression for the patient and doctor. We briefly present adjunctive tools in the workup including the use of a bladder scan and bladder diary, whereas urodynamics are described in a later chapter.

HISTORY TAKING

The history is rarely explained in detail, and a framework on how to gather information is helpful (Table 19.1).

CURRENT URINARY SYMPTOMS
Start the history with the patient's current urinary symptoms, as these symptoms are often related to their chief complaint.

PERTINENT REVIEW OF SYMPTOMS
BLADDER FUNCTION
The interview continues by focusing on bladder, bowel, and sexual function. We can divide questions about bladder function into both storage and emptying symptoms (Table 19.2).

In terms of storage symptoms, it is important to assess the presence of urinary urgency, frequency, nocturia, and incontinence.[4,5] The questions listed in

Table 19.3 are helpful in elucidating this information. Patients are often unable to distinguish between the sensation of urge and that of bladder fullness.[6] If the pelvic nerves or the sacral segments are not functioning, the desire to void is absent, however sensation of bladder fullness is caused by distention of the peritoneum covering the bladder, which is felt even when the bladder afferents are damaged.[7]

Similarly, the feeling of urgency or imminence, or that one needs to urinate immediately, also relies on proprioception of the pelvic musculature conducted by the pelvic and pudendal nerves. Therefore, you should ask if they have a feeling or sensation that they are about to urinate and if that sensation differs from that before their diagnosis.

When assessing emptying symptoms (Table 19.4), one must inquire how urination is initiated by the patient and if the patient uses physical maneuvers to initiate flow. A decreased force of stream may be due to many causes including obstruction, detrusor-sphincter dyssynergia, or poor bladder contractility.

AUTONOMIC DYSREFLEXIA
Additional questions should be asked to determine if the patient exhibits signs or symptoms of autonomic dysreflexia such as hypertension, reflexive bradycardia, diaphoresis, facial flushing, altered mental status, and headache.

BLADDER DIARY
A bladder diary is a helpful tool to objectively capture a patient's fluid intake and urine output over a 3-day course. A bladder diary may help identify many causes for lower urinary tract symptoms (LUTS) including nocturnal polyuria (defined as greater than one-third of the total urine production overnight) and excessive fluid or caffeine intake.[9,10]

BOWEL FUNCTION
Similar to the assessment of bladder function, when we ask patients about their bowels, we ask about sensation and symptoms (Table 19.5). Again, you want to ask if their sensation differs from before their injury or diagnosis. The ability to sense the passage of stool or gas through the rectum depends on the

Table 19.1 History and Physical Exam Framework

History	Physical Exam

• History of present illness
  • Current urinary symptoms
• Pertinent review of symptoms
  • Bladder function
  • Bowel function
  • Sexual function
    • Gynecologic history
  • History of neurologic disease
  • Medications
  • Past medical and surgical history
  • Family history
  • Social history
    • Occupation, dexterity, impact on activities of daily living
  • Allergies
	• Gross motor function
	  • Mobility
	  • Dexterity
	  • Spasticity
	• Abdominal exam
	• Reflex testing
	  • Lower extremity
	    • Babinski
	    • Ankle (plantar)
	    • Patellar (knee jerk)
	  • Genital
	    • Cremasteric
	    • Bulbocavernosus
	    • Anal
	• Sacral sensitivity testing
	• Genitourinary exam
	  • Male
	  • Female
	• Rectal examination

Table 19.2 Bladder Function

Storage Symptoms	Emptying Symptoms
• Urgency • Frequency • Nocturia • Incontinence	• Hesitancy • Straining • Decreased force of stream • Intermittency

Table 19.3 Questions to Assess Bladder Function: Storage Symptoms

- *Do you experience an urge to urinate?*
  - *Different from before diagnosis or injury?*
    - Absent if
      - Pelvic nerves or sacral segments are nonfunctioning
      - Interrupted pathway between the cerebral and sacral segments
    - Bladder fullness prompted by distension of peritoneum over the bladder
      - Lesion below T10—sensation of suprapubic fullness remains present
      - Lesion close to T6 or above—sensation of fullness less localized
- *Do you have a feeling or sensation that you are about to urinate?*
  - *Different from before diagnosis or injury?*
    - Dependent on proprioception of the pelvic musculature
    - Conducted by pelvic and pudendal nerves
- *How often do you urinate during the day and night?*
- *Do you leak urine?*
  - Urge, stress, mixed, overflow, functional

Table 19.4 Questions to Assess Bladder Function

- *How do you initiate urination?*
  - Voluntary, precipitously, reflexively, strain/Credé
- *Do you have to wait for the urinary stream to start?*
- *Have you noticed a decrease in force of your urinary stream?*
- *Is your flow continuous or intermittent during urination?*
  - *Do you have to strain or "bear down" during urination? Do you ever press on your abdomen to help you urinate?*

Table 19.5 Questions to Assess Bowel Function

- *Do you feel a sensation to move your bowels?*
- *Frequency of bowel movements?*
- *History of constipation?*
  - Less than 3 bowel movements/week
- *Need for medications, enemas, or digital manipulation?*
- *Control of stool and/or gas (incontinence episodes)*

should be queried. Constipation may contribute to obstructive symptoms or urinary retention.[11]

SEXUAL FUNCTION

Sexual dysfunction is common among men and women with neurologic conditions. Men may suffer from neurogenic erectile dysfunction and/or ejaculatory problems. Erections may be absent or, if present, only be achieved either psychogenically or reflexively. It is important to note that ejaculation is a reflex composed of emission via sympathetic hypogastric nerves followed by expulsion due to contractions of the bulbocavernosus muscle via somatic pudendal nerves.

rectal autonomic nerve supply and on the pudendal nerves that conduct proprioception of the rectal sphincter. Frequency of bowels is also a key factor, and the presence of constipation or fecal incontinence

Table 19.6 Sexual Function Questions for Men and Women

Male	Female
• Libido • Erection • Absent? • Present? (psycogenic versus reflexive)? • Orgasm • Ejaculation • Absent versus dribbles versus projectile	• Libido • Vaginal lubrication • Orgasm • Dyspareunia

Asking about the force of ejaculation can give clues to the extent of the patient's nervous injury.

The key aspects of sexual function for the female patient differ from those of a male patient (Table 19.6). While some of her function may be dependent on whether she is neurologically intact, some function may also depend on portions of her gynecologic history. It is therefore helpful to ask about pregnancies and deliveries, if she has had a hysterectomy, and previous pelvic surgeries. In addition, we ask the patient if she is sexually active and if she has any discomfort with vaginal intercourse. Previous surgical history, menopausal status, and neurologic history may all contribute to pelvic floor dysfunction.

MEDICATIONS
As noted in Table 19.7, many medications commonly prescribed for adults have significant effects on urinary function. Thorough evaluation of a patient's current medications may offer insight to potentially overlooked factors contributing to their urinary complaints.[12]

CONSIDERATIONS FOR THE PHYSICAL EXAMINATION

As noted earlier, the physical evaluation should include inspection of the patient's gross motor function, which includes the patient's mobility, dexterity, and degree of spasticity, followed by a standard abdominal exam. The rest of the neuro-urological evaluation focuses mainly on the lower extremities and pelvis and is broken down into further sensory, motor, and reflex testing. The preferred order of examination may alternate among these components, with the intention of following a flow of less to more invasive. As such, the genitourinary exam, focusing on male or female anatomic findings and rectal examination, is performed last.

GROSS MOTOR FUNCTION
The focused neuro-urological exam begins with evaluation of the patient's gross motor function. Much of a patient's gross motor function can typically be assessed during initial inspection of the patient as the patient enters the room. *Are they sitting in a wheelchair or have a walker or cane nearby? Do they exhibit obvious contractures of their upper or lower extremities? Were they able to use a pen or pencil to fill out standardized questionnaires?*

Begin the gross motor exam by assessing the lower extremities. If the patient is capable of standing, observe the lower back for signs of previous surgery, muscle asymmetry, and possibly a dimple or tuft of hair over the spinal column as a sign of

Table 19.7 Evaluation of Current Medications

Medication	Effects	Types of Incontinence
Diuretics	Increased urine production, frequency, urgency	Urge and stress incontinence
Muscle relaxants and sedatives	Urethral relaxation, sedation, drowsiness; lack of concern to void	Stress and functional incontinence
Narcotics	Bladder relaxation, sedation, obstructive symptoms	Urinary retention, overflow, and functional incontinence
Antihistamines	Reduced bladder contractions	Urinary retention, overflow incontinence
Alpha-adrenergic antagonists	Bladder outlet muscle relaxation	Stress incontinence (mostly women)
Cholinesterase inhibitors	Increased bladder contractions	Urge incontinence
Calcium channel blockers	Reduced bladder contractions, constipation	Urinary retention, overflow incontinence
Anticholinergic agents	Reduced bladder contractions, constipation, impaired cognition	Urinary retention, overflow incontinence
Tricyclic antidepressants and antipsychotics	Reduced bladder contractions, sedation	Urinary retention, overflow and functional incontinence
Selective serotonin reuptake inhibitors	Increased bladder contractions, sedation	Urge and functional incontinence

myelodysplasia. If the patient is able, have them walk a short distance across the room and take a deep bend at the knee.

ABDOMINAL EXAM

Inspection and palpation of the patient's abdomen is a necessary component of the physical exam. While the patient is in the supine position, sensation of the thoracic dermatomes can be assessed. The physician should note abdominal scars from previous surgeries, rule out hernias, and note if the patient has any discomfort upon palpation, such as a full palpable bladder in the suprapubic region. Sensitivity testing is reviewed later, but if a patient has a cervical or thoracic lesion, level of sensation may be assessed at this point.

If the patient has voided or self-catheterized prior to the examination, a bladder scan can be performed at this point to measure postvoid residual and provide further information about the patient's ability to empty their bladder.

REFLEX TESTING

Testing the patient's lower extremity reflexes is another important component of the neuro-urologic exam that is often overlooked and underestimated. Abnormal reflexes of the lumbosacral spinal cord are often present in patients with neuro-urologic disorders and may help elucidate the level of the lesion. The absence of certain reflexes may also offer insight into the patient's possible bladder and bowel function (Figure 19.1).

First, examine the patient's lower extremity reflexes. This includes the patellar, ankle, and Babinski reflexes. The cremasteric, bulbocavernosus, and anal reflex testing will be performed later in the exam once the patient is in dorsal lithotomy position and after sacral sensitivity testing is performed, as we leave more invasive testing for last.

The lower spinal cord reflexes to be integrated into the neuro-urologic exam and how to perform them are listed in Table 19.8.[13]

It is important to note whether reflexes are increased, normal, reduced, or absent. For instance, if you find that there is an absent or weak patellar reflex, there is a possible nerve root injury at L3 and a weak or absent ankle jerk reflex could mean a possible nerve root injury at S1. An upgoing toe during Babinski testing may indicate corticospinal motor systems failure.

SACRAL SENSITIVITY TESTING

Sacral sensitivity testing is an important component of the neuro-urologic physical exam as abnormal findings can suggest a lesion of a lumbosacral segment.[14] Sacral sensitivity testing utilizes light touch, pinprick, and proprioceptive maneuvers to stimulate three different nerve pathways including the anterior and lateral spinothalamic tracts as well as the dorsal columns, respectively.[15] Mapping out distinct areas of sensory impairment helps localize the lesion.

Stimuli from the sacral dermatomes are conveyed to the spinal cord via afferent fibers in the sacral roots. Afferent fibers from the bladder join these sacral roots before they enter the sacrum. Therefore, missing sensation in a specific sacral dermatome can indicate that the relevant afferent nerves are damaged in the periphery rather than the spinal cord (Figures 19.2 and 19.3).[16]

Reduced or absent sensation indicates damage along the sacral nerves and corresponding spinal pathways. If you have peripheral bladder denervation, such as an injury after pelvic surgery, the sensitivity in the sacral dermatomes is still intact.

If the patient reports the feeling of bladder fullness but cannot sense pinprick or gentle brushing to the

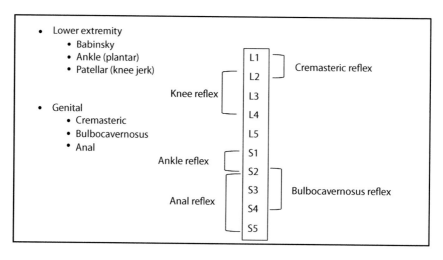

Figure 19.1   Reflex testing.

Table 19.8   Lower Spinal Cord Reflexes

Reflex	Nerve Level	Afferent Nerve	Efferent Nerve	Description
Cremasteric	L1-L2	Femoral branch of genitofemoral n. Ileoinguinal n.	Genital branch of genitofemoral n.	*Action*: Briskly stroke the medial thigh *Reaction*: Contraction of the cremasteric muscle that pulls the testicle closer to the external inguinal ring
Patellar (knee jerk)	L2-L4	Femoral n.	Femoral n.	*Action*: Strong tap on the patellar tendon while the leg dangles at a 90° angle *Reaction*: Sudden contraction of the quadriceps muscle with lower leg extension
Ankle (plantar reflex)	S1-S2	Tibial n.	Tibial n.	*Action*: Striking the Achilles tendon with a reflex hammer *Reaction*: Plantar flexion
Babinski (adults)	L5-S1	S1 dermatome to tibial n.	Tibial n. (flexion) or deep peroneal nerve (extension)	*Action*: Rub the lateral sole of the foot with a blunt instrument from the heel to the toes *Reaction*: Normal is flexion of the hallux (downward great toe); abnormal is extension of the hallux (upward great toe) due to loss of suppression of the extensor withdrawal
Bulbocavernosus	S2-S4	Dorsal branch of pudendal n.	Perineal branch of pudendal n.	*Action*: Gentle squeezing of the glans penis or clitoris, or gently tugging on an indwelling urethral catheter *Reaction*: Contraction of the anal sphincter
Anal	S2-S5	Pudendal n.	S2-S4	*Action*: Stroke skin around the anus *Reaction*: Contraction of the external anal sphincter

sacral dermatome, the damage is along the afferent pathway from the sacral dermatome prior to reaching the sacral root.

Alternately, if the patient denies feelings of bladder urge or fullness but can sense pinprick or gentle brushing to a sacral dermatome, the damage is along the afferent pathway from the bladder to the sacrum, prior to reaching the sacral roots.

Lumbosacral sensitivity testing is performed by placing the patient in the lithotomy position. Once completed, proceed with the more invasive evaluation including the male and female pelvic exams, genital reflex testing, and rectal exam. To perform the sacral sensitivity testing, we use a Q-tip that is broken in half. The sharp side is used to assess pinprick, while the soft side is used to assess light touch. Demonstrate the difference on a part of the body where the patient feels sensation, such as the patient's hand. Then, use both sides of the Q-tip to assess the patient's perception of pain and light touch on the various sacral dermatomes.

Note again that light touch ascends in the anterior spinothalamic tract. Pinprick ascends in the lateral

spinothalamic tract. L2 through S1 dermatomes are tested in the anterior and posterior thigh, lower legs, and lateral and medial aspects of both feet. Lumbar dermatome distribution extends from the suprapubic region to the feet in a V-shaped pattern.

PELVIC EXAM
FEMALE PELVIC EXAM
The female pelvic exam emphasizes anatomic findings such as genital tissue integrity, pelvic organ position, and urethral mobility.[17] A woman's level of atrophy should also be appreciated if she is in a postmenopausal state.

With the patient in the lithotomy position, one should observe the presence or absence of any indwelling catheters. During bimanual exam using well-lubricated fingers, palpate all portions of the vagina to assess for pelvic floor pain and muscle tension. Ask the patient to contract the pelvic floor and note whether the contraction is strong, medium, weak, or absent. Pelvic floor muscle contraction is mediated by the perineal nerve. A half speculum is then inserted into the vagina to assess for pelvic organ prolapse, vaginal atrophy, bleeding, or discharge. The patient

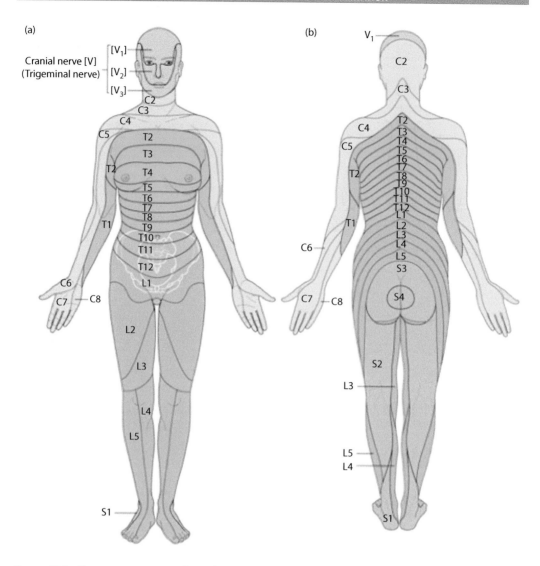

Figure 19.2 Dermatome map, anterior and posterior views. (Courtesy of *Gray's Anatomy for Students*, Drake, Richard L., PhD, FAAA; Vogl, A. Wayne, PhD, FAAA; Mitchell, Adam W.M., MBBS, FRCS, FRCR. Published January 1, 2020. Pages 1–48. © 2020. Fig. 1.39 Dermatomes. A. Anterior view. B. Posterior view.)

is asked to cough to demonstrate if she has stress urinary incontinence or urethral hypermobility.

MALE PELVIC EXAM

Similarly, with the male patient in the lithotomy position, one should observe the presence or absence of any indwelling catheters. Palpate the shaft of the penis and inspect the glans and foreskin if present, making sure to look for urethral meatus stenosis or traumatic hypospadias.

PELVIC AND GENITAL REFLEX TESTING

Next, test the genital reflexes including the bulbocavernosus and anal reflex while the patient is in the lithotomy position, since the exam should flow from least to most invasive. In the male patient, we can also check the cremasteric reflex first. The

bulbocavernosus reflex is important to assess since it is one of the first reflexes to return in patients with spinal shock after their injury (Table 19.9).[8]

A positive or present bulbocavernosus reflex is a normal finding in neurologically intact patients but can correlate with a suprasacral spinal cord lesion and may be present along with detrusor-sphincter dyssynergia. An absent reflex is abnormal and indicates a defect in the sacral reflex arc, specifically in L5 through S5. In a female patient, this part of the exam can be performed as part of the vaginal exam before proceeding to the rectal exam. In a male, this reflex should be tested during the rectal exam.

RECTAL EXAM

The rectal exam is typically the last component to be assessed during a physical exam as it is the most

(a)

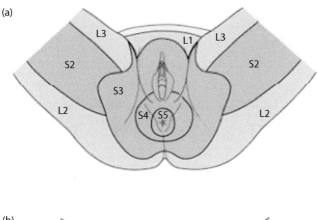

(b)

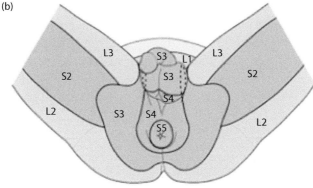

Figure 19.3 Dermatomes of the perineum. (Courtesy of *Gray's Anatomy for Students*, Drake, Richard L., PhD, FAAA; Vogl, A. Wayne, PhD, FAAA; Mitchell, Adam W.M., MBBS, FRCS, FRCR. Published January 1, 2020. Pages 413–524.e5. © 2020. Fig. 5.14 Dermatomes of the perineum. A. In women. B. In men.)

invasive. The rectal exam is a key component of the physical exam for all urologic patients, including assessment of the prostate in males. During the exam, size, symmetry, and texture of the prostate are detected as well as the presence of hemorrhoids, bleeding, and sphincter tone (Table 19.10).

There are some unique aspects of the rectal exam that pertain to the neurologic patient. It is important to note the configuration of the anus, specifically if it is patulous, as well as if the sphincter tone is normal, spastic, or flaccid. We examine these things because voluntary contraction and relaxation of the anus allow for suppression of bladder and bowel urgency and imply an intact pathway. This starts with the patient's ability to activate relevant cortical areas with

complete signal transmission down the pyramidal tract to the pudendal nerve nuclei within the anterior horn of the sacral cord and then to the peripheral pudendal nerve.

Table 19.9 Bulbocavernosus Reflex

- Positive bulbocavernosus reflex correlates with:
  - A suprasacral spinal cord lesion
  - Detrusor-sphincter/bladder neck dyssynergia
- Negative bulbocavernosus reflex indicates a defect in the sacral reflex arc:
  - On the afferent side of the pudendal nerve
  - In the spinal cord segments L5 through S5
  - On the efferent side of the pudendal nerve

Table 19.10 Rectal Examination

Standard	Neurogenic/Lower Urinary Tract Dysfunction

• Size, symmetry, and consistency of prostate
  • Tender, boggy, indurated
• Presence of hemorrhoids
• Anal sphincter tone
	• Configuration of anus
	  • Normal or patulous
	• Anal sphincter tone
	  • Normal, spastic, or flaccid
	• Anal contractility
	  • Ability to voluntarily contract and relax sphincter
	• Presence of impacted stool
	  • Indication of neurogenic bowel

Additionally, preserved ability for voluntary contraction and relaxation is a good prognostic sign to achieve continence with bladder retraining programs

CONCLUSION

The history and physical exam for the neuro-urologic patient should be performed in a stepwise fashion. With the aging of our population and widening spectrum of diseases, we have an increasing number of patients with lower urinary tract symptoms and neurologic conditions. The patient presenting to the office with a possible neurologic condition will likely need additional testing to clarify the diagnosis, but a thorough history and physical exam is paramount to understanding the relationship between the patient's urologic complaint and the patient's neurologic condition.

REFERENCES

1. Bors E and Turner RD. History and physical examination in neurological urology. *J Urol.* 1960;83:759–67. http://dx.doi.org/10.1016/s0022-5347(17)65794-x
2. Drake MJ, Apostolidis A, Cocci A et al. Neurogenic lower urinary tract dysfunction: Clinical management recommendations of the Neurologic Incontinence committee of the fifth International Consultation on Incontinence 2013. *Neurourol Urodyn.* 2016;35:657–65. http://dx.doi.org/10.1002/nau.23027
3. Panicker JN, Fowler CJ, and Kessler TM. Lower urinary tract dysfunction in the neurological patient: Clinical assessment and management. *Lancet Neurol.* 2015;14:720–32.
4. Unger CA, Tunitsky-Bitton E, Muffly T et al. Neuroanatomy, neurophysiology, and dysfunction of the female lower urinary tract. *Female Pelvic Med Reconstructive Surg* 2014;20:65–75. http://dx.doi.org/10.1097/spv.0000000000000058
5. Nitti VW. Evaluation of the female with neurogenic voiding dysfunction. *Int Urogynecol J Pelvic Floor Dysfunct.* 1999;10:119–29. http://dx.doi.org/10.1007/s001920050031
6. Drake MJ, Fowler CJ, Griffiths D et al. Neural control of the lower urinary and gastrointestinal tracts: Supraspinal CNS mechanisms. *Neurourol Urodyn.* 2010;29:119–27. http://dx.doi.org/10.1002/nau.20841
7. Bors E and Estin Comarr A. Neurological Urology: Physiology of Micturition, Its Neurological Disorders and Sequelae. Basel, Switzerland: S.Karger; 1971.
8. Wyndaele JJ and De Sy WA. Correlation between the findings of a clinical neurological examination and the urodynamic dysfunction in children with myelodysplasia. *J Urol* 1985;133:638–40.
9. Ku JH, Jeong IG, Lim DJ et al. Voiding diary for the evaluation of urinary incontinence and lower urinary tract symptoms: Prospective assessment of patient compliance and burden. *Neurourol Urodyn.* 2004;23:331–5. http://dx.doi.org/10.1002/nau.20027
10. Naoemova I, De Wachter S, Wuyts FL et al. Reliability of the 24-h sensation-related bladder diary in women with urinary incontinence. *Int Urogynecol J Pelvic Floor Dysfunct.* 2008;19:955–59.
11. Pannek J, Göcking K, and Bersch U. "Neurogenic" urinary tract dysfunction: Don't overlook the bowel! *Spinal Cord.* 2009;47:93–4. http://dx.doi.org/10.1038/sc.2008.79
12. Benson JT, Thomas Benson J, and Walters MD. Neurophysiology and pharmacology of the lower urinary tract. *Urogynecol Reconstr Pelvic Surg.* 2007:31–43.
13. Palleschi G, Pastore AL, Stocchi F et al. Correlation between the overactive bladder questionnaire (OAB-q) and urodynamic data of Parkinson disease patients affected by neurogenic detrusor overactivity during antimuscarinic treatment. *Clin Neuropharmacol.* 2006;29:220–9. http://dx.doi.org/10.1097/01.wnf.0000228177.75711.0f
14. Groen J, Pannek J, Castro Diaz D et al. Summary of European Association of Urology (EAU) guidelines on Neuro-Urology. *Eur Urol.* 2016;69:324–33.
15. Schurch B, Schmid DM, and Kaegi K. Value of sensory examination in predicting bladder function in patients with T12-L1 fractures and spinal cord injury. *Arch Phys Med Rehabil.* 2003;84:83–89.
16. Philo R. *Gray's Anatomy for Students*, 2nd ed. by Richard L. Drake, A. Wayne Vogl, and Adam W M. Mitchell. *Clin Anat.* 2009;22:846–7. http://dx.doi.org/10.1002/ca.20863
17. Yang CC and Cardenas DD. Bladder management in women with neurologic disabilities. *Phys Med Rehabil Clin N Am.* 2001;12:91–110.

Chapter 20

PATIENT-REPORTED OUTCOME MEASURES IN NEUROGENIC BLADDER

Blayne Welk

INTRODUCTION

The field of measurement involves assigning values (often numerical ones) to a trait. In many cases this is quite intuitive, such as measuring the length of an object using a ruler and then describing it using the metric system. In other cases, it can be challenging and involve more complex traits (such as degree of urinary incontinence), or abstract ideas such as health-related or disease-specific quality of life (QOL). Almost all clinical trials now include a QOL outcome, and reporting standards have highlighted the importance of these outcomes.[1] The contemporary practice of patient-centered medicine emphasizes understanding and optimizing the QOL of the patient. In order to do this in a neuro-urology practice, the healthcare professional must be able to understand, elicit, and integrate a patient's feelings, values, and expectations into the medical care. Patient-reported outcome measures (PROMs) are the most common, standardized way to do this. This chapter reviews PROMs that are relevant to neuro-urology.

GENERAL OVERVIEW OF PATIENT-REPORTED OUTCOME MEASURES

When selecting a PROM to use in clinical practice or for a research study, or if you are reading the results of a study that used a PROM, it is important to consider the intended purpose of the PROM. Some may be for specific conditions (e.g., the impact of incontinence on QOL), or they may be for specific diseases (e.g., a general QOL measure for patients with a spinal cord injury [SCI]). Using a PROM assesses QOL from perhaps the most important viewpoint: that of the patient. The complex, multisystem morbidity inherent to many patients with neurogenic bladder means that a general QOL measure may not be sensitive to important bladder changes[2]; however, condition-specific QOL can be problematic to define from a theoretical perspective.[3]

PROMs have different potential applications. They may have been designed to look at patients at one point in time (cross-sectional), predict things like a clinical improvement, or demonstrate a change over time.[4] To ensure a PROM is appropriate for use in clinical research, it should be assessed for its internal validity (using psychometric properties such as Cronbach's alpha), external validity (how well it demonstrates hypothetical relationships with other related PROMs or clinical traits), reliability (how consistent the results are when they are repeated in an unchanged patient), and in some cases responsiveness (which represents how well the PROM score can prove a real change has occurred in a patient or a group of patients).[5]

A systematic review published in 2016 summarized the PROMs that have been used in the published neuro-urology literature between 2000 and 2014.[6] Most studies involved patients with SCI or multiple sclerosis (MS), and a variety of PROMs were used. The majority of PROMs were not designed for neuro-urology patients or validated for use in the neuro-urology population. Examples include common questionnaires such as the Incontinence Impact Questionnaire 7 (IIQ-7) and the Kings Health Questionnaire Lower Urinary Tract (KHQ-LUTS), which were not specifically assessed for their appropriateness in patients with neurogenic bladder. In many cases, overall QOL tools, such as SF-36, were used. This PROM assesses overall mental and physical health and would be unlikely to capture specific neuro-urology concerns.

A subsequent systematic review identified 18 general PROMs that were validated for patients with a neurologic condition; the questionnaires usually covered multiple health domains, but all had at least one item related to bladder function.[7] In most of these cases, the PROMs addressed overall QOL for people with MS or SCI and had only a few questions devoted to bowel and bladder management. This means that the scores of these instruments would not be expected to change significantly with most neuro-urologic interventions, or necessarily represent bladder-specific QOL very well. However, they do include general questions about avoidance/limiting behavior, energy, mobility, cognition, household functioning, hand function, and social and economic supports, which may be indirectly affected by bladder management. A similar review focused specifically on QOL measures in SCI patients with neurogenic bladder[8]; these authors concluded that the best assessment of QOL likely requires multiple, complementary PROMs that address both objective and subjective measures of QOL and are designed and appropriately validated for patients with neurogenic bladder. This highlights the fact that subjective and objective QOL measures are different, and the scores from such measures can vary significantly. As an example, a subjective question might ask them to rate how they perceive their bladder function in relation to others, while an objective question might ask them whether incontinence has caused them skin problems. Therefore, consistent results across different QOL instruments provide the highest degree of evidence when QOL is a key outcome of interest, although for most research projects a single, well-selected, appropriately validated QOL measure is likely sufficient.

SPECIFIC PATIENT-REPORTED OUTCOME MEASURES IN NEURO-UROLOGY

QUALIVEEN

The Qualiveen was developed with the support of Coloplast in 2001 and represents one of the first bladder-specific QOL tools designed for neuro-urology (in this case patients with SCI).[9] It includes 30 items that cover four domains (limitations, constraints, fears, and feelings). A short form has been developed which has only eight questions.[10] It has also been validated among patients with MS.[11] It is valid, reliable, and responsive to change, and an excellent choice for quickly assessing bladder-related QOL in patients with SCI and MS. It is well suited for both clinical practice and for research studies. Additional studies of the measurement characteristics of the Qualiveen have been conducted, including determination of the minimally important difference, and a secondary validation using Rasch analysis.[12,13] Several validation studies of different cultural/language adaptations are available including English, Persian, French, Spanish, German, Portuguese, Dutch, and Italian.

I-QOL

The Incontinence-QOL PROM was originally developed in 1999 to assess the impact of urinary incontinence on QOL in women.[14] It includes 22 items, with three domains (avoidance and limiting factors, psychosocial impact, and social embarrassment). In 2007 it was studied in a population of predominately

patients with SCI with neurogenic urinary incontinence.[15] It demonstrated good validity, reliability, and responsiveness, particularly as a single overall score (rather than individual domain scores). Numerous different culture/language validation studies have been published given its popularity in the nonneurogenic bladder incontinence literature (including French, Spanish, Swedish, German, and Italian).

SCI-QOL

The SCI-QOL is a set of QOL questionnaires that assess various aspects of life after a SCI.[16] As part of this process, two bladder-specific modules were published in 2015: the SCI-QOL bladder management difficulties and the SCI-QOL bladder complications scale.[17] Item-response theory was used to develop computer adaptive test versions of each of these scales, and paper-based complete and short forms versions are also available. The SCI-QOL bladder management difficulties module includes 15 questions covering topics such as worries about bladder management and incontinence, and the impact of bladder management daily activities. The SCI-QOL bladder complications module asks six questions about the impact of urinary infection symptoms and their effect on daily activities. They are available through the National Institutes of Health toolbox, and as an added convenience they are preprogrammed into the REDCap common library.

NBSS

The Neurogenic Bladder Symptom Score (NBSS) was published in 2014.[18] Its primary purpose is to assess the urologic symptom burden of patients with SCI, MS, or spina bifida across different bladder management strategies. It includes 22 items that cover three symptom domains (incontinence, storage and voiding, and consequences). There is an additional nonscored question to stratify patients based on their bladder management method, and there is a single stand-alone QOL question. It is valid, reliable, and responsive to change,[19,20] and some cultural/language adaptions are available (French, Portuguese, Russian, Polish, Greek and Italian).

QUALAS-A

The QUAlity of Life Assessment in Spina bifida for Adults (QUALAS-A) is a health-related QOL measure for patients with spina bifida.[21] It was specifically developed for use among people born with spina bifida and has 15 questions divided among three domains (health and relationships, esteem and sexuality, and bladder/bowel). The bladder/bowel domain assesses the bother and impact of urinary incontinence and has reasonable domain-specific measurement characteristics. Analogous versions of this PROM have been developed for children and adolescents.

ABSST-SF

The Actionable Bladder Symptom Screening Tool-Short Form (ABSST-SF) has a different purpose than the previously discussed PROMs.[22] It was developed to identify patients with MS with urinary symptoms who may benefit from a more detailed urologic evaluation or a formal referral to a urologist. It has eight questions that can quickly and easily be administered during a clinic visit and would likely be used as a screening tool during clinical practice in a MS speciality clinic. It has been translated into Dutch and Spanish.

LUTS-TCA

The Lower Urinary Tract Symptoms Treatment Constraints Assessment (LUTS-TCA) PROM was developed in patients with MS, SCI, and Parkinson's disease (published in 2018).[23] This PROM looks at symptoms and QOL a bit differently: rather than consider the positive aspects of treatment, it measures the limitations imposed by different bladder management options (such as medications, intravesical botulinum toxin, neuromodulation, and intermittent catheters) using 22 questions. An important point to remember is that this PROM is assessing constraints due to treatment and management, and not the underlying neurogenic bladder symptoms or complications.

USQNB-IC

The Urinary Symptom Questionnaire for individuals with Neuropathic Bladder using Intermittent Catheterization (USQNB-IC) was developed using a novel patient-centered approach (published in 2018). It included patients with either SCI or spina bifida, as well as nonneurogenic bladder populations who acted as negative controls.[24] As the name suggests, this PROM describes the urinary signs and symptoms in patients with neurogenic bladder who use intermittent catheters. The eventual goal of the authors is to create a score that can be used to follow urinary signs and symptoms, and possibly identify urinary infections in this patient population. Further work is necessary to understand how to use this PROM.

ICIQ-LTCQOL

The International Consultation on Incontinence Questionnaire-Long Term Catheter quality of life tool (ICIQ-LTCqol, published in 2016)[25] is an evolution of previous work by some of the same authors who created the C-IQOL[26] (a modification of the I-QOL questionnaire for indwelling catheter patients). It includes 16 items with two main domains: lifestyle impact and catheter function and concern. There are additional unclassified questions about pain, bladder spasms, bypassing, and prevention of sexual activity. The patient population used to create this PROM was not explicitly described; however, it likely includes patients with neurogenic bladder dysfunction given their previous study populations.

CONCLUSION

Over the last 20 years, the study of QOL among patients with neurogenic bladder has moved forward significantly with the development and publication of several PROMs specific to this population. Hopefully the addition of these new PROMs that address neurogenic bladder-specific QOL, urinary symptoms, intermittent catheter symptoms, and indwelling catheter QOL will add to our understanding of neurogenic bladder, and how it changes with the various medical, procedural, and surgical options. Researchers and clinicians now have several potential PROMs that can be used both in the clinic and when designing prospective research studies.

REFERENCES

1. Calvert M, Blazeby J, Altman DG et al. Reporting of patient-reported outcomes in randomized trials: The CONSORT PRO extension. *Am Med Assoc.* 2013;309:814–22. doi:10.1001/jama.2013.879
2. Noonan VK, Kopec JA, Zhang H, and Dvorak MF. Impact of associated conditions resulting from spinal cord injury on health status and quality of life in people with traumatic central cord syndrome. *YAPMR.* 2008;89(6):1074–82. doi:10.1016/j.apmr.2007.10.041
3. Dijkers M. "What's in a name?" The indiscriminate use of the "Quality of life" label, and the need to bring about clarity in conceptualizations. *Int J Nurs Stud.* 2007;44(1):153–5. doi:10.1016/j.ijnurstu.2006.07.016
4. Wright JG, McLeod RS, Lossing A, Walters BC, and Hu X. Measurement in surgical clinical research. *Surgery.* 1996;119(3):241–4.
5. Clark R and Welk B. Patient reported outcome measures in neurogenic bladder. *Transl Androl Urol.* 2016;5(1):22–30. doi:10.3978/j.issn.2223-4683.2015.12.05
6. Patel DP, Elliott SP, Stoffel JT, Brant WO, Hotaling JM, and Myers JB. Patient reported outcomes measures in neurogenic bladder and bowel: A systematic review of the current literature. *Neurourol Urodyn.* 2016;35(1):8–14. doi:10.1002/nau.22673
7. Tsang B, Stothers L, Macnab A, Lazare D, and Nigro M. A systematic review and comparison of questionnaires in the management of spinal cord injury, multiple sclerosis and the neurogenic bladder. *Neurourol Urodyn.* 2016;35(3):354–64. doi:10.1002/nau.22720
8. Best KL, Ethans K, Craven BC, Noreau L, and Hitzig SL. Identifying and classifying quality of life tools for neurogenic bladder function after spinal cord injury: A systematic review. *J Spinal Cord Med.* 2016;7(3):1–25. doi:10.1080/10790268.2016.1226700
9. Costa P, Perrouin-Verbe B, Colvez A et al. Quality of life in spinal cord injury patients with urinary difficulties. Development and validation of Qualiveen. *Eur Urol.* 2001;39(1):107–13.

10. Bonniaud V, Bryant D, Parratte B, and Guyatt G. Development and validation of the short form of a urinary quality of life questionnaire: SF-Qualiveen. *J Urol.* 2008;180(6):2592–8. doi:10.1016/j.juro.2008.08.016

11. Bonniaud V, Bryant D, Parratte B, Gallien P, and Guyatt G. Qualiveen: A urinary disorder-specific instrument for use in clinical trials in multiple sclerosis. *Arch Phys Med Rehabil.* 2006;87(12):1661–3. doi:10.1016/j.apmr.2006.08.345

12. Milinis K, Tennant A, and A Young C, TONiC Study Group. Rasch analysis of SF-Qualiveen in multiple sclerosis. *Neurourol Urodyn.* 2017;36(4):1161–6. doi:10.1002/nau.23081

13. Bonniaud V, Bryant D, Parratte B, and Guyatt G. Qualiveen, a urinary-disorder specific instrument: 0.5 corresponds to the minimal important difference. *J Clin Epidemiol.* 2008;61(5):505–10. doi:10.1016/j.jclinepi.2007.06.008

14. Patrick DL, Martin ML, Bushnell DM, Yalcin I, Wagner TH, and Buesching DP. Quality of life of women with urinary incontinence: Further development of the incontinence quality of life instrument (I-QOL). *Urology.* 1999;53(1):71–6.

15. Schurch B, Denys P, Kozma CM, Reese PR, Slaton T, and Barron R. Reliability and validity of the Incontinence Quality of Life questionnaire in patients with neurogenic urinary incontinence. *Arch Phys Med Rehabil.* 2007;88(5):646–52. doi:10.1016/j.apmr.2007.02.009

16. Tulsky DS, Kisala PA, Victorson D et al. Developing a contemporary patient-reported outcomes measure for spinal cord injury. *Arch Phys Med Rehabil.* 2011;92(10 Suppl):S44–51. doi:10.1016/j.apmr.2011.04.024

17. Tulsky DS, Kisala PA, Tate DG, Spungen AM, and Kirshblum SC. Development and psychometric characteristics of the SCI-QOL Bladder Management Difficulties and Bowel Management Difficulties item banks and short forms and the SCI-QOL Bladder Complications scale. *J Spinal Cord Med.* 2015;38(3):288–302. doi:10.1179/20457723 15Y.0000000030

18. Welk B, Morrow S, Madarasz W, Baverstock R, Macnab J, and Sequeira K. The validity and reliability of the neurogenic bladder symptom score. *J Urol.* 2014;192(2):452–7. doi:10.1016/j.juro.2014.01.027

19. Welk B, Lenherr S, Elliott S et al. The Neurogenic Bladder Symptom Score (NBSS): A secondary assessment of its validity, reliability among people with a spinal cord injury. *Spinal Cord.* 2018;56(3):259–64. doi:10.1038/s41393-017-0028-0

20. Welk B, Carlson K, and Baverstock R. A pilot study of the responsiveness of the Neurogenic Bladder Symptom Score (NBSS). *Can Urol Assoc J.* 2017;11(12):376–8. doi:10.5489/cuaj.4833

21. Szymanski KM, Misseri R, Whittam B et al. QUAlity of Life Assessment in Spina bifida for Adults (QUALAS- A): Development and international validation of a novel health-related quality of life instrument. *Qual Life Res.* 2015;24(10):2355–64. doi:10.1007/s11136-015-0988-5

22. Bates D, Burks J, Globe D et al. Development of a short form and scoring algorithm from the validated actionable bladder symptom screening tool. *BMC Neurol.* 2013;13:78. doi:10.1186/1471-2377-13-78

23. Turmel N, Lévy P, Hentzen C et al. Lower urinary tract symptoms treatment constraints assessment (LUTS-TCA): A new tool for a global evaluation of neurogenic bladder treatments. *World J Urol.* 2018;61(1):37–9. doi:10.1007/s00345-018-2580-4

24. Tractenberg RE, Groah SL, Rounds AK, Ljungberg IH, and Schladen MM. Preliminary validation of a Urinary Symptom Questionnaire for individuals with Neuropathic Bladder using Intermittent Catheterization (USQNB-IC): A patient-centered patient reported outcome. *PLOS ONE.* 2018;13(7):e0197568. doi:10.1371/journal.pone.0197568

25. Cotterill N, Fowler S, Avery M et al. Development and psychometric evaluation of the ICIQ-LTCqol: A self-report quality of life questionnaire for long-term indwelling catheter users. *Neurourol Urodyn.* 2016;35(3):423–8. doi:10.1002/nau.22729

26. Wilde MH, Getliffe K, Brasch J, McMahon J, Anson E, and Tu X. A new urinary catheter-related quality of life instrument for adults. *Neurourol Urodyn.* 2010;29(7):1282–5. doi:10.1002/nau.20865

Chapter 21

ENDOSCOPIC EVALUATION OF NEUROGENIC BLADDER

Romain Caremel and Jacques Corcos

INTRODUCTION

Urethrocystoscopy is very instrumental in the assessment of lower urinary tract anatomy, helping in the appraisal of urethral and bladder anatomic anomalies, most of the time secondary to complications such as urethral strictures, trabeculations, bladder stones, and diverticula.

EQUIPMENT

Different companies offer different types and sizes of extremely well-designed, rigid urethrocystoscopes (Figure 21.1), some with fixed lens (12°–70°), others with exchangeable lens (0°, 30°, 70°, 120°). The choice of lens depends on the segment of urinary tract that we want to study: 0° or 30° for the urethra and 70° or 120° for the bladder in general. Since sensitivity is often not a problem in patients with neurogenic bladder, rigid urethrocystoscopes are often preferred. They give a much better optical field than flexible cystoscopes (Figure 21.2) and allow various manipulations through a bigger working channel (irrigation, washing, small-stone extraction, etc.). Flexible cystoscopes are mainly used in men with preserved sensitivity, and the test is usually much less painful than with a rigid instrument. One of the biggest advantages of these cystoscopes is the possibility of introducing them in a supine as well as in a sitting position. Because of their deflection abilities, they allow a retrograde view of the bladder neck as well as the complete exploration of diverticula, whatever the position.

TECHNIQUE

Most of the time, the patient is installed in the lithotomy position, but, as mentioned earlier, a supine or a sitting position can be used with a flexible cystoscope. After the usual disinfection of the genitalia with a nonalcoholic solution, draping creates a sterile field around the genitalia. In our experience, we do not use any local anesthetic but only lubricating jelly. Others prefer to inject 2% Xylocaine (lidocaine) jelly transurethrally 2–4 minutes before the procedure.[1]

Once the patient is informed of the beginning of the examination, the cystoscope, lubricated with sterile jelly, is very gently introduced into the meatus. A global view of the urethra permits the confirmation of penile urethra integrity in men. The cystoscope is then pushed forward into the membranous urethra, making the external sphincter visible. This concentric muscle closes the urethra and can usually be passed by gentle pressure on the cystoscope. The prostatic urethra is then observed, and the anatomy of the prostate is then noted, mainly the size of the lateral lobes and the presence or absence of a median lobe.

Once into the bladder, the technique is slightly different, depending on the type of cystoscope. With a rigid cystoscope, we normally use a 70° or 120° lens. The instrument will have only in-and-out and rotating motions, allowing a complete view of the bladder without bending the unit, which may cause unnecessary pain and discomfort. With a flexible cystoscope, the same in-and-out motion is applied, but the rotation motion is replaced by deflections of the instrument's tip, which gives a complete view of the bladder wall. Observation of the ureteral orifices, urine efflux from these orifices, and exploration of bladder diverticula may be necessary. Washings, biopsies, and so on are performed at that time if indicated. Once the test is completed, the instrument is gently withdrawn after emptying the bladder (when using a rigid instrument). Drinking up to 6–8 glasses of water per day for 3 days is usually recommended, and the patient is discharged. No antibiotics are required unless the patient has an artificial heart valve or they are considered necessary by the physician.

URETHROCYSTOSCOPIC FINDINGS

URETHRAL ABNORMALITIES
URETHRAL STRICTURES
Indwelling catheters, multiple endoscopic manipulations, intermittent catheterizations, and

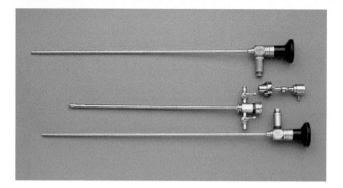

Figure 21.1   Rigid cystoscope.

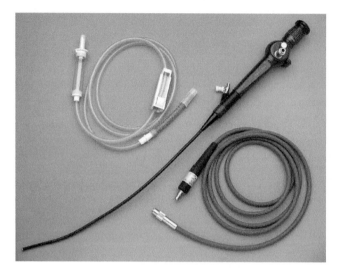

Figure 21.2   Flexible cystoscope.

neurogenic trophicity changes lead to frequent urethral strictures and false passages (Figures 21.3 and 21.4). For instance, a study was carried out to identify complications of clean intermittent catheterization in males and young boys with neurogenic bladder dysfunction. Major urethral lesions were seen on cystoscopy and included urethral stricture, false passages, and meatal stenosis.[2]

BLADDER NECK CYSTOSCOPIC EVALUATION

The degree of opening of the neurogenic bladder neck cannot be adequately evaluated by cystoscopy. False results can be induced by irrigation flow. These changes are dynamic and not anatomic. They should be evaluated by videourodynamicor simple voiding cystogram. In fact, a voiding cystourethrogram (VCUG) might provide a tremendous amount of information useful in identifying multiple complications such as trabeculations, sacculations, diverticulae, vesicoureteric reflux, and postvoid residual, as well as the bladder's ability to empty.[3] However, after bladder neck incision or resection to decrease bladder neck resistance, bladder neck strictures can be easily seen by cystoscopy, but here

again, their real impact on bladder function can be assessed only by voiding cystogram.

ENDOSCOPIC EVALUATION OF URETHRAL STENTS

Sphincterotomies are rarely used. Some patients have received in the past endoluminal stents instead (i.e., Urolume—AMS). These stents are no longer available. It is usually easy to introduce a flexible cystoscope through these stents, which "disappear" completely after a few months as the device is epithelialized through and in between its pores: 90%–100% of epithelialization of the stent has been demonstrated in 47.1% of cases 3 months after insertion, and in 87.7% of cases 12 months after insertion. Mild epithelial hyperplasia can occur (34%–44.4%) after stent insertion and may look like an obstructed urethra. Much less frequently, these strictures are severe (3.1%), requiring urethrotomy or sometimes laser resection of the excess tissue.[3] Occasionally, however, and even several years later, part of the stent may remain visible but usually does not cause any problem. Calcifications of the stents are rare. No stone formation has been reported.[4]

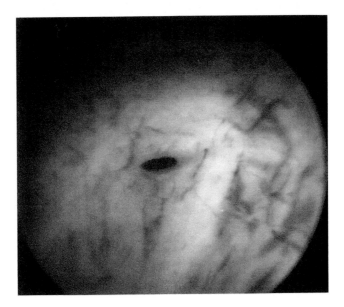

Figure 21.3   Urethral stricture.

STRUCTURAL BLADDER ANOMALIES

The well-balanced bladder of a patient compliant with therapy looks normal (Figure 21.5) most of the time. However, it may show significant changes because of patient noncompliance with intermittent catheterization, medication, and so on, or because these treatments may have no effect.

BLADDER WALL ABNORMALITIES

Often associated with chronic infections but also often not related to any obvious disease, cystitis glandularis (Figure 21.6) and cystitis follicularis (Figure 21.7) can be found during systematic cystoscopic evaluation.

BLADDER WALL TRABECULATIONS

There is no consensus in the literature regarding the significance of bladder wall trabeculations (Figures 21.8 through 21.11). O'Donnell[5] suggested that they could be related to high bladder pressure.[3] To Brocklehurst,[6] McGuire,[7] Shah,[8] and O'Reilly,[9] they are secondary to an infravesical obstruction. More authors believe that trabeculations reflect bladder overactivity and uninhibited contractions (Figure 21.12).

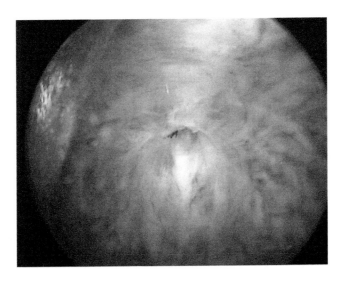

Figure 21.4   Very tight urethral stricture.

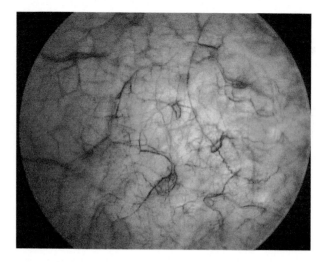

Figure 21.5   Normal bladder mucosa.

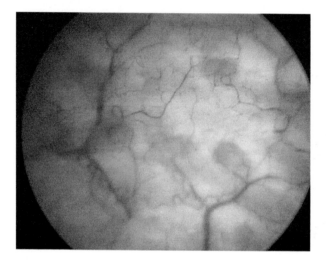

Figure 21.6   Cystitis glandularis.

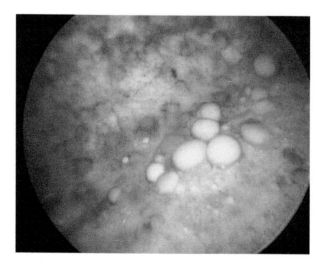

Figure 21.7   Cystitis follicularis.

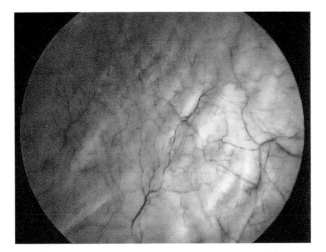

Figure 21.8   Trabeculation grade 1.

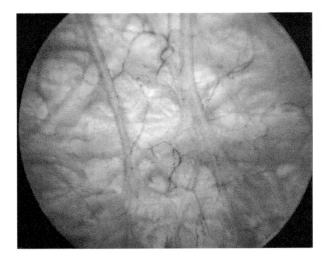

Figure 21.9   Trabeculation grade 2.

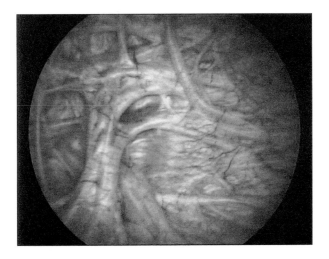

Figure 21.10   Trabeculation grade 3.

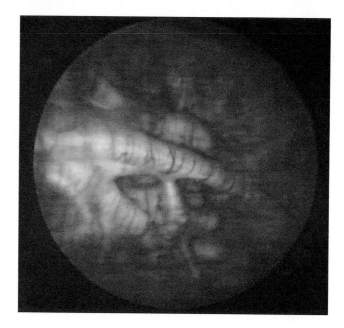

Figure 21.11   Trabeculation grade 4.

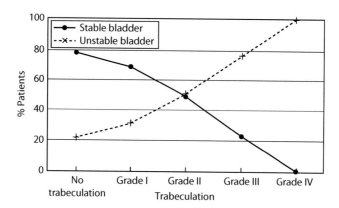

Figure 21.12   Correlation between the trabeculation grade and percentage of unstable bladders.

URETERAL ORIFICES

High bladder pressure, recurrent infections, and changes in bladder wall thickness may provoke alterations in the shape of the ureteral orifices. In some cases, they can look wide open. Their appearance cannot preclude the efficacy of the intramural ureteral valve mechanism and the presence of reflux. Reflux can be diagnosed only by cystogram with a contrast agent or a radioisotope fluid. Ureterocele can be of variable size (Figure 21.13).

TUMORS, STONES, AND FOREIGN BODIES

BLADDER STONES

Usually secondary to infections, bladder stones are frequent findings in neurogenic patients. They must be suspected in cases of recurrent *Proteus mirabilis* infections, increased spasticity, increased autonomic dysreflexia or incontinence, or elimination of small calcified fragments. They are easy to diagnose by cystoscopy and sometimes can be crushed for removal in the same setup. Their aspects are extremely variable, from small, round, single, or multiple stones to huge "egglike" stones (Figures 21.14 and 21.15).

BLADDER TUMORS

Patients with chronic indwelling catheters must undergo annual cystoscopic evaluation. Usually, this routine starts after 5 years of continuous indwelling catheterization. Cystoscopy remains the only way (with cytology) to detect suspicious lesions such as bladder carcinoma. Usually, these lesions start at the level of the trigone, where the

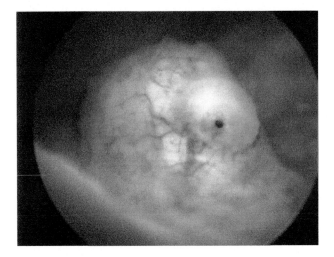

Figure 21.13   Ureterocele.

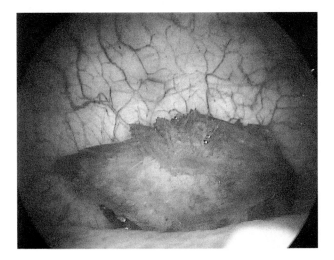

Figure 21.14   Bladder stone.

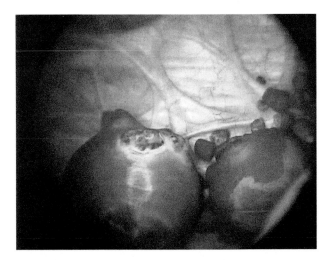

Figure 21.15   Multiple bladder stones.

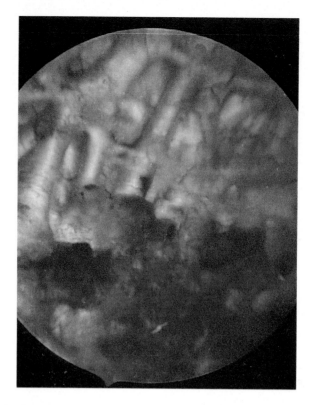

Figure 21.16   Mucosal catheter reaction.

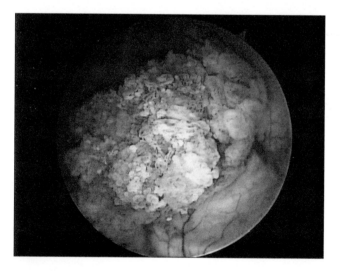

Figure 21.17   Bladder papillary tumor (partially calcified).

catheter and the balloon lie down. In these patients, there is almost always a small reddish area, which is difficult to differentiate from an early carcinoma (Figure 21.16). Biopsy of these lesions is a simple way of reassuring the physician and patient. Bladder tumors can be located anywhere in the bladder and have different aspects, but most frequently papillary (Figure 21.17). Much less frequent are urethral tumors (Figure 21.18).

FOREIGN BODIES

Foreign bodies are rare. Not infrequently, hairs can be found in patients with intermittent catheterization. Sometimes, they start to be calcified, and they always have to be removed. Even less frequently found are iatrogenic foreign bodies. Pieces of Foley catheter balloons or sutures from urologic or nonurologic procedures are eroded into the bladder (Figures 21.19 and 21.20).

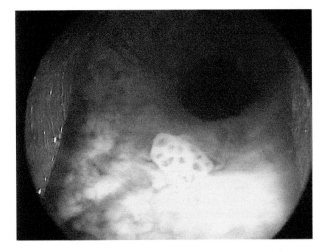

Figure 21.18   Urethral papillary tumor.

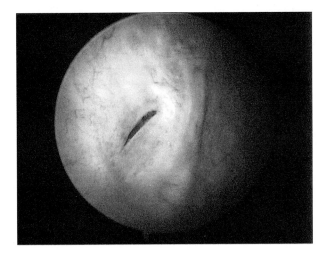

Figure 21.19   Stitch eroding the bladder wall.

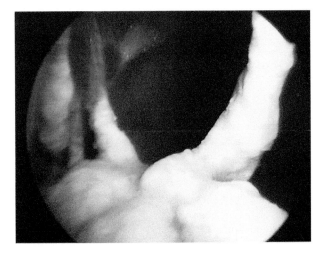

Figure 21.20   Calcified stitch into the bladder.

SPECIAL CONSIDERATIONS

SUPRAPUBIC TUBES

Patients with urinary drainage from a suprapubic catheter deserve special mention based on the additional clinical scenarios and technical aspects associated with evaluation of the lower urinary tract. Indications for cystourethroscopy include regular inspection for bladder stones and surveillance for bladder tumors in patients with suprapubic catheters for more than 5–10 years. Endoscopy may be performed per urethra (when patent) or through the suprapubic tract. Navigation and visualization of the suprapubic tract are usually straightforward in patients with normal body habitus and a mature urinary tract. Rigid cystoscopes may fit into large, mature urinary tracts and are advantageous when ancillary procedures are indicated, but they may be difficult to maneuver in long urinary tracts. Flexible cystoscopes offer improved maneuverability and may fit into smaller urinary tracts. Identification of the ureteral orifices may be challenging owing to edema related to the indwelling catheter or to the angle of vision through the tract.

CONTINENT URINARY DIVERSIONS

Continent urinary diversion is a common urinary reconstructive technique used after cystectomy. Diversions can be categorized as cutaneous continent diversions or orthotopic diversions. In cutaneous continent urinary diversions, detubularized bowel is arranged to create a urinary reservoir with a catheterizable limb anastomosed to the umbilicus or another site on the abdominal wall that provides access for drainage. In orthotopic diversions, the urinary reservoir is anastomosed to the urethra, allowing for volitional voiding. Detailed understanding of the diversion construction is crucial before any endoscopic intervention. Key elements include the type and location of the ureteroenteric anastomosis, the presence or absence of an afferent limb, and the continence mechanism used. Many neobladders have an afferent limb extending from the reservoir to which the ureters are anastomosed. In orthotopic neobladders, the continence mechanism is the external urinary sphincter. Typical continence mechanisms in cutaneous catheterizable diversions include the tunneled appendix (Mitrofanoff), the tapered/imbricated terminal ileum and ileocecal valve, and the intussuscepted nipple valve. The Mitrofanoff and tapered/imbricated ileal continence mechanisms are fragile, and aggressive manipulation can lead to stomal stenosis and/or loss of urinary continence. In these cases, simple visualization and reservoir

filling through the catheterizable channel may be performed with small-caliber flexible endoscopes (e.g., a flexible ureteroscope), but if ancillary procedures are indicated, percutaneous access should be used. Similarly, percutaneous access for interventions other than simple diagnostic procedures in orthotopic neobladders may avoid the risk of bladder neck contracture or sphincteric damage. In both types of diversions, orientation and visualization can be impaired by mucus and debris, bowel peristalsis, mucosal folding, and tortuous afferent limbs. Steps to overcome these difficulties include thorough irrigation and use of fluoroscopy with intravesical administration of a contrast agent to identify the os of the afferent limb and guide endoscope advancement. When present, afferent limbs are best visualized with flexible endoscopes because they are best suited to navigate limb folding, kinking, and tortuosity.

CONCLUSION

Urethrocystoscopy is important in follow-up, surveillance and diagnosis of complications of neurogenic bladders. It often allows us to understand the patient's worsening lower urinary tract function. For now, and for most of the changes and abnormalities found by cystoscopy, no other test can replace it with the same accuracy and reliability.

REFERENCES

1. Tzortzis V, Gravas S, Melekos MM, and de la Rosette JJ. Intraurethral lubricants: A critical literature review and recommendations. *J Endourol.* 2009;23(5):821–6.
2. Lindehall B, Abrahamsson K, Hjalmas K et al. Complications of clean intermittent catheterization in boys and young males with neurogenic bladder dysfunction. *J Urol.* 2004;172:1686–8.
3. Palmer LS. Pediatric urologic imaging. *Urol Clin N Am.* 2006;33:409–23.
4. Rivas DA and Chancelor MB. Sphincterotomy and sphincter stent prosthesis. In: Corcus J, and Schick E, eds. *The Urinary Sphincter.* New York, NY: Marcel Dekker; 2001:565–82.
5. O'Donnell P. Water endoscopy. In: Raz S, ed. *Female Urology.* Philadelphia, PA: WB Saunders; 1983:51–60.
6. Brocklehurst JC. The genitourinary system. In: Brocklehurst JC, ed. *Textbook of Geriatric Medicine and Gerontology.* New York, NY: Churchill Livingstone; 1978:306–25.
7. McGuire EJ. Normal function of lower urinary tract and its relation to neurophysiology. In: Libertino IA, ed. *Clinical Evaluation and Treatments of Neurogenic*

Vesical Dysfunction. International Perspectives in Urology. Baltimore, MD: Williams & Wilkins; 1984:1–15.

8. Shah PJR. Clinical presentation and differential diagnosis. In: Fitzpatrick JM, and Krane RJ, eds. *The Prostate.* Edinburgh: Churchill Livingstone; 1989:91–102.

9. O'Reilly PH. The effect of prostatic obstruction on the upper urinary tract. In: Fitzpatrick JM, and Krane RJ, eds. *The Prostate.* Edinburgh: Churchill Livingstone; 1989:111–18.

Chapter 22

EVALUATION OF NEUROGENIC LOWER URINARY TRACT DYSFUNCTION
Urodynamics

Frank C. Lin and Victor W. Nitti

CLASSIFICATION OF NEUROGENIC LOWER URINARY TRACT DYSFUNCTION

The evaluation of patients suspected of having neurogenic lower urinary tract dysfunction (NLUTD) has two goals: first, to elucidate the process resulting in signs or symptoms of dysfunction, and second, to determine if the upper and lower urinary tracts are at risk for damage. The ultimate aims are to prevent renal compromise and treat bothersome symptoms. Wein's "Functional Classification" of NULTD provides a framework to conceptualize the underlying pathology in patients with NULTD and also allows for a practical guide to management.[1] The lower urinary tract has two basic functions: storage of adequate volume of urine at low pressures, and voluntary and complete evacuation of urine from the bladder. When function is normal there must be proper coordination of the bladder and bladder outlet (bladder neck, urethra, external sphincter). Hence, NLUTD can be classified under the following rubrics: "failure to store" (storage abnormality), "failure to empty" (emptying abnormality), or a combination of both. Each type of "failure" can result from bladder dysfunction, bladder outlet dysfunction, or a combination of both (Table 22.1).

Patients with NLUTD can further be classified as at risk or not at risk for upper urinary tract damage/decompensation. At-risk patients are prone to high storage pressures, usually associated with incomplete bladder emptying. This usually occurs with high outlet resistance, e.g., detrusor-sphincter dyssynergia (DSD) (external sphincter or bladder neck) in patients with suprasacral spinal cord lesions (spinal cord injury, transverse myelitis, myelodysplasia). Patients with incomplete bladder emptying in the absence of DSD can also be at risk if storage pressures are high or postvoid residuals are excessive.

URODYNAMIC ASSESSMENT OF NEUROGENIC LOWER URINARY TRACT DYSFUNCTION

Not all NLUTD is the same, and different patients require different degrees of evaluation depending on the underlying neurologic disease and the symptoms present. In certain scenarios of NLUTD, serious urinary tract and/or renal function damage can result in the absence of symptoms.[2,3] In other instances, symptoms are obvious and difficult to control. In this chapter we do not focus on urodynamic study (UDS) manifestation of specific neurologic conditions, but rather on the use of UDS in general. Specific guidelines for the use of UDS in NLUTD from the European Association of Urology (EAU) are available online (https://uroweb.org/guideline/neuro-urology).

There are several scenarios where UDS is critical to the patient with NLUTD:

1. The patient who demonstrates or is at risk for upper urinary tract decompensation.

2. The patient in whom it is important to establish baseline function, e.g., initial recovery of bladder function after spinal shock.

3. The patient who is not at risk for upper tract damage, in whom symptoms are not well controlled, despite appropriate empiric therapy, for example, a woman with multiple sclerosis who has urgency incontinence but empties normally and has failed medical therapy.

4. The patient who has a nonneurologic condition that can cause lower urinary tract dysfunction, in addition to a neurologic condition, and the cause of symptoms is unclear, for example, a man with refractory urgency incontinence with benign prostatic hyperplasia (BPH) and Parkinson's disease.

Table 22.1   Functional classification of voiding disorders with examples of dysfunction

Failure to Store	
• Bladder dysfunction	Neurogenic DO, impaired compliance
• Bladder outlet dysfunction	Neurogenic intrinsic sphincter deficiency
• Combined dysfunction of bladder and bladder outlet	
Failure to Empty	
• Bladder dysfunction	Detrusor underactivity, acontractile detrusor
• Bladder outlet dysfunction	DESD, DISD
• Combined dysfunction of bladder and bladder outlet	

Abbreviations: DESD, detrusor external sphincter dyssynergia; DISD, detrusor internal sphincter dyssynergia; DO, detrusor overactivity.

5. The patient in whom less invasive testing has obligated a need for more precise diagnosis, for example, a patient not at risk for DSD, who has a significantly elevated postvoid residual (PVR) and/or hydronephrosis.

6. The patient in whom consequences of neurologic disease may affect the outcome of treatment for a nonneurologic disease, for example, a man with benign prostatic obstruction and a history of stroke prior to a transurethral resection of the prostate.

The following are several simple tests that can help determine the need for UDS.

- *Postvoid Residual (PVR).* PVR is considered a standard part of the assessment during initial urologic evaluation of patients with suspected NULTD.[3] While it does not determine the underlying dysfunction, documentation of bladder emptying ability is vital and can be tracked over time. Incomplete emptying can be a sign of suspected or unsuspected DSD or can prompt UDS evaluation as to its cause in the patient not at risk for DSD. In addition, the presence or absence of incomplete emptying can prompt further testing such as UDS.

- *Noninvasive Uroflow.* Similarly, noninvasive uroflowmetry, used in conjunction with PVR, can be used as a screening test for voiding phase dysfunction but is also nonspecific as to cause. It is important to look at both flow rate and the shape of the flow curve. For example, a woman with multiple sclerosis and urgency incontinence who has a normal uroflow and PVR unlikely has significant DSD and may not require UDS.

- *Renal Ultrasound.* The upper urinary tract can be adversely affected by vesicoureteral reflux (VUR), ascending infection, hydronephrosis, or stones.[4] In a patient with NLUTD and hydroureteronephrosis, UDS or videourodynamics (VUDS) may be helpful in determining the etiology.

- *Bladder Diary.* A fluid intake and voiding diary including frequency/volume of voids or log of catheterized volumes can reveal more information about fluid consumption, functional bladder capacity, and characteristics of urine output over a 24-hour period.[5,6] Abnormalities or concerns about diary data may prompt UDS investigation. Diary data can also be used for tracking treatment progress.[7]

Multichannel UDS and VUDS are the mainstays of evaluation in patients with NULTD. UDS has an important role because the presenting symptoms and physical examination findings do not always correlate with the type or extent of the disease/injury or risk of deterioration to the upper tracts. Spinal cord injury level is not always predictive of UDS findings.[8-14]

The goals of UDS in patients with neurologic bladder dysfunction are as follows:

1. To reproduce and document the effect of neurologic disease on the LUT

2. To correlate patient symptoms with urodynamic events

3. To assess for the presence of urologic risk factors (DSD, poor bladder compliance, sustained high-pressure detrusor contractions, and VUR)

The urodynamic evaluation consists of several components including cystometrogram (CMG), abdominal pressure monitoring, electromyography (EMG), uroflowmetry, and voiding pressure-flow studies. Simultaneous fluoroscopic imaging of the entire urinary tract during UDS (VUDS) is extremely useful in cases of known or suspected neurogenic voiding dysfunction. In these complicated cases, UDSs may need to be repeated several times to fulfill the objectives. The entire evaluation can be thought to be in two parts: storage and voiding.

CYSTOMETROGRAM

The CMG assesses the bladder's filling and storage of urine, while the pressure-volume relationship within the bladder is recorded.[8] Starting with an empty bladder, filling should ideally commence with body-temperature fluid at a relatively physiologic filling rate to minimize provoking artificial detrusor overactivity, and bladder compliance tends to be more physiologic and reproducible. Bladder sensation, capacity, the presence of involuntary detrusor contractions, and storage pressures should be documented. When involuntary detrusor contractions are seen in the setting of a relevant neurologic condition, this is referred to as neurogenic detrusor overactivity (DO) according to the International Continence Society (ICS) (Figure 22.1).[15] The intensity, frequency, and timing of DO should be noted.

The following are important points regarding DO:

1. Ensure that the contraction is indeed involuntary. Patients may become confused during the study and actually void as soon as they feel the desire.

2. Determine whether or not a patient's symptoms are reproduced during the involuntary contraction. However, in cases of neurologic disease, DO can occur without symptoms and should not be discounted.

3. The volume at which contractions occur and the pressure/intensity of the contractions should be recorded.

4. Consider repeating the CMG at a slower filling rate if the patient experiences uncharacteristic symptoms (e.g., early fullness, incontinence, or spasms) associated with DO.

5. Incontinence during DO should be documented. Sometimes DO will bring on involuntary voiding to completion (precipitant micturition).[16]

STORAGE PARAMETERS: DETRUSOR OVERACTIVITY, COMPLIANCE, AND LEAK POINT PRESSURES

Bladder compliance is a critical component of the LUT evaluation, especially in patients with advanced neurologic disease. It is calculated as the change in bladder volume and change in detrusor pressure ($\Delta_{volume}/\Delta_{pressure}$) and is measured in milliliters per centimeters (mL/cm) H_2O.[17] According to ICS standards, this calculation should be carried out at the start of bladder filling and at cystometric capacity. Both points are measured excluding any detrusor contraction. The second point can be more difficult to define in patients with NLUTD with phasic detrusor overactivity that results in significant leakage of urine. This may require repeated filling cycles to ensure an adequate bladder volume is achieved.

Impaired compliance leads to high bladder storage pressures and is potentially hazardous. The degree of impaired compliance in NULTD is usually dependent on outlet resistance (e.g., DSD); however, poor compliance can also occur with chronically catheterized bladders (Figure 22.2). The calculated value of compliance is probably less

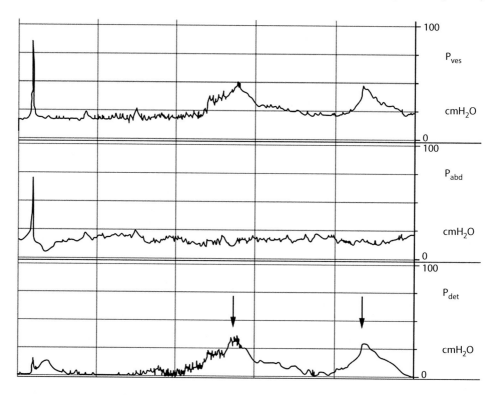

Figure 22.1 Filling phase of a urodynamic study in a 68-year-old woman with urgency incontinence after cerebrovascular accident. Note the involuntary detrusor contractions (arrows). There is a rise in total bladder pressure (P_{ves}) and detrusor pressure (P_{det}), but no change in abdominal pressure (P_{abd}).

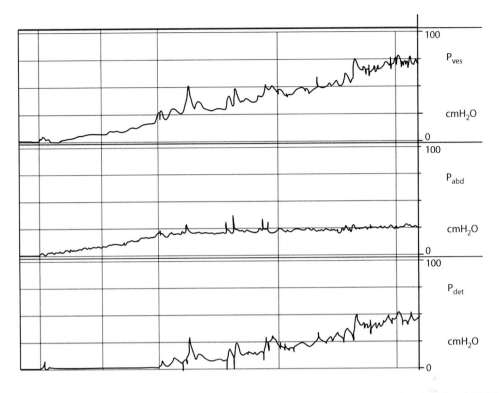

Figure 22.2 Impaired compliance in a 35-year-old male with a T8 spinal cord injury. Note that there is an initial rise in both total vesical pressure (P_{ves}) and abdominal pressure (P_{abd}), but the P_{ves} and, thus, the detrusor pressure (P_{det}) continue to rise to pressures exceeding 40 cm H_2O.

important than the actual bladder pressure during filling as the calculated compliance value can vary, depending on the volume over which it is calculated. Normal compliance is difficult to establish, and when calculated on a volume curve it becomes a "static" property that oversimplifies the concept of compliance.[18] Bladder pressures can sometimes be affected by filling rate during UDS; overly rapid filling rates may produce erroneously lower compliance values. Finally, neurogenic DO can mimic impaired compliance; two methods of differentiating these two entities are (1) stopping the infusion rate and, if necessary, (2) having the patient perform a sustained Kegel maneuver to suppress a possible involuntary contraction.

The determination of bladder storage pressures is critical in patients with NULTD. McGuire demonstrated that myelodysplastic patients with detrusor leak point pressures greater than 40 cm H_2O risked upper tract changes.[19] While this value is often used as a cut point of concern because of risk for upper urinary tract damage (i.e., renal failure), the actual "danger level" in a particular patient may be lower.

During the filling portion of UDS, continence status should be assessed. Urinary leakage can be secondary to a bladder dysfunction (DO or impaired compliance) and/or bladder outlet dysfunction (intrinsic sphincter deficiency).

The detrusor leak point pressure (DLPP) measures the lowest detrusor pressure required to cause urinary incontinence in the absence of increased abdominal pressure. According to ICS, standard DLPP should be measured in the absence of a detrusor contraction.[15] DLPP should not be confused with the abdominal leak point pressure (ALPP), which is defined by the ICS as the intravesical pressure at which urine leakage occurs due to the increased abdominal pressure in the absence of a detrusor contraction. ALPP is a measure of outlet resistance during storage. DLPP is a reflection of the bladder's response to increased outlet resistance during emptying (voluntary or involuntary); high outlet resistance (e.g., DSD) can cause changes in compliance resulting in high storage pressures. The higher the DLPP (which reflects the pressure pop-off mechanism at the urethra), the higher the detrusor pressure will go; this pressure can ultimately be transferred to the upper urinary tracts causing renal deterioration (Figure 22.3). Determination of DLPP and the volume at which it occurs is useful as it allows the clinician to determine when detrusor pressure reaches dangerous levels. The DLPP value does not indicate the amount of time that the urinary tract is exposed to the elevated pressure,

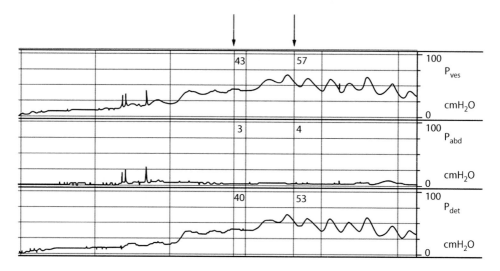

Figure 22.3 Detrusor overactivity occurring in the face of impaired compliance in a teenage girl with myelomeningocele. The left arrow indicates where detrusor pressure equals and then exceeds 40 cm H_2O. The right arrow indicates where leakage occurs—at a bladder leak point pressure of 53 cm H_2O. P_{abd}, abdominal pressure; P_{det}, detrusor pressure; P_{ves}, total vesical pressure.

or if excessive pressure is experienced during involuntary contractions, which also has a critical role in management options.

Urinary leakage secondary to sphincteric dysfunction is measured by ALPP (sometimes referred to as Valsalva LPP).[15] The ALPP is an indirect measure of the ability of the urethra to resist changes in abdominal pressure as an expulsive force.[20] Clinically, it is used to determine the presence of stress urinary incontinence and the abdominal pressure at which it occurs (Figure 22.4). Normally, there is no physiologic abdominal pressure that should cause incontinence;

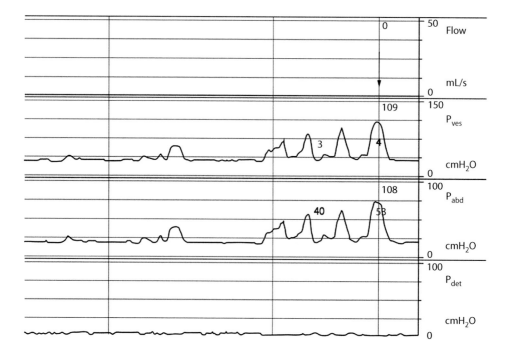

Figure 22.4 Urodynamic tracing of woman with stress incontinence. Tracing shows progressive Valsalva maneuvers until leakage occurs (arrow) at an abdominal pressure of 109 cm H_2O, which is the abdominal leak point pressure (ALPP). Note that there is no rise in detrusor pressure. P_{abd}, abdominal pressure; P_{det}, detrusor pressure; P_{ves}, total vesical pressure.

Table 22.2   Basic Urodynamic Finding Based On Level Of Lesion Or Area Affected By Neurologic Disease

Lesion Location	
Above the brainstem	Common to see DO. Depends on (1) lesion nature (destructive or irritative) and (2) area affected (normally inhibitory or stimulatory). Rare to see DESD (if ever)
Between brainstem and sacral cord	Often see DO ± DESD. Can see DISD (sympathetic, smooth muscle) if complete transection and above T6
Sacral cord and distal	Typically a highly compliant acontractile bladder. External sphincter is functional with preservation of continence

Source: Adapted from Wein, AJ, *Voiding Dysfunction in Neurologic Injury and Disease*, 2012.
Abbreviations: DESD, detrusor external sphincter dyssynergia; DISD, detrusor internal sphincter dyssynergia; DO, detrusor overactivity.

therefore, there is no "normal ALPP." Unlike the DLPP, an elevated ALPP does not indicate potential danger to the kidneys.

VOIDING PHASE

During the voiding phase of UDS the presence, strength, and duration of the detrusor contraction during emptying are measured. Detrusor contractility may be impaired (detrusor underactivity) in particular types of neurologic disease, particularly with lower motor neuron lesions. Outlet resistance can also be measured while voiding. While DSD is commonly seen in patients with NULTD (with suprasacral cord lesions), obstruction can occur anywhere distal to the bladder. Several nomograms and formulas exist to categorize pressure-flow relationships in terms of nonobstructed, obstructed, or equivocal in NULTD patients.[21–25] If DO occurs and causes significant emptying the bladder prematurely, this pressure-flow relationship should

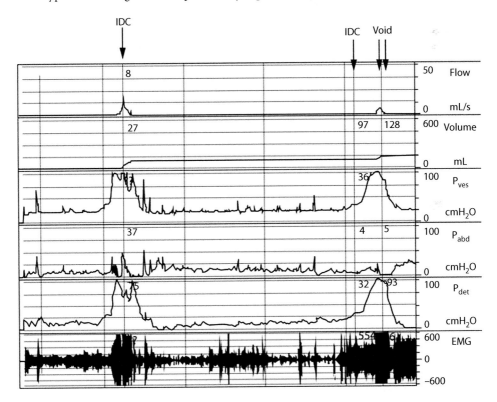

Figure 22.5   Urodynamic tracing of an 18-year-old woman with frequency, urgency, and urge incontinence, who was diagnosed with a tethered cord. Note detrusor overactivity (involuntary detrusor contraction [IDC], arrow) associated with high-volume urine loss as registered in the flow meter. There is increased sphincter activity, as demonstrated by increased electromyograph (EMG) activity consistent with detrusor-external sphincter dyssynergia. On the second fill there is again an IDC, but this time the patient is instructed to void (double void). Note that there is increased EMG activity throughout the IC and "voluntary void." Detrusor pressures with DO are quite high because of the resistance of the contracting striated sphincter. P_{abd}, abdominal pressure; P_{det}, detrusor pressure; P_{ves}, total vesical pressure.

not be interpreted as normal physiologic voiding (though it may be "normal" emptying for a specific patient with NULTD).

EMG evaluates the striated sphincter function during micturition.[8] Surface patch electrodes are most often used but are prone to motion artifact.[26] Needle electrodes permit more accurate recordings but are more invasive. Normal voluntary voiding is preceded by a complete relaxation of the striated sphincter. DESD refers to "a detrusor contraction concurrent with an involuntary contraction of the urethral and/or periurethral striated muscle," which results in a functional obstruction.[15] True DESD can be seen in patients with lesions between the brainstem and sacral spinal cord (Table 22.2 and Figure 22.5).

VIDEOURODYNAMICS

VUDS is the most comprehensive and accurate way of assessing NULTD.[27] It is the test of choice for patients with advanced NULTD at risk for upper tract decompensation. During the filling phase, VUDS can determine the presence of vesicoureteral reflux and the pressure and volume at which this occurs. Elevated bladder pressures may be masked secondary to a "pop-off valve" phenomenon into the upper tracts. In that case, detrusor pressure and

compliance calculations do not accurately reflect the pressure experienced by the upper urinary tracts. Moreover, assessment of the DLPP or ALPP is facilitated as fluoroscopy is often more sensitive than direct observation of urinary leakage. VUDS also permits the radiographic evaluation of the internal urethral sphincter or bladder neck during storage and helps determine the level of continence. It is also useful to determine DSD and has been shown to be more accurate than EMG.[26] Additionally, other abnormalities such as bladder and urethral diverticula and fistula can be seen. During the voiding phase, fluoroscopy can elucidate the site of obstruction when high pressure/low flow exists. VUDS is the only test to determine the presence of detrusor-internal sphincter (bladder neck) dyssynergia by the lack of opening of the bladder neck on fluoroscopy during a detrusor contraction[28] (Figure 22.6).

CONCLUSION

UDS can be useful and in some cases critical in evaluating patients with neurologic disease to improve quality of life and to prevent any deleterious

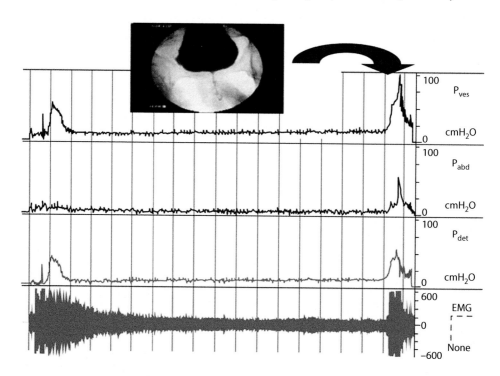

Figure 22.6 Detrusor external sphincter dyssynergia (DESD) and detrusor internal sphincter dyssynergia (DISD) in a 35-year-old male with a high cervical spinal cord injury. There are two episodes of DO with associated increased electromyographic (EMG) activity consistent with DESD. However, the fluoroscopic picture taken at the time of the second episode of DO shows an incompletely opened bladder neck consistent with DISD. This patient underwent a striated sphincterotomy as well as a bladder neck incision to facilitate emptying and lower pressures. P_{abd}, abdominal pressure; P_{det}, detrusor pressure; P_{ves}, total vesical pressure.

effect on the urinary tract ultimately leading to renal failure. It may be needed in asymptomatic patients as the effects on the urinary tract can be clinically silent. Patients without a history of neurologic disease, whose urologic evaluation is suspicious for NLUTD, should be evaluated for occult neurologic disease.

REFERENCES

1. Wein AJ. Classification of neurogenic voiding dysfunction. *J Urol.* 1981;125(5):605–9.
2. Nitti VW. Evaluation of the female with neurogenic voiding dysfunction. *Int Urogynecol J Pelvic Floor Dysfunct.* 1999;10:119–29.
3. Panicker JN, De Sèze M, Fowler CJ. Neurogenic lower urinary tract dysfunction. *Handb Clin Neurol.* 2013;110:209–20.
4. Shenot PJ, Moy ML. Office-based care of the neurogenic bladder patient. *Curr Bladder Dysfunct Rep.* 2011; 6: 74–80.
5. Stöhrer M, Goepel M, Kondo A et al. The standardization of terminology in neurogenic lower urinary tract dysfunction: With suggestions for diagnostic procedures. International Continence Society Standardization Committee. *Neurourol Urodyn.* 1999;18:139–58.
6. de SÈZE M, Ruffion A, Denys P et al. The neurogenic bladder in multiple sclerosis: Review of the literature and proposal of management guidelines. *Mult Scler.* 2007;13:915–28.
7. Pannek J, Einig E-M, and Einig W. Clinical management of bladder dysfunction caused by sexual abuse. *Urol Int.* 2009;82:420–5.
8. Winters JC, Dmochowski RR, Goldman HB et al. Urodynamic studies in adults: AUA/SUFU Guideline. *J Urol.* 2012;188:2464–72.
9. Bunts RC. Management of urological complication in 1000 paraplegics. *JURO.* 1958;79:733–1.
10. Delnay KM, Stonehill WH, Goldman H et al. Bladder histological changes associated with chronic indwelling urinary catheter. *J Urol.* 1999;161:1106–9.
11. Kaufman JM, Fam B, Jacobs SC et al. Bladder cancer and squamous metaplasia in spinal cord injury patients. *JURO.* 1977;118:967–71.
12. Jacobs SC and Kaufman JM. Complications of permanent bladder catheter drainage in spinal cord injury patients. *JURO.* 1978;119:740–1.
13. Wein AJ. Voiding Dysfunction in Neurologic Injury and Disease. PowerPoint presentation, 2012.
14. Weld KJ and Dmochowski RR. Association of level of injury and bladder behavior in patients with post-traumatic spinal cord injury. *Urology.* 2000;55:490–4.
15. Abrams P, Cardozo L, Fall M et al. The standardisation of terminology in lower urinary tract function: Report from the standardisation sub-committee of the International Continence Society. *Urology.* 2003;61:37–49.
16. Nitti VW. Cystometry and abdominal pressure monitoring. In: Nitti VW, ed. *Practical Urodynamics.* Philadelphia, PA: WB Saunders; 1998:38–51.
17. Toppercer A and Tetreault JP. Compliance of the bladder: An attempt to establish normal values. *Urology.* 1979;14:204–5.
18. Gilmour RF, Churchill BM, Steckler RE et al. A new technique for dynamic analysis of bladder compliance. *JURO.* 1993;150:1200–3.
19. MCGuire EJ, Woodside JR, Borden TA, and Weiss RM. Prognostic value of urodynamic testing in myelodysplastic patients. *J Urol.* 1981;126:205–9.
20. McGuire EJ, Cespedes RD, and O'Connell HE. Leak-point pressures. *Urol Clin N Am.* 1996;23:253–62.
21. Abrams PH and Griffiths DJ. The assessment of prostatic obstruction from urodynamic measurements and from residual urine. *Br J Urol.* 1979;51:129–34.
22. Schäfer W. Principles and clinical application of advanced urodynamic analysis of voiding function. *Urol Clin North Am.* 1990;17:553–66.
23. Abrams P. Bladder outlet obstruction index, bladder contractility index and bladder voiding efficiency: Three simple indices to define bladder voiding function. *BJU Int.* 1999;84:14–5.
24. Blaivas JG and Groutz A. Bladder outlet obstruction nomogram for women with lower urinary tract symptomatology. *Neurourol Urodyn.* 2000; 19:553–64.
25. Lemack GE and Zimmern PE. Pressure flow analysis may aid in identifying women with outflow obstruction. *J Urol.* 2000;163:1823–8.
26. Brucker BM, Fong E, Shah S et al. Urodynamic differences between dysfunctional voiding and primary bladder neck obstruction in women. *Urology.* 2012;80:55–60.
27. Blaivas JG. Videourodynamics studies. In: Nitti VW, ed. *Practical Urodynamics.* Philadelphia, PA: WB Saunders; 1998:78–93.
28. Watanabe T and Chancellor M. Neurogenic voiding dysfunction. In: Nitti VW, ed. *Practical Urodynamics.* Philadelphia, PA: WB Saunders; 1998:142–55.

Chapter 23

ELECTROPHYSIOLOGIC EVALUATION
Basic Principles and Clinical Applications

Melita Rotar and David B. Vodušek

INTRODUCTION

Electrophysiologic (= neurophysiologic) testing of nerves and muscles is used in the assessment of patients with (suspected) nervous system lesions. It may be indicated in selected patients for a more precise diagnosis of muscle and nervous system dysfunction. The results of testing need to be interpreted in the clinical context (after a thorough history and physical investigation) with the awareness of the pathophysiologic meaning of the test results and the limitations of individual tests.

BASIC PRINCIPLES

Clinical neurophysiologic tests evaluate all parts of the neuromuscular system and may be divided into electromyography and tests of conduction, assessing striated muscles and motor and sensory pathways, respectively (Table 23.1).

ELECTROMYOGRAPHY

Electromyography (EMG) is the recording of muscle electrical activity generated by the excitable membranes of muscle cells (usually called fibers). The normal EMG signal consists of potentials generated by motor units (a motor unit is the assembly of muscle fibers innervated by one lower motor neuron) (Figure 23.1). Pathologic changes in muscle are either "myopathic" (due to muscle disease) or "neuropathic" (due to a lesion or disease of the lower motor neuron). These changes are reflected in the EMG as abnormal spontaneous activity and/or changes in the number and shape of motor unit potentials (MUPs).

EMG may be performed for two quite distinct although complementary purposes. On the one hand, the "quantity" of the EMG signal is an indicator of the activity of muscle; or the EMG signal is analyzed and conveys information whether the muscle is normal, myopathic, or denervated/reinnervated. The former has been called "kinesiological EMG" and the latter

"concentric needle" EMG, but often this division is not specified and both types of examination are just called "EMG," which can confuse the uninitiated.

TESTS OF CONDUCTION

Tests of conduction rely on the principle that the nervous system has excitable membranes and can be depolarized by an electric current. Electrical stimulation (or stimulation using a changing magnetic field, which induces electric currents) can be applied to different parts of the central and peripheral nervous systems (Figure 23.2). The depolarization spreads along the nervous pathways. Thus, the depolarization after stimulation of a sensory nerve can be recorded along the particular afferent pathway. (It also elicits reflex responses.) Stimulation of motor pathways causes activation of striated muscles, which can be recorded as an evoked compound muscle potential.

Classified anatomically, the conduction tests can be divided into motor, sensory, and autonomic. Recording reflexes is testing conduction, too.

Technically, it is easy to measure the latency of responses obtained on stimulation. Latency correlates with the speed of conduction of the action potentials along the nervous pathway. If the consequence of disease is demyelination (as in multiple sclerosis or Guillain-Barré syndrome), the conduction velocity will be slowed (and latencies delayed).

If the pathologic process, however, affects partial axon loss (as in the majority of nervous lesions), the conduction of the preserved axons will remain normal, and the measurement of latencies will not reveal the abnormality. Axonal loss is reflected in the diminished amplitude of the evoked response, but amplitudes are technically difficult to record accurately and are less specific indicators of abnormality.

As electrical stimulation preferentially depolarizes the thickest myelinated nerve fibers, the conduction tests do not provide information on thin nerve fibers (important for pain perception).

Details of the methods mentioned in this text (and of their application) are extensively described in textbooks on clinical neurophysiology.[1]

Table 23.1   Unique Information Provided By Electrophysiological Tests

Information	Structure	Method	Finding
Neuronal integrity preserved	Lower motor neuron	CNEMG	Absent spontaneous denervation activity, continuous MUP firing during relaxation
	Lower and upper motor neuron	CNEMG	Dense IP on voluntary activation
	Sacral reflex arc	CNEMG sacral reflex	Dense IP on reflex activation by touch; brisk responses of normal latency
	Somatosensory pathways	Pudendal SEP	Normal shape and latency of responses
Localization of neuronal lesions	Root versus plexus/nerve	CNEMG	Paravertebral denervation activity in neighboring myotomes
		SNAP	Normal (penile) SNAP with impaired (penile) skin sensation
Severity of neuronal lesions	Complete versus partial	CNEMG	Profuse spontaneous denervation activity absent MUPs
	Severe versus moderate	Sacral reflex	Response nonelicitable
Type of neuronal lesion	Conduction block versus axonotmeisis	CNEMG	Absent/sparse spontaneous denervation activity
	Axonotmeisis versus neurotmesis	CNEMG	Appearance of nascent MUPs after complete muscle denervation

Source: Corcos J, and Schnick E, *Textbook of the Neurogenic Bladder*. Informa Healthcare UK, London, United Kingdom, 2008.
Abbreviations: CNEMG, concentric needle electromyography; IP, interference pattern; MUP, motor unit potential; SEP, somatosensory evoked potential; SNAP, sensory nerve action potential.

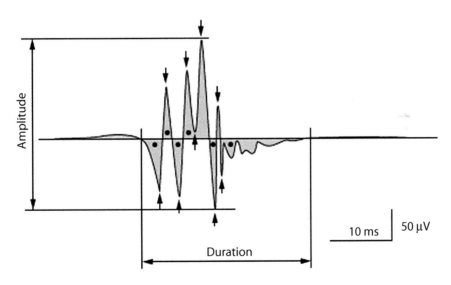

Figure 23.1   Motor unit potential (MUP) parameters. Amplitude is the voltage difference (μV) between the most positive and most negative points of the MUP trace. The MUP duration is the time (ms) between the first deflection and the point when the MUP waveform finally returns to baseline. The number of MUP phases (small circles) is defined by the number of MUP areas alternatively below and above the baseline and can be counted as the "number of baseline crossings plus one." Turns (arrows) are defined as changes in direction of the MUP trace that are larger than the specified amplitude (e.g., 50 μV) but not crossing the baseline. MUP area measures the integrated surface of the MUP waveform (shaded). (From Corcos, J, and Schnick E, *Textbook of the Neurogenic Bladder*. Informa Healthcare UK, London, United Kingdom, 2008.)

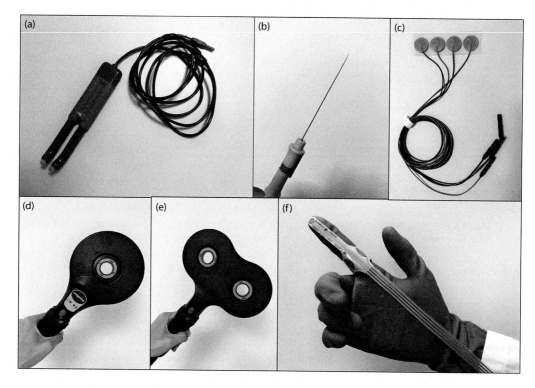

Figure 23.2 Different electrodes used in electrophysiological testing. (a) Surface stimulation electrode: it is placed over the stimulated nerve and delivers electical stimuli; (b) concentric needle electrode consists of an insulated platinum wire that is inserted through a steel cannula and detects muscle activity up to 2.5 mm from the electrode tip; (c) surface recording electrodes: disposable adhesive prewired discs with added silver/silver-chloride conductive layer, which ensures low impedance and enables optimal signal recording; (d) round and (e) figure-eight-shaped metal coil for transcutaneous magnetic stimulation. A short and strong current is passed through it. This creates a time-variable magnetic field, which induces an electrical field; (f) St. Mark's electrode for pudendal nerve terminal motor latency measurement. The electrode consists of a bipolar stimulating part at the tip of the finger and a recording pair of electrodes 8 cm proximally (at the base of the index finger).

ROUTINELY USED ELECTROPHYSIOLOGIC TESTS IN CLINICAL PRACTICE

KINESIOLOGIC ELECTROMYOGRAPHY

The purpose of kinesiologic EMG is assessment of the pattern of activity of a particular muscle. In patients with lower urinary tract (LUT) dysfunction, kinesiologic EMG is used for assessing pelvic floor muscle (PFM) activity during bladder filling and emptying, particularly in the case of neurogenic LUT dysfunction and in patients with dysfunctional voiding. (It may also be called "urodynamic EMG.")[2–4] Surface electrodes or indwelling electrodes may be used. The latter record a better-defined EMG signal with less artifacts, and the recording is more selective for deeper or small muscles. Surface electrodes are preferred in practice because they are not invasive.

The information from kinesiologic EMG is on the intensity and time course of the muscle activity and may be used for both diagnostic and therapeutic use (biofeedback).

Aim:

- Assessment of intensity and time course of the activity of chosen muscles
- Monitoring of sphincter function during storage and voiding
- Providing biofeedback therapy in LUT dysfunction

Drawback:

- Not applicable for detection of reinnervation changes in muscle
- No detection of signs of denervation in muscle

CONCENTRIC NEEDLE ELECTROMYOGRAPHY

Concentric needle EMG (CNEMG) takes the name from the fact that a particular standardized type of needle electrode is used for detection of the EMG signal. This way of recording from muscle allows straightforward EMG signal analysis and the differentiation between normal striated muscle, primary muscle disease, and denervation/reinnervation in patients with suspected neuromuscular disorders. In patients with suspected lesions in the lower sacral segments (which include innervation of pelvic organs), it is the most useful technique to detect abnormalities of the peripheral innervation of PFM. The practical signature muscle to be examined is the external anal sphincter (EAS), because it is easily accessible and has sufficient muscle bulk.[5] EAS is a skeletal muscle under voluntary control, but it differs from most other skeletal muscles by the presence of continuous firing of low-threshold MUPs at rest. During voluntary and reflex activation, high-threshold MUPs are recruited, which are typically larger than the continuously firing MUPs.[6] The CNEMG includes assessment of insertion activity, tonic activity, voluntary and reflex activation of motor units, detection of pathologic spontaneous ("denervation") activity, qualitative assessment of the interference pattern, and quantitative MUP analysis. Signs of denervation (positive sharp waves, fibrillation potentials) are as a rule linked to recent (or progressive) denervation (Figure 23.3). Reinnervation produces long, polyphasic, and high-amplitude MUPs. Repetitive discharges may be found in chronically denervated muscle (but also in the external urethral sphincter of women with chronic urinary retention—Fowler's syndrome [Figure 23.4]).[7,8]

Motor unit loss is assessed by evaluating the reduction in the number of activated motor units, which fire at a faster rate. There are also several automated programs available to quantitatively assess the interference pattern.[9] Individual MUPs can be analyzed by computer programs. (We prefer quantitative MUP analysis.)[10] The program extracts and averages obtained MUPs, calculates MUP duration, area, amplitude, and number of phases and turns. The most significant findings on CNEMG are pathologic spontaneous activity and/or changes in the mean duration of MUPs (Figure 23.5).

To summarize, an axonal lesion in the peripheral motor innervation of PFM (recent or in the past) will be revealed by CNEMG.

There are advances in the EMG signal analysis as recorded with surface electrodes,[11,12] but for the diagnosis of denervation/reinnervation of striated muscles in individual patients, these methods are not (yet) useful.

Aim:

- Diagnosis of lesions of the pudendal nerve, sacral plexus, cauda equina, sacral roots, and conus medullaris
- Determination of Onuf's nucleus degeneration in degenerative diseases
- Diagnosis of nonneurogenic urinary retention in young women (Fowler's syndrome)
- Clues provided of possible suprasegmental nervous system lesions

Drawback:

- Invasive

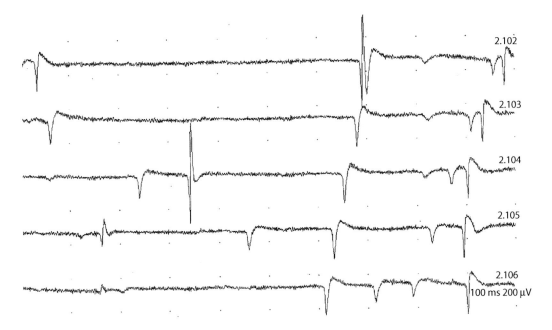

Figure 23.3 Activity recorded after recent denervation of muscle. Bulbospongiosus muscle concentric needle electromyography in 31-year-old male patient 4 weeks after acute total cauda equina lesion. The bulbospongiosus muscle has no tonic activity, and pathologic spontaneous (denervation) activity in the form of positive sharp waves (b) and fibrillation potentials (a) can be dependably demonstrated. There was no voluntary or reflex activation of motor units.

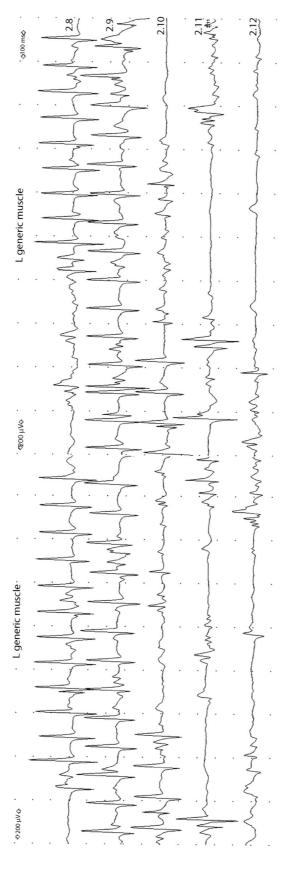

Figure 23.4 Fowler's syndrome. Concentric needle electromyography of external urethral sphincter in a 32-year-old woman who presented with urinary retention. Continuous electromyographic trace showing repetitive discharges.

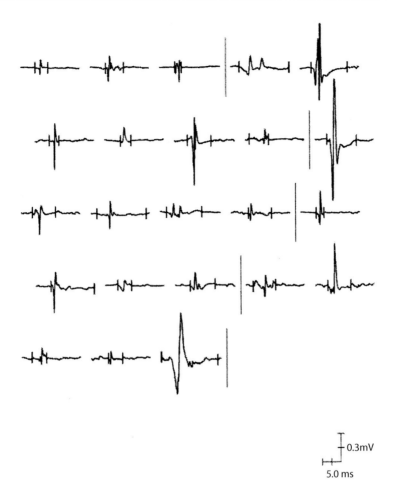

0.3mV

5.0 ms

Figure 23.5 Multi-motor unit potential (MUP) analysis of external anal sphincter (EAS) concentric needle electromyography signal in a 72-year-old patient with clinically possible multiple system atrophy with erectile dysfunction and urinary urgency. A computer program was used to automatically extract MUPs from a 4.8-second period of the signal. Repeatingly firing MUPs were averaged and presented separately. The computer algorithm set take-off and end points of MUPs and calculated MUP duration, area, amplitude, number of phases, and turns. In this patient, several MUPs are of high amplitude, have long duration, and are polyphasic, which is a sign of chronic reinnervation.

BULBOCAVERNOUS REFLEX

Neurophysiologically, the bulbocavernous reflex (BCR) is elicited by applying a mechanical, magnetic, or electrical stimulus to the penis/clitoris and recording the activation of the target muscles (bulbospongiosus muscle, EAS) using needle or surface electrodes.[13] Electrical stimulation of the dorsal nerve of the penis/clitoris yields two reflex components of the BCR, the first being stable and nonhabituable at latencies about 35 ms, and the second that is more variable and represents a polysynaptic reflex at latencies above 50 ms.[14] The only measured parameter of the BCR is the onset latency of the early component (Figure 23.6).[15,16]

The BCR may be analyzed separately for the left and right sides of the EAS or bulbospongiosus muscle. Interside latency difference helps to identify the presence of asymmetric lesions. Short latency of the BCR may be due to a low position of the conus medullaris as in tethered cord syndrome[17] or a suprasegmental cord lesion.[18] A normal reflex latency does not exclude the presence of a partial axonal lesion, nor is an abnormal latency necessarily indicative of pelvic organ dysfunction.

Aim:

- To demonstrate the presence of the reflex (which is often clinically ambiguous)
- To evaluate conduction along the sacral reflex arc

Drawback:

- A normal reflex latency does not exclude a partial axonal lesion

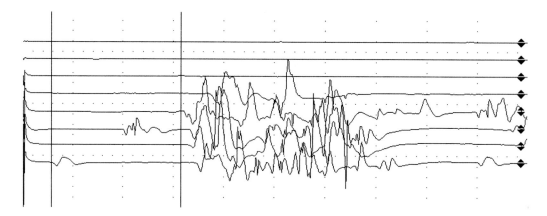

Figure 23.6 Electrophysiologic measurement of the bulbocavernous reflex (BCR) in a 71-year-old male patient with urinary urgency and nocturia. BCR was elicited by applying electrical stimulus with surface electrode to the dorsal nerve of the penis. Strong stimulus starts at the fourth ray. Response is detected with a concentric needle electromyography electrode in right bulbospongiosus muscle. The minimal latency is set at 31.6 ms.

- An abnormal reflex latency cannot be equated with organ dysfunction (incontinence, etc.)

OTHER ELECTROPHYSIOLOGIC TESTS USED IN SPECIAL CLINICAL CIRCUMSTANCES

PUDENDAL SOMATOSENSORY EVOKED POTENTIALS

The pudendal somatosensory evoked potentials (pSEP) can be recorded with electrical stimulation of the dorsal nerve of the penis or clitoris and detection of the response with disk electrodes fixed to the scalp at the central detection site (Cz - 2 cm) of the International 10–20 electroencephalography system (Figure 23.7).[19] "Dermatomal" electrical stimulation (in the perianal region, intraurethrally, in the bladder— see page 178) also elicits cortical SEPs.

SEPs assess the conduction along the somatosensory pathways from the periphery to the cerebral cortex and may be abnormal in patients with spinal cord lesions, cauda equina lesions, and peripheral nerve lesions,[20] but the test is not sensitive to partial axonal lesions (Figure 23.8).

Aim:

- To objectively investigate the conduction in afferent neural pathways from the periphery to the sensory cortex

Drawback:

- Test is not sensitive to partial axonal lesions and may be "normal" in patient with partial perineal sensory loss
- Investigation adds little to the clinical examination

SACRAL MOTOR EVOKED POTENTIALS

Conduction in the central motor pathways is assessed by transcutaneous magnetic stimulation of motor cortex and recording of the response of the skeletal muscle. By separately stimulating the motor cortex

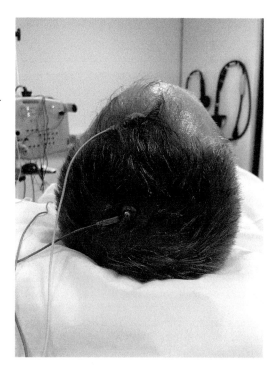

Figure 23.7 Electrode placement for somatosensory evoked potential (SEP) detection. The pudendal SEP can be recorded with electrical stimulation of the dorsal nerve of the penis or clitoris. Detection of the response is with eletrodes fixed to the scalp at the central detection site (Cz - 2 cm) of the International 10–20 electroencephalograpy system with the Fz reference.

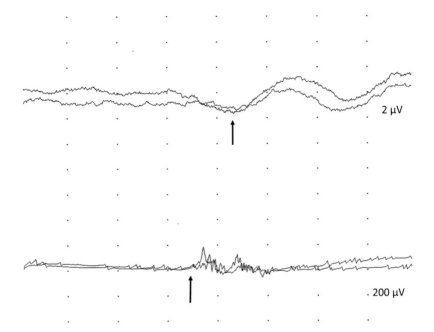

2 µV

. 200 µV

Figure 23.8 Cerebral somatosensory evoked potential (SEP) (above) and bulbocavernosus reflex (below) on stimulation of the dorsal nerve of the penis in a 42-year-old healthy man. SEP is recorded with surface electrodes (Cz –2 cm: Fz); the bulbocavernosus reflex is recorded from the bulbospongiosus muscle with needle electrode; the dorsal nerve of the penis is stimulated with disposable adhesive electrodes. Two consecutive averages of 100 responses are superimposed. The P40 of the SEP and the first component of the bulbocavernosus reflex are indicated with arrows.

and ventral spinal roots, and subtracting the latencies, the "central motor conduction" time can be calculated.

To obtain pelvic floor MEP, stimulation is applied over the vertex (primary motor center in the precentral gyrus) and to the upper lumbar spine (exit of the sacral roots from the conus medullaris).[21] Magnetic stimulation evokes responses from several adjacent muscles; therefore, in the case of striated sphincter MEP detection, a selective response is obtained only by using a concentric needle electrode.[22] The reported mean latencies from EAS were 25–30 ms without facilitation and shorter with facilitation; mean central motor conduction time is 16 ms without facilitation and 13 ms with facilitation.[21]

Aim:
- Evaluation of the central and peripheral motor conduction to the individual pelvic floor muscles
- Demonstration of a lesion in the motor pathway

Drawback:
- Poor sensitivity to partial axonal lesions
- Investigation adds as a rule little to clinical examination

SACRAL SYMPATHETIC SKIN RESPONSE

Sympathetic skin response (SSR) is a reflex consisting of myelinated sensory afferent fibers and complex central transduction and sympathetic efferent fibers. It can be elicited by using an electrical pulse

delivered to a limb or the sacral region and recorded from perineal skin or penis. Responses are variable, dependent on various factors, and habituate rapidly; therefore, only the absence of a response is considered abnormal.[23]

Aim:
- Assessment of neuropathies of unmyelinated nerve fibers
- Assessment of thoracolumbar sympathetic pathways

Drawback:
- Variable responses

OTHER INVESTIGATIONS

SINGLE-FIBER ELECTROMYOGRAPHY

Single-fiber EMG (SFEMG) is a technique of needle EMG and records action potentials of single muscle cells (fibers). It is mostly used to diagnose muscle end-plate pathology (myasthenia gravis). It can also detect changes in muscle due to reinnervation. "Fiber density" is defined as the mean number of muscle fiber potentials per detection site (normally below 2); higher values correlate with reinnervation.[24] SFEMG of EAS has been of value in research; the gold standard in diagnostics of patients with lesions of the sacral nervous system in clinical practice is, however, CNEMG with concomitant recording of BCR.[25]

Aim:

- To detect changes in striated muscle due to reinnervation

Drawback:

- Lacks the ability to detect abnormal spontaneous activity

PUDENDAL NERVE TERMINAL MOTOR LATENCY

Due to the anatomic position of the pudendal nerve, the nerve is not accessible for classical recording of conduction velocity. The pudendal nerve terminal motor latency (PNTML) represents only the conduction of the fastest conducting fibers of the distal part of the pudendal nerve (Figure 23.9). PNTML is measured with a special stimulation/recording electrode assembly fixed onto a gloved index finger of the examiner (St. Mark's electrode). The electrode consists of a stimulating part at the tip of the finger and a recording pair of (surface) electrodes at the base of the index finger, which has to be inserted into the rectum.[26] Prolongation or asymmetry of PNTML has been claimed to diagnose pudendal neuropathy, but the validity of the test is controversial, and no correlation was found between PNTML value and either EAS EMG or anorectal manometry parameters. In contrast, EMG strongly correlated with squeeze pressure measured by anorectal manometry and was more closely related to the anal functional status than PNTML.[27]

Aim:

- To detect (asymmetry of) pudendal nerve conduction
- To determine the presence of motor response in patients with suspected complete denervation in the lower sacral myotomes

Drawback:

- It is not sensitive to partial axonal loss
- Prolongation of the latency is not a measure of denervation
- The validity of the test is controversial

NEUROGRAPHY OF DORSAL PENILE NERVE

By stimulating at the glans and detecting the sensory action potential at the base of the penis, a sensory action potential can be recorded.[28]

Aim:

- Demonstration of a normal amplitude response in a hypesthetic penis locates the lesion proximal to the sensory ganglion

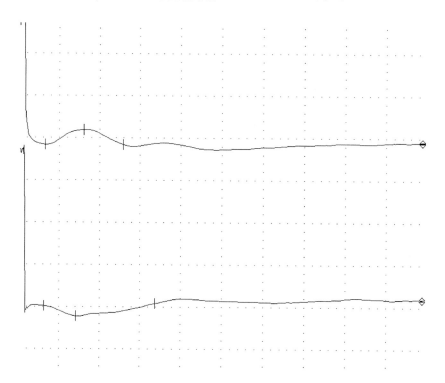

Figure 23.9 Pudendal nerve terminal motor latency in a 38-year-old male patient with perineal pain and no voiding dysfunction. Motor response of the right (top) and left (bottom) pudendal nerves. For stimulation the St. Mark's electrode was used. The latency of the response is 1.3 and 1.2 ms, respectively.

Drawback:

- Sensory velocity calculation is imprecise as the length of the nerve tested is difficult to measure precisely

SOMATOSENSORY EVOKED POTENTIAL ON STIMULATION OF THE BLADDER AND URETHRA

Sensory pathways from the bladder (or urethra) can be assessed by applying electrical stimulation to either of them by using special catheters[29] and detecting cortical responses from the scalp.

Aim:

- To test sensory pathways from bladder/urethra

Drawback:

- Technically difficult; unrecordable responses in some normal subjects

BLADDER SMOOTH MUSCLE ELECTROMYOGRAPHY

In assessment of sacral parasympathetic function, some circumstantial information is provided by cystometry. Definitive evaluation of detrusor innervation should be obtained by detrusor EMG, but the methods used at present provide controversial results.

Aim:

- To assess parasympathetic innervation of the bladder

Drawback:

- No replicable recording protocols

PATIENT GROUPS IN WHOM ELECTROPHYSIOLOGICAL TESTING IS OF CLINICAL VALUE

Electrophysiological tests have been found to add little to clinical diagnosis in patients with neurogenic LUT dysfunction due to a central nervous system lesion (excluding here kinesiologic EMG measured simultaneously with a pressure flow study). Sensory and motor evoked potentials are, however, useful in intraoperative monitoring (not discussed here, see Vodusek and Deletis[30]).

If in a patient there is, however, a need to substantiate a suspicion of a peripheral nervous system lesion causing LUT symptoms, or better define such a lesion (as in patients with dysraphism, tethered cord syndrome, cauda equina lesions, sacral plexus lesions, or neurodegenerative diseases involving the Onuf's nucleus), performing a CNEMG and BCR will provide useful information.

REFERENCES

1. Dumitru D, Amato A, and Zwartz M. *Electrodiagnostic Medicine*. 2nd ed. Philadelphia, PA: Hanley & Belfus; 2002.
2. De EJ, Patel CY, Tharian B, Westney OL, Graves DE, and Hairston JC. Diagnostic discordance of electromyography (EMG) versus voiding cystourethrogram (VCUG) for detrusor-external sphincter dyssynergy (DESD). *Neurourol Urodyn*. 2005;24:616–21.
3. Groutz A, Blaivas JG, Pies C, and Sassone AM. Learned voiding dysfunction (non-neurogenic, neurogenic bladder) among adults. *Neurourol Urodyn*. 2001;20:359–68.
4. Deindl FM, Vodusek DB, Bischoff C, Hofmann R, and Hartung R. Dysfunctional voiding in women: Which muscles are responsible? *BJU*. 1998;82:814–9.
5. Podnar S, and Vodusek DB. Protocol for clinical neurophysiologic examination of pelvic floor. *Neurourol Urodyn*. 2001;20:669–82.
6. Podnar S and Vodusek DB. Standardisation of anal sphincter EMG: Low and high threshold motor units. *Clin Neurophysiol*. 1999;110:1488–91.
7. Fowler CJ, Kirby RS, and Harrison MJ. Decelerating burst and complex repetitive discharges in the striated muscle of the urethral sphincter, associated with urinary retention in women. *J Neurol Neurosurg Psychiatry*. 1985;48:1004–9.
8. Fitzgerald MP, Blazek B, and Brubaker L. Complex repetitive discharges during urethral sphincter EMG: Clinical correlates. *Neurourol Urodyn*. 2000;19:557–83.
9. Nandedkar SD, Sanders DB, and Stalberg EV. Automatic analysis of the electromyographic interference pattern. Part II: Findings in control subjects and in some neuromuscular disease. *Muscle Nerve*. 1986;9:491–500.
10. Stalberg E, Falk B, Sonoo M, Stalberg S, and Astrom M. Multi-MUP EMG analysis—A two year experience in daily clinical work. *Electroencephalogr Clin Neurophysiol*. 1995;97:145–54.
11. Merletti R, Bottin A, Cescon C et al. Multichannel surface EMG for the non-invasive assessment of the anal sphincter muscle. *Digestion*. 2004;69;112–22.
12. Drusany Starič K, Bukovec P, Jakopič K, Zdravevski E, Trajkovik V, and Lukanović A. Can we predict obstetric anal sphincter injury? *Eur J Obstet Gynecol Reprod Biol*. 2017;210:196–200.
13. Ertekin C and Reef F. Bulbocavernous reflex in normal men and in patients with neurogenic bladder and/or impotence. *J Neurol Sci*. 1976;28:1–15.
14. Vodusek DB and Janko M. The bulbocavernous reflex a single motor neuron study. *Brain*. 1990;113:813–20.
15. Vodusek DB, Amarenco G, Batra A et al. Clinical neurophysiology. In: Abrams P, Cardozo L, Khoury S, and Wein A, eds. *Incontinence*. Plymouth, UK: Health Publication Ltd; 2005:675–706.
16. Nikifordis G, Koutsojannis C, Giannoulis S, and Barbalias G. Reduced variance of latencies in pudendal evoked potentials after normalisation for body height. *Neurourol Urodyn*. 1995;14:239–51.
17. Hanson P, Rigaux P, and Biset E. Sacral reflex latencies in tethered cord syndrome. *Am J Phys Med Rehabil*. 1993;72:39–43.
18. Bilkey WJ, Awad EA, and Smith AD. Clinical application of sacral reflex latency. *J Urol*. 1983;129:1187–9.

19. Haldeman S, Bradley WE, and Bhatia N. Evoked responses from the pudendal nerve. *J Urol.* 1982;128:974–80.

20. Niu X, Shao B, Ni P et al.. Bulbocavernosus reflex and pudendal nerve somatosensory-evoked potentials responses in female patients with nerve system diseases. *J Clin Neurophysiol.* 2010;27:207–11.

21. Brostrøm S. Motor evoked potentials from the pelvic floor. *Neurourol Urodyn.* 2003;22:620–37.

22. Brostrom S, Jennum P, and Lose G. Motor evoked potentials from the striated urethral sphincter: A comparison of concentric needle and surface electrodes. *Neurourol Urodyn.* 2003;22:123–9.

23. Daffertshofer M, Linden D, Syren M, Junemann KP, and Berlit P. Assessment of local sympathetic function in patients with erectile dysfunction. *Int J Impot Res.* 1994;6:213–25.

24. Jameson JS, Chia YW, Kamm MA, Speakman CT, Chye YH, and Henry MM. Effect of age, sex and parity on anorectal function. *Br J Surg.* 1994;81:1689–92.

25. Vodusek DB, Janko M, and Lokar J. EMG, single fibre EMG and sacral reflexes in assessment of sacral nervous system lesions. *J Neurol Neurosurg Psychiatry.* 1982;45:1064–6.

26. Kiff ES and Swash M. Normal proximal and delayed distal conduction in the pudendal nerves of patients with idiopathic (neurogenic) faecal incontinence. *J Neurol Neurosurg Psychiatry.* 1984;47:820–3.

27. Thomas C, Lefaucheur JP, Galula G, de Parades V, Bourguignon J, and Atienza P. Respective value of pudendal nerve terminal motor latency and anal sphincter electromyography in neurogenic fecal incontinence. *Neurophysiol Clin.* 2002;32:85–90.

28. Bradley WE, Lin JT, and Johnson B. Measurement of conduction velocity of the dorsal nerve of the penis. *J Urol.* 1984;131:1127–9.

29. Hansen MW, Ertekin C, and Larsson LE. Cerebral evoked potentials after stimulation of the posterior urethra in man. *Electroencephalogr Clin Neurophysiol.* 1990;77:52–8.

30. Vodusek DB and Deletis V. Sacral roots and nerves, and monitoring for neuro-urologic procedures. In: Nuwer MR, ed. *Intraoperative Monitoring of Neural Function (Handbook of Clinical Neurophysiology, Vol. 8).* Amsterdam: Elsevier; 2008:423–33.

31. Corcos J and Schnick E, Textbook of the Neurogenic Bladder. *Informa Healthcare UK, London, United Kingdom,* 2008.

Chapter 24

NEUROIMAGING IN THE EVALUATION OF NEUROGENIC BLADDER DYSFUNCTION

Ulrich Mehnert

Neuroimaging is the umbrella term for all imaging methods that are able to visualize neuronal activity of the central and/or peripheral nervous system.

There are several imaging modalities available that all have their advantages, disadvantages, and limits, but not all play a role in the evaluation of neurogenic bladder dysfunction. Hence, this chapter focuses on the most commonly used techniques in the context of neurogenic bladder dysfunction. The neuronal structure in focus, so far, is almost exclusively the brain as a whole or specific parts of it.

In general, neuroimaging modalities are great tools to assess neuronal processes in humans *in vivo* which would otherwise not be possible. Neuroimaging is a huge and dynamic area of neuroscientific research with constant improvement and development of image acquisition and analysis techniques. However, to adequately use these tools and interpret the outcome, several aspects in study design, data acquisition, and analysis in relation to the selected imaging modality have to be understood and respected. It would exceed the scope of this chapter to go into all these details for each imaging modality. However, a short summary on the basic methodological background of each imaging method is described to allow for an impression on what is actually measured to visualize the neural activity, and appropriate references are provided.

WHY IS NEUROIMAGING RELEVANT IN THE EVALUATION OF NEUROGENIC BLADDER DYSFUNCTION?

It is well known from numerous animal studies that the lower urinary tract (LUT) is controlled by a complex, multilevel network of different peripheral and central neuronal structures and pathways to enable proper execution of the two opposing functions of urine storage and voiding.[20–22] When talking about neurogenic bladder dysfunction in our patients, we at least suspect that a neuronal lesion, disease, or dysfunction interferes with this complex control and is the cause for their LUT problems.

However, we often do not know how exactly and to what extent a neurologic lesion or disorder affects the LUT control network and consequently causes the dysfunction and symptoms. Animal models of certain diseases or dysfunction can only incompletely explain the processes in humans, and translation, specifically in the context of neurogenic bladder dysfunction, remains a challenge. Assessment of neuronal structures and processes in humans *in vivo* using neuroimaging is a great advantage that finally allows us to shed light on the possible locations where the underlying etiology of neurogenic bladder dysfunction is located or at least suspected. Therefore, neuroimaging has great potential to further improve our understanding of neurogenic bladder dysfunction in more detail, which may enable us to develop more targeted and effective therapies. In addition, neuroimaging can help us to better define neurogenic bladder dysfunction in those patients who are currently labeled "idiopathic" but most probably have some kind of disturbance of the LUT control network that cannot be assessed by the current neurologic or urologic standard diagnostic tools.

PRELIMINARY WORKING MODEL OF SUPRASPINAL LUT CONTROL

The available literature on neuroimaging in regard to LUT function is constantly increasing and impressively demonstrating how much this field has already influenced our idea of supraspinal LUT control in humans (Figure 24.1).

Based on previous neuroimaging findings, current working models on supraspinal LUT control (Figure 24.1) suggest that the ascending signals form the LUT are relayed through the periaqueductal gray (PAG) and thalamus to cortical areas that further process the information and that are involved in appropriate decision-making and action-taking processes.[1–3] These cortical areas specifically comprise the insula, the prefrontal cortex, and the anterior cingulate cortex (ACC). The insula as primary interoceptive

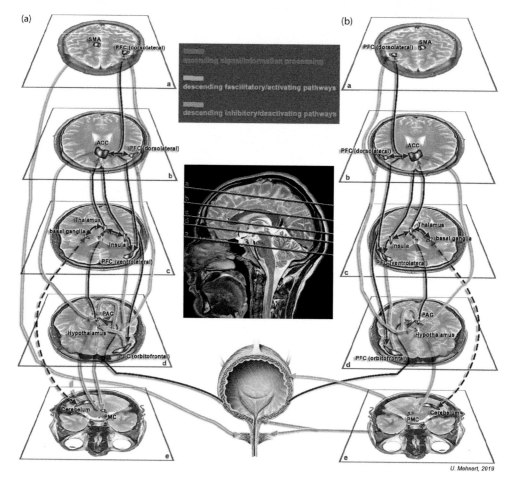

Figure 24.1 Preliminary working model of supraspinal lower urinary tract (LUT) control during urine storage (a) and voiding (b).

cortex is supposed to be involved in a first-order mapping of visceral signals (e.g., bladder distention) with second-order regions such as the prefrontal cortex and the ACC which are involved in the subjective awareness and feeling of the visceral signal (e.g., desire to void).[1,4,5] The prefrontal cortex (PFC) is involved in planning complex cognitive and appropriate social behavior (e.g., handling of strong desire to void in different circumstances) as well as attention and response-selection mechanisms (e.g., postponement of micturition), which are essential for the volitional control of the LUT.[2,6–8] The PFC has strong and multiple connections to the cingulate cortex and hypothalamus which are part of the limbic system and considered to provide emotional and motivational input to the prefrontal decision-making process. The ACC in the example is thought to modulate how much attention is provided to signals coming from the bladder and how one reacts to them.[1] The hypothalamus, which is also associated with autonomic control due to its projections to all autonomic preganglionic motor neurons in the

spinal cord, including the sacral parasympathetic and sphincter motor nuclei, is one of the few regions that has direct afferent projections to the pontine micturition center (PMC).[1,3] This connection has been interpreted as an additional "layer of control" that permits micturition in healthy subjects only if it is judged "safe" to do so. The supplementary motor area (SMA) has been mainly observed in association with pelvic floor muscle contractions and may serve as an additional continence mechanism in situations of strong desire to void or urgency to prevent premature leakage.[9,10] Although previous studies have reported cerebellar and basal ganglia activity in response to different LUT conditions, their role in LUT control is not yet clear.[10,11] Both structures are known to be involved in motor activity but also in other functions such as cognition, attention, emotion, and behavior.[12–14] Lesions or disorders of basal ganglia and cerebellum seem to frequently result in LUT dysfunction, predominantly detrusor overactivity and detrusor-sphincter dyssynergia.[15–19] Both structures seem to contribute facilitatory but also inhibitory input to LUT control and may be involved in level-setting and fine-tuning processes of LUT control.

The neuroimaging data supporting the up-to-date working models are mainly from healthy subjects and patients with overactive bladder (OAB).[1,22,23] Interestingly, the latter group is commonly declared as having idiopathic or nonneurogenic OAB. However, considering their neuroimaging findings with altered brain activity and/or connectivity compared to healthy controls in relation to LUT function, most of them should be reconsidered as neurogenic.[25,26]

NEUROIMAGING TECHNIQUES AND THEIR ROLE IN NEUROGENIC BLADDER DYSFUNCTION

The studies on adult patients with classical neurogenic bladder dysfunction from Parkinson's disease (PD), multiple sclerosis (MS), spinal cord injury (SCI), etc., are summarized in this chapter according to the imaging technique used to investigate supraspinal LUT control.

ELECTROENCEPHALOGRAPHY

Electroencephalography (EEG) was one of the first neuroimaging methods used to improve our understanding of neuronal processes in the brain. It is also one of the few methods that allow direct recording of neuronal activity, which results in a good temporal resolution of neuronal events. However, the spatial resolution of EEG is rather low compared to other imaging methods, such as magnetic resonance imaging (MRI), and mainly confined to the cortex from where signals are taken up by the EEG electrodes. Nevertheless, as for most imaging methods, analyses tools of EEG data have reasonably improved during the last decades, allowing for the extraction of more information from the recorded data, such as source localization and topographical analysis.[27]

In regard to LUT control, EEG has been used since the 1950s to primarily investigate EEG patterns in patients with nocturnal or ictal enuresis.[28,29] The altered patterns that could be observed in the EEG traces of enuretic patients were interpreted as global maturation deficiency and/or dyssynchronization of neural activity between different areas involved in LUT control.[30-32] In addition, specific sleep disturbances could be detected, indicating deficiencies in arousal that may as well contribute to enuresis.[33]

In the more recent decades, EEG has been eclipsed by positron emission tomography (PET) and MRI techniques in regard to investigations of brain-bladder interactions. However, EEG has its advantages (noninvasive, high temporal resolution, portable, inexpensive), and several groups still use it in the context of LUT dysfunction to investigate emotional processing in children with daytime incontinence,[34] to measure/analyze evoked potentials to evaluate brainstem dysfunction involved in childhood enuresis,[35] and to evaluate LUT afferent processing.[36-38] The full potential of this technique seems not yet fully explored and utilized in the field of adult neurogenic LUT dysfunction. Specifically in combination with other imaging modalities such as MRI, EEG might be of value to better describe temporal aspects of the supraspinal processes involved in LUT control.

SINGLE-PHOTON EMISSION COMPUTED TOMOGRAPHY AND POSITRON EMISSION TOMOGRAPHY

For single-photon emission computed tomography (SPECT), a γ-emitting radionuclide is applied intravenously, and the emitted γ-rays of the decaying radionuclide are recorded with a special camera.[39] For the purpose of functional brain imaging, the radionuclide technetium ^{99m}Tc is attached to hexamethylpropylene amine oxime (HMPAO) or ethyl cysteinate dimer (EDA), which are taken up by brain tissue in a proportion that corresponds to the blood flow to that brain tissue.[40]

For PET imaging, a positron emitting radionuclide on a tracer molecule is intravenously applied prior to the PET scan.[39] When the emitted positrons collide with electrons within the tissue of the investigated body area, annihilation (= γ-) radiation emits in 180° opposite directions and can be detected as coincidences by the PET scanner. There are different radionuclides available, which are chosen based on their specific characteristics and the purpose of investigation. For PET investigation of supraspinal LUT control, mainly the ^{15}O radionuclide in conjunction with hydrogen (= $H_2{}^{15}O$) is used due to its short half-life of about 2 minutes. This allows for repetitive scans of different or similar conditions (e.g., empty bladder, full bladder, micturition) within a shorter time span. The accumulation of the applied radionuclide and amount of recorded annihilations correspond to the blood flow to the brain tissue.

Hence, what is actually measured using PET or SPECT is not direct neuronal activity but regional changes of cerebral blood flow that are correlating to increased neuronal activity in this area.[39]

SPECT and PET studies were first evaluated in the late 1990s to visualize the human brain areas involved in LUT control; prior to these studies, this had only been evaluated in animal studies.[41,42] Based on the first PET studies, Kavia et al. presented an initial summary describing the supraspinal LUT control network: anterior cingulate cortex (ACC), insula, periaqueductal gray (PAG), pons, prefrontal cortex (PFC), and thalamus.[7]

In relation to neurogenic LUT dysfunction, Sakakibara et al., using SPECT, demonstrated that deficient cerebellar activity, compared to a healthy control group, is involved in the storage and voiding symptoms in patients with multiple system atrophy (MSA).[17] Despite the fact that the exact role of the cerebellum in LUT control is still poorly understood, such results are of interest as they allow recognition that the cerebellum might be involved in LUT control, which is in line with many subsequent neuroimaging studies that described cerebellar activity in the context of different LUT tasks.[3]

Sakakibara et al. also investigated patients with idiopathic normal-pressure hydrocephalus (iNPH) using SPECT to explore the pathophysiologic background of urinary dysfunction in this patient population.[46] They could demonstrate that lower urinary tract symptoms (LUTS) were related to a significant decrease in tracer activity in the right-side-dominant bilateral frontal cortex and the left inferior temporal gyrus. Following shunt surgery for iNPH, patients with improved LUT function showed increased bilateral midcingulate, parietal, and left frontal blood flow, whereas in patients with unchanged or worsened bladder function after surgery, no such increased cerebral blood flow was observed.[47]

Sakakibara et al. demonstrated that the presence of LUTS in patients with PD was associated with a larger reduction of brain activity in the caudate nucleus and putamen compared to patients with PD without LUTS.[48] Similar results were presented by Winge et al., who demonstrated in a SPECT study that patients with PD and LUTS had significant less uptake of radiotracer in the striatum (= caudate nucleus + putamen) than those without LUTS.[49] In addition, patients with severe LUT dysfunction had a positive correlation of symptoms and the putamen/caudate ratio. These results indicate a contribution of basal ganglia, specifically the striatum, to LUT control and the degree of degeneration of nigrostriatal dopaminergic neurons to and in the caudate nucleus seems to determine the presence and severity of LUTS, respectively.[49] This appears comprehensible, considering that the dopaminergic neurons of the substantia nigra (pars compacta) largely project to the striatum, which is an important relay structure to all other basal ganglia and subsequently the basal ganglia-thalamocortical circuitry.[50] In addition, the striatum has been found to be a multizone structure that is coupled to multiple functional networks within the cerebral cortex, including *inter alia* the prefrontal cortex, anterior cingulate cortex, supplementary motor area, and brainstem, which are brain regions found to be involved in LUT control.[51] For some time, the influence of the basal ganglia on the LUT control circuitry has been discussed in relation to PD including two potential mechanisms[49,52]: (1) Dopamine release in response to substantia nigra (pars compacta) neuronal firing activates the dopamine D1-GABAergic direct pathway, which has inhibitory input to the brainstem centers controlling micturition, i.e., PAG and pontine micturition center (PMC). Lack of this inhibitory pathway in PD may lead to detrusor overactivity (DO) and urgency/frequency. (2) Dopaminergic neurons of the ventral tegmentum area (VTA) seem to strongly influence supraspinal centers of LUT control, i.e., hypothalamus, via D1 (inhibitory) and D2 (excitatory) receptors. An imbalance between the potentially more severely damaged inhibitory dopaminergic neurons from the substantia nigra and the less severely damaged excitatory dopaminergic neurons from the VTA in PD may result in DO and urgency/frequency.

Herzog et al. used PET to investigate the effect of subthalamic nucleus deep brain stimulation (STN-DBS) on LUT function in patients with PD.[53] They demonstrated that STN-DBS specifically modulated activity in the ACC and lateral frontal cortex (LFC). Switching the STN-DBS "on" decreased ACC and LFC activity and increased the cystometric volume at perception of the urge to void, whereas switching the STN-DBS "off" caused an increase in ACC and LFC activity and corresponded to a decrease in cystometric volume at perception of the urge to void. The exact mechanism by which STN-DBS is inducing such effects is unclear, but it is assumed that STN-DBS improves basal ganglia function that in turn facilitates LUT afferent signal processing from the PAG to other areas such as the thalamus. In a subsequent study, Herzog et al. demonstrated that STN-DBS increased activity in core areas of LUT sensory perception (i.e., PAG, thalamus, and insula) specifically during bladder filling, which was interpreted as further evidence for the enhancing effect of STN-DBS on afferent urinary bladder information processing.[54]

Using PET scanning during DO in patients with PD, Kitta et al. demonstrated a slightly different supraspinal activation pattern with a lack of pontine and ACC activity compared to a previously investigated healthy group.[55] This was speculated to be part of the pathophysiology leading to LUT dysfunction in PD. On the one hand, this finding could be in line with the concept of altered sensory processing related to the impaired basal ganglia-thalamocortical circuitry with reduced interaction between basal ganglia and ACC and PMC. On the other hand, it appears contradictory to the findings from Herzog and the consideration that DO in PD may result from a lacking inhibition on brainstem structures such as PAG and PMC. In contrast to the SPECT study of Sakakibara et al. in patients with MSA, cerebellar vermis activity was strong in patients with PD.[17,55] Assuming an involvement of the cerebellum in external urethral sphincter coordination as part of its motor control abilities, this finding may be related to the signs of sphincter denervation specifically found in MSA but not PD.[56]

Last, Perneczky et al. investigated patients with frontotemporal lobe degenerations using PET and identified significantly less activity in premotor/ anterior cingulate cortex and the putamen/ claustrum/insula regions in those patients with concomitant urinary incontinence.[57]

MAGNETIC RESONANCE IMAGING

MRI is currently one of the most important and frequently used techniques for neuroimaging in general and specifically for the investigation of supraspinal LUT control (Figure 24.2).

The advantage of MRI compared to PET is that it is noninvasive and does not expose the patient to radioactivity or radiation. If the security rules related to the strong magnetic field of the scanner are strictly followed, it is a very safe diagnostic tool without known adverse events. In addition, it is a technique that becomes more and more readily available and is continuously being improved.

Functional assessments have been primarily performed using blood-oxygen-level-dependent (BOLD)-MRI during a paradigm of repetitive tasks of LUT and/or pelvic floor stimulation, such as bladder filling/emptying through a catheter, voiding,

and pelvic floor muscle contractions/relaxations. The BOLD signal is based on a hemodynamic response driven by the need of active neurons for (more) energy. This results in a regional change of blood oxygenation that can be detected using MRI due to the different magnetic properties of oxy- and deoxyhemoglobin. Thus, BOLD-MRI displays neuronal activity indirectly through changes in regional blood oxygenation levels. Due to the relatively small signal amplitude, several repetitions and statistical analyses are required to detect those neuronal structures that show the most activity during the investigated task compared to a control condition (i.e., rest or another task).[58]

This method has very good spatial resolution down to a millimeter. However, since the hemodynamic response is much slower (seconds) than the effective neural activity (milliseconds), the temporal resolution is very limited.

Beyond BOLD-MRI, there are further MRI-based imaging modalities that have been recently evaluated for the investigation of specific structural (e.g., diffusion weighted imaging, voxel-based morphometry) and functional (e.g., resting-state or task-based functional connectivity) aspects of supraspinal LUT control.

In patients with incomplete SCI, Zempleni et al. demonstrated in a BOLD-MRI study that some supraspinal representation of the bladder-filling sensation is preserved ($p \leq 0.001$ uncorrected).[59] However, right prefrontal responses were decreased, whereas left prefrontal responses were increased, which was interpreted as correlates of the altered supraspinal LUT control with compensatory

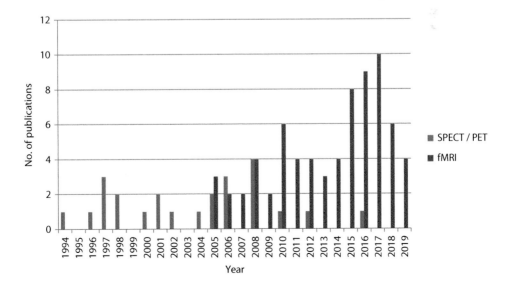

Figure 24.2 Development of number of publications for single-photon emission computed tomography/positron emission tomography and functional magnetic resonance imaging studies on supraspinal lower urinary tract control since the first study.

reorganization. Pudendal stimulation training for 2 weeks induced significant changes, predominantly signal increases, in the normal cortical network of bladder control but most prominently in the right posterior insula. These findings corresponded with improvements in bladder function after the pudendal stimulation training and thus may reflect the neuromodulative effect at the supraspinal level.[59]

Even in patients with complete SCI, Krhut et al. demonstrated in a BOLD-MRI study significant ($p \leq$ 0.001 uncorrected) supraspinal responses toward bladder filling in the nucleus of the solitary tract (NTS), parabrachial nucleus (PBN), hypothalamus, thalamus, amygdala, insular lobe, ACC, and PFC.[60] Most of these areas have been described as relevant components of the homeostatic afferent system, which is essential for the maintenance of cardiovascular, respiratory, energy, and fluid balances.[61] Specifically, activations in the NTS and PBN were attributed to vagal nerve activity. Extra- or paraspinal autonomic pathways bypassing the spinal cord lesion may explain brain activity in response to bladder filling despite a complete SCI.

In patients with MS, Khavari et al. investigated brain activity in response to bladder filling and voiding using BOLD-MRI.[62] Patients with MS demonstrated significant activity ($p \leq 0.05$ uncorrected) in the frontal gyrus, lentiform nucleus, anterior and posterior cingulate cortex, parietal lobules, precuneus, and subcallosal gyrus associated with a strong desire to void. At the initiation of voiding, patients with MS showed significant activity ($p \leq 0.05$ uncorrected) in the middle and medial frontal gyrus, supplementary motor area, left lentiform nucleus, cingulate cortex, insula, parahippocampal gyrus, subcallosal gyrus, thalamus, and cerebellum. Compared to a previously investigated group of healthy controls, patients with MS appear to demonstrate lower and more diffuse supraspinal activation.[62,63]

In another recent study using BOLD-MRI in patients with MS, Khavari et al. demonstrated that patients with enhanced MS lesions had less supraspinal functional connectivity.[64] In addition, patients with MS with preserved ability of spontaneous voiding showed a much higher functional connectivity than those patients without this ability, which may indicate that a certain communication between the supraspinal areas is prerequisite to orchestrate voluntary micturition. Khavari et al. also investigated the effect of onabotulinumtoxinA intradetrusor injections for neurogenic OAB on supraspinal activity in patients with MS.[65] Supraspinal activity ($p \leq .05$ uncorrected) in response to bladder filling appeared to increase after treatment, which may have been confounded by larger filling volumes due to the onabotulinumtoxinA effect on the bladder.

Using diffusion-weighted MRI, Roy et al. investigated in patients with PD brainstem diffusivity in relation to their LUTS severity.[66] The mean diffusivity (MD) is an unspecific but sensitive marker for the impairment of barriers that restrict motion of water molecules in tissue such as axonal/neuronal membranes. MD in areas close to the pontine continence center correlated significantly with LUTS severity, indicating that degenerative changes in the pontine continence center may be involved in the pathogenesis of LUTS in PD.

Khoo et al. investigated default mode network connectivity using resting state functional MRI (fMRI) in patients with iNPH and demonstrated that the default mode network (DMN) connectivity was reduced in patients with iNPH compared to healthy controls.[67] However, in the iNPH group, DMN connectivity was positively correlated with the clinical symptom scores. DMN connectivity seems to be altered in patients with iNPH and may serve as a marker for severity of clinical symptoms.

NEAR-INFRARED SPECTROSCOPY

Near-infrared spectroscopy (NIRS) is an optical imaging method that uses light near the infrared spectrum (650–950 nm). Based on the different optical absorption characteristics of different tissues and structures, it can be used to assess regional concentration and oxygenation of hemoglobin in the brain, which are associated with neural activity.[68]

Similar to EEG, NIRS is an inexpensive, portable, and noninvasive imaging method but also has limited depth sensitivity, which allows for cortical brain imaging only. The temporal resolution is around 100 Hz and thus much better than that of MRI or PET. It can be used complementary to MRI.

So far, there are very few studies using NIRS in the context of functional neuroimaging of supraspinal LUT control. Of those studies, none investigated patients with neurogenic bladder dysfunction. In healthy subjects or patients with nonneurogenic OAB, results from other imaging modalities could be reproduced with increased levels of oxyhemoglobin in the bilateral frontal cortex with increasing bladder filling.[44,45,69,70]

CONCLUSION

Neuroimaging mainly using PET, and more recently BOLD-MRI, enables us to identify certain brain areas that respond to LUT stimulation tasks and thus seem to be involved in supraspinal LUT control: ACG, cerebellum, IFG, insula, PAG, pons, and thalamus.[24,43]

On a group level, functional neuroimaging, specifically fMRI, has been used to demonstrate differences in supraspinal LUT control between healthy volunteers and patients with LUT dysfunction, which may explain part of the underlying neuropathophysiology causing the LUT dysfunction. Patients with neurogenic bladder dysfunction seem to have generally less and/or altered supraspinal activity with reduced connectivity. The altered supraspinal activity may represent compensatory mechanisms to maintain at least some control or result directly from the neurologic deficit. In addition, functional neuroimaging seems, at least on group level, to reflect supraspinal responses to therapeutic interventions, which in some studies correlated with the clinical improvement.

However, despite these achievements, the use of neuroimaging in the evaluation of neurogenic bladder dysfunction is still in its infancy, and there are still many lessons to be learned. Results often originate from rather small group sizes ($n < 20$) and are presented on low significance levels (e.g., $p \leq 0.05$ uncorrected). There is a large heterogeneity of applied methodology/protocols, analysis, and outcome reporting that hamper a reasonable comparison of studies. Study conclusions often remain vague and do not progress to the level of explaining the meaning of the findings in the pathophysiologic context of the investigated LUTD. Currently, functional neuroimaging is a pure research tool without clear or significant clinical implications, which is also due to the fact that results are not conclusive on a single subject level. Due to the rather limited reliability of BOLD-MRI and the large number of confounding factors, evaluation of treatment effects should be interpreted with great caution.

Nevertheless, neuroimaging in neuro-urology is a challenging approach, and the pioneers in this area are to be congratulated as we have learned from previous experiences to further assess and improve the use of neuroimaging techniques for the purpose of understanding bladder-brain interaction and LUT control in our patients.

Pure BOLD-MRI or PET investigations may show us the involved brain areas, but this does not help in understanding how such areas communicate and what each area is contributing to LUT control. Hence, analysis of structural and functional connectivity as well as multimodal imaging approaches, i.e., EEG-fMRI, may bring more insight into how the brain is controlling the LUT and to verify or to adapt the proposed working models. Longitudinal studies of neurologic patients, i.e., MS and PD, when LUTS are not yet present until LUTS develop are worthwhile to be considered to better understand what kind of changes are specifically related to the start of symptoms. However, to provide a solid basis in order to achieve the envisioned improvements and

conduct meaningful studies, it will be necessary to optimize scanning parameters and protocols and to standardize analysis pathways and outcome reporting to enable larger multicenter studies and comparison between studies.

Last but not least, due to the complexity of neuroimaging methods, it is advisable to perform such studies in a multidisciplinary team of neuroscientists, physicists, and clinicians to generate meaningful protocols and study outcomes.

REFERENCES

1. Fowler CJ, Griffiths D, and de Groat WC. The neural control of micturition. *Nat Rev Neurosci.* 2008;9(6):453–66.
2. Fowler CJ and Griffiths DJ. A decade of functional brain imaging applied to bladder control. *Neurourol Urodyn.* 2010;29(1):49–55.
3. Griffiths D and Tadic SD. Bladder control, urgency, and urge incontinence: Evidence from functional brain imaging. *Neurourol Urodyn.* 2008;27(6):466–74.
4. Craig AD. How do you feel? Interoception: The sense of the physiological condition of the body. *Nat Rev Neurosci.* 2002;3(8):655–66.
5. Craig AD. How do you feel—now? The anterior insula and human awareness. *Nat Rev Neurosci.* 2009;10(1):59–70.
6. Bechara A, Damasio H, and Damasio AR. Emotion, decision making and the orbitofrontal cortex. *Cereb Cortex.* 2000;10(3):295–307.
7. Kavia RB, Dasgupta R, and Fowler CJ. Functional imaging and the central control of the bladder. *J Comp Neurol.* 2005;493(1):27–32.
8. Pardo JV, Fox PT, and Raichle ME. Localization of a human system for sustained attention by positron emission tomography. *Nature.* 1991;349(6304):61–4.
9. Griffiths D, Clarkson B, Tadic SD, and Resnick NM. Brain mechanisms underlying urge incontinence and its response to pelvic floor muscle training. *J Urol.* 2015;194(3):708–15.
10. Zhang H, Reitz A, Kollias S, Summers P, Curt A, and Schurch B. An fMRI study of the role of suprapontine brain structures in the voluntary voiding control induced by pelvic floor contraction. *Neuroimage.* 2005;24(1):174–80.
11. Seseke S, Baudewig J, Kallenberg K, Ringert RH, Seseke F, and Dechent P. Voluntary pelvic floor muscle control—An fMRI study. *Neuroimage.* 2006;31(4):1399–407.
12. D'Angelo E. Physiology of the cerebellum. *Handb Clin Neurol.* 2018;154:85–108.
13. Florio TM, Scarnati E, Rosa I et al. The Basal Ganglia: More than just a switching device. *CNS Neurosci Ther.* 2018;24(8):677–84.
14. Wolf U, Rapoport MJ, and Schweizer TA. Evaluating the affective component of the cerebellar cognitive affective syndrome. *J Neuropsychiatry Clin Neurosci.* 2009;21(3):245–53.
15. Chou YC, Jiang YH, Harnod T, and Kuo HC. Characteristics of neurogenic voiding dysfunction in cerebellar stroke: A cross-sectional, retrospective video urodynamic study. *Cerebellum.* 2013;12(5):601–6.

16. Dietrichs E and Haines DE. Possible pathways for cerebellar modulation of autonomic responses: Micturition. *Scand J Urol Nephrol Suppl.* 2002(210):16–20.

17. Sakakibara R, Uchida Y, Uchiyama T, Yamanishi T, and Hattori T. Reduced cerebellar vermis activation during urinary storage and micturition in multiple system atrophy: 99mTc-labelled ECD SPECT study. *Eur J Neurol.* 2004;11(10):705–8.

18. Sakakibara R, Uchiyama T, Yamanishi T, Shirai K, and Hattori T. Bladder and bowel dysfunction in Parkinson's disease. *J Neural Transm (Vienna).* 2008;115(3):443–60.

19. Winge K, Skau AM, Stimpel H, Nielsen KK, and Werdelin L. Prevalence of bladder dysfunction in Parkinson's disease. *Neurourol Urodyn.* 2006;25(2):116–22.

20. de Groat WC. Integrative control of the lower urinary tract: Preclinical perspective. *Br J Pharmacol.* 2006;147(Suppl 2):S25–40.

21. Blok BF and Holstege G. The neuronal control of micturition and its relation to the emotional motor system. In: Holstege G, Bandler R, and Saper CB, eds. *Progress in Brain Research*, Vol 107. New York, NY: Elsevier Science; 1996:113–26.

22. Kinder MV, Bastiaanssen EH, Janknegt RA, and Marani E. Neuronal circuitry of the lower urinary tract; central and peripheral neuronal control of the micturition cycle. *Anat Embryol (Berl).* 1995;192(3):195–209.

23. de Groat WC, Griffiths D, and Yoshimura N. Neural control of the lower urinary tract. *Compr Physiol.* 2015;5(1):327–96.

24. Harvie C, Weissbart SJ, Kadam-Halani P, Rao H, and Arya LA. Brain activation during the voiding phase of micturition in healthy adults: A meta-analysis of neuroimaging studies. *Clin Anat.* 2019;32(1):13–9.

25. Griffiths D, Derbyshire S, Stenger A, and Resnick N. Brain control of normal and overactive bladder. *J Urol.* 2005;174(5):1862–7.

26. Nardos R, Karstens L, Carpenter S et al. Abnormal functional connectivity in women with urgency urinary incontinence: Can we predict disease presence and severity in individual women using Rs-fcMRI. *Neurourol Urodyn.* 2016;35(5):564–73.

27. Niedermeyer E and Lopes da Silva F. *Electroencephalography: Basic Principles, Clinical Applications, and Related Fields.* 5th ed. Philadelphia, PA: Lippincott Williams & Wilkins; 2004.

28. Gunnarson S and Melin KA. The electroencephalogram in enuresis. *Acta Paediatr.* 1951;40(4):496–501.

29. Turton EC and Spear AB. EEG findings in 100 cases of severe enuresis. *Arch Dis Child.* 1953;28(140):316–20.

30. Valentino RJ, Wood SK, Wein AJ, and Zderic SA. The bladder-brain connection: Putative role of corticotropin-releasing factor. *Nat Rev Urol.* 2011;8(1):19–28.

31. DiBianco JM, Morley C, and Al-Omar O. Nocturnal enuresis: A topic review and institution experience. *Avicenna J Med.* 2014;4(4):77–86.

32. Hallioglu O, Ozge A, Comelekoglu U et al. Evaluation of cerebral maturation by visual and quantitative analysis of resting electroencephalography in children with primary nocturnal enuresis. *J Child Neurol.* 2001;16(10):714–8.

33. Kawauchi A, Imada N, Tanaka Y, Minami M, Watanabe H, and Shirakawa S. Changes in the structure of sleep spindles and delta waves on electroencephalography in patients with nocturnal enuresis. *Br J Urol.* 1998;81(Suppl 3):72–5.

34. Niemczyk J, Equit M, Rieck K, Rubly M, Wagner C, and von Gontard A. EEG measurement of emotion processing in children with daytime urinary incontinence. *Z Kinder Jugendpsychiatr Psychother.* 2018;46(4):336–41.

35. Freitag CM, Rohling D, Seifen S, Pukrop R, and von Gontard A. Neurophysiology of nocturnal enuresis: Evoked potentials and prepulse inhibition of the startle reflex. *Dev Med Child Neurol.* 2006;48(4):278–84.

36. Gregorini F, Knupfer SC, Liechti MD et al. Sensory evoked potentials of the bladder and urethra in middle-aged women: The effect of age. *BJU Int.* 2015;115(Suppl 6):18–25.

37. Gregorini F, Wollner J, Schubert M, Curt A, Kessler TM, and Mehnert U. Sensory evoked potentials of the human lower urinary tract. *J Urol.* 2013;189(6):2179–85.

38. Knupfer SC, Liechti MD, van der Lely S et al. Sensory evoked cortical potentials of the lower urinary tract in healthy men. *Neurourol Urodyn.* 2018;37(8):2614–24.

39. Council NR. *Mathematics and Physics of Emerging Biomedical Imaging.* Washington, DC: National Academies Press; 1996.

40. Pupi A, Castagnoli A, De Cristofaro MT, Bacciottini L, and Petti AR. Quantitative comparison between 99mTc-HMPAO and 99mTc-ECD: Measurement of arterial input and brain retention. *Eur J Nucl Med.* 1994;21(2):124–30.

41. Blok BFM, Willemsen ATM, and Holstege G. A PET study on brain control of micturition in humans. *Brain.* 1997;120(1):111–21.

42. Fukuyama H, Matsuzaki S, Ouchi Y et al. Neural control of micturition in man examined with single photon emission computed tomography using 99mTc-HMPAO. *Neuroreport.* 1996;7(18):3009–12.

43. Arya NG, Weissbart SJ, Xu S, and Rao H. Brain activation in response to bladder filling in healthy adults: An activation likelihood estimation meta-analysis of neuroimaging studies. *Neurourol Urodyn.* 2017;36(4):960–5.

44. Sakakibara R, Tsunoyama K, Takahashi O et al. Real-time measurement of oxyhemoglobin concentration changes in the frontal micturition area: An fNIRS study. *Neurourol Urodyn.* 2010;29(5):757–64.

45. Matsumoto S, Ishikawa A, Matsumoto S, and Homma Y. Brain response provoked by different bladder volumes: A near infrared spectroscopy study. *Neurourol Urodyn.* 2011;30(4):529–35.

46. Sakakibara R, Uchida Y, Ishii K et al. SINPHONI. Correlation of right frontal hypoperfusion and urinary dysfunction in iNPH: A SPECT study. *Neurourol Urodynam.* 2012;31(1):50–5.

47. Sakakibara R, Uchida Y, Ishii K et al. Bladder recovery relates with increased mid-cingulate perfusion after shunt surgery in idiopathic normal-pressure hydrocephalus: A single-photon emission tomography study. *Int Urol Nephrol.* 2016;48(2):169–74.

48. Sakakibara R, Shinotoh H, Uchiyama T, Yoshiyama M, Hattori T, and Yamanishi T. SPECT imaging of the dopamine transporter with [(123)I]-beta-CIT reveals marked decline of nigrostriatal dopaminergic function in Parkinson's disease with urinary dysfunction. *J Neurol Sci.* 2001;187(1–2):55–9.

49. Winge K, Friberg L, Werdelin L, Nielsen KK, and Stimpel H. Relationship between nigrostriatal dopaminergic degeneration, urinary symptoms, and bladder control in Parkinson's disease. *Eur J Neurol.* 2005;12(11):842–50.

50. DeLong M and Wichmann T. Update on models of basal ganglia function and dysfunction. *Parkinsonism Relat Disord.* 2009;15(Suppl 3):S237–40.

51. Choi EY, Yeo BT, and Buckner RL. The organization of the human striatum estimated by intrinsic functional connectivity. *J Neurophysiol.* 2012;108(8):2242–63.

52. Sakakibara R, Tateno F, Kishi M, Tsuyuzaki Y, Uchiyama T, and Yamamoto T. Pathophysiology of bladder dysfunction in Parkinson's disease. *Neurobiol Dis.* 2012;46(3):565–71.

53. Herzog J, Weiss PH, Assmus A et al. Subthalamic stimulation modulates cortical control of urinary bladder in Parkinson's disease. *Brain.* 2006;129(Pt 12):3366–75.

54. Herzog J, Weiss PH, Assmus A et al. Improved sensory gating of urinary bladder afferents in Parkinson's disease following subthalamic stimulation. *Brain.* 2008;131(Pt 1):132–45.

55. Kitta T, Kakizaki H, Furuno T et al. Brain activation during detrusor overactivity in patients with Parkinson's disease: A positron emission tomography study. *J Urol.* 2006;175(3 Pt 1):994–8.

56. Sakakibara R, Hattori T, Uchiyama T, and Yamanishi T. Videourodynamic and sphincter motor unit potential analyses in Parkinson's disease and multiple system atrophy. *J Neurol Neurosurg Psychiatry.* 2001;71(5):600–6.

57. Perneczky R, Diehl-Schmid J, Forstl H, Drzezga A, May F, and Kurz A. Urinary incontinence and its functional anatomy in frontotemporal lobar degenerations. *Eur J Nucl Med Mol Imaging.* 2008;35(3):605–10.

58. Huettel SA, Song AW, and McCarthy G. *Functional Magnetic Resonance Imaging.* 2nd ed. Sunderland, MA: Sinauer; 2008.

59. Zempleni MZ, Michels L, Mehnert U, Schurch B, and Kollias S. Cortical substrate of bladder control in SCI and the effect of peripheral pudendal stimulation. *Neuroimage.* 2010;49(4):2983–94.

60. Krhut J, Tintera J, Bilkova K et al. Brain activity on fMRI associated with urinary bladder filling in patients with a complete spinal cord injury. *Neurourol Urodyn.* 2017;36(1):155–9.

61. Craig AD. Interoception: The sense of the physiological condition of the body. *Curr Opin Neurobiol.* 2003;13(4):500–5.

62. Khavari R, Karmonik C, Shy M, Fletcher S, and Boone T. Functional magnetic resonance imaging with concurrent urodynamic testing identifies brain structures involved in micturition cycle in patients with multiple sclerosis. *J Urol.* 2017;197(2):438–44.

63. Shy M, Fung S, Boone TB, Karmonik C, Fletcher SG, and Khavari R. Functional magnetic resonance imaging during urodynamic testing identifies brain structures initiating micturition. *J Urol.* 2014;192(4):1149–54.

64. Khavari R, Elias SN, Boone T, and Karmonik C. Similarity of functional connectivity patterns in patients with multiple sclerosis who void spontaneously versus patients with voiding dysfunction. *Neurourol Urodynam.* 2019;38(1):239–47.

65. Khavari R, Elias SN, Pande R, Wu KM, Boone TB, and Karmonik C. Higher neural correlates in patients with multiple sclerosis and neurogenic overactive bladder following treatment with intradetrusor injection of onabotulinumtoxinA. *J Urol.* 2019;201(1):135–40.

66. Roy HA, Griffiths DJ, Aziz TZ, Green AL, and Menke RAL. Investigation of urinary storage symptoms in Parkinson's disease utilizing structural MRI techniques. *Neurourol Urodynam.* 2019;14:14.

67. Khoo HM, Kishima H, Tani N et al. Default mode network connectivity in patients with idiopathic normal pressure hydrocephalus. *J Neurosurg.* 2016;124(2):350–8.

68. Boas DA and Franceschini MA. Near infrared imaging. *Scholarpedia.* 2009;4:6997.

69. Jiang CP, Sun CW, Tong YP, and Cheng CL, *IEEE. Study of Brain Responses to Changes in Bladder Continence and Micturition Using Near Infrared Spectroscopy.* New York, NY: IEEE; 2004:173–4.

70. Matsumoto S, Ishikawa A, Kume H, Takeuchi T, and Homma Y. Near infrared spectroscopy study of the central nervous activity during artificial changes in bladder sensation in men. *Int J Urol.* 2009;16(9):760–4.

Chapter 25

PRACTICAL GUIDE TO DIAGNOSIS AND FOLLOW-UP OF PATIENTS WITH NEUROGENIC BLADDER DYSFUNCTION

Jacques Corcos

INTRODUCTION

This chapter aims to summarize the knowledge developed in detail in previous chapters. It may be useful for a quick overview of current recommended management in terms of the use of diagnostic tools and planning of follow-up.

GENERAL REMARKS ON DIAGNOSIS AND FOLLOW-UP

Most traumatic, congenital, neoplastic, or degenerative neurologic pathologies have direct consequences on vesicourethral function. Diagnosis of these complex urologic conditions will be based on a good history and evaluation of quality of life impact. Physical examination, including motor and sensory testing, is essential in initial evaluation. Imaging techniques (upper tract ultrasound, abdominal computed tomography [CT] scan, and nuclear scans) will give information on the anatomic and morphologic status of the urinary tract. Endoscopy will provide further anatomic information, such as mucosal appearance, tumors, urethral stricture, degree of prostatic enlargement, and bladder stones. Urodynamics is the only diagnostic tool that allows functional evaluation of the lower urinary tract. It does not replace any of the other diagnostic modalities, but rather it complements them. It plays a major role in therapeutic decisions and during follow-up.

Urologic surveillance of patients with neurogenic bladder dysfunction in different countries has been described by only a few authors,[1–4] mainly in patients with spinal cord injuries (SCIs). In the United States,[1] most physicians (85%) favor yearly renal ultrasound for routine surveillance of the upper urinary tract,

and 65% performed urodynamic studies annually or every other year for evaluation of the lower urinary tract. In the United Kingdom and Ireland,[2] upper urinary tract screening and urodynamics are performed from annually to every 3 years by the majority of physicians. In Japan,[3] surveillance of the urinary tract is performed on a yearly basis by almost half (46.2%) of the 333 physicians involved in the surveillance and management of patients with SCIs who responded to a nationwide questionnaire. The majority (71.8%) preferred abdominal ultrasound for the upper urinary tract. In Canada,[4] 80% of urologists who treated patients with neurogenic bladder dysfunction favored yearly renal ultrasound and urodynamic studies.

NEUROGENIC BLADDER DYSFUNCTION AFTER TRAUMA

Traumatic injury to the central nervous system (cerebral or spinal) is often followed by the so-called spinal shock phase (see also Chapter 7). The bladder is hypotonic during this phase, which may last from 2 weeks to 8 weeks[5,6] but sometimes up to 1 year.[7,8] Formal urodynamic evaluation during this period does not add anything to the management.[9] Intermittent catheterization is considered the best treatment modality even if it is not supported by strong evidence. In the case of an incomplete spinal cord lesion, the reappearance of bladder sensation will indicate the end of the spinal shock phase. In the case of a complete lesion, reappearance of osteotendinous reflexes, urine spillage around the urethral catheter if it was left in place, and incontinence episodes between intermittent catheterizations will suggest the presence of bladder activity, which will have to be demonstrated by urodynamics. The first urodynamic evaluation is made at this time (Figure 25.1). The site of the neurologic lesion will give some indication as to the type of neurogenic bladder function to expect.

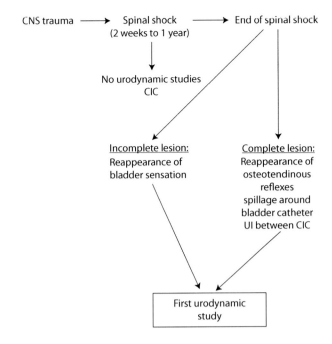

Figure 25.1 Initial evaluation and management of patients with central nervous system trauma. CIC, clean intermittent catheterization; CNS, central nervous system; UI, urinary incontinence.

Suprasacral lesions result in detrusor overactivity, whereas lesions at T11 or below result in a hypotonic bladder.[8]

The presence of detrusor-sphincter dyssynergia is more difficult to predict because only two-thirds of overactive detrusors will be accompanied by dyssynergic voiding. In general, it is associated with suprasacral cord lesions.[9]

NEUROGENIC BLADDER DYSFUNCTION AFTER NONTRAUMATIC NEUROLOGIC PATHOLOGY

Usually, the urologist will see these patients with a well-defined neurologic diagnosis. Urinary symptoms can appear any time during the course of the disease and may be constant or intermittent as well as stable or progressive, depending on the primary neurologic disorder.

The extent of the urologic evaluation will depend on the severity of urinary symptoms and the response to initial management. In general, modalities such as urine analysis and culture; ultrasonographic imaging of the upper urinary tract; free flowmetry, when possible; and postvoid residual assessment are done routinely at initial evaluation and during follow-up. An important issue is the always possible concomitance of voiding dysfunctions related and not related to the neurogenic condition. For example, a male patient with Parkinson's disease may also have voiding dysfunction related to a prostate hypertrophy. A female patient with multiple sclerosis may also have stress urinary incontinence not related to her neurologic condition. It then becomes important to analyze the symptoms and testing results to optimize management of the lower urinary tract symptoms.

AUTONOMIC DYSREFLEXIA

Autonomic dysreflexia (AD) is an exaggerated sympathetic response to afferent stimulation when SCI is at the level of T6 or above (see also Chapter 6). Acute, life-threatening AD episodes are not exceptional with urologic maneuvers (cystoscopy, botulinum A injection, suprapubic catheter insertion, etc.). It can be controlled by a quick reduction of the nociceptive stimuli (empty the bladder, stop injections, etc.). However, if none of these measures are effective and systolic blood pressure is greater than 150 mm Hg, 1 inch of Nitropaste should be applied to a hairless part of the upper body. If blood pressure is not improved after 15 minutes, then another inch is placed. Nitropaste has an onset of action of typically 9–11 minutes, and full clinical effectiveness is in 14–20 minutes. If the two applications of Nitropaste have not relieved the AD, then 10 mg of oral hydralazine can be given. Any patient who received Nitropaste or oral hydralazine should be monitored for several hours for recurrence of the hypertension but also hypotension.[10]

RENAL SURVEILLANCE

In a follow-up study by Donelly et al.[11, 12] of paraplegics from World War II, renal disease was the most common cause of death in the first 20 years after the injury, accounting for 40% of all deaths. More recently, in a series of 406 consecutive patients with SCI followed for 15 years, Webb et al.[13] reported a secondary death rate of 0.5% (2/406) from renal complications. This highlights the importance of dedicated follow-up to significantly reduce kidney-related mortality in these patients. Renal ultrasound[14] combined with plain radiography of the abdomen when stones are detected are the routine tests used.[15,16] Color flow Doppler ultrasound could eventually replace retrograde cystography in the detection of vesicourethral reflux. Papdaki et al.[17] reported that color Doppler ultrasonography diagnosed all grade IV and V, 87.5% of grade III, 83.3% of grade II, and 57.4% of grade I refluxes.

The frequency of upper tract ultrasound will depend on the evaluated deterioration risk. Urodynamics gives information on pressure conditions in the bladder. With a high-pressure system, the upper urinary tract is at high risk for deterioration, and upper tract monitoring should be more frequent (every 6–12 months). In the case of a low-pressure system, this danger is only relative, and we undertake renal ultrasound study approximately every 2–3 years if no change in clinical symptoms suggests modification of the bladder's pressure status.

ROLE OF URODYNAMICS

Urodynamics is the cornerstone in the diagnosis and management of neurogenic bladder dysfunction (see also Chapter 22). In this respect, the main parameters that require special attention are high detrusor pressure during the filling or storage phase of the bladder (decreased bladder wall compliance and/or sustained detrusor contraction) and detrusor-external sphincter dyssynergia during micturition. Well-conducted, multichannel videourodynamic evaluation will highlight these conditions and consequently allow the initiation of appropriate therapeutic measures that should ideally transform a high-pressure system to a low-pressure system.

As previously mentioned, repetition of these essential tests for an accurate evaluation of neurogenic bladders will depend not only on individual practices but

also on risk evaluation and continence status. Some patients with high detrusor pressures and/or poor continence, despite treatments, may require more frequently repeated urodynamic testing. A continent patient with a low-pressure bladder can be mainly followed clinically with occasional urodynamics done routinely or because of recurrent urinary tract infections or any other unexplained clinical changes.

PLACE OF ENDOSCOPY

Cystoscopy is an important, office-based evaluation of the lower urinary tract. It can detect bladder outlet obstruction due to urethral stricture or prostatic hypertrophy, and bladder abnormalities such as bladder tumor, trabeculation, and bladder stones, although the value of cystoscopy at initial evaluation has been questioned.[18–22] We recommend doing cystoscopy at initial evaluation, and as a diagnostic tool for patients who present with difficult catheterization to diagnose urethral stricture and false passage, or when presenting with recurrent urinary tract infection, increased incontinence, bladder spasticity, and/or dysreflexia for the possibility of finding a bladder stone. It should be noted that cystoscopy is a mandatory investigation for hematuria workup.[23] Screening cystoscopy for patients on a chronic indwelling catheter is recommended for early diagnosis of bladder cancer, although the value of such an approach has not been proven.[24]

REFERENCES

1. Razdan S, Leboeuf L, Meinbach DS, Weinstein D, and Gousse AE. Current practice patterns in the urologic surveillance and management of patients with spinal cord injury. *Urology.* 2003;61:893–6.
2. Bycroft J, Hamid R, Bywater H, Patki P, and Shah J. Variation in urological practice amongst spinal injuries unites in the UK and Eire. *Neurourol Urodyn.* 2004;23:252–6.
3. Kitahara S, Iwatsubo E, Yasuda K et al. Practice patterns of Japanese physicians in urologic surveillance and management of spinal cord injury patients. *Spinal Cord.* 2006;44:362–8.
4. Blok BF, Karsenty G, and Corcos J. Urological surveillance and management of patients with neurogenic bladder: Results of a survey among practicing urologists in Canada. *Can J Urol.* 2006;13:3239–43.
5. Light JK, Faganel J, and Beric A. Detrusor areflexia in suprasacral spinal cord injuries. *J Urol.* 1985;134:295–7.
6. Chancellor MB, and Kiilholma P. Urodynamic evaluation of patients following spinal cord injury. *Semin Urol.* 1992;10:83–94.
7. Wheeler JS Jr and Walter JW. Acute urologic management of the patient with spinal cord injury: Initial hospitalisation. *Urol Clin N Am.* 1993;20:403–11.

8. Perlow DL and Diokno AC. Predicting lower urinary tract dysfunctions in patients with spinal cord injury. *Urology*. 1981;18:531–5.

9. Chancellor MB. Urodynamic evaluation after spinal cord injury. *Phys Med Rehab Clin N Am*. 1993;4:273–98.

10. Solinsky R, Bunnell AE, Linsenmeyer TA, Svircev JN, Engle A, and Burns SP. Pharmacodynamics and effectiveness of topical nitroglycerin at lowering blood pressure during autonomic dysreflexia. *Spinal Cord*. 2017;55(10):911–4.

11. McGuire EJ. Immediate management of the inability to void. In: Parsons FK, and Fitzpatrick JM, eds. *Practical Urology in Spinal Cord Injury*. London, UK: Springer Verlag; 1991:5–10.

12. Donelly J, Hackler RH, and Bunts RC. Present urologic status of the World War II paraplegic: 25-Year follow-up. Comparison with status of the 20-year Korean War paraplegic and the 5-year Vietnam paraplegic. *J Urol*. 1972;108:558–62.

13. Webb DR, Fitzpatrick JM, and O'Flynn JD. A 15-year follow-up of 406 consecutive spinal cord injuries. *Br J Urol*. 1984;56:614–7.

14. Bodley R. Imaging in chronic spinal cord injury—Indications and benefits. *Eur J Radiol*. 2002;42:135–53.

15. Morcos SK and Thomas DG. A comparison of real-time ultrasonography with intravenous urography in the follow-up of patients with spinal cord injury. *Clin Radiol*. 1988;39:49–50.

16. Chagnon S, Vallée C, Laissy JP, and Blery M. Ultrasonographic evaluation of the urinary tract in patients with spinal cord injuries. Systematic comparison with intravenous urography in 50 cases. *J Radiol (Paris)*. 1985;66:801–6.

17. Papdaki PJ, Vlychou MK, Zavras GM et al. Investigation of vesicourethral reflux with colour Doppler sonography in adult patients with spinal cord injury. *Eur Radiol*. 2002;12:366–70.

18. Phillips JP, Jadvar H, Sullivan G et al. Effect of radionuclide reno-grams on treatment of patients with spinal cord injury. *Am J Roentgenol*. 1997;169:1045–7.

19. Kavanagh A, Baverstock R, Campeau L et al. Canadian Urological Association guidelines: Diagnosis, management, and surveillance of neurogenic lower urinary tract dysfunction—Full text. *Can Urol Assoc J*. 2019;13(6):E157–76.

20. Welk B, Schneider MP, Thavaseelan J, Traini LR, Curt A, and Kessler TM. Early urological care of patients with spinal cord injury. *World J Urol*. 2018;36(10):1537–44.

21. Groen J, Pannek J, Castro Diaz D et al. Summary of European Association of Urology (EAU) guidelines on neuro-urology. *Eur Urol*. 2016; 69(2):324–33.

22. Welk B, Liu K, and Shariff SZ. The use of urologic investigations among patients with traumatic spinal cord injuries. *Res Rep Urol*. 2016;8:27–34.

23. Yoshimura N, Jeong JY, Kim DK, and Chancellor MB. Integrated physiology of the lower urinary tract. In: Corcos J, Ginsburg D, and Karsenty G, eds. *Textbook of the Neurogenic Bladder*, 3rd ed. Boca Raton, FL: CRC Press, Taylor & Francis Group; 2016:33–47.

24. Welk B, McIntyre A, Teasell R et al. Bladder cancer in individuals with spinal cord injuries. *Spinal Cord*. 2013;51:516–21.

Part IV

CLASSIFICATION

Chapter 26

CLASSIFICATION OF LOWER URINARY TRACT DYSFUNCTION

Jan Groen and Bertil F.M. Blok

The innervation of the lower urinary tract seems to be complex. Providing a classification system of its dysfunction might be therefore a complicated matter and is necessarily based on a schematization of the innervation. A crucial role is played by the pontine micturition center (PMC).[1] This center is inhibited during urine storage by suprapontine input, from both cortical and subcortical areas. In addition, the smooth detrusor muscle of the urinary bladder is inhibited by spinal mechanisms during urine storage. Bladder pressure thus remains low during bladder filling due to sympathetic activity from preganglionic motoneurons in T10 through L2, that is mostly conveyed by the hypogastric nerves.[2] Continence is maintained by continuous contraction of the striated external urethral sphincter (EUS). When the urinary bladder is fuller, the bladder neck (smooth muscle internal urethral sphincter) contracts also, and the detrusor muscle relaxes actively by activation of the sympathetic system. The EUS is innervated via the pudendal nerves by fibers originating from Onuf's nucleus in S1 through S3. The EUS contracts continuously and involuntarily due to excitation by the so-called pontine storage center (PSC).[1] The EUS is also under conscious control via the primary motor cortex, but this conscious control does not play a role in normal urinary storage and continence.[1,3] When a person decides to void and experiences a sense of safe environment, the PMC is activated, and the external urethral sphincter relaxes via interneuronal inhibition of the motoneurons in Onuf's nucleus followed by a contraction of the detrusor muscle via excitation of the detrusor motoneurons in S2 through S4. Once initiated, voiding progresses automatically via the spinobulbospinal reflex pathway. Ascending afferent input from the spinal cord reaches the PMC after relay in the periaqueductal gray (PAG).[4,5] The PMC is the area where the coordination between the excitation of the detrusor motoneurons and the inhibition of the motoneurons in Onuf's nucleus occurs.[6–8]

Based on this schematization, four levels of origin of neurologic lower urinary tract dysfunction can be discerned that determine the functional consequences of the lesion: (a) suprapontine lesions, (b) pontine and suprasacral spinal lesions, (c) sacral lesions, and (d) infrasacral lesions.[9]

SUPRAPONTINE LESIONS

Suprapontine lesions and diseases that may affect lower urinary tract function include cerebrovascular accidents, dementias, parkinsonian syndromes, brain tumors, traumatic brain injury, cerebral palsy, and normal pressure hydrocephalus. If the extension of these abnormalities is such that they affect the pathways involved in bladder control, the inhibitory signals to the PMC are disturbed, so that involuntary detrusor contractions occur, which in turn can result in urinary frequency, urgency, urinary incontinence, nocturia, and even uninhibited voiding; that is, in the neurogenic overactive bladder (OAB) syndrome. As the pons is unaffected, there is no impact on the coordination between the contraction of the detrusor muscle and the relaxation of the internal and external urinary sphincters, so that the micturition process itself occurs in a normal fashion. A postvoid residual volume is therefore not to be expected, at least not on neurologic grounds.

PONTINE AND SUPRASACRAL SPINAL LESIONS

Multiple system atrophy and pontine infarction are examples of diseases that can be located in the pons. Suprasacral spinal lesions include spinal cord injury (SCI), multiple sclerosis (MS), myelitis and other demyelinating disorders, and myelodysplasia (spina bifida). Lesions in the pons and the suprasacral part of the spinal cord can affect both the storage and the voiding phase of the micturition cycle. As in suprapontine lesions, involuntary detrusor contractions may occur. The nature of the detrusor overactivity is, however, different. The normally present inhibition of the sacral detrusor motoneurons at the spinal level has been inactivated by the occurrence of segmental reflexes mediated by C-fiber afferents, which are silent under normal circumstances. This can be considered as the reemergence of primitive, infantile voiding reflexes.[10]

Acute SCI does not immediately result in detrusor overactivity. There is initially a phase of spinal shock of several weeks, that is characterized by a loss of muscle tone and segmental spinal reflexes such as the anal reflex and the bulbocavernosus reflex, and by acontractility of the detrusor. Detrusor overactivity emerges after about 6 weeks.[11]

Disruption of the spinobulbospinal reflex pathway involved in voiding results in the loss of coordination of the activation of the detrusor motoneurons and the inhibition of Onuf's nucleus. This results in a simultaneous contraction of the detrusor muscle and the external urethral sphincter, a condition called detrusor-sphincter dyssynergia (DSD). DSD may lead to obstructed voiding, high intravesical pressures, and incomplete bladder emptying.

LESIONS AT OR ABOVE T6
Special attention should be paid to patients with SCI with lesions at or above T6. In these patients, autonomic dysreflexia may occur. This phenomenon can be life-threatening and may be triggered by noxious and nonnoxious stimuli below the level of injury. It is defined by a more than 20 mm Hg rise in systolic blood pressure. Its signs and symptoms include headache, flushing, piloerection, stuffy nose, sweating above the level of the lesion, vasoconstriction below the level of the lesion, and cardiac dysrhythmias.[12] Relevant triggers from a urologic point of view include bladder distension, instrumentation of the lower urinary tract, urinary tract infections, and sexual activity.

SACRAL LESIONS

The conus medullaris is the place where upper and lower motor neurons involved in the function of the lower urinary tract connect. Damage to this structure can consequently result in a variety of clinical manifestations that are characteristic for suprasacral lesions (see the previous paragraph) and infrasacral lesions (see the next paragraph). When the motoneurons of the external urethral sphincter are damaged at S1 and S2, patients will present with stress urinary incontinence. Damage of the preganglionic parasympathetic motoneurons of the detrusor muscle will result in an underactive bladder and possible urinary retention. Conus lesions may be due to congenital causes, lumbar disk herniation, tumors, and trauma.

INFRASACRAL LESIONS

The cauda equina and peripheral nerves convey fibers originating from the detrusor motoneurons and Onuf's nucleus. Lesions at this level can consequently result in a weakly contracting or even noncontracting detrusor, that is, in an underactive or acontractile detrusor, and urinary retention or a significant postvoid residual volume. Impaired innervation of the external urethral sphincter implies weakening of its function. Involvement of the sympathetic hypogastric nerve fibers implies bladder neck weakness and possibly also impaired bladder compliance. It is obvious from this summary that stress urinary incontinence and overflow incontinence may be predominant symptoms in patients with infrasacral lesions.

Infrasacral lesions can be due to many different causes. Iatrogenic causes include prostatectomy, hysterectomy, colorectal surgery, and radiotherapy.[9]

LIMITATIONS OF THE CLASSIFICATION SYSTEM

The classification system described, namely directly above this new section can aid in deciding on the appropriate therapeutic approach. It does, however, have its limitations.

RENAL FUNCTION
One of the main goals in the treatment of patients with a neurogenic bladder is preservation of renal function. The classification system does not predict which patients are at risk for upper urinary tract damage. In a retrospective study on 42 children with myelodysplasia, McGuire et al. found a higher rate of hydronephrosis and vesicoureteral reflux in those who had urethral leakage at detrusor pressures greater than 40 cm H_2O during a urodynamic examination.[13] This cut-off value of the detrusor leak point pressure (DLPP) has been accepted by many authors as an objective measure for the safety of the upper urinary tract.[14] However, the evidence for this cut-off value was considered low, at least in adult patients, in a systematic review.[15] In addition to patients with spina bifida, patients with SCI have a substantially higher risk of developing renal failure compared with the general population. By contrast, the prevalence of upper urinary tract damage and renal failure is low in patients with slowly progressive nontraumatic neurologic disorders that can also demonstrate elevated detrusor pressures, such as multiple sclerosis and Parkinson's disease.[16] Not surprisingly, Musco et al. concluded in a systematic review that the statement that a DLPP greater than 40 cm H_2O is a risk factor for upper urinary tract deterioration should not be extended to all ages and neurologic populations. They confirmed, however, that a high DLPP is a major risk factor for such a deterioration, in addition to low compliance.[14]

SENSORY FUNCTION

The classification system is based on the behavior of the detrusor muscle and the urethral sphincters, that is, on the motor function of the lower urinary tract; it ignores its sensory function. The afferent fibers of the lower urinary tract follow the same pathways as the efferent fibers. Those of the bladder run in the parasympathetic pelvic and sympathetic hypogastric nerves. The somatic afferents from the urethra run with the pudendal nerves. The afferent fibers run to the spinal segments T10 through L2 and S2 through S4. At these segments, some of the afferent fibers synapse with efferent fibers, while the remainder ascend the spinal cord to the brainstem and higher centers.[17] Despite the common pathways, neurogenic motor dysfunction of the lower urinary tract does not necessarily reflect its sensory dysfunction, and vice versa. This depends on the type, location, and extension of the lesion involved. The extreme of such a discrepancy is a condition that has been called "sensory neurogenic bladder."[18] In this condition, the sensory fibers between the bladder and the spinal cord or the fibers ascending to the brain are selectively interrupted. The most common diseases causing this situation are diabetes mellitus, tabes dorsalis, and pernicious anemia. The consequences of impaired bladder sensation may be overdistension, detrusor underactivity, and significant amounts of postvoid residual urine.

CONCLUSION

A classification system of lower urinary tract dysfunction was described that was based on the location of the lesion. This location was used to predict the motor function of the detrusor muscle and the urethral sphincters, especially the striated sphincter, from the organization of the nervous system. Thus, dysfunction of the storage and voiding phase of the micturition cycle can be understood. In clinical practice, however, damage of the nervous system is often not restricted to one specific level, and its severity may vary. A thorough clinical evaluation, including a urodynamic examination, is therefore indispensable to optimize therapy in these patients and to identify those who are at risk for upper urinary tract deterioration.

REFERENCES

1. Blok BF. Central pathways controlling micturition and urinary continence. *Urology.* 2002;59(5 Suppl 1):13.

2. Vaughan CW and Satchell PM. Role of sympathetic innervation in the feline continence process under natural filling conditions. *J Neurophysiol.* 1992;68:1842.

3. Fowler CJ, Griffiths D, and de Groat WC. The neural control of micturition. *Nat Rev Neurosci.* 2008;9:453.

4. Blok BF, and Holstege G. Direct projections from the periaqueductal gray to the pontine micturition center (M-region). An anterograde and retrograde tracing study in the cat. *Neurosci Lett.* 1994;166:93.

5. Blok BF, De Weerd H, and Holstege G. Ultrastructural evidence for a paucity of projections from the lumbosacral cord to the pontine micturition center or M-region in the cat: A new concept for the organization of the micturition reflex with the periaqueductal gray as central relay. *J Comp Neurol.* 1995;359:300.

6. Blok BF and Holstege G. Ultrastructural evidence for a direct pathway from the pontine micturition center to the parasympathetic preganglionic motoneurons of the bladder of the cat. *Neurosci Lett.* 1997;222:195.

7. Blok BF, de Weerd H, and Holstege G. The pontine micturition center projects to sacral cord GABA immunoreactive neurons in the cat. *Neurosci Lett.* 1997;233:109.

8. Blok BF, van Maarseveen JT, and Holstege G. Electrical stimulation of the sacral dorsal gray commissure evokes relaxation of the external urethral sphincter in the cat. *Neurosci Lett.* 1998;249:68.

9. Apostolidis A, Drake MJ, Emmanuel A et al. Committee 10. Neurologic urinary and faecal incontinence. In: Abrams P, Cardozo L, Wagg A, and Wein A, eds. *Incontinence,* 6th ed. Tokyo: 6th International Consultation on Incontinence; 2017:1093–1308.

10. de Groat WC. Plasticity of bladder reflex pathways during postnatal development. *Physiol Behav.* 2002;77:689.

11. Panicker JN, Fowler CJ, and Kessler TM. Lower urinary tract dysfunction in the neurological patient: Clinical assessment and management. *Lancet Neurol.* 2015;14:720.

12. Krassioukov A, Biering-Sørensen F, Donovan W et al. International standards to document remaining autonomic function after spinal cord injury. *J Spinal Cord Med.* 2012;35:201.

13. McGuire EJ, Woodside JR, Borden TA, and Weiss RM. Prognostic value of urodynamic testing in myelodysplastic patients. *J Urol.* 1981;126:205.

14. Musco S, Padilla-Fernández B, Del Popolo G et al. Value of urodynamic findings in predicting upper urinary tract damage in neuro-urological patients: A systematic review. *Neurourol Urodyn.* 2018;37:1522.

15. Veenboer PW, Bosch JLHR, van Asbeck FWA, and de Kort LMO. Upper and lower urinary tract outcomes in adult myelomeningocele patients: A systematic review. *PLOS ONE* 2012;7(10):e48399.

16. Lawrenson R, Wyndaele JJ, Vlachonikolis I, Farmer C, and Glickman S. Renal failure in patients with neurogenic lower urinary tract dysfunction. *Neuroepidemiology.* 2001;20:138.

17. Mundy AR and Thomas PJ. Clinical physiology of the bladder, urethra and pelvic floor. In: Mundy AR, Stephenson TP, and Wein AJ, eds. *Urodynamics: Principles, Practice and Application,* 2nd ed. New York, NY: Churchill Livingstone; 1994:15–27.

18. Lapides J. Neuromuscular, vesical and ureteral dysfunction. In: Campbell MF, and Harrison JH, eds. *Urology.* Philadelphia, PA: WB Saunders; 1970:1343–79.

Part V

TREATMENT

Chapter 27

CONSERVATIVE TREATMENT

Samer Shamout and Lysanne Campeau

INTRODUCTION (PRINCIPLES OF MANAGEMENT)

Conservative treatment remains the cornerstone for urologic management of the neurologically impaired patient. The principal goals of bladder management in individuals with neurogenic lower urinary tract dysfunction (NLUTD) are to preserve kidney function, achieve urinary continence, minimize urologic complications, and improve quality of life.[1] The approach to treatment of the NLUTD should address both voiding and storage dysfunction. Treatment is directed at maintaining a low detrusor pressure and ensuring complete bladder emptying. (Table 27.1). In this chapter, we present an abridged overview of the available techniques applied in conservative treatment, including behavioral therapy, physiotherapy, and catheterization.

BEHAVIORAL THERAPY

TRIGGERED REFLEX VOIDING

Triggering the bladder reflex achieves voiding through a nonphysiologic mechanism that elicits a reflex detrusor contraction through activation of C-fibers. The most frequently applied maneuver includes suprapubic tapping, an average of seven to eight percussions every 3 seconds until voiding starts. It is essential to perform an early urodynamic study before starting triggered voiding in order to avoid high-pressure development due to detrusor sphincter dyssynergia. Bladder outlet obstruction should be managed in all patients with triggered voiding to improve emptying and prevent harmful high pressure. Evidence based on four recent systematic reviews supports the use of clean intermittent catheterization (IC) as the mainstay of bladder management before considering bladder reflex triggering (Table 27.2).[2]

BLADDER EXPRESSION (CREDÉ AND VALSALVA)

Bladder expression involves several maneuvers intended to increase intravesical pressure to enable or to facilitate emptying of urine. The most commonly used are the Valsalva (abdominal straining) and the Credé (manual compression of the lower abdomen) maneuvers. It is generally recommended to avoid bladder expression.[3]

Bladder expression can only be considered in individuals with lower motor neuron lesions or sacral spinal cord injury (SCI), resulting in a combination of an areflexic bladder with an underactive or anatomic incompetent urethral sphincter. Although bladder expression enables many patients to empty their bladder even incompletely, over 50% of patients had influx into the prostate and the seminal vesicles along with other adverse events such as upper urinary tract reflux, hemorrhoids, genital prolapse, and infections.[4]

Table 27.1 Principles of Conservative Management of Neurogenic Lower Urinary Tract Dysfunction (NLUTD)

Types of NLUTD	Treatment Modalities
Detrusor overactivity with detrusor-sphincter dyssynergia	• Intermittent catheterization ± pharmacotherapy • Indwelling catheter ± pharmacotherapy
Detrusor overactivity with negligible postvoid residual and no detrusor-sphincter dyssynergia	According to cooperation and mobility • Behavioral, bladder relaxant drugs, intermittent catheterization • Triggered voiding (if urodynamically safe) • External appliances • Indwelling catheter + pharmacotherapy
Detrusor underactivity with postvoid residual	• Intermittent catheterization • α-Adrenergic antagonist
Stress urinary incontinence due to sphincter incompetence	• Behavioral/timed voiding and external appliances

Source: Adapted from Wyndaele J-J. *Eur Urol Suppl.* 2008;7(8):557–65.

Table 27.2 Contraindication to Triggered Voiding

Inadequate upper extremity function
Weak detrusor contraction
Unbalanced voiding
Upper urinary tract reflux
Reflux in the seminal vesicles or in the vas
Uncontrollable autonomic dysreflexia
Unresolved recurrent urinary tract infections (UTIs)

BEHAVIORAL TRAINING/TOILETING ASSISTANCE

Behavioral training comprises several approaches[5,6] and often necessitates support from caregivers and treating physicians for successful outcomes. It may be more valuable to address functional incontinence* that is often present in neurogenic patients.[7]

- *Timed voiding* involves scheduled voiding at fixed intervals between toilet visits and can be utilized to prevent episodes of urge incontinence and decreasing postvoid residual volume. Timed voiding is useful as adjunctive treatment to IC and/or tapping or Credé maneuver and/ or in patients with partially preserved bladder control.[8] It is also of value in diabetic patients with impaired bladder sensation.[4]
- *Prolonging voiding intervals* to minimize frequency.
- *Bladder training/drill* is characterized by training the bladder to hold more urine in an effort to increase capacity and control bladder urgency.
- *Habit retraining* involves the development of a toileting schedule specific to the needs of each patient depending on usual voiding pattern. This technique helps patients to maintain voluntary bladder emptying and is mainly suitable for institutionalized patients.
- *Prompted voiding* and positive reinforcement through request for help might be useful in improving bladder control.
- *Lifestyle modification* includes modifying drinking habits and avoiding caffeinated beverages. Evaluating drug intake is important, especially if it induces diuresis and/or affects bladder function. Other physical or psychologic conditions such as constipation and depression should be managed. All are important measures to promote optimal lower urinary tract (LUT) function.
- *Keeping a voiding diary* is important for treatment adjustment and also has a direct therapeutic effect. It is very useful in early and institutional care.[6,94]

* Functional incontinence: Complaint of involuntary loss of urine that results from an inability to reach the toilet due to cognitive, functional, or mobility impairments in the presence of an intact lower urinary tract.[7]

PHYSIOTHERAPY

Pelvic floor muscle training (PFMT) has been shown to be beneficial in multiple sclerosis (MS) populations (predominantly female patients) with detrusor overactivity. This approach resulted in significant improvements in the following parameters after 1 month of treatment: urinary frequency, number of incontinence episodes per day, and mean cystometric capacity.[9] McClurg et al. explored a combined approach using PFMT, intravaginal electrical stimulation, and electromyography (EMG) biofeedback in the treatment of bladder dysfunction related to MS. They reported statistically significant improvements related to number of leaks and pad weight.[10] PFMT and biofeedback can have successful outcomes in patients with at least partly preserved voluntary and/or sensory function (Table 27.3).

INTERMITTENT BLADDER CATHETERIZATION

Since its introduction in 1972,[11] intermittent self-catheterization (ISC) is the standard treatment for patients with neurogenic voiding dysfunction. It enables complete bladder emptying and thus avoids consequent risks for upper tract damage and infections. It also facilitates appropriate urine storage, which helps to achieve social continence. It gives the patient a complete autonomy that a third part IC would not.

The time to institute IC depends on the physician's practice patterns and the medical condition of the patient.[12] Early institution of IC seems to diminish catheter-related complications and decrease the incidence of bacteriuria.[13]

Table 27.3 Key Ooints (Behavioral and Physiotherapy)

- Morbidity occurs more frequently during early treatment course. This includes deterioration of bladder function, renal damage, infection, stones, and unresolved incontinence.
- Long-term complications are hardly avoidable, making regular follow-up a necessity.
- Bladder expression is potentially dangerous and should be avoided.
- Behavioral training techniques are used in many rehabilitation settings to improve continence. However, the evidence supporting these techniques is lacking, and the management efficiency is low.
- Pelvic floor muscle training aims to improve continence. It may be helpful in selected patients with *neurogenic lower urinary tract dysfunction* with voluntary control of the lower urinary tract.

CHOICE OF CATHETERS

Many types of catheters can be used in clinical practice: in terms of catheter material (PVC versus silicone or rubber), coating (hydrophilic coated versus uncoated), method single-use versus multiple-use, and catheter design (standard versus compact). Choices depend on patients' individual anatomy, hand dexterity, availability, and social and financial resources.[14]

Hydrophilic lubricated catheters are associated with significantly lower risk of urinary tract infection (UTI) and urethral trauma and improved patient's satisfaction and quality of life.[15] However, financial limitations can limit hydrophilic catheter use in different communities. Certain patients may wish to use a single-use disposable catheter over repeated multiple uses.[16] Reused catheters do not appear to be associated with increased likelihood of UTI.[17,18]

CATHETERIZATION TECHNIQUE

There are two main techniques regarding sterility and IC: sterile approach[19] (nontouch technique where sterility is maintained) and clean approach[11] (where only general hygiene practices are followed). The sterile technique is associated with high cost and mostly used in a hospital setting. In the majority of cases, a clean catheterization technique is employed. This technique is found to be easily used and reduced urologic complications in patients with SCI.[14] The ongoing debate on the optimal IC technique does not appear to change the practical outcome of IC given that general rules are applied: adequate patient education and training, clean and nontraumatic catheterization, adequate number of catheterizations, and long-term patient compliance.[20] For patients with catheterization difficulty due to DSD, botulinum toxin injection in the striated sphincter can be useful.[21]

CATHETERIZATION FREQUENCY

The required number of catheterizations per day depends on many factors, such as fluid intake, bladder capacity, and urodynamic measures (filling and voiding pressure). The average frequency of catheterizations is four to six times a day. Considering IC is the only technique of emptying urine, patients will need to maintain this frequency of catheterization. Less frequent catheterization in 24 hours is associated with a higher risk of symptomatic UTIs.[22–24]

Adjunctive measures should be considered to overcome high detrusor pressure and OAB, and achieve continence: oral drugs (anticholinergics, β_3-agonists), botulinum toxin injections, or surgical interventions as with bladder augmentation may be necessary to achieve these goals.[25,26] If nighttime overdistension is noted due to high diuresis

and variation of antidiuretic hormone, DDAVP (desmopressin) is safe and effective.[27,28]

CATHETERIZATION COMPLICATIONS

Despite being the preferred method of management for patients with NLUTD, IC is not without its complications, namely, bacteriuria, UTI, and urethral trauma.

Asymptomatic bacteriuria is a frequent finding in patients with NLUTD using IC.[29] The incidence of bacteriuria is 1%–3% per catheterization.[30] It is estimated that one to four episodes of bacteriuria occur for 100 days of IC,[31] with significant bacteriuria defined as urine culture with more than 10^2 cfu/mL. Asymptomatic bacteriuria only require treatment for patients undergoing surgical or endoscopic interventions and during pregnancies.[32–35]

Recurrent symptomatic UTIs are the most common complication observed among patients with NLUTD and those who perform IC. Incidence of UTI varies widely in the literature, for many reasons: inconsistent definition of UTI, different techniques of IC, variability in the frequency of urine analysis, and methods applied for evaluation.

The most important measures to minimize UTI risk are appropriate technique, education on hygiene, prevention of bladder overdistention, and maintenance of a low-pressure bladder.[36]

Urethritis and epididymo-orchitis occurs in 2%–28.5% of patients on IC. Use of smaller-sized catheters, lubricants, and hydrophilic catheters can all reduce this risk.[37,38] Prostatitis is often difficult to diagnose and treat in patients with NLUTD and could be a source of recurrent UTIs. Overall incidence reaches 33%, although previous report is thought to be around 5%–18%.[39–41]

Urethral stricture rates rise after 5 years[29] up to 4%–25% despite using hydrophilic-coated catheters.[42,43]

QUALITY OF LIFE AND COMPLIANCE

ISC leads to high patient satisfaction and significant improvement in quality of life. Kessler et al. showed that 60% of IC cohorts reported improved quality of life, and the majority (78.3%) found this technique to be very easy with no interference with life activities.[44] On the other hand, IC by attendant was reported to negatively affect quality of life.[45]

It is known that some patients may give up IC to try other modalities.[46] The main reasons for stopping IC were recurrent UTIs, incontinence, dependence on caregivers, and urethral strictures. All of these reasons can be related to inappropriate bladder management with persistence of high pressure and/or urgency/incontinence, or to inappropriate situations to implement SIC (impaired upper limb function, difficulty to reach urethra, etc.).

INDWELLING CATHETERS

While clinical guidelines recommend IC for routine long-term treatment of NLUTD, IC is not an optimal technique for patients with impaired dexterity and without a caregiver, urethral abnormalities, poor cognition, reluctance of the patient, lack of financial support, or persistent incontinence.[47,48]

INDWELLING URETHRAL CATHETERS

Indwelling urethral catheterization is generally considered during the initial management of NLUTD after spinal injury.[49] Urethral catheters should be inserted with a strict aseptic technique and changed regularly every 4–6 weeks in a chronic patient with NLUTD; catheter sizes between 12 and 14 Fr are commonly used with 10cc balloons positioned in the bladder. The use of large-caliber catheters is associated with a high risk for urethral erosion and discomfort and proved ineffective in preventing pericatheter urinary leakage, which is mostly related to neurogenic detrusor overactivity. Proper education on daily cleanliness and hygiene for patient and caregiver is important to avoid complications related to blockage, overdistension, or infection. Consider the use of anticholinergic drugs in individuals with neurogenic bladder overactivity to prevent the development of hydronephrosis and poor compliance.[50]

Indwelling catheterization is associated with a higher rate of complications compared to IC. It significantly increases the risk of acute and chronic UTI (sixfold higher risk of UTI in patients with indwelling catheters compared to IC[51,52]). Routine antimicrobial prophylaxis is, however, not recommended.[53] IC also promotes stone formation, urethral trauma, fistula formation, periurethral abscess, and strictures.[54–56]

The presence of a long-term indwelling catheter, whether transurethral or suprapubic, is associated with increased risk of squamous cell carcinoma of the bladder (2.3%–10%[57,58]).

Therefore, urethral catheterization should be reserved for individuals who are not suitable candidates for IC or who are contraindicated to other bladder management strategies such as suprapubic catheter (SPC) or condom drainage (Table 27.4).

SUPRAPUBIC CATHETERS

A SPC may serve as a practical option for carefully selected patients with neurogenic voiding dysfunction, because it significantly reduces the complications related to urethral trauma and stricture formation. In addition, it maximizes patient independence and facilitates engagement in sexual activities.[1,59] This strategy has been used successfully in patients with poor hand dexterity or who are unwilling to perform IC, independent of attendant care, at an

Table 27.4 Key Points (Intermittent and Indwelling Catheters)

- Intermittent catheterization (IC) is the first-choice treatment for patients with neurogenic lower urinary tract dysfunction.
- Patient education and teaching are necessary to prevent and reduce complications.
- Patients should be instructed regarding frequency of catheterization and a nontraumatizing technique.
- The most widely used technique is "clean" IC.
- The most common complications associated with IC are recurrent urinary tract infection (UTI) and urethral trauma.
- Indwelling urethral catheterization should be used only exceptionally due to the high rate of complications (infections, epididymitis, periurethral abscess, erosion).
- In some selected patients, it could be the only noninvasive option. In such cases, the risk/benefit balance between indwelling catheterization and more invasive options (diversions) should be discussed (patient and family/physician/caregivers).
- Indwelling catheterization is frequently associated with UTI, stones, and renal impairment.
- Urethral trauma is much more prevalent with indwelling urethral catheter than IC.
- Silicone or hydrogel-coated indwelling catheters are recommended and should be changed *every 4–6 weeks*.
- Suprapubic catheter has the advantage of preventing urethral injury and is overall better tolerated.

early treatment phase of SCI, with persistent urinary incontinence, urethral damage, or stricture disease, with spasticity, or neurologic disease progression.[60–64]

The main disadvantage with SPC is that it requires a minimally invasive surgical intervention for insertion. Complications related to SPC insertion include potential injury to adjacent structures, infection, bleeding, and inability to pass the catheter into the bladder.[65,66] Regular follow-up and surveillance are needed to minimize associated morbidity and improve prognosis.

APPLIANCES (CONDOM CATHETERS AND PENILE CLAMPS)

Condom catheters are suitable for male patients with NLUTD who use reflex voiding or bladder expression and are incontinent. This approach should be avoided in patients with retracted penis, skin/penile lesion, confusion/dementia, or urinary retention.[67] More than 50% of patients may develop bacteriuria with prolonged use of condom catheters.[68] However, the

Table 27.5   Medications Promoting Storage

Class	Drug	Dose Range	Pharmacology	Adverse Events
Nonselective anticholinergics	Propantheline	Up to 90 mg daily	Nonselective antimuscarinic	Constipation, dry mouth, tachycardia, hypersensitivity to light
	Oxybutynin	Immediate release 5–30 mg thrice daily (up to 45 mg daily tolerated)	Nonselective antimuscarinic	Dry mouth, dry eyes, blurred vision, constipation, headache, sleep disturbance, diarrhea, worst cognitive
	Oxybutynin	Extended release 10–30 mg daily	Slower breakdown of the capsule allows slower release Reduced side-effect profile	Dry mouth, dry eyes, constipation, headache, sleep disturbance, diarrhea, worst cognitive
	Oxybutynin	Transdermal patch (Oxytrol) 3.9 mg/ patch every 3–4 days	Bypasses first-pass hepatic metabolism	Itching and local skin reaction, dry mouth, dry eyes, constipation, headache, sleep disturbance, diarrhea, worst cognitive
	Oxybutynin	Topical gel (Gelnique) 3% (84 mg) daily	Bypasses first-pass hepatic metabolism	Skin reaction, dry mouth, constipation, headache, sleep disturbance
	Tolterodine	Immediate release 2–8 mg twice daily Extended release 2–8 mg/day	Noncompetitive antimuscarinic	Dry mouth, dry eyes, constipation, headache, sleep disturbance
	Propiverine	Up to 90 mg daily	Calcium agonist with moderate anticholinergic effects	Dry mouth, dry eyes, constipation, headache, sleep disturbance, diarrhea, restlessness, dizziness, vertigo, speech disorders
	Trospium	Immediate release 20–60 mg twice daily Extended release 20–60 mg daily (up to 120 mg)	Quaternary ammonium derivative with antimuscarinic action	Dry mouth, dry eyes, dry nose, constipation, headache, sleep disturbance, diarrhea
	Fesoterodine	Extended release 4–8 mg daily	Dose adjustment with hepatic/renal impairment and with CYP3A4 inhibitors	Dry mouth, dry eyes, dry skin, constipation, back pain
Selective anticholinergics	Solifenacin	Extended release 7.5–15 mg daily	M3 antagonist	Most constipation of any in class, headache, dizziness, dry eyes, dry mouth
	Darifenacin	Extended release 5–10 mg daily	M3 antagonist	Most constipation of any in class, headache, dizziness, dry eyes, dry mouth
β3-selective adrenergic agonist	Mirabegron	25–50 mg daily	β_3-agonist CYP2D6 inhibitor	Tachycardia, hypertension, nasopharyngitis
Alpha-blockers	Table 27.6	Table 27.6	Alpha-receptor blockade at α_{1A}, α_{1D} receptors	Table 27.6
Tricyclic antidepressants	Imipramine	10–45 mg twice or thrice daily	Anticholinergic and serotonin reuptake inhibitor	Dizziness, drowsiness, dry mouth, constipation, blurred vision, nightmares, breast swelling, lethal cardiac arrhythmia at high doses (overdose)

rate for UTI is lower than with indwelling catheters and similar to IC.[4,52] Patients with incontinence have better quality of life with condom catheter use than wearing absorbent pads.[69]

Patients with NLUTD are not recommended to use penile clamps because they are associated with increased risk of urethral and skin lesions.

ORAL PHARMACOTHERAPY

In patients with NLUTD, drugs are prescribed to decrease detrusor storage pressure, increase bladder capacity, improve urinary incontinence, or influence urethral resistance.

Frequently used medications are summarized in Table 27.5.

ANTICHOLINERGICS (ANTIMUSCARINIC)

Anticholinergic agents have proven effective to improve LUT symptoms in patients with SCI (anticholinergic 63% versus placebo 22%).[70] A meta-analysis of 960 patients from 16 randomized controlled trials (RCTs) showed significant improvement in urodynamic parameters compared to placebo, especially with regard to decreased maximum detrusor pressure (by 38.30 cm/H_2O; 95% confidence interval, 53.17–23.43). There is limited evidence supporting the superiority of one antimuscarinic over the others in terms of health-related quality of life and cost to the healthcare system.[71,72] The choice of optimal antimuscarinic agent should be individualized, taking into account the safety and tolerability profiles for each drug.[73] Dose escalation may be required to enhance symptomatic or urodynamic improvement taking into consideration patient tolerance, with potential chance of more dose-related adverse events.[74–77]

β₃-ADRENERGIC AGONIST THERAPY

β_3-Adrenergic receptor agonist mirabegron (Myrbetriq™ in North America and Betmiga™ in Europe) evolves as a future alternative in the management of NDO. Although mirabegron avoids antimuscarinic-related adverse events such as dry mouth, constipation, and cognitive impairment, it increases the risk of certain cardiovascular system side effects. Current evidence is insufficient to support effectiveness of mirabegron over anticholinergic agents in this population due to the lack of efficacy to improve urodynamic parameters.[78–81]

DESMOPRESSIN (DDAVP)

Desmopressin is a synthetic analog of arginine vasopressin; it has been used to treat urinary frequency or nocturia in patients with NLUTD.[82,83] Desmopressin is also helpful with nocturnal polyuria

Table 27.6   Alpha-Blocker Medications

Medication	Dose Range (mg Daily)	Common Side Effects
Alpha-blockers	–	Rhinitis, postural hypotension, dizziness, abnormal ejaculation
Alfuzosin	5–10	Less ejaculatory problems and less dizziness/postural hypotension
Doxazosin	2–8	Most dizziness and postural hypotension—dose escalation required
Terazosin	2–10	Most dizziness and postural hypotension—dose escalation required
Tamsulosin	0.4–0.8	High risk of ejaculatory problems
Silosodin	8	Lowest rate of ejaculatory problems and hypotension

shown to decrease a number of catheterizations overnight.[84] This has proved effective in small numbers and necessitates close monitoring.[85] Desmopressin should be carefully considered in patients above 65 years or with dependent leg edema due to the risk of congestive heart failure or hyponatraemia.[28]

α-ADRENERGIC ANTAGONISTS

α-Adrenergic antagonists facilitate bladder emptying by reducing bladder outlet resistance and detrusor pressure and are useful in the prevention of autonomic dysreflexia.[86–89] In patients with multiple

Table 27.7   Key Points (Oral Pharmacotherapy)

- Long-term efficacy and safety of anticholinergics for *neurogenic lower urinary tract dysfunction* (NLUTD) is adequately documented.
- Anticholinergic medications improve bladder storage function and decrease lower urinary tract symptoms and upper tract deterioration in patients with intermittent catheterization or indwelling catheters.
- The extended-release preparations have considerably fewer side effects.
- There is limited evidence supporting the use of mirabegron as an alternative or in combination with antimuscarinics in NLUTD.
- Alpha-blockers can facilitate voiding in patients with spinal cord injury and improve bladder capacity and compliance in combination with anticholinergics.
- Desmopressin is effective in treating nocturnal polyuria in patients with spinal cord injury, but additional studies are needed.

sclerosis, comparing tamsulosin to placebo improved the maximum and average flow rate and residual volume significantly after treatment.[90] When given in combination with anticholinergic therapy, alpha-blockers act in a synergistic pathway and have proven to be more effective than monotherapy with either agent.[91–93] Commonly used alpha-blockers are listed in Table 27.6. Table 27.7 summarizes key points related to use of oral pharmacology for NLUTD.

REFERENCES

1. Weld KJ, and Dmochowski RR. Effect of bladder management on urological complications in spinal cord injured patients. *J Urol.* 2000;163(3):768–72.
2. Groen J, Pannek J, Diaz DC et al. Summary of European Association of Urology (EAU) guidelines on neuro-urology. *Eur Urol.* 2016;69(2):324–33.
3. EAU Guidelines on Neuro-Urology. Paper presented at *EAU Annual Congress Barcelona 2019.*
4. Wyndaele J-J. Conservative treatment of patients with neurogenic bladder. *Eur Urol Suppl.* 2008;7(8): 557–65.
5. Hadley EC. Bladder training and related therapies for urinary incontinence in older people. *JAMA.* 1986;256(3):372–9.
6. Dowd T, Kolcaba K, and Steiner R. Using cognitive strategies to enhance bladder control and comfort. *Holist Nurs Pract.* 2000;14(2):91–103.
7. Abrams P, Cardozo L, Wagg A, and Wein A. *Incontinence 6th Edition ICI-ICS.* Bristol, UK: International Continence Society; 2017.
8. Ersoz M, and Akyuz M. Bladder-filling sensation in patients with spinal cord injury and the potential for sensation-dependent bladder emptying. *Spinal Cord.* 2004;42(2):110.
9. De DR, Vermeulen C, Ketelaer P, Van HP, and Baert L. Pelvic floor rehabilitation in multiple sclerosis. *Acta Neurol Belg.* 1999;99(1):61–4.
10. McClurg D, Ashe R, Marshall K, and Lowe-Strong A. Comparison of pelvic floor muscle training, electromyography biofeedback, and neuromuscular electrical stimulation for bladder dysfunction in people with multiple sclerosis: A randomized pilot study. *Neurourol Urodynam Off J Int Continence Soc.* 2006;25(4):337–48.
11. Lapides J, Diokno AC, Silber SJ, and Lowe BS. Clean, intermittent self-catheterization in the treatment of urinary tract disease. *J Urol.* 1972;107(3):458–61.
12. Linsenmeyer T, Bodner D, Creasey G et al. Bladder management for adults with spinal cord injury: A clinical practice guideline for health-care providers. *J Spinal Cord Med.* 2006;29(5):527–73.
13. Zermann D-H, Wunderlich H, Derry F, Schröder S, and Schubert J. Audit of early bladder management complications after spinal cord injury in first-treating hospitals. *Eur Urol.* 2000;37(2):156–60.
14. Wyndaele J. Intermittent catheterization: Which is the optimal technique? *Spinal Cord.* 2002; 40(9):432.
15. Shamout S, Biardeau X, Corcos J, and Campeau L. Outcome comparison of different approaches to self-intermittent catheterization in neurogenic patients: A systematic review. *Spinal Cord.* 2017. July;55(7):629-643.
16. Christison K, Walter M, Wyndaele J-JJ et al. Intermittent catheterization: The devil is in the details. *J Neurotrauma.* 2018;35(7):985–9.
17. Champion VL. Clean technique for intermittent self-catheterization. *Nurs Res.* 1976;25(1):13–8.
18. Silbar EC, Cicmanec JF, Burke BM, and Bracken RB. Microwave sterilization: A method for home sterilization of urinary catheters. *J Urol.* 1989; 141(1):88–90.
19. Guttmann L, and Frankel H. The value of intermittent catheterisation in the early management of traumatic paraplegia and tetraplegia. *Paraplegia.* 1966;4(2):63–84.
20. Wyndaele J, Madersbacher H, and Kovindha A. Conservative treatment of the neuropathic bladder in spinal cord injured patients. *Spinal Cord.* 2001;39(6):294.
21. Wheeler Jr JS, Walter JS, Chintam RS, and Rao S. Botulinum toxin injections for voiding dysfunction following SCI. *J Spinal Cord Med.* 1998;21(3):227–9.
22. Wyndaele JJ. Complications of intermittent catheterization: Their prevention and treatment. *Spinal Cord.* 2002;40(10):536–41.
23. Bakke A, Digranes A, and Høisœter P. Physical predictors of infection in patients treated with clean intermittent catheterization: A prospective 7-year study. *Br J Urol.* 1997;79(1):85–90.
24. Sauerwein D. Urinary tract infection in patients with neurogenic bladder dysfunction. *Int J Antimicrob Agents.* 2002;19(6):592–7.
25. Schurch B, Stohrer M, Kramer G, Schmid DM, Gaul G, and Hauri D. Botulinum-A toxin for treating detrusor hyperreflexia in spinal cord injured patients: A new alternative to anticholinergic drugs? Preliminary results. *J Urol.* 2000;164(3 Pt 1):692–7.
26. Mast P, Hoebeke P, Wyndaele J, Oosterlinck W, and Everaert K. Experience with augmentation cystoplasty. A review. *Spinal Cord.* 1995;33(10):560.
27. Kilinc S, Akman M, Levendoglu F, and Özker R. Diurnal variation of antidiuretic hormone and urinary output in spinal cord injury. *Spinal Cord.* 1999;37(5):332.
28. Chancellor MB, Rivas DA, and Staas Jr WE. DDAVP in the urological management of the difficult neurogenic bladder in spinal cord injury: Preliminary report. *J Am Paraplegia Soc.* 1994;17(4):165–7.
29. Perrouin-Verbe B, Labat J, Richard I, De La Greve IM, Buzelin J, and Mathe J. Clean intermittent catheterisation from the acute period in spinal cord injury patients. Long term evaluation of urethral and genital tolerance. *Spinal Cord.* 1995;33(11):619.
30. Warren JW. Catheter-associated urinary tract infections. *Int J Antimicrob Agents.* 2001;17(4):299–303.
31. Goldmark E, Niver B, and Ginsberg DA. Neurogenic bladder: From diagnosis to management. *Curr Urol Rep.* 2014;15(10):448.
32. Lewis RI, Carrion HM, Lockhart JL, and Politano VA. Significance of asymptomatic bacterium in neurogenic bladder disease. *Urology.* 1984;23(4):343–7.
33. Nicolle LE, Bradley S, Colgan R, Rice JC, Schaeffer A, and Hooton TM. Infectious Diseases Society of America guidelines for the diagnosis and treatment of asymptomatic bacteriuria in adults. *Clin Infect Dis.* 2005;40:643–54.
34. Michau A, Dinh A, Denys P et al. Control cross-sectional study evaluating an antibiotic prevention strategy in 30 pregnancies under clean intermittent self-catheterization and review of literature. *Urology.* 2016;91:58–63.

35. Hooton TM, Bradley SF, Cardenas DD et al. Diagnosis, prevention, and treatment of catheter-associated urinary tract infection in adults: 2009 International Clinical Practice Guidelines from the Infectious Diseases Society of America. *Clin Infect Dis*. 2010;50(5):625–63.

36. Chhabra H. *ISCoS Text Book on Comprehensive Management of Spinal Cord Injuries*. New Delhi, India: Wolters Kluwer; 2015.

37. Vaidyanathan S, Soni B, Dundas S, and Krishnan K. Urethral cytology in spinal cord injury patients performing intermittent catheterisation. *Spinal Cord*. 1994;32(7):493.

38. Ku JH, Jung T, Lee J, Park W, and Shim H. Influence of bladder management on epididymo-orchitis in patients with spinal cord injury: Clean intermittent catheterization is a risk factor for epididymo-orchitis. *Spinal Cord*. 2006;44(3):165.

39. Krebs J, Bartel P, and Pannek J. Bacterial persistence in the prostate after antibiotic treatment of chronic bacterial prostatitis in men with spinal cord injury. *Urology*. 2014;83(3):515–20.

40. Siroky MB. Pathogenesis of bacteriuria and infection in the spinal cord injured patient. *Am J Med*. 2002;113(1):67–79.

41. Wyndaele J. Chronic prostatitis in spinal cord injury patients. *Paraplegia*. 1985;23(3):164–9.

42. Cornejo-Dávila V, Durán-Ortiz S, and Pacheco-Gahbler C. Incidence of urethral stricture in patients with spinal cord injury treated with clean intermittent self-catheterization. *Urology*. 2017;99:260–4.

43. Krebs J, Wollner J, and Pannek J. Urethral strictures in men with neurogenic lower urinary tract dysfunction using intermittent catheterization for bladder evacuation. *Spinal Cord*. 2015;53(4):310–3.

44. Kessler TM, Ryu G, and Burkhard FC. Clean intermittent self-catheterization: A burden for the patient? *Neurourol Urodynam Off J Int Continence Soc*. 2009;28(1):18–21.

45. Akkoç Y, Ersöz M, Yıldız N et al. Effects of different bladder management methods on the quality of life in patients with traumatic spinal cord injury. *Spinal Cord*. 2013;51(3):226.

46. Afsar S, Yemisci O, Cosar S, and Cetin N. Compliance with clean intermittent catheterization in spinal cord injury patients: A long-term follow-up study. *Spinal Cord*. 2013;51(8):645.

47. Feifer A, and Corcos J. Contemporary role of suprapubic cystostomy in treatment of neuropathic bladder dysfunction in spinal cord injured patients. *Neurourol Urodynam Off J Int Continence Soc*. 2008;27(6):475–9.

48. Cameron AP, Wallner LP, Tate DG, Sarma AV, Rodriguez GM, and Clemens JQ. Bladder management after spinal cord injury in the United States 1972 to 2005. *J Urol*. 2010;184(1):213–7.

49. Abrams P, Agarwal M, Drake M et al. A proposed guideline for the urological management of patients with spinal cord injury. *BJU Int*. 2008;101(8):989–94.

50. Kim YH, Bird ET, Priebe M, and Boone TB. The role of oxybutynin in spinal cord injured patients with indwelling catheters. *J Urol*. 1997;158(6):2083–6.

51. Shekelle PG, Morton SC, Clark KA, Pathak M, and Vickrey BG. Systematic review of risk factors for urinary tract infection in adults with spinal cord dysfunction. *J Spinal Cord Med*. 1999;22(4):258–72.

52. Esclarín de ruz A, García Leoni E, and Herruzo Cabrera R. Epidemiology and risk factors for urinary tract infection in patients with spinal cord injury. *J Urol*. 2000;164(4):1285–9.

53. Biering-Sørensen F, Bagi P, and Høiby N. Urinary tract infections in patients with spinal cord lesions. *Drugs*. 2001;61(9):1275–87.

54. Turi MH, Hanif S, Fasih Q, and Shaikh MA. Proportion of complications in patients practicing clean intermittent self-catheterization (CISC) vs indwelling catheter. *JPMA*. 2006;56(401).

55. Cameron AP, Wallner LP, Forchheimer MB et al. Medical and psychosocial complications associated with method of bladder management after traumatic spinal cord injury. *Arch Phys Med Rehabil*. 2011;92(3):449–56.

56. Bennett CJ, Young MN, Adkins RH, and Diaz F. Comparison of bladder management complication outcomes in female spinal cord injury patients. *J Urol*. 1995;153(5):1458–60.

57. Kaufman JM, Fam B, Jacobs SC et al. Bladder cancer and squamous metaplasia in spinal cord injury patients. *J Urol*. 1977;118(6):967–71.

58. Bejany DE, Lockhart JL, and Rhamy RK. Malignant vesical tumors following spinal cord injury. *J Urol*. 1987;138(6):1390–2.

59. Sugimura T, Arnold E, English S, and Moore J. Chronic suprapubic catheterization in the management of patients with spinal cord injuries: Analysis of upper and lower urinary tract complications. *BJU Int*. 2008;101(11):1396–400.

60. Barnes D, Shaw P, Timoney A, and Tsokos N. Management of the neuropathic bladder by suprapubic catheterisation. *Br J Urol*. 1993;72(2):169–72.

61. MacDiarmid S, Arnold E, Palmer N, and Anthony A. Management of spinal cord injured patients by indwelling suprapubic catheterization. *J Urol*. 1995;154(2):492–4.

62. Nomura S, Ishido T, Teranishi J-I, and Makiyama K. Long-term analysis of suprapubic cystostomy drainage in patients with neurogenic bladder. *Urol Int*. 2000;65(4):185–9.

63. Böthig R, Hirschfeld S, and Thietje R. Quality of life and urological morbidity in tetraplegics with artificial ventilation managed with suprapubic or intermittent catheterisation. *Spinal Cord*. 2012;50(3):247.

64. Peatfield R, Burt A, and Smith P. Suprapubic catheterisation after spinal cord injury: A follow-up report. *Paraplegia*. 1983;21(4):220–6.

65. Hamid R, Peters J, and Shah P. Pitfall in insertion of suprapubic catheter in patients with spinal cord injuries. *Spinal Cord*. 2002;40(10):542.

66. Morse RM, Spirnak JP, and Resnick MI. Iatrogenic colon and rectal injuries associated with urological intervention: Report of 14 patients. *J Urol*. 1988;140(1):101–3.

67. Smart C. Urinary sheaths for male incontinence. *Br J Nurs*. 2014;23(12):650–2.

68. Newman E, and Price M. External catheters: Hazards and benefits of their use by men with spinal cord lesions. *Arch Phys Med Rehabil*. 1985;66(5):310–3.

69. Chartier-Kastler E, Ballanger P, Petit J et al. Randomized, crossover study evaluating patient preference and the impact on quality of life of urisheaths vs absorbent products in incontinent men. *BJU Int*. 2011;108(2):241–7.

70. Stöhrer M, Madersbacher H, Richter R, Wehnert J, and Dreikorn K. Efficacy and safety of propiverine in SCI-patients suffering from detrusor hyperreflexia—A double-blind, placebo-controlled clinical trial. *Spinal Cord*. 1999;37(3):196.

71. Madhuvrata P, Singh M, Hasafa Z, and Abdel-Fattah M. Anticholinergic drugs for adult neurogenic detrusor overactivity: A systematic review and meta-analysis. *Eur Urol*. 2012;62(5):816–30.

72. Athanasopoulos A, and Giannitsas K. An overview of the clinical use of antimuscarinics in the treatment of overactive bladder. *Adv Urol.* 2011;2011:820816.

73. Jost WH. Urological problems in Parkinson's disease: Clinical aspects. *J Neural Transm.* 2013;120(4):587–91.

74. Madersbacher H, Mürtz G, and Stöhrer M. Neurogenic detrusor overactivity in adults: A review on efficacy, tolerability and safety of oral antimuscarinics. *Spinal Cord.* 2013;51(6):432.

75. Horstmann M, Schaefer T, Aguilar Y, Stenzl A, and Sievert K. Neurogenic bladder treatment by doubling the recommended antimuscarinic dosage. *Neurourol Urodynam Off J Int Continence Soc.* 2006;25(5):441–5.

76. Nardulli R, Losavio E, Ranieri M et al. Combined antimuscarinics for treatment of neurogenic overactive bladder. *Int J Immunopathol Pharmacol.* 2012;25(1 Suppl):35–41.

77. Amend B, Hennenlotter J, Schäfer T, Horstmann M, Stenzl A, and Sievert K-D. Effective treatment of neurogenic detrusor dysfunction by combined high-dosed antimuscarinics without increased side-effects. *Eur Urol.* 2008;53(5):1021–8.

78. Chapple CR, Cardozo L, Nitti VW, Siddiqui E, and Michel MC. Mirabegron in overactive bladder: A review of efficacy, safety, and tolerability. *Neurourol Urodyn.* 2014;33(1):17–30.

79. Wöllner J, and Pannek J. Initial experience with the treatment of neurogenic detrusor overactivity with a new β-3 agonist (mirabegron) in patients with spinal cord injury. *Spinal Cord.* 2016;54(1):78.

80. Welk B, Hickling D, McKibbon M, Radomski S, and Ethans K. A pilot randomized-controlled trial of the urodynamic efficacy of mirabegron for patients with neurogenic lower urinary tract dysfunction. *Neurourol Urodyn.* 2018;37(8):2810–7.

81. Krhut J, Borovička V, Bílková K et al. Efficacy and safety of mirabegron for the treatment of neurogenic detrusor overactivity—Prospective, randomized, double-blind, placebo-controlled study. *Neurourol Urodyn.* 2018;37(7):2226–33.

82. Bosma R, Wynia K, Havlikova E, De Keyser J, and Middel B. Efficacy of desmopressin in patients with multiple sclerosis suffering from bladder dysfunction: A meta-analysis. *Acta Neurol Scand.* 2005;112(1):1–5.

83. Valiquette G, Herbert J, and Meade-D'Alisera P. Desmopressin in the management of nocturia in patients with multiple sclerosis: A double-blind, crossover trial. *Arch Neurol.* 1996;53(12):1270–5.

84. Szollar S, North J, and Chung J. Antidiuretic hormone levels and polyuria in spinal cord injury. A preliminary report. *Spinal Cord.* 1995;33(2):94.

85. Panicker JN, Fowler CJ, and Kessler TM. Lower urinary tract dysfunction in the neurological patient: Clinical assessment and management. *Lancet Neurol.* 2015;14(7):720–32.

86. Linsenmeyer TA, Horton J, Benevento J. Impact of α-blockers in men with spinal cord injury and upper tract stasis. *J Spinal Cord Med.* 2002;25(2):124–8.

87. Abrams P, Amarenco G, Bakke A et al. Tamsulosin: Efficacy and safety in patients with neurogenic lower urinary tract dysfunction due to suprasacral spinal cord injury. *J Urol.* 2003;170(4 Part 1):1242–51.

88. Al-Ali M, Salman G, Rasheed A et al. Phenoxybenzamine in the management of neuropathic bladder following spinal cord injury. *Aust N Z J Surg.* 1999;69(9):660–3.

89. Swierzewski III SJ, Gormley EA, Belville WD, Sweetser PM, Wan J, and Mcguire EJ. The effect of terazosin on bladder function in the spinal cord injured patient. *J Urol.* 1994;151(4):951–4.

90. Kakizaki H, Ameda K, Kobayashi S, Tanaka H, Shibata T, and Koyanagi T. Urodynamic effects of α1-blocker tamsulosin on voiding dysfunction in patients with neurogenic bladder. *Int J Urol.* 2003;10(11):576–81.

91. Ruggieri MR Sr, Braverman AS, and Pontari MA. Combined use of α-adrenergic and muscarinic antagonists for the treatment of voiding dysfunction. *J Urol.* 2005;174(5):1743–8.

92. Wada N, Shimizu T, Takai S et al. Combinational effects of muscarinic receptor inhibition and β3-adrenoceptor stimulation on neurogenic bladder dysfunction in rats with spinal cord injury. *Neurourol Urodyn.* 2017;36(4):1039–45.

93. Yamanishi T, Yasuda K, Kamai T et al. Combination of a cholinergic drug and an α-blocker is more effective than monotherapy for the treatment of voiding difficulty in patients with underactive detrusor. *Int J Urol.* 2004;11(2):88–96.

94. Diaz Dc, Robinson D, Bosch R, et al. Initial assessment of urinary incontinence in adult male and female patients. In: Abrams P, Cardozo L, Wagg A, Wein A, eds. *Incontinence. Vol 6th International Consultation on Incontinence. Tokyo* 2017:517.

Chapter 28

SYSTEMIC, INTRATHECAL, AND INTRAVESICAL PHARMACOLOGIC TREATMENT OF NEUROGENIC LOWER URINARY TRACT DYSFUNCTION

Christopher S. Elliott

INTRODUCTION

The genitourinary problems associated with neurogenic lower urinary tract dysfunction (NLUTD) typically result from a failure of the bladder to store urine at low pressures or properly empty, sometimes in combination.[1] While the pathophysiology of a failure to store and empty are described elsewhere in this textbook, the resultant sequelae include, but are not limited to, urinary frequency, urgency, incontinence, an increased susceptibility to urinary tract infection, and in some cases, upper tract deterioration. Most patients with NLUTD are managed via systemic, intravesical, or intrathecal pharmacology either alone or in combination with other bladder management modalities (i.e., catheterization).[2]

SYSTEMIC THERAPIES

TO INCREASE BLADDER STORAGE
ANTIMUSCARINIC MEDICATIONS

Classically, antimuscarinic medications are the first-line systemic therapy to increase bladder storage capacity and decrease bladder storage pressures in those with NLUTD. The currently available antimuscarinic medications include darifenacin, fesoterodine, imidafenacin, oxybutynin, propiverine, solifenacin, tolterodine, and trospium chloride.[3] As a class, antimuscarinics act to block cholinergic stimulation of the detrusor and its neuronal innervation.[4] Antimuscarinic medications can be administered via oral routes (tablet), transdermal routes (patch and gel applications), or intravesical routes with the differing routes affecting their metabolism. The varying antimuscarinic medications also have differing molecular sizes (tertiary amine versus quaternary amine), which affect their absorption and their passage through the blood-brain barrier. Both intermediate-release and extended-release versions of certain antimuscarinics are available. Coupled with the varying muscarinic receptor subtype selectivity (M1-M5) (Table 28.1), the differences in molecular size and absorption alter the side-effect profile for one agent versus another (with the common side effects being visual disturbances, dry mouth, and constipation).[5,6]

Overall, it is well documented that antimuscarinics significantly reduce maximal detrusor pressure with parallel increases in maximum cystometric bladder capacity and bladder-specific quality of life. To date, no particular drug or dosage has been found to be superior to another in a head-to-head comparison in those with NLUTD. As a result, most practitioners should aim to find antimuscarinics with acceptable side-effect profiles that afford patient tolerability (i.e., extended-release preparations over immediate-release preparations).[7,8]

β₃-RECEPTOR AGONIST

Approved for use in 2012 by the U.S. Food and Drug Administration, Mirabegron (the only currently approved β_3-receptor agonist) has become a widely used systemic therapy for NLUTD, though data on its efficacy in this population is limited. Like antimuscarinic agents, β_3-receptor agonists act to increase bladder storage capacity and decrease detrusor storage pressures via activation of β_3 receptors on the detrusor, promoting relaxation during the storage phase of bladder filling. Compared to placebo, no significant adverse events are noted in users of β_3-agonist medications (including similar rates of cardiovascular-related events compared to placebo), though it is advised that periodic blood pressure measurements be made in patients taking the drug, as blood pressure may increase in some individuals.[9–11] The small risk of increased blood pressure may also theoretically worsen the effects of autonomic dysreflexia in susceptible patients; however, to date there is no evidence to either support or refute this concern.

When compared to antimuscarinic medications, similar outcomes in bladder-specific measures have been noted in persons with NLUTD.[12] To date, no specific head-to-head comparisons of antimuscarinic

Table 28.1 Pharmacokinetic Profiles of the Different Antimuscarinic Drugs

	Molecular Weight	Chemical Structure	Lipophilicity	Polarity	Metabolizing Enzymes	Receptor Selectivity
Oxybutynin	393.9	Tertiary amine	Lipophilic	Natural	CYP3A4	M1, M2 ≥ M3
Tolterodine	475.6	Tertiary amine	Slightly lipophilic	Positive	CYP2D6	No
Propiverine	404	Benzylic acid	NA	NA	CYP2D6	No
Trospium	428	Quaternary amine	Lipophobic	Highly positive	Ester hydrolysis	No
Darifenacin	507.5	Tertiary amine	Highly lipophilic	Positive	CYP2D6, CYP3A4	M3
Solifenacin	480.55	Tertiary amine	NA	NA	CYP3A4	M3 ≥ M2, M1
Fesoterodine	527.66	Hydrogen fumarate salt	Low lipophilicity	NA	Nonspecific esterase	No

drugs versus β_3 agonists have been published in those with NLUTD. As a result, whether an antimuscarinic medication or a β_3 agonist should be used as initial therapy remains unclear and should be decided based on side-effect profile and formulary coverage. Most importantly, given the different end targets of antimuscarinic and β_3-agonist medications, the ability to use the medications concurrently is an option for patients not achieving a desired result with one agent alone. Combination therapy using both Mirabegron and an antimuscarinic agent has been shown to have additive effects with increases in cystometric capacity and bladder compliance compared to monotherapy alone.[13]

TO INCREASE BLADDER EMPTYING
SYMPATHOMIMETICS AND α-ANTAGONISTS
Theoretically, improved bladder emptying is possible with systemic therapy via either increasing detrusor contraction pressure or decreasing bladder outlet resistance. To date, the use of the parasympathomimetic medication, Bethanechol, to improve detrusor contraction strength, is largely anecdotal with no significant data available to support its use in those with NLUTD. Interestingly, even in patients with underactive bladder who do not have neurologic conditions, parasympathomimetic agents (while occasionally used) fail to show significant differences in effect when compared to placebo.[14] Likewise, medications to decrease bladder neck and urethral resistance (i.e., alpha blockers) have not been shown to significantly decrease urethral resistance in a manner that promotes volitional voiding in those with NLUTD.[15] Interestingly, despite not being common practice, several studies suggest that α-blockade may warrant further consideration.[16-18]

INTRATHECAL THERAPY

To date, the most commonly studied intrathecal therapy for NLUTD has been carried out in patients with baclofen pumps. Baclofen is thought to inhibit spinal cord transmission via its activation of γ-aminobutyric acid (GABA) receptors. In those with neurologic disability, baclofen is used primarily to control skeletal muscle spasticity.[19] A noted concurrent effect is a decrease in external striated sphincter activity, which allows some patients, whose prior spasticity prevented catheter passage, to perform intermittent catheterization with greater ease.[20] Unfortunately, however, the practical use of baclofen to decrease bladder outlet resistance and promote volitional voiding in those with detrusor-sphincter dyssynergia is limited by the concurrent side effects of ever-increasing doses (i.e., drowsiness and weakness) and is not of practical use.[21]

INTRAVESICAL THERAPY

TO INCREASE BLADDER STORAGE
ANTIMUSCARINIC MEDICATIONS
Intravesical antimuscarinic administration, though not widely used, is an alternative measure to promote bladder storage in persons performing intermittent catheterization who are either unable to tolerate the side effects of oral/transdermal antimuscarinic administration or have poor absorption (intestinal or skin).[22] As described, oxybutynin immediate-release tablets are crushed and mixed into a small solution of saline to create a slurry. The medication slurry is then instilled into the bladder following catheterization and left to dwell. Direct intravesical antimuscarinic instillation is thought to decrease the first-pass metabolism associated with systemic administration and potentially to have a local anesthetic effect on the mucosal lining of the bladder.[23] Much like systemic administration via pills, patches, and gels, increases in cystometric capacity and decreases in bladder storage pressures are observed with intravesical antimuscarinic therapy.[24] A downside to intravesical antimuscarinic installation is the lack of convenient,

commercially available preparations.[25] Hence, patients generally are required to prepare their own instillations, and the dropout rate over time is thought to be higher compared to oral antimuscarinic administration.[26]

BOTULINUM TOXIN

Since its introduction in the year 2000, cystoscopic injection of botulinum toxin into the detrusor has rapidly become a mainstay in the treatment of NLUTD, with resultant increases in bladder storage capacity and decreases in detrusor pressure.[27] Botulinum toxin exerts its therapeutic effect by inhibiting the release of acetylcholine vesicles at presynaptic cholinergic neuromuscular junctions in peripheral nerve endings, resulting in temporary muscle paralysis. In addition to the inhibition of detrusor contraction, it is generally thought that botulinum toxin affects sensory nerve conduction as well.[28] The commercially available forms of botulinum toxin include onabotulinumtoxinA (Botox), abobotulinumtoxinA (Dysport), incobotulinumtoxinA (Xeomin), and rimabotulinumtoxinB (Myobloc), though only onabotulinumtoxinA (Botox) and abobotulinumtoxinA (Dysport) have adequate clinical data to support their use for the treatment of NLUTD, and only onabotulinumtoxinA (Botox) has been approved for neurogenic detrusor overactivity by the U.S. Food and Drug Administration.[29,30]

Typically, onabotulinumtoxinA (Botox) is dosed at either 100 units for those who are volitionally voiding or 200 units for those who are catheterization dependent (with abobotulinumtoxinA [Dysport] being dosed at 250 units or 500 units for volitional voiding and catheterization-dependent patients, respectively).[31-33] When first introduced, most practitioners performed botulinum toxin administration via 20–30 injection sites within the bladder. However, subsequent studies have demonstrated that utilizing fewer injection sites appears to be as efficacious at drug delivery, and it is currently common for practitioners to use ten or fewer sites[34] (Figure 28.1). Similarly, botulinum toxin, whether injected into the detrusor or the submucosal layer, appears to result in similar outcomes.[35,36] In addition, the inclusion of trigone injecting techniques are gaining favor as studies have shown improved bladder storage outcomes with no increase in urinary reflux.[37] As opposed to skeletal muscle injections that may only last for 1–2 months, injections into the detrusor (smooth muscle) typically last anywhere from 4 to 12 months before needing to be repeated.[33,38,39] Several studies demonstrate that serial injections of botulinum toxin into those with NLUTD are successful long term, with a rare risk of antibody development to the toxin or ultrastructural changes to the detrusor[38-42] (Figure 28.2).

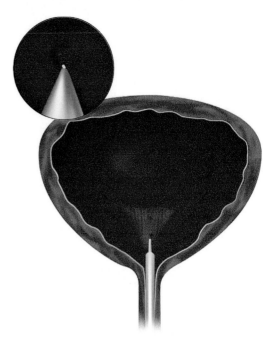

Figure 28.1 Modified ten-point onabotulinumtoxinA injection technique within the bladder trigone and base used successfully in spontaneously voiding patients with mild to moderate overactive bladder symptoms. (Reprinted from Smith CP and Chancellor MB. *J Endourol.* 2005;19[7]:880–2. With permission.)

The risk of botulinum toxin injection therapy is limited in most patients. Approximately 50% of patients are noted to develop a symptomatic urinary tract infection, the risk of bleeding is negligible, and in those patients who are volitionally voiding, a 5%–10% risk of symptomatic urinary retention is known to occur with dosing of 100 units.[43,44] In rare instances, botulinum toxin injections have been associated with systemic weakness, though these reports are rare compared to the number of NLUTD patients receiving Botox injections and self-limiting when appropriate dosing regimens are followed.[45,46]

One current iteration of botulinum toxin administration that is under development is a catheter-based, gel-based delivery system that obviates the need for cystoscopic instrumentation and needle administration. To date, several small studies have been conducted in persons with overactive bladder and interstitial cystitis/painful bladder syndrome with varying success (though with seemingly less efficacious outcomes compared to cystoscopic injection).[47,48] While not commercially available at this time, gel-based instillation therapies, specifically for individuals who are already intermittently catheterizing their bladder, would decrease the need for office-based injections and promote on-demand botulinum toxin administration.

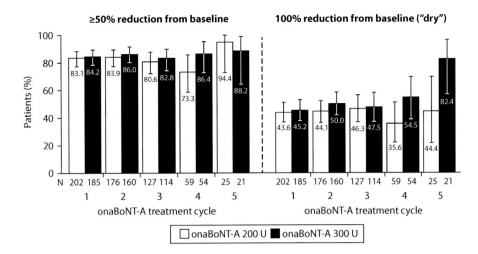

Figure 28.2 Number of patients who achieved greater than or equal to 50% reduction or 100% reduction (total continence) of urinary incontinence episodes. (Reprinted from Kennelly et al. *Urology.* 2013;81[3]:491–7. With permission.)

Much like systemic drug administration, botulinum toxin injections can likely be combined with other bladder-based therapies for increased effect. The need for possible combination therapy is evidenced by the fact that approximately 50% of patients with neurogenic detrusor overactivity will discontinue intradetrusor onabotulinumtoxinA injections in the long term and is further supported by randomized trial data showing that only 35%–45% achieve complete urinary continence.[43,49,50] However, for a large majority of patients, the introduction of botulinum toxin injection into the bladder has provided an avenue to obtain satisfactory continence short of needing a more invasive enterocytoplasty operation.[51,52] In addition, even in those with a prior enterocystoplasty surgery, botulinum toxin administration can play a role, specifically in those patients who have continued urinary incontinence postoperatively. In this specific population, injection of botulinum toxin, either into the detrusor or the augmented bowel segment, increases cystometric capacity and decreases urinary leakage.[53]

TO INCREASE BLADDER EMPTYING
BOTULINUM TOXIN
Attempts to inactivate the external urethral sphincter via direct botulinum toxin injection (with the primary aim of replacing traditional surgical sphincterotomy in a reversible manner) predates the use of botulinum in the bladder.[54] In multiple small trials, administration of 50–100 units of botulinum toxin into the external sphincter has been shown to decrease maximal urethral closure pressure, postvoid residual, and voiding pressure. Unfortunately, chemical sphincterotomy with botulinum toxin is subject to variable lengths of action, requires revision every 2–6 months, and is burdened by a significant

follow-up regimen to ensure that unsafe voiding parameters do not return in between treatments. As a result, despite initial enthusiasm for the technique, it is not employed by most practitioners to date.[55]

REFERENCES

1. Wein AJ and Rovner ES. *Pathophysiology and Classification of Voiding Dysfunction.* Totowa, NJ: Humana Press; 2000.
2. Romo PGB, Smith CP, Cox A et al. Non-surgical urologic management of neurogenic bladder after spinal cord injury. *World J Urol.* 2018;36:1555.
3. Groen J, Pannek J, Castro Diaz D, Del Popolo G, Gross T, Hamid R, Karsenty G, Kessler TM, Schneider M, 't Hoen L, Blok B. Summary of European Association of Urology (EAU) Guidelines on Neuro-Urology. *Eur Urol.* 2016 Feb;69(2):324–33. doi: 10.1016/j.eururo.2015.07.071. Epub 2015 Aug 22.
4. Andersson KE and Wein AJ. Pharmacology of the lower urinary tract: Basis for current and future treatments of urinary incontinence. *Pharmacol Rev.* 2004;56:581.
5. Abrams P and Andersson KE. Muscarinic receptor antagonists for overactive bladder. *BJU Int.* 2007;100:987.
6. Jirschele K and Sand PK. Oxybutynin: Past, present, and future. *Int Urogynecol J.* 2013;24:595.
7. Madersbacher H, Murtz G and Stohrer M. Neurogenic detrusor overactivity in adults: A review on efficacy, tolerability and safety of oral antimuscarinics. *Spinal Cord.* 2013;51:432.
8. Madhuvrata P, Singh M, Hasafa Z and Abdel-Fattah M. Anticholinergic drugs for adult neurogenic detrusor overactivity: A systematic review and meta-analysis. *Eur Urol.* 2012;62:816.
9. Nitti VW, Auerbach S, Martin N et al. Results of a randomized phase III trial of mirabegron in patients with overactive bladder. *J Urol.* 2013;189:1388.

10. Khullar V, Amarenco G, Angulo JC et al. Efficacy and tolerability of mirabegron, a beta(3)-adrenoceptor agonist, in patients with overactive bladder: Results from a randomised European-Australian phase 3 trial. *Eur Urol.* 2013;63:283.

11. Nitti VW, Khullar V, van Kerrebroeck P et al. Mirabegron for the treatment of overactive bladder: A prespecified pooled efficacy analysis and pooled safety analysis of three randomised, double-blind, placebo-controlled, phase III studies. *Int J Clin Pract.* 2013;67:619.

12. Wollner J and Pannek J. Initial experience with the treatment of neurogenic detrusor overactivity with a new beta-3 agonist (mirabegron) in patients with spinal cord injury. *Spinal Cord.* 2016;54:78.

13. Han SH, Cho IK, Jung JH et al. Long-term efficacy of Mirabegron add-on therapy to antimuscarinic agents in patients with spinal cord injury. *Ann Rehabil Med.* 2019;43:54.

14. Barendrecht MM, Oelke M, Laguna MP et al. Is the use of parasympathomimetics for treating an underactive urinary bladder evidence-based? *BJU Int.* 2007;99:749.

15. Kakizaki H, Ameda K, Kobayashi S et al. Urodynamic effects of α1-blocker Tamsulosin on voiding dysfunction in patients with neurogenic bladder. *Int J Urol.* 2003;10:576.

16. Cameron AP, Clemens JQ, Latini JM et al. Combination drug therapy improves compliance of the neurogenic bladder. *J Urol.* 2009;182:1062.

17. Abrams P, Amarenco G, Bakke A et al. Tamsulosin: Efficacy and safety in patients with neurogenic lower urinary tract dysfunction due to suprasacral spinal cord injury. *J Urol.* 2003;170:1242.

18. Schneider MP, Tornic J, Sykora R et al. Alpha-blockers for treating neurogenic lower urinary tract dysfunction in patients with multiple sclerosis: A systematic review and meta-analysis. A report from the Neuro-Urology Promotion Committee of the International Continence Society (ICS). *Neurourol Urodyn.* 2019;38:1482.

19. Coffey JR, Cahill D, Steers W et al. Intrathecal baclofen for intractable spasticity of spinal origin: Results of a long-term multicenter study. *J Neurosurg.* 1993;78:226.

20. Kilicarslan H, Ayan S, Vuruskan H et al. Treatment of detrusor sphincter dyssynergia with baclofen and doxazosin. *Int Urol Nephrol.* 2006;38:537.

21. Rigal L, Legay Hoang L, Alexandre-Dubroeucq C et al. Tolerability of high-dose baclofen in the treatment of patients with alcohol disorders: A retrospective study. *Alcohol Alcohol.* 2015;50:551.

22. Madersbacher H and Jilg G. Control of detrusor hyperreflexia by the intravesical instillation of oxybutynine hydrochloride. *Paraplegia.* 1991;29:84.

23. Di Stasi SM, Giannantoni A, Navarra P et al. Intravesical oxybutynin: Mode of action assessed by passive diffusion and electromotive administration with pharmacokinetics of oxybutynin and N-desethyl oxybutynin. *J Urol.* 2001;166:2232.

24. Guerra LA, Moher D, Sampson M et al. Intravesical oxybutynin for children with poorly compliant neurogenic bladder: A systematic review. *J Urol.* 2008;180:1091.

25. Reitz A and Schurch B. Intravesical therapy options for neurogenic detrusor overactivity. *Spinal Cord.* 2004;42:267.

26. Palmer LS, Zebold K, Firlit CF et al. Complications of intravesical oxybutynin chloride therapy in the pediatric myelomeningocele population. *J Urol.* 1997;157:638.

27. Schurch B, Schmid DM and Stohrer M. Treatment of neurogenic incontinence with botulinum toxin A. *N Engl J Med.* 2000;342:665.

28. Cooley LF and Kielb S. A review of botulinum toxin A for the treatment of neurogenic bladder. *PM R.* 2019;11:192.

29. Chancellor MB, Elovic E, Esquenazi A et al. Evidence-based review and assessment of botulinum neurotoxin for the treatment of urologic conditions. *Toxicon.* 2013;67:129.

30. Orasanu B and Mahajan ST. The use of botulinum toxin for the treatment of overactive bladder syndrome. *Indian J Urol.* 2013;29:2.

31. Cruz F, Herschorn S, Aliotta P et al. Efficacy and safety of onabotulinumtoxinA in patients with urinary incontinence due to neurogenic detrusor overactivity: A randomised, double-blind, placebo-controlled trial. *Eur Urol.* 2011;60:742.

32. Ginsberg D, Gousse A, Keppenne V et al. Phase 3 efficacy and tolerability study of onabotulinumtoxinA for urinary incontinence from neurogenic detrusor overactivity. *J Urol.* 2012;187:2131.

33. Kennelly M, Dmochowski R, Ethans K et al. Long-term efficacy and safety of onabotulinumtoxinA in patients with urinary incontinence due to neurogenic detrusor overactivity: An interim analysis. *Urology.* 2013;81:491.

34. Liao CH, Chen SF and Kuo HC. Different number of intravesical onabotulinumtoxinA injections for patients with refractory detrusor overactivity do not affect treatment outcome: A prospective randomized comparative study. *Neurourol Urodyn.* 2016;35:717.

35. Krhut J, Samal V, Nemec D et al. Intradetrusor versus suburothelial onabotulinumtoxinA injections for neurogenic detrusor overactivity: A pilot study. *Spinal Cord.* 2012;50:904.

36. Samal V, Mecl J and Sram J. Submucosal administration of onabotulinumtoxinA in the treatment of neurogenic detrusor overactivity: Pilot single-centre experience and comparison with standard injection into the detrusor. *Urol Int.* 2013;91:423.

37. Jo JK, Kim KN, Kim DW et al. The effect of onabotulinumtoxinA according to site of injection in patients with overactive bladder: A systematic review and meta-analysis. *World J Urol.* 2018;36:305.

38. Ginsberg DA, Drake MJ, Kaufmann A et al. Long-term treatment with onabotulinumtoxinA results in consistent, durable improvements in health related quality of life in patients with overactive bladder. *J Urol.* 2017;198:897.

39. Kennelly M, Dmochowski R, Schulte-Baukloh H et al. Efficacy and safety of onabotulinumtoxinA therapy are sustained over 4 years of treatment in patients with neurogenic detrusor overactivity: Final results of a long-term extension study. *Neurourol Urodyn.* 2017;36:368.

40. Giannantoni A, Mearini E, Del Zingaro M et al. Six-year follow-up of botulinum toxin A intradetrusorial injections in patients with refractory neurogenic detrusor overactivity: Clinical and urodynamic results. *Eur Urol.* 2009;55:705.

41. Haferkamp A, Schurch B, Reitz A et al. Lack of ultrastructural detrusor changes following endoscopic injection of botulinum toxin type A in overactive neurogenic bladder. *Eur Urol.* 2004;46:784.

42. Rovner E, Kohan A, Chartier-Kastler E et al. Long-term efficacy and safety of onabotulinumtoxinA in patients with neurogenic detrusor overactivity who completed 4 years of treatment. *J Urol.* 2016;196:801.

43. Ginsberg D, Cruz F, Herschorn S et al. OnabotulinumtoxinA is effective in patients with urinary incontinence due to neurogenic detrusor overactivity [corrected] regardless of concomitant anticholinergic use or neurologic etiology. *Adv Ther.* 2013;30:819.

44. Li GP, Wang XY and Zhang Y. Efficacy and safety of onabotulinumtoxinA in patients with neurogenic detrusor overactivity caused by spinal cord injury: A systematic review and meta-analysis. *Int Neurourol J.* 2018;22:275.

45. Crowner BE, Torres-Russotto D, Carter AR et al. Systemic weakness after therapeutic injections of botulinum toxin A: A case series and review of the literature. *Clin Neuropharmacol.* 2010;33:243.

46. Wyndaele JJ and Van Dromme SA. Muscular weakness as side effect of botulinum toxin injection for neurogenic detrusor overactivity. *Spinal Cord.* 2002;40:599.

47. Krhut J, Navratilova M, Sykora R et al. Intravesical instillation of onabotulinum toxin A embedded in inert hydrogel in the treatment of idiopathic overactive bladder: A double-blind randomized pilot study. *Scand J Urol.* 2016;50:200.

48. Rappaport YH, Zisman A, Jeshurun-Gutshtat M et al. Safety and feasibility of intravesical instillation of botulinum toxin-A in hydrogel-based slow-release delivery system in patients with interstitial cystitis-bladder pain syndrome: A pilot study. *Urology.* 2018;114:60.

49. Baron M, Peyronnet B, Auble A et al. Long-term discontinuation of botulinum toxin A intradetrusor injections for neurogenic detrusor overactivity: A multicenter study. *J Urol.* 2019;201:769.

50. Leitner L, Guggenbuhl-Roy S, Knupfer SC et al. More than 15 years of experience with intradetrusor onabotulinumtoxinA injections for treating refractory neurogenic detrusor overactivity: Lessons to be learned. *Eur Urol.* 2016;70:522.

51. Schlomer BJ, Saperston K and Baskin L. National trends in augmentation cystoplasty in the 2000s and factors associated with patient outcomes. *J Urol.* 2013;190:1352.

52. Biers SM, Venn SN, Greenwell TJ. The past, present and future of augmentation cystoplasty. *BJU Int.* 2012;109:1280.

53. Michel F, Ciceron C, Bernuz B et al. Botulinum toxin type A injection after failure of augmentation Enterocystoplasty performed for neurogenic detrusor overactivity: Preliminary results of a salvage strategy. The ENTEROTOX study. *Urology.* 2019;129:43–7.

54. Dykstra DD, Sidi AA, Scott AB et al. Effects of botulinum A toxin on detrusor-sphincter dyssynergia in spinal cord injury patients. *J Urol.* 1988;139:919.

55. Seth J, Rintoul-Hoad S and Sahai A. Urethral sphincter injection of botulinum toxin A: A review of its application and outcomes. *Low Urin Tract Symptoms.* 2018;10:109.

Chapter 29

MANAGEMENT OF AUTONOMIC DYSREFLEXIA

François Hervé, Christina W. Agudelo, and Karel Everaert

INTRODUCTION

Autonomic dysreflexia (AD) is a frequent, dangerous, and avoidable complication found in patients with spinal cord injury (SCI) at T6 or above characterized by sudden spikes in blood pressure. The incidence of AD for individuals with SCI above T6 is between 50% and 70%.[1-3] AD is more pronounced in patients with complete SCI than with incomplete SCI and cervical lesions compared to thoracic.[4,5]

This phenomenon is a medical emergency, and late recognition or inappropriate management can result in life-threatening complications, including intracerebral hemorrhage, myocardial infarct, and hypertensive encephalopathy.[6-10]

The aim of this chapter is to improve the knowledge of healthcare providers involved in the care of patients with SCI in order to better diagnose the signs and symptoms of this dangerous condition and identify the potential triggers of AD. This chapter also aims to explain how to manage acute episodes of AD.

PATHOPHYSIOLOGY AND ETIOLOGIES

AD is the result of an uncontrolled sympathetic response secondary to a noxious stimulus below the level of the spinal cord lesion. This response leads to vasoconstriction of vascular, muscular, and splanchnic beds. A compensatory response, aiming to counteract the massive sympathetic overactivity, induces vasodilatation above the level of the SCI (see Part II, Chapter 6).

Bladder distension is found in 75%–85% of the cases, and it represents the primary cause of AD.[3]

Fecal impaction, a relatively frequent condition in neurogenic patients who often suffer from constipation, is the second cause of AD (20% of AD patients).[11]

Some other urinary tract precipitants that may be encountered include urinary tract infection, bladder calculi, urethral distention, testicular torsion, and instrumentation.

Many other precipitating factors can also be responsible for AD, including pressure ulcers, bedsores, burns, ingrown toenails, and bone fracture. Sexual activity, erection, orgasm, or electroejaculation, and labor and delivery are also listed among the causative factors of AD.[12,13]

DIAGNOSIS OF AUTONOMIC DYSREFLEXIA

A typical clinical description of AD is presented in Figure 29.1.[14,15]

Subacute AD presentations do exist, with minimal or absent signs and symptoms of AD, despite elevated blood pressure. Because of cognitive and verbal communication impairments, patients with SCI might have difficulty disclosing their symptoms when AD presents.[15]

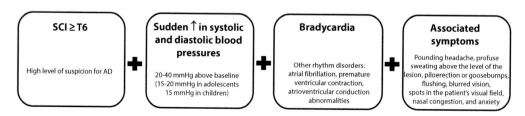

Figure 29.1 Typical clinical description of AD.

For this reason, any caregiver or relative involved in the care of patients with SCI should be fully educated regarding AD.

Also, patients often feel their AD coming on when the bladder is full, and consequently, they will empty their bladder before a full-blown episode occurs.

ACUTE TREATMENT OF AUTONOMIC DYSREFLEXIA

LIFE-SAVING MEASURES

Prompt management of AD is extremely important. The first step is to place the patient upright in the seated position, with his or her legs down in order to provoke an orthostatic drop in blood pressure by allowing pooling in the lower extremities.[15]

During an AD episode, the patient should be monitored closely, every 2–5 minutes, until the blood pressure has stabilized.[14–17]

REMOVAL OF TRIGGER RESPONSIBLE FOR AUTONOMIC DYSREFLEXIA

Elimination of the trigger is the cornerstone of the management of AD, otherwise the patient is at risk of further episodes. By eliminating the noxious stimulus, we aim to suppress the "irritative stitch" responsible for the onset of AD.

AVOID BLADDER DISTENSION

Bladder distension is the most common cause of AD. If the patient does not have an indwelling catheter, a catheter should be immediately placed in the bladder.[14,15]

If the patient has an indwelling catheter, the system should be checked for obstruction or kinks and eventually changed. If AD occurs during a cystoscopy, the procedure should be interrupted and the bladder emptied.

Both large volumes and cold irrigation solutions should be avoided because they can also exacerbate AD. Irrigation with lidocaine solution may help decrease sensory input from the bladder.

AVOID FECAL IMPACTION

If the blood pressure remains elevated after bladder catheterization, fecal impaction should be suspected as it is the second most common cause of AD. Impaction reversal can be accomplished by introducing intrarectal lidocaine jelly 2% for at least 2 minutes and checking for stool impaction. If AD worsens during rectal manipulation, the manual evacuation should be stopped and rechecked after 20 minutes.[15]

AVOID OTHER "IRRITATIVE STITCHES"

Avoid vibration, electroejaculation, or sexual activity.

If the precipitating trigger has still not been identified, a thorough exploration for the cause must be initiated. The blood pressure should be monitored for at least 2 hours after resolution of the symptoms of an AD episode, and the patient should be instructed to monitor his or her symptoms to identify a possible recurrence.[15]

PHARMACOTHERAPY TO LOWER BLOOD PRESSURE

Antihypertensive drugs with rapid onset and short duration of action should be used in the management of acute AD episodes.[15] The Consortium for Spinal Cord Medicine[15] recommends that if non-pharmacologic measures fail and arterial blood pressure remains 150 mm Hg or greater, pharmacologic management should be initiated. However, the consortium does not preferentially identify any particular medication for acute AD management. Numerous pharmacologic agents (e.g., nifedipine, nitrates, captopril, terazosin, prazosin, phenoxybenzamine, prostaglandin E2, and sildenafil) have been proposed for the management of AD episodes.[14,15,18] The majority of these recommendations are based on experience and studies on the clinical management of hypertensive crises in able-bodied populations.[19]

NITRATES (NITROGLYCERINE, DEPO-NIT, NITROSTAT, NITROL, AND NITRO-BID)

Nitrates cause relaxation of vascular smooth muscle by producing vasodilator effects on peripheral arteries and veins, promoting blood pressure lowering (preload and after-load).

Nitrates are the most commonly used agents in the management of AD in individuals with SCI[14,16,20]; however, there are no clinical studies supporting the use of nitrates in the acute management of AD post-SCI, only expert opinions[14,16] (level 5 evidence).

Nitrates are available through different administration modalities: IV, sublingual, ointments, and transdermal.[20] Transdermal application has the advantage that the paste can be wiped off once the therapeutic effect has been achieved. The main problem with nitrates is that they often cause headache, which is one of the main symptoms guiding clinical response to therapy.

CAVEAT: Before nitrates are administered, a person with a SCI presenting with acute AD should be questioned regarding his or her use of sildenafil. If this agent has been used within the past 24 hours, nitrates are contraindicated because of the risk of severe hypotension.

PRAZOSIN (MINIPRESS)

Prazosin is a postsynaptic α_1-adrenoceptor blocker, which lowers blood pressure by relaxing blood vessels. It has a negligible effect on cardiac function due to its α_1-receptor selectivity and does not excessively lower baseline blood pressure.

There is one randomized controlled trial[21] that showed that prazosin is superior to placebo in the prophylactic management of AD (level 1 evidence).

Phillips et al.[22] reported that prazosin decreased the level of blood pressure recorded during electrical ejaculation (stimulation for sperm retrieval).

NIFEDIPINE (ADALAT AND PROCARDIA)

Nifedipine is a calcium channel blocker that selectively inhibits calcium ion influx across the cell membrane of cardiac and vascular smooth muscle. Nifedipine causes decreased peripheral vascular resistance and a modest fall in systolic and diastolic pressures (5–10 mm Hg systolic), though the drop in blood pressure can sometimes be more dramatic.

Two controlled trials[23,24] showed that nifedipine is useful for preventing dangerous blood pressure reactions during cystoscopy and other diagnostic or therapeutic procedures in patients with SCI with AD.

However, there is clinical consensus that the potential exists for serious adverse events (severe drop in blood pressure) with this drug, based on what has been reported in other, non-SCI populations.[25] For this reason, the cardiorenal Advisory Committee of the U.S. Food and Drug Administration advised against the use of nifedipine for hypertensive emergencies (level 2 evidence).[26]

CAPTOPRIL

Captopril is a specific competitive inhibitor of the angiotensin I-converting enzyme. During an acute episode of AD, 25 mg of captopril is often administered sublingually. In one study (n=26),[27] captopril was safe and effective for AD management in four out of five episodes. This prospective, open-labeled study and numerous expert opinions support the use of captopril as a primary medication in the management of AD (level 4 evidence).[14,28,29]

OTHER PHARMACOLOGIC AGENTS TESTED FOR THE MANAGEMENT OF AUTONOMIC DYSREFLEXIA

The use of other pharmacologic agents for the management of AD in individuals with SCI has been reported in the literature (e.g., expert opinion and case reports), but the evidence is insufficient to warrant their recommendation (phenazopyridine[30] magnesium sulfate for AD associated with labor[31] or life-threatening AD in intensive care,[32] and diazoxide [Hyperstat][33] for acute AD episodes). The results are conflicting (phenoxybenzamine for AD in patients with SCI[24,34]) or no effect on blood pressure has been demonstrated during episodes of AD (Sildenafil[35]). In addition, there have been reports on the use of beta-blockers,[36] mecamylamine (Inversine),[16] and hydralazine (Apresoline)[33] for the general management of AD symptoms in individuals with SCI.

MANAGING SECONDARY HYPOTENSION

After the removal of the trigger responsible for AD or pharmaceutical treatment of elevated blood pressure, the blood pressure should be monitored closely for possible hypotension. If hypotension ensues, the patient should be placed lying down with the legs elevated. Volume repletion with intravenous fluids and the administration of an adrenergic agonist can also be considered if the hypotension is symptomatic or refractory. The ability to wipe off transdermal nitrates once the AD has been treated, and thus potentially avoid secondary hypotension, is one reason many practitioners prefer transdermal nitrates as their initial therapy for an acute AD episode.

PREVENTION AND PROPHYLACTIC TREATMENT OF AUTONOMIC DYSREFLEXIA

EDUCATION
Structured education for all patients, their families, and healthcare professionals, as soon as possible, is an important aspect in the management of SCI and in the prevention of the acute crisis of AD.

Patients at risk should be advised to hold in their wallets an "Autonomic Dysreflexia medical card"[12,26] summarizing normal blood pressure, previous AD episodes, including signs and symptoms at presentation, the trigger responsible for the acute event, and the treatment instituted.[15]

It is important to mention that the "normal" blood pressure of many patients with SCI is very low at baseline; therefore, an AD blood pressure might not be as elevated as suspected.

PHARMACEUTICAL PREVENTION

An α-adrenoceptor blocker, terazosin 5 mg or tamsulosin 0.8 mg, may reduce the frequency, severity, and bother of AD in patients at risk.[37,38]

As acute AD may be precipitated by surgical, cystoscopic, urodynamic, and radiologic procedures, prophylactic pharmaceutical management with nifedipine 10 mg or nitropaste 2% can be given shortly before the procedure.

Recently, a small study demonstrated that botulinum toxin (BTX) injected into the detrusor muscle to treat neurogenic bladder[39] could be a promising way to reduce bladder-related AD and its severity in adults.[40] One paper reported the successful use of BTX to abort persistent AD in a pediatric patient.[41]

Prophylactic treatments do not eliminate the need for careful monitoring during procedures and the need for appropriate care for the genitourinary, gastrointestinal, and other systems to eliminate avoidable triggers.[7,15–17,37,38]

ANESTHETIC CONSIDERATIONS IN AUTONOMIC DYSREFLEXIA

Most AD episodes are triggered by a urologic manipulation or surgery. Anesthetic techniques for controlling AD include topical application for cystoscopy, general anesthesia, and spinal and epidural anesthesia. Lidocaine jelly may decrease the sensation and relax the sphincter during cystoscopy.

Spinal anesthesia has been reported to give excellent control for the prevention of an AD episode and has also been recommended in acute AD refractory to medical management.[42–51]

When a dysreflexic episode occurs during a procedure in a patient under general anesthesia, the first step in management is to increase the depth of anesthesia.[51] In patients known to have had a previous AD episode or at high risk for a dysreflexic event, intraoperative and postoperative cardiac monitoring are warranted because AD may occur up to a few days after surgery.

AUTONOMIC DYSREFLEXIA TREATMENT DURING PREGNANCY AND LABOR

AD is a common complication of pregnancy in SCI. Prevention remains the most important factor in AD management to avoid morbidity and mortality in patients or their fetus. AD during pregnancy has the same pathophysiology and requires the same methods of management as in nonpregnant patients. An important differential diagnosis to an AD episode during pregnancy in women with SCI is preeclampsia.

A complete anesthesia consultation should be undertaken prior to labor. AD can be controlled during labor by epidural block,[42] and placement of an epidural catheter should be done at the first sign of labor.[45] Because AD may occur up to 48 hours after delivery, maintenance of epidural anesthesia for that period is usually recommended.[47] Oral nifedipine, intravenous hydralazine, or trimethaphan have been suggested to control extremely high blood pressure in this population during labor. Intravenous nitroprusside is not generally recommended during pregnancy or labor out of concern for elevation of fetal cyanide levels. Ganglionic blocking agents with a short duration of action, such as a 0.1% solution of trimethaphan in 5% dextrose by intravenous drip, can be administered in refractory AD cases during labor that are not adequately controlled by regional anesthesia.[49,52]

CONCLUSION

AD is a medical emergency often related to urologic, gastrointestinal, and gynecologic problems or manipulations. Its management starts primarily with its prevention. Identification and avoidance of noxious stimuli can often be managed by adequate bladder, bowel, and skin care.

Healthcare providers should also be informed about this pathology to promptly recognize and treat AD. Physicians must be aware of the procedures and treatment cascades that can be undertaken to avoid the possibly devastating consequences of acute AD.

REFERENCES

1. Shergill IS, Arya M, Hamid R, Khastgir J, Patel HRH, and Shah PJR. The importance of autonomic dysreflexia to the urologist. *BJU Int*. 2004;93(7):923–6. http://doi.wiley.com/10.1111/j.1464-410X.2003.04756.x

2. Karlsson AK. Autonomic dysreflexia. *Spinal Cord.* 1999;37(6):383–91. http://www.ncbi.nlm.nih.gov/pubmed/10432257

3. Lindan R, Joiner E, Freehafer AA, and Hazel C. Incidence and clinical features of autonomic dysreflexia in patients with spinal cord injury. *Spinal Cord.* 1980;18(5):285–92. http://www.ncbi.nlm.nih.gov/pubmed/7443280

4. Kewalramani LS. Autonomic dysreflexia in traumatic myelopathy. *Am J Phys Med.* 1980;59(1):1–21. http://www.ncbi.nlm.nih.gov/pubmed/6986791

5. Trop CS, and Bennett CJ. Autonomic dysreflexia and its urological implications: A review. *J Urol.* 1991;146(6):1461–9. http://www.jurology.com/doi/10.1016/S0022-5347%2817%2938140-5

6. Kursh ED, Freehafer A, and Persky L. Complications of autonomic dysreflexia. *J Urol.* 1977;118(1 Part 1):70–2. http://www.jurology.com/doi/10.1016/S0022-5347%2817%2957892-1

7. Eltorai I, Kim R, Vulpe M, Kasravi H, and Ho W. Fatal cerebral hemorrhage due to autonomic dysreflexia in a tetraplegic patient: Case report and review. *Spinal Cord.* 1992;30(5):355–60. http://www.nature.com/articles/sc199282

8. Pine ZM, Miller SD, and Alonso JA. Atrial fibrillation associated with autonomic dysreflexia. *Am J Phys Med Rehabil.* 1991;70(5):271–3. http://www.ncbi.nlm.nih.gov/pubmed/1910653

9. Vallès M, Benito J, Portell E, and Vidal J. Cerebral hemorrhage due to autonomic dysreflexia in a spinal cord injury patient. *Spinal Cord.* 2005;43(12):738–40. http://www.ncbi.nlm.nih.gov/pubmed/16010281

10. Pan S-L, Wang Y-H, Lin H-L, Chang C-W, Wu T-Y, and Hsieh E-T. Intracerebral hemorrhage secondary to autonomic dysreflexia in a young person with incomplete C8 tetraplegia: A case report. *Arch Phys Med Rehabil.* 2005;86(3):591–3. https://linkinghub.elsevier.com/retrieve/pii/S0003999304004009

11. Lindan R, Joiner E, Freehafer AA, and Hazel C. Incidence and clinical features of autonomic dysreflexia in patients with spinal cord injury. *Paraplegia.* 1980;18(5):285–92.

12. Cherian J, Thwaini A, Rao A, Arya N, Shergill IS, and Patel HRH. Autonomic dysreflexia: Emergency. *Clin Features.* 2005;66(5):294–6.

13. Wanner MB, Rageth CJ, and Zäch GA. Pregnancy and autonomic hyperreflexia in patients with spinal cord lesions. *Spinal Cord.* 1987;25(6):482–90. http://www.ncbi.nlm.nih.gov/pubmed/3324019

14. Blackmer J. Rehabilitation medicine: 1. Autonomic dysreflexia. *CMAJ.* 2003;169(9):931–5. https://www.ncbi.nlm.nih.gov/pubmed/?term=Blackmer+J.+Rehabilitation+medicine%3A+1.+Autonomic+dysreflexia

15. Consortium for Spinal Cord Medicine. Acute management of autonomic dysreflexia: Individuals with spinal cord injury presenting to health-care facilities. *J Spinal Cord Med.* 2002;25(Suppl 1):S67–88. http://www.ncbi.nlm.nih.gov/pubmed/12051242

16. Braddom RL and Rocco JF. Autonomic dysreflexia. A survey of current treatment. *Am J Phys Med Rehabil.* 1991;70(5):234–41. http://www.ncbi.nlm.nih.gov/pubmed/1910647

17. Dykstra DD, Sidi AA, and Anderson LC. The effect of nifedipine on cystoscopy-induced autonomic hyperreflexia in patients with high spinal cord injuries. *J Urol.* 1987;138(5):1155–7. http://www.jurology.com/doi/10.1016/S0022-5347%2817%2943533-6

18. Naftchi NE and Richardson JS. Autonomic dysreflexia: Pharmacological management of hypertensive crises in spinal cord injured patients. *J Spinal Cord Med.* 1997;20(3):355–60. http://www.ncbi.nlm.nih.gov/pubmed/9261783

19. Eldahan KC and Rabchevsky AG. Autonomic dysreflexia after spinal cord injury: Systemic pathophysiology and methods of management. *Auton Neurosci.* 2018;209:59–70. http://www.ncbi.nlm.nih.gov/pubmed/28506502

20. Caruso D, Gater D, and Harnish C. Prevention of recurrent autonomic dysreflexia: A survey of current practice. *Clin Auton Res.* 2015;25(5):293–300. http://www.ncbi.nlm.nih.gov/pubmed/26280219

21. Krum H, Louis WJ, Brown DJ, and Howes LG. A study of the alpha-1 adrenoceptor blocker prazosin in the prophylactic management of autonomic dysreflexia in high spinal cord injury patients. *Clin Auton Res.* 1992;2(2):83–8. http://www.ncbi.nlm.nih.gov/pubmed/1353386

22. Phillips AA, Elliott SL, Zheng MMZ, and Krassioukov AV. Selective alpha adrenergic antagonist reduces severity of transient hypertension during sexual stimulation after spinal cord injury. *J Neurotrauma.* 2015;32(6):392–6. http://www.ncbi.nlm.nih.gov/pubmed/25093677

23. Steinberger RE, Ohl DA, Bennett CJ, McCabe M, and Wang SC. Nifedipine pretreatment for autonomic dysreflexia during electroejaculation. *Urology.* 1990;36(3):228–31. http://www.ncbi.nlm.nih.gov/pubmed/2392813

24. Lindan R, Leffler EJ, and Kedia KR. A comparison of the efficacy of an alpha-I-adrenergic blocker in the slow calcium channel blocker in the control of autonomic dysreflexia. *Paraplegia.* 1985;23(1):34–8. http://www.nature.com/articles/sc19856

25. Furlan JC and Fehlings MG. Cardiovascular complications after acute spinal cord injury: Pathophysiology, diagnosis, and management. *Neurosurg Focus.* 2008;25(5):E13. https://thejns.org/view/journals/neurosurg-focus/25/5/article-pE13.xml

26. Khastgir J, Drake MJ, and Abrams P. Recognition and effective management of autonomic dysreflexia in spinal cord injuries. *Expert Opin Pharmacother.* 2007;8(7):945–56.

27. Esmail Z, Shalansky KF, Sunderji R, Anton H, Chambers K, and Fish W. Evaluation of captopril for the management of hypertension in autonomic dysreflexia: A pilot study. *Arch Phys Med Rehabil.* 2002;83(5):604–8. http://www.ncbi.nlm.nih.gov/pubmed/11994798

28. Frost F. Antihypertensive therapy, nifedipine, and autonomic dysreflexia. *Arch Phys Med Rehabil.* 2002;83(9):1325–6; author reply 1326. http://www.ncbi.nlm.nih.gov/pubmed/12235621

29. Anton HA and Townson A. Drug therapy for autonomic dysreflexia. *CMAJ.* 2004;170(8):1210; author reply 1210. http://www.ncbi.nlm.nih.gov/pubmed/15078832

30. Paola FA, Sales D, and Garcia-Zozaya I. Phenazopyridine in the management of autonomic dysreflexia associated with urinary tract infection. *J Spinal Cord Med.* 2003;26(4):409–11. https://www.tandfonline.com/doi/full/10.1080/10790268.2003.11753714

31. Maehama T, Izena H, and Kanazawa K. Management of autonomic hyperreflexia with magnesium sulfate during labor in a woman with spinal cord injury. *Am J Obstet Gynecol.* 2000;183(2):492–3. https://linkinghub.elsevier.com/retrieve/pii/S0002937800879715

32. Jones NA and Jones SD. Management of life-threatening autonomic hyper-reflexia using

magnesium sulphate in a patient with a high spinal cord injury in the intensive care unit. *Br J Anaesth.* 2002;88(3):434–8. https://linkinghub.elsevier.com/retrieve/pii/S0007091217365170

33. Erickson RP. Autonomic hyperreflexia: Pathophysiology and medical management. *Arch Phys Med Rehabil.* 1980;61(10):431–40. http://www.ncbi.nlm.nih.gov/pubmed/6107074

34. McGuire J, Wagner FM, and Weiss RM. Treatment of autonomic dysreflexia with phenoxybenzamine. *J Urol.* 1976;115(1):53–5. http://www.ncbi.nlm.nih.gov/pubmed/1246113

35. Sheel AW, Krassioukov AV, Inglis JT, and Elliott SL. Autonomic dysreflexia during sperm retrieval in spinal cord injury: Influence of lesion level and sildenafil citrate. *J Appl Physiol.* 2005;99(1):53–8. http://www.physiology.org/doi/10.1152/japplphysiol.00154.2005

36. Pasquina PF, Houston RM, and Belandres PV. Beta blockade in the treatment of autonomic dysreflexia: A case report and review. *Arch Phys Med Rehabil.* 1998;79(5):582–4. http://www.ncbi.nlm.nih.gov/pubmed/9596403

37. Vaidyanathan S, Soni BM, Sett P, Watt JW, Oo T, and Bingley J. Pathophysiology of autonomic dysreflexia: Long-term treatment with terazosin in adult and paediatric spinal cord injury patients manifesting recurrent dysreflexic episodes. *Spinal Cord.* 1998;36(11):761–70. http://www.ncbi.nlm.nih.gov/pubmed/9848483

38. Abrams P, Amarenco G, Bakke A et al. Tamsulosin: Efficacy and safety in patients with neurogenic lower urinary tract dysfunction due to suprasacral spinal cord injury. *J Urol.* 2003;170(4 Part 1):1242–51. http://www.ncbi.nlm.nih.gov/pubmed/14501734

39. Schurch B, Schmid DM, and Stöhrer M. Treatment of neurogenic incontinence with botulinum toxin A. *N Engl J Med.* 2000;342(9):665. http://www.ncbi.nlm.nih.gov/pubmed/10702067

40. Fougere RJ, Currie KD, Nigro MK, Stothers L, Rapoport D, and Krassioukov AV. Original articles reduction in bladder-related autonomic dysreflexia after onabotulinumtoxin a treatment in spinal cord injury. *J Neurotrauma.* 2016;33:1651–7. https://www.ncbi.nlm.nih.gov/pmc/articles/PMC5035837/pdf/neu.2015.4278.pdf

41. Lockwood G, Durkee C, and Groth T. Intravesical botulinum toxin for persistent autonomic dysreflexia in a pediatric patient. *Case Rep Urol.* 2016;2016:1–4. http://www.ncbi.nlm.nih.gov/pubmed/27006855

42. Burns AS and Jackson AB. Gynecologic and reproductive issues in women with spinal cord injury. *Phys Med Rehabil Clin N Am.* 2001;12(1):183–99. http://www.ncbi.nlm.nih.gov/pubmed/11853036

43. Greenspoon JS and Paul RH. Paraplegia and quadriplegia: Special considerations during pregnancy and labor and delivery. *Am J Obstet Gynecol.* 1986;155(4):738–41. https://linkinghub.elsevier.com/retrieve/pii/S0002937886800102

44. Burns R and Clark VA. Epidural anaesthesia for caesarean section in a patient with quadriplegia and autonomic hyperreflexia. *Int J Obstet Anesth.* 2004;13(2):120–3. https://linkinghub.elsevier.com/retrieve/pii/S0959289X03001821

45. Kobayashi A, Mizobe T, Tojo H, and Hashimoto S. Autonomic hyperreflexia during labour. *Can J Anaesth.* 1995;42(12):1134–6. http://link.springer.com/10.1007/BF03015101

46. Gunaydin B, Akcali D, and Alkan M. Epidural anaesthesia for caesarean section in a patient with Devic's syndrome. *Anaesthesia.* 2001;56(6):565–7. http://www.ncbi.nlm.nih.gov/pubmed/11412164

47. Murphy DB, McGuire G, and Peng P. Treatment of autonomic hyperreflexia in a quadriplegic patient by epidural anesthesia in the postoperative period. *Anesth Analg.* 1999;89(1):148–9. https://insights.ovid.com/crossref?an=00000539-199907000-00025

48. Colachis SC. Autonomic hyperreflexia with spinal cord injury. *J Am Paraplegia Soc.* 1992;15(3):171–86. http://www.ncbi.nlm.nih.gov/pubmed/1500943

49. Tabsh KM, Brinkman CR, and Reff RA. Autonomic dysreflexia in pregnancy. *Obstet Gynecol.* 1982;60(1):119–22. http://www.ncbi.nlm.nih.gov/pubmed/7088442

50. Cross LL, Meythaler JM, Tuel SM, and Cross AL. Pregnancy, labor and delivery post spinal cord injury. *Spinal Cord.* 1992;30(12):890–902. http://www.ncbi.nlm.nih.gov/pubmed/1287543

51. Hambly PR and Martin B. Anaesthesia for chronic spinal cord lesions. *Anaesthesia.* 1998;53(3):273–89. https://onlinelibrary.wiley.com/doi/abs/10.1046/j.1365-2044.1998.00337.x

52. Ravindran RS, Cummins DF, and Smith IE. Experience with the use of nitroprusside and subsequent epidural analgesia in a pregnant quadriplegic patient. *Anesth Analg.* 1981;60(1):61–3. http://www.ncbi.nlm.nih.gov/pubmed/7192952

PERIPHERAL AND INTRAVESICAL ELECTRICAL STIMULATION OF THE BLADDER TO RESTORE BLADDER FUNCTION

Karl-Dietrich Sievert

INTRODUCTION

Electrical devices for the control of bladder management have a number of potential benefits over alternative methods, such as mechanical devices, pharmaceuticals, and surgical interventions.[1] Electrical stimulation techniques can provide immediate, reversible effect. This on-demand function returns control of the bladder based on individual needs, goals, and lifestyles without the known systemic side effects of other treatment options. Some of the challenges of electrical device development for bladder function include electrode design, surgical implantation, and tuning stimulation parameters to effect.

Electrodes are designed to optimize reliability, stability, and control of the spread of electrical current to activate target neurons without coactivating or activating nontarget neurons. Implantation techniques should be minimally invasive while still allowing access to target neurons for electrical activation. Finally, many stimulation techniques require careful tuning of stimulation parameters, such as frequency, amplitude, and more. Achieving this parameter tuning in each individual can take time.

DIFFERENT TYPES OF STIMULATION

GENITAL NERVE STIMULATION
Bladder inhibition has been demonstrated in acute studies using electrical stimulation of the genital nerve (GN). Genital nerve stimulation (GNS) is a more direct, defined neural pathway than sacral foramen stimulation, which does not activate a consistent or defined set of fibers in the sacral root to inhibit bladder contraction.[17,18] Wheeler et al., using surface electrodes to stimulate the GN, showed significant increases in bladder filling volume during cystometrography[58] with a carry-on effect.[59] As a result, the indications were expanded to patients with SCI (Figure 30.1)[60–65] and those with MS.[66] The effect on blood pressure was excluded,[67] but a possible associated risk of autonomic dysreflexia for patients with spinal cord lesions above T6 has been reported.[68]

GNS acts by both somatic-parasympathetic and somatic-sympathetic pathways contained in the spinal cord.[59,69,70] The GN is very superficial and can be stimulated easily with skin electrodes. Because the GN is primarily a sensory nerve, higher stimulation amplitudes can be used without causing unwanted muscle movement, particularly those without sensation. GNS may lead to more predictable results and benefit a higher percentage of patients than sacral nerve stimulation (SNM) or foramen stimulation, where multiple motor and sensory components are stimulated, making it difficult to predict or control which pathways are involved. Although GNS has been demonstrated to be effective in an acute environment, few groups have tested this approach chronically.[71–74]

INTRAURETHRAL STIMULATION
Gustafson et al. used mounted electrodes on urinary catheters and successfully activated urethral sensory afferents in humans.[20] These reports provided evidence for a urethral pudendal micturition reflex pathway in humans as in cats. They confirmed that the bladder pressures resulting from intraurethral neuromodulation depend on bladder volume.[19] Stimulation of sensory afferents in the pudendal nerve may provide a minimally invasive approach to restoring voiding function.[16]

INTRAVESICAL ELECTRICAL STIMULATION
Almost 100 years after the initial publication,[2–4] Ebner et al. investigated the working mechanism in rodents and cats.[5] They concluded the direct activation through the mechanoreceptor afferents may elicit reflexive detrusor contractions (Figure 30.2).

Intravesical electrical stimulation (IVES) activates an excitatory bladder reflex to promote voiding. However, if a spinal lesion disrupts this reflex, it may compromise its effectiveness. Cortically evoked

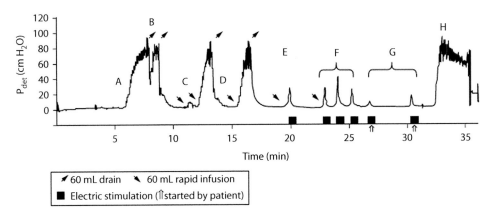

Figure 30.1   Bladder pressure recordings with and without genital nerve stimulation during rapid bladder filling. The subject demonstrated reflexive bladder contractions during normal bladder infusion (a and b). Reproducible reflexive contractions were produced in response to rapid filling (c and d). Further reflexive contractions were diminished with genital nerve stimulation (e, f, and g). No stimulation was provided during a final contraction (h), which showed a return of reflexive bladder activity in the absence of stimulation. Stimulation periods underneath the open braces (f and g) were initiated by the study participant. In the absence of stimulation, reflexive bladder contractions are not suppressed. (From Lee Y et al. *Arch Phys Med Rehabil.* 2003;84[1]:136–40.)

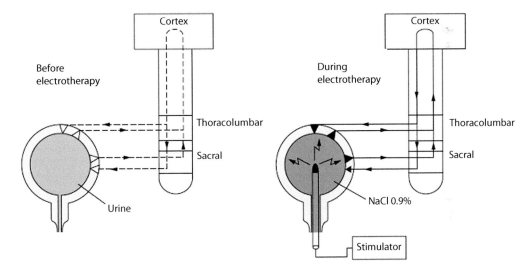

Figure 30.2   Intravesical electrical stimulation activation and contractions.

urothelium potentials may be used to assess the degree of the afferent lesion to predict the outcome of IVES. Both afferent and efferent pathways can be compromised by neurogenic issues, and deficits can affect the sensory and/or the motor function of the detrusor. The primary reason to use IVES is to restore micturition. Hagerty described a benefit to improve bladder compliance and bladder sensation in children.[6,7] The efficacy of IVES was investigated in patients with acute prolonged bladder overdistension and was proven in those patients with a residual detrusor function.

IVES remains a controversial therapy. Some have reported regained detrusor activity and sensation

of bladder filling after IVES, while others have reported negative findings.[8–11] In the comparison of IVES versus sacral neuromodulation (SNM), a strict correlation of clinical and urodynamic patterns was demonstrated in patients with incomplete spinal cord injury (SCI) and without a lower urinary tract (LUT) obstruction but for IVES only short-term voiding improvement.[12] Deng reviewed retrospectively 89 patients with detrusor underactivity (DU): 47.2% (42/89) were responders, and greater than 50% achieved a reduction in the postvoid residual (PVR). PVR reduction (greater than 80%) occurred in 27% (24/89) of the patients. Voiding Efficiency (VE) developed in 76.4% (68/89) of the patients, and 30.3%

(27/89) of the patients experienced a greater than 50% increase. Based on the questionnaire, bladder sensation was regained in 44.8% (43/96) of the patients.[13] Besides the indication to treat Neurogenic Detrusor Underactivity (nDU) in neurogenic patients, IVES has been investigated in those patients with overactive bladder (OAB).[14] Further, IVES remains labor intensive and material consuming. The option of using home-based treatments requires patient endurance and discipline and is often unrealistic and unattainable.

BLADDER WALL STIMULATION

In 1950, direct bladder wall stimulation was the most intuitive approach to evoke detrusor contractions and bladder voiding.[21] However, this approach has demonstrated limited effectiveness due to a number of challenges.[22,23] Nonetheless, this approach remains a potential alternative if these challenges can be overcome, especially for individuals with lower motor neuron lesions that might not benefit from sacral root stimulation.[24]

PELVIC NERVE STIMULATION STIMULATION/ MODULATION

Pelvic nerve stimulation (PNS) should cause more complete detrusor contraction than bladder wall stimulation and at lower stimulation amplitudes.[23] In practice, PNS results in detrusor contraction and in coactivation of the urethral sphincter, hampering effective voiding.[15] This sphincter activation is likely a reflexive response to activation of the bladder and urethral sensory afferents also passing through the pudendal nerve (PN). Further, surgical placement of the electrodes is challenging (laparoscopic) compared to other electrode sites, such as sacral root implants.[25,26]

In 2005, Spinelli et al.[27] performed the first PNM in 15 patients (8 males and 7 females) with a traumatic or nontraumatic SCI, which resulted in neurogenic detrusor overactivity (NDO) and urinary incontinence. Patients evaluated the pelvic nerve modulation (PNM) to be superior to the previous sacral neuromodulation, although the micturition diary did not demonstrate any superiority. In another evaluation, compared to baseline, no significant benefit was noted using nerve modulation.[28] Recently, with drugs administered into the bladder (PGE1), voiding efficiency increased, and external urethral sphincter (EUS) electromyographic (EMG) activity increased at a specific stimulation condition (1 mA at 10 Hz), which might provide further options in patient modalities.[29]

CONUS MEDULLARIS STIMULATION

Nashold and Friedman developed an approach whereby stimulation through electrodes implanted in the conus medullaris might achieve this coordinated micturition response—a strong bladder contraction

concomitant with relaxation of the urethra and sphincter.[30–32] The challenges to stimulate the relevant nuclei and avoid the costimulation of continence-related areas (sphincter contraction) were so far the primary reasons why this approach has not been further investigated.

SACRAL ANTERIOR ROOT STIMULATION FOR EMPTYING THE PARALYZED BLADDER

After Alexander and Rowan demonstrated evidence that PNS can lead to voiding,[33] Brindley specified sacral anterior root stimulation (SARS) further for the sacral anterior roots (S1–S2) in the primate resulting in the Finetech-Brindley stimulator (Figure 30.3: Finetech Medical Limited, Welwyn Garden City, United Kingdom) to preserve continence.[34] The development of the implant was adapted to be implanted in humans, which caused a sequence of single micturitions, interrupted by fatiguing sphincter contractions (poststimulus-void).[35]

With the further surgical approach (sacral deafferentation of the posterior nerve roots of S2-S4 [SDAF]) of Sauerwein, the remaining high-pressure detrusor was overcome, even at lower bladder urine volumes. More than 90% of patients were continent and able to have a bladder capacity of more than 500 mL,[37,38] in addition to the further reduction of the required amplitude.

SARS can also be used to aid in bowel evacuation (approximately 50% of the patients) and produce implant-driven erections in males. The Finetech-Brindley device has been used successfully in many countries throughout the world. The implant significantly improved patient quality of life, although the number of devices implanted has decreased over the years.[39]

Possover et al. described a laparoscopic technique to access the pelvic autonomic plexus to revise the existing intrathecal or extradural electrodes to regain the use of a Finetech-Brindley bladder stimulator.[41] Although the Finetech-Brindley stimulator has excellent longevity and outcomes in terms of bladder[40] and bowel management, the use of SDAF, with its possible consequent loss of reflex erections, reflex ejaculation, bowel problems, and potential pelvic floor weakness, can be a challenge for male patients.[39] Besides the additional drug treatment to reach a more acceptable treatment level, there might be an alternative solution to SDAF, which involves stimulation of these afferent pathways (nerve block), rather than cutting them to suppress reflex incontinence.

TECHNIQUES FOR STIMULATION AND BLOCKING OF SACRAL ROOTS TO PREVENT DETRUSOR-SPHINCTER DYSSYNERGIA

Sacral anterior roots contain both the large somatic nerves to the urethral striated sphincter and the small

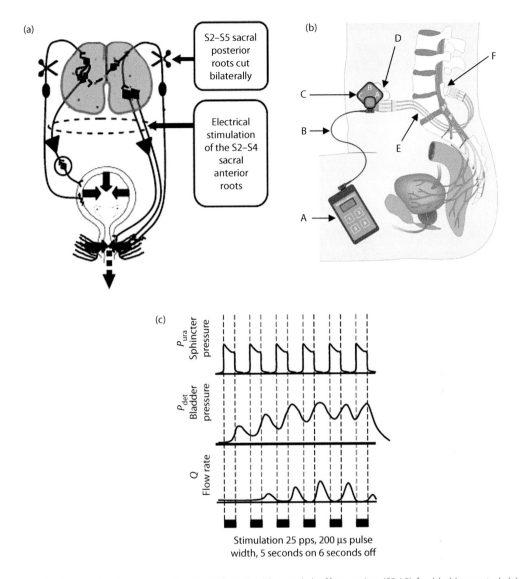

Figure 30.3 Sacral anterior root stimulation (SARS) with sacral deafferentation (SDAF) for bladder control. (a) Finetech-Brindley SARS implantable stimulator uses bilaterally placed intrathecal or extradural electrodes on the S2 through S4 sacral roots to activate the preganglionic parasympathetic pathway to produce efficient bladder emptying. A rhizotomy of the corresponding posterior roots (sensory) prevents neurogenic detrusor overactivity, dyssynergia of the sphincter, and incontinence. (b) Anatomic configuration of the Finetech-Brindley implant. The user selects one of the stimulation programs. The external controller (A) sends power and control signals to the transmitter block via the transmitter lead (B). The user holds the transmitter block (C) over the site of the implant receiver (D). The implant receiver converts the signals from the transmitter block into electrical impulses. The impulses travel via extremely flexible cables (E) to the electrodes (F). The electrodes transfer the impulses to the nerves causing the appropriate muscles to contract at the appropriate time.[36] (c) Bursts of stimulation activate simultaneously the striated sphincter muscle and the detrusor smooth muscle resulting in poststimulus voiding. During the intervals between the bursts, the sphincter relaxes rapidly to leave a low urethral resistance, while the detrusor is still contracting slowly to a higher pressure so as to enable very efficient voiding.

preganglionic parasympathetic nerves to the bladder detrusor smooth muscle. Consequently, during SARS, bladder emptying is impaired by coactivation of both nerve qualities (Figure 30.3). This is the cause of poststimulus voiding,[43] which is the result of rapid fatiguing of the sphincter and the delayed oncoming detrusor contraction leading to bladder emptying. This type of voiding is not particularly physiologic but effective. However, in the presence of intact sacral reflexes (i.e., no sacral deafferentation), the dyssynergia persists in the gap between the bursts of stimulation to prevent efficient emptying, especially when stimulation is applied to the mixed nerve roots.[105]

To overcome this problem, different approaches are available: cold temperature, nerve blocking (anode block), and high-frequency block to block the sphincter, resulting in a more physiologic bladder evacuation.[44,45] The proof of principle has been performed in the animal model, although this additional step will reach a more physiological void, but this has not been included in a standard clinical procedure.[46]

POSTERIOR TIBIAL NERVE STIMULATION

Posterior tibial nerve stimulation (PTNS) has an efferent motor effect and an afferent sensory effect. Stimulation of the posterior tibial nerve results in great toe flexion or fanning of the toes. The sensory effect is a radiating tickling sensation of the sole of the foot. McGuire explored this in 15 neurologic patients with detrusor overactivity (DO).[47] Inspired by this work, Stoller initiated research on PTNS as a neuromodulative treatment in lower urinary tract dysfunction.[48]

A 34-gauge stainless steel needle is inserted approximately three fingers above the cephalad to the medial malleolus (between the posterior margin of the tibia and soleus muscle). A surface electrode is placed near the arch of the ipsilateral foot. At a tolerated amplitude intensity, the stimulation is applied for 30 minutes once a week for 3 months. If a good response occurs, the patient is offered chronic treatment.[49] PTNS is suitable for neurogenic patients because of several advantages: remote from the pelvis, easy access, and no continuous stimulation.

PTNS is easy to apply, and it does not interfere with any medication patients are taking.[50–53] It is also possible to apply transcutaneous TNS instead of PTNS, although data are limited.[54]

Recently, PTNS became possible to be performed using a chronic implant. However, PTNS has not been investigated over the long term.[55] In the comparison of PTNS versus electrical stimulation with pelvic floor muscle training, PTNS demonstrated more improvements in the treatment for OAB.[56] StimWave has sustained CE approval for a wireless and full-body magnetic resonance imaging (MRI) (1.5 and 3 T) sacral stimulator, where data have been published at international meetings. Further, additional transcutaneous TNS devices have become available.[57]

SACRAL NEUROMODULATION

Modulation of the extradural sacral roots, which activates sensory afferents in the posterior roots, was introduced by Tanagho and Schmidt to control continence.[75,76] They found that stimulation at low frequencies and low amplitudes produced reflexive sphincter contractions without detrusor activation. Indeed, stimulation of the external urethral sphincter can result in inhibition of the detrusor, thus improving urine retention. The market has changed with the increasing competition of new devices that has in turn stimulated the development of new and enhanced devices.

INTERSTIM BY MEDTRONIC

The initial commercially available device for SNM was called Interstim (Medtronic, Minneapolis, Minnesota) (Figure 30.4). The device is used to reduce

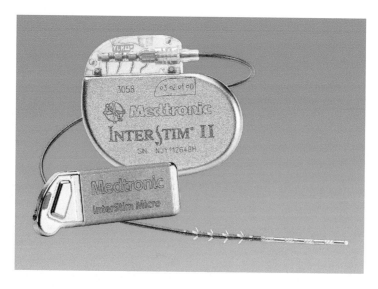

Figure 30.4 Interstim. The rechargeable implant (InterStim Micro) of Medtronic is available in addition to the well-known Interstim. Implantable pulse generators (IPGs) and leads (InterStim SureScan magnetic resonance imaging [MRI] leads) are planned to be full-body MRI (1.5 and 3 T) approved. (From De Wachter S et al. *Adv Ther.* 2020;37[2]:637–643.)

incontinence, reduce urge frequency, and increase bladder capacity.[75] Using the self-anchoring tined lead electrode minimizes invasiveness and recovery times.[77,78] Several studies examined the safety of implants for electrical interfaces. Although bacterial colonization has been observed (40%), there has been no effect on the outcome of the SNM implants or even a need for infection-related explanation.[79]

SNM has been tested in individuals with a wide variety of non- and neurogenic urinary incontinence. This population includes individuals with spinal cord injuries, stroke, and OAB due to age or postpartum changes in the lower urinary tract.[81,82] Especially in persons with SCI, SNM has been demonstrated to be effective in a subset of that population.[83] Therefore, before implantation of the Interstim system, patients are prescreened to assess their responses to stimulation through a percutaneous sacral electrode and an external stimulator.[84] We would like to add that the Medtronic patient does have now full body approved implants (IPG and electrode) for the interstim II and the rechargeable (Interstim Micro) (1.5 and 3 T). This has importance, especially in patients who will have to undergo after implantation and MIR investigations on a regular base (like MS patients). This was a hurdle for all the previous years and either withheld the patients from receiving an implant or it was explanted.

SACRAL NEUROMODULATION IN EARLY SPINAL CORD INJURY

The mechanism of this "neuromodulatory" action has yet to be determined, but one theory suggests that neuromodulation involves inhibitory action by pudendal afferent (sensory, S2 through S4) nerve stimulation on pelvic nerve motor pathways to the bladder through spinal cord circuits.[7,80,85,86] Electrical stimulation of purely afferent pathways depends essentially on the stimulation level diminishing when stimulation is switched off (Figure 30.5).[87–89] Interestingly, intermittent stimulation also appears to lead to good results, although the ideal interval between bursts has yet to be determined to suppress every NDO contraction reliably while preserving the battery life of the stimulator.[47]

One strategy is to attempt to prevent or reduce the occurrence of detrusor-sphincter dyssynergia (DSD). Sievert and colleagues[90] investigated patients with complete SCI who were in the early, areflexic stages following injury. They demonstrated that those treated with SNM had fewer incidents of urinary tract infection (UTI), greater urinary continence with higher bladder capacities, and improved bowel control, contributing to their increased quality of life.

The occurrence of DSD and DO following SCI is poorly understood. One theory favoring the use of

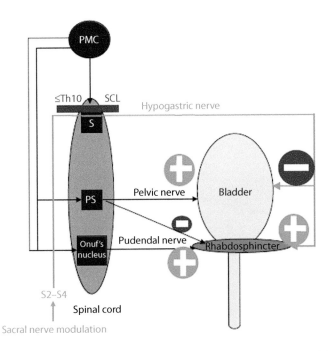

Figure 30.5   Effect of spinal cord injury versus the influence of early applied sacral neuromodulation in this patient group. The pontine micturition center normally regulates activity in Onuf's nucleus, as well as the sympathetic (S) and parasympathetic (PS) drives. Following a spinal cord lesion (SCL, red bar), this control is lost and the parasympathetic pathway can reflexively excite the bladder (+) and inhibit the sphincter (–). Sacral nerve modulation activates sympathetic pathways to promote urinary continence by inhibiting the parasympathetic drive to inhibit the bladder and excite the sphincter.

early SNM is that the return of reflexive autonomic activity in the months following SCI may also represent the development of irreversible autonomic malfunctions. This early stage of SCI presents an opportunity for preventive treatment, taking advantage of the neuroplasticity and the reforming spinal circuits to avoid the development of OAB or DSD (Figure 30.6).

In ongoing experimental research in the large animal model, it was possible to demonstrate regeneration in the damaged area of the spine using SNM with the bilateral sacral root stimulation; but this was not seen in pudendal nerve stimulation.[91, 92, 106] Recently, Redshaw et al. initiated a follow-up trial to investigate the effect of early SNM on SCI in a multicenter study.[93] In comparison to the initial study by Sievert et al.,[90] patients with both complete and incomplete SCI will be accepted (inclusion criteria: acute SCI ≥T12, ASIA scale A or B) in addition to other criteria. It needs to be seen if such a heterogenous group can reflect the initial reported results of the highly selective inclusion criteria.

INSITE

The InSite trial (prospective, multicenter, U.S. Food and Drug Administration–mandated postapproval study, comparison of the SNM against standard medical therapy [SMT]) demonstrated superiority in the 5-year follow-up. The 6-year follow-up is expected to be completed by early 2020.[98,99]

AXIONICS

One of the first rechargeable implants (Axonics®) (Figure 30.6) received permission to begin post-market testing in Europe of a rechargeable SNM system claiming a 15-year battery life.[94–96] The

initial data of the RELAX-OAB study was recently published and demonstrated clinically significant improvements in OAB with an easy and acceptable recharging experience (for <2 h every 1–3 weeks).[97] The implant is currently only approved for head MRIs (1.5 and 3 T).

OTHER DEVICES

Further devices have been evaluated in clinical studies including a multi-canal device to be more selective, but no data have been published. In other studies using noninvasive multi-pulse magnetic stimulation over the sacrum to stimulate the mixed extradural sacral roots (S2 through S4), the authors demonstrated that the increase in bladder capacity can be brought about with the suppression of NDO in patients with SCI.[100]

CONDITIONAL NEUROMODULATION FOR AUTOMATIC CONTROL OF REFLEX INCONTINENCE

A conditional system that detects the onset of NDO contractions and then suppresses them has a number of theoretical advantages. Although continuous neuromodulation is an effective and simple way to increase bladder capacity in people with SCI or other neurogenic indications (e.g., MS),[49,50,89] in many situations it may not be ideal, not least of which is because of the effects of reflex habituation.[101]

The aim would be a complex implant facilitating neuromodulation only when necessary in the most effective way and providing feedback about bladder filling to the patient to signal the optimal point at which to evacuate the bladder to have the best effect of the stimulation and to avoid incontinence. This functionality might become available in its complexity

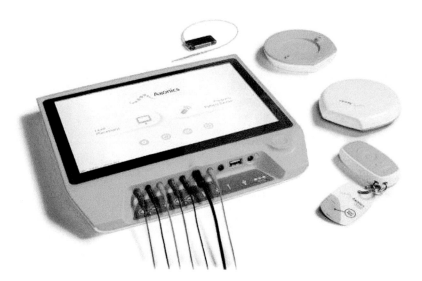

Figure 30.6   Axonics hardware (rechargeable implant and external device). (From Axonics, https://www.fda.gov/medical-devices/recently-approved-devices/axonics-sacral-neuromodulation-snm-system-urinary-control-p180046)

using additional tools (implantable devices) that can build a complex interacting platform.[102,103]

COMBINED BLADDER EMPTYING AND INHIBITION OF NEUROGENIC DETRUSOR OVERACTIVITY BY PUDENDAL NEVER STIMULATION

De Groat described the excitatory perineal-to-bladder reflex, which seems to be suppressed late in development.[107] The spinal reflexes of the lower urinary tract undergo significant plasticity.[108] Some research suggests that this situation leads to the restoration of the initial reflex—at least in several animal models.[104,108] From a clinical aspect, neurogenic bladder overactivity can be influenced in patients after incomplete SCI resulting in increased bladder capacity if an amplitude is applied to GN stimulation (greater than or equal to twice the threshold).[109]

This principle has been taken into clinical practice as a proof of principal evaluation. Knight et al. demonstrate a developed Knight et al. developed a transrectal device (CARM®).[110] The device (Figure 30.7) is placed rectally close to the pudendal nerves, detecting the EAS EMG as a reliable indicator of NDO contraction—actuating stimulation (frequency: 15 pulse/s and pulse width: 200 μs; applied in 60-second periods).

The neurogenic detrusor contractions are supposed to be suppressed resulting in an increased bladder capacity with lower detrusor pressure. This seems to be a huge step in providing neurogenic patients with an effective noninvasive device to influence DSD.[110]

With further development to pick up signals, which transfer acute functional information to operate the related stimulation/modulation, this will give us the opportunity to develop hardware to control such a complex function of storage/micturition in the most functional sequence.

PROSPECTS FOR COMPLETE RESTORATION OF BLADDER CONTROL

The treatment to improve motor function after SCI has made major progress (Figure 30.8). In addition to neurostimulation, a surgical procedure for contralateral seventh cervical nerve (C7) transfer from the nonparalyzed side to the paralyzed side was performed.[111] With additional modified neuromodulation, further improved motor control was gained.[111] This can be enhanced by selective reinnervated peripheral nerve input to the brain as well as visual motor feedback to the patient to promote brain reorganization, which seems to be critical for functional recovery.[112-114] In addition to nerve transfer, implantable new devices for multisite optogenetic stimulation of peripheral nerves, neurostimulation, demonstrate further improved function without any sign of pain.[115]

These encouraging results need to be confirmed in clinical trials and evaluated for autonomous organs like the lower urinary tract, which might be another challenge. Initial steps have been made to register the current status, which needs to be compared to a "normal functioning" autonomous organ, as there are storage areas of the urinary bladder with the optimum filling points that need to be emptied. The process needs to be "communicated" to the patient in order to ensure the patient has the opportunity to reach a toilet to evacuate the bladder via stimulus, initiate the time of the optimum possible bladder contraction, as well as relax the "closing/continence" structure—the inner and outer urinary sphincter.

We partially addressed these issues as early stimulation to avoid, like DSD,[116] and sensing the filling that needs to be working in one interface to support low-pressure storage[42] and allow evacuation at a chosen time and location.

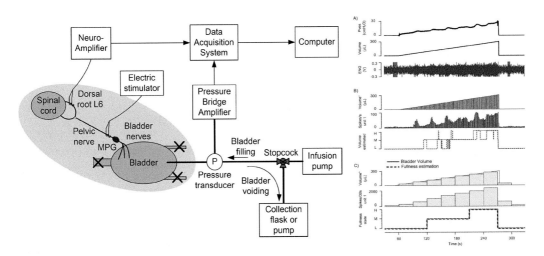

Figure 30.7 Conditional neuromodulation for the automatic control of reflex incontinence.

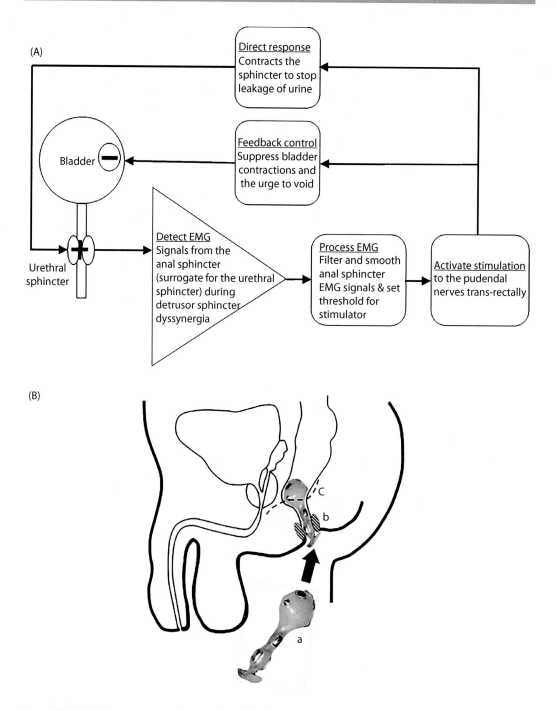

Figure 30.8 Bladder response and contractions. (A) Diagrammatic representation of conditional neuromodulation control in the CARM device. (B) The CARM device was manufactured from medical-grade silicone rubber and shaped for conformity within the anal canal into which the device was inserted with the aid of electrode gel (a). The electromyographic recording electrodes were located equidistant around the circumference to ensure best contact with the anal sphincter (b). The stimulating electrodes were designed as a bipolar pair bilaterally and directed toward the trajectory of the pudendal nerves (c) through Alcock's canal located near the anorectal junction. A reference electrode was located at an electrically inactive position on the stem of the device. (From Brindley GS, Polkey CE, and Rushton DN. *Paraplegia*. 1982;20[6]:365–81.)

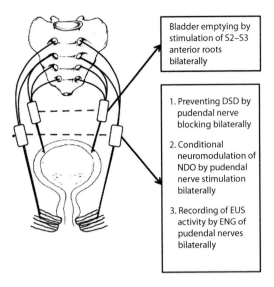

Bladder emptying by stimulation of S2–S3 anterior roots bilaterally

1. Preventing DSD by pudendal nerve blocking bilaterally

2. Conditional neuromodulation of NDO by pudendal nerve stimulation bilaterally

3. Recording of EUS activity by ENG of pudendal nerves bilaterally

Figure 30.9 Full restoration of bladder control to the neurogenic bladder. Possible techniques to overcome problems of the neurogenic bladder in spinal cord injury. With the combination of pudendal nerve blocking and sacral nerve stimulation is supposed to result in stimulation induced "voiding" in SCI patients (Boger AS, Bhadra N, Gustafson KJ. High frequency sacral root nerve block allows bladder voiding. *Neurourol Urodyn.* 2012; 31(5):677–682.). DSD, detrusor-sphincter dyssynergia; ENG, electroneurography; EUS, external urethral sphincter; NDO, neurogenic detrusor overactivity.

SUMMARY

Ultimately, it is hoped that we can initiate permanent registration impulses received from the bladder and compare them to the "normal" signal by combining conditional neuromodulation with selective neurostimulation to obtain an "almost" physiologic storage and evacuation. The big challenge will probably be to overcome the DSD resulting from the emergence of aberrant reflexes following SCI, but new techniques of nerve blocking may provide the solution.

REFERENCES

1. Gaunt RA, Prochazka A, Mushahwar VK, Guevremont L, and Ellaway PH. Intraspinal microstimulation excites multisegmental sensory afferents at lower stimulus levels than local alpha-motoneuron responses. *J Neurophysiol.* 2006;96(6):2995–3005.
2. Saxtorph, Chirurgiske Forelæsninger. Clinisk Chirurgi, Supplement 1878.
3. Katona F. Stages of vegetative afferentation in reorganization of bladder control during intravesical electrotherapy. *Urol Int.* 1975;30:192–203.
4. Madersbacher. Intravesical electrical stimulation for the rehabilitation of the neuropathic bladder. *Paraplegia* 1990;28:349–52.
5. Ebner ER, Kiss G, Berger T, Rehder P, and Madersbacher H. The value of intravesical electrostimulation in the treatment of acute prolonged bladder overdistension. *J Urol.* 1992;148:920–4.
6. Hagerty JA, Richards I, and Kaplan WE. Intravesical electrotherapy for neurogenic bladder dysfunction: A 22-years experience. *J Urol.* 2007;178(4 Suppl): 1680–3.
7. Huber ER, Kiss G, Berger T, Rehder P, and Madersbacher H. The value of intravesical electrostimulation in the treatment of acute prolonged bladder overdistension. *Urologe.* 2007;46:662–6.
8. Madersbacher H, Pauer W, Reiner E, Hetzel H, and Spanudakis S. Rehabilitation of micturition in patients with incomplete spinal cord lesions by transurethral electrostimulation of the bladder. *Eur Urol.* 1982;8:111–6.
9. Primus G, Kramer G, and Pummer K. Restoration of micturition in patients with acontractile and hypocontractile detrusor by transurethral electrical bladder stimulation. *Neurourol Urodyn.* 1996;15:489–97.
10. Boone TB, Roehrborn C, and Hurt G. Transurethral intravesical electrotherapy for neurogenic bladder dysfunction in children with myelodysplasia: A prospective, randomized clinical trial. *J Urol.* 1992;148:550–4.
11. Madersbacher H. Intravesical electrostimulation (IVES). In: Liao L, and Madersbacher H, eds. *Neurourology.* 2019, Dordrecht: Springer.
12. Lombardi G, Musco S, Celso M et al. Intravesical electrostimulation versus sacral neuromodulation for incomplete spinal cord patients suffering from neurogenic non-obstructive urinary retention. *Spinal Cord.* 2013;51(7):571–8.
13. Han Deng M, Liao L, Wu J et al. Clinical efficacy of intravesical electrical stimulation on detrusor underactivity 8 years of experience from a single center. *Medicine (Baltimore).* 2017;96(38):e8020.
14. Joshua Yune JKS, Pierce MA, Hardesty JS, Kim J, and Siddighi S. Intravesical electrical stimulation treatment for overactive bladder: An observational study. *Investig Clin Urol.* 2018;59(4):246–51.
15. Bruns TM, Bhadra N, and Gustafson KJ. Variable patterned pudendal nerve stimuli improves reflex bladder activation. *IEEE Trans Neural Syst Rehabil Eng.* 2008;16(2):140–8.
16. Bruns TM, Bhadra N, and Gustafson KJ. Intraurethral stimulation for reflex bladder activation depends on stimulation pattern and location. *Neurourol Urodyn.* 2009;28:561–6.
17. Woock JP, Yoo P, and Grill WM. Activation and inhibition of the micturition reflex by penile afferents in the cat. *Am J Physiol Regul Integr Comp Physiol.* 2008;294(6):R1880–9.
18. Yoo PB, Woock J, and Grill WM. Bladder activation by selective stimulation of pudendal nerve afferents in the cat. *Exp Neurol.* 2008;212(1):218–25.
19. Yu T, Liao L, and Wyndaele JJ. Can intraurethral stimulation inhibit micturition reflex in normal female rats? *Int Braz J Urol.* 2016;42(3):608–13.
20. Gustafson KJ, Creasey G, and Grill WM. A urethral afferent mediated excitatory bladder reflex exists in humans. *Neurosci Lett.* 2004;360(1–2):9–12.
21. Boyce WH, Lathem J, and Hunt LD. Research related to the development of an artificial electrical stimulation for the paralyzed human bladder: A review. *J Urol.* 1964;91:41–51.

22. Bradley WE, Chou SN, and French LA. Further experience with the radio transmitter receiver unit for the neurogenic bladder. *J Neurosurg.* 1963;20:953–60.

23. Hald T, Maier W, Khalili A, Agrawal G, Benton JG, and Kantrowitz A. Clinical experience with a radio-linked bladder stimulator. *J Urol.* 1967;97(1):73–8.

24. Walter JS, Wheeler J, Cai W, King WW, and Wurster RD. Evaluation of a suture electrode for direct bladder stimulation in a lower motor neuron lesioned animal model. *IEEE Trans Rehabil Eng.* 1999;7(2):159–66.

25. Burghele Th. Electrostimulation of the neurogenic urinary bladder. In: Lutzmeyer W, ed. *Urodynamics. Upper and Lower Urinary Tract.* Berlin, Germany: Springer-Verlag; 1973:319–22.

26. Kaeckenbeeck B. Electrostimulation of the bladder in paraplegia. Method of Burghele-Ichim-Demetrescu. *Acta Urol Belg.* 1979;47:139–40.

27. Spinelli M, Giardiello G, Lazzeri M, Tarantola J, and Van Den Hombergh U. A new minimally invasive procedure for pudendal nerve stimulation to treat neurogenic bladder: Description of the method and preliminary data. *Neurourol Urodyn.* 2005;24(4):305–9.

28. McCoin JL, Bhadra N, and Gustafson KJ. Electrical stimulation of sacral dermatomes can suppress aberrant urethral reflexes in felines with chronic spinal cord injury. *Neurourol Urodyn.* 2013;32(1):92–7.

29. Langdale CL, Hokanson J, Sridhar A, and Grill WM. Stimulation of the pelvic nerve increases bladder capacity in the prostaglandin E2 rat model of overactive bladder. *Am J Physiol Renal Physiol.* 2017;313(3):F657–65.

30. Friedman H, Nashold BS Jr, and Senechal P. Spinal cord stimulation and bladder function in normal and paraplegic animals. *J Neurosurg.* 1973;36:430–7.

31. Nashold BS Jr, Friedman H, and Grimes J. Electrical stimulation of the conus medullaris to control the bladder in the paraplegic patient. A 10-year review. *Appl Neurophysiol.* 1981;44:225–32.

32. Nashold BS Jr, Friedman H, Glenn JF, Grimes JH, Barry WF, and Avery R. Electromicturition in paraplegia. Implantation of a spinal neuroprosthesis. *Arch Surg.* 1972;104:195–202.

33. Alexander SR and Rowan D. Electrical control of urinary incontinence by radio implant. A report of 14 patients. *Br J Surg.* 1968;55:358–64.

34. Brindley GS. An implant to empty the bladder or close the urethra. *J Neurol Neurosurg Psychiatry.* 1977;40:358–69.

35. Brindley GS, Polkey CE, and Rushton DN. Sacral anterior root stimulators for bladder control in paraplegia. *Paraplegia.* 1982;20(6):365–81.

36. Finetech-Brindley. https://finetech-medical.co.uk/products/finetech-brindley-bladder-control-system/

37. Sauerwein D. Die operative Behandlung der spastischen Blasenlähmung bei Querschnittslähmung. *Urol A.* 1990;29(4):196–203.

38. Sauerwein DI, Fischer W, Madersbacher J et al. Extradurale implantation of sacral anterior root stimulators. *Neurol Neurosurg Psychiatry.* 1990;53(8):681–4.

39. Krasmik D, Krebs J, van Ophoven A, and Pannek J. Urodynamic results, clinical efficacy, and complication rates of sacral intradural deafferentation and sacral anterior root stimulation in patients with neurogenic lower urinary tract dysfunction resulting from complete spinal cord injury. *Neurourol Urodyn.* 2014;33(8):1202–6.

40. Cardozo L, Krishnan K, Polkey CE, Rushton DN, and Brindley GS. Urodynamic observations on patients with sacral anterior root stimulators. *Paraplegia* 1984;22(4):201–9.

41. Possover M, Baekelandt J, Kaufmann A, and Chiantera V. Laparoscopic endopelvic sacral implantation of a Brindley controller for recovery of bladder function in a paralyzed patient. *Spinal Cord.* 2008;46(1):70–3.

42. Karam R, Bourbeau D, Majerus S et al. Real-time classification of bladder events for effective diagnosis and treatment of urinary incontinence. *IEEE Trans Biomed Eng.* 2016;63(4):721–9.

43. Jonas U and Tanagho EA. Studies on feasibility of urinary bladder evacuation by direct spinal cord stimulation II. Poststimulus voiding: A way to overcome outflow resistance. *Invest Urol.* 1975;13(2):151–3.

44. Gleason CA, Jünemann K, Alken P, and Tanagho EA. Physiologic bladder evacuation with selective sacral root stimulation: Sinusoidal signal and organ-specific frequency. *Neurourol Urodyn.* 2002;21(1):80–91.

45. Boger AS, Bhadra N, and Gustafson KJ. High frequency sacral root nerve block allows bladder voiding. *Neurourol Urodyn.* 2012;31(5):677–82.

46. Boger A, Bhadra N, and Gustafson KJ. Different clinical electrodes achieve similar electrical nerve conduction block. *J Neural Eng.* 2013;10(5):056016.

47. McGuire EJ, Zhang S, Horwinski ER, and Lytton B. Treatment of motor and sensory detrusor instability by electrical stimulation. *J Urol.* 1983;129(1):78–9.

48. Cooperburg MR, and Stoller M. Percutaneous neuromodulation. *Urol Cllin North Am.* 2005;32(1):71–8, vii.

49. Govier FE, Litwiller S, Nitti V et al. Percutaneous afferent neuromodulation for the refractory overactive bladder: Results of a multicenter study. *J Urol.* 2001;165:1193–8.

50. van Balken MR, Vandoninck V, Gisolf KW et al. Posterior tibial nerve stimulation as neuromodulative treatment of lower urinary tract dysfunction. *J Urol.* 2001;166:914–8.

51. Vandoninck V, Van Balken M, Finazzi Agró E et al. Posterior tibial nerve stimulation in the treatment of urge incontinence. *Neurourol Urodyn.* 2003;22:17–23.

52. Klingler HC, Pycha A, Schmidbauer J, and Marberger M. Use of peripheral neuromodulation of the S3 region for treatment of detrusor overactivity: A urodynamic-based study. *Urology.* 2000;56:766–71.

53. Hentzen C, Haddad R, Sheikh Ismaël S, Chesnel C, Robain G, Amarenco G, and GRAPPPA, Clinical research Group of perineal dysfunctions in older adults. Efficacy of posterior tibial nerve stimulation (PTNS) on overactive bladder in older adults. *Eur Geriatr Med.* 2018;9:249–253.

54. Guidelines EAU, Neuro-Urology 2020. https://uroweb.org/guideline/neuro-urology/

55. Tutolo M, Ammirati E, Heesakkers J et al. Efficacy and safety of sacral and percutaneous tibial neuromodulation in non-neurogenic lower urinary tract dysfunction and chronic pelvic pain: A systematic review of the literature. *Eur Urol.* 2018;73(3):406–18.

56. Scaldazza CV, Morosetti C, Giampieretti R, Lorenzetti R, and Baroni M. Percutaneous tibial nerve stimulation versus electrical stimulation with pelvic floor muscle training for overactive bladder syndrome in women: Results of a randomized controlled study. *Int Braz J Urol.* 2017;43(1):121–6.

57. Seth JH, Gonzales G, Haslam C et al. Feasibility of using a novel non-invasive ambulatory tibial nerve stimulation device for the home-based treatment of overactive bladder symptoms. *Transl Adrol Urol.* 2018;7(6):912–9.

58. Wheeler JS Jr, Walter J, and Zaszczurynski PJ. Bladder inhibition by penile nerve stimulation in spinal cord injury patients. *J Urol.* 1992;147(1):100–3.

59. Craggs M and McFarlane J. Neuromodulation of the lower urinary tract. *Exp Physiol.* 1999;84(1):149–60.

60. Kirkham AP, Shah N, Knight SL, Shah PJ, and Craggs MD. The acute effects of continuous and conditional neuromodulation on the bladder in spinal cord injury. *Spinal Cord.* 2001;39(8):420–8.

61. Dalmose AL, Rijkhoff N, Kirkeby HJ, Nohr M, Sinkjaer T, and Djurhuus JC. Conditional stimulation of the dorsal penile/clitoral nerve may increase cystometric capacity in patients with spinal cord injury. *Neurourol Urodyn.* 2003;22(2):130–7.

62. Hansen J, Media S, Nohr M, Biering-Sorenson F, Sinkjaer T, and Rijkhoff NJ. Treatment of neurogenic detrusor overactivity in spinal cord injured patients by conditional electrical stimulation. *J Urol.* 2005;173(6):2035–9.

63. Opisso E, Borau A, Rodríguez A, Hansen J, and Rijkhoff NJ. Patient controlled versus automatic stimulation of pudendal nerve afferents to treat neurogenic detrusor overactivity. *J Urol.* 2008;180(4):1403–8.

64. Horvath EE, Yoo P, Amundsen CL, Webster GD, and Grill WM. Conditional and continuous electrical stimulation increase cystometric capacity in persons with spinal cord injury. *Neurourol Urodyn.* 2010;29(3):401–7.

65. Lee YH, Kim J, Im HT, Lee KW, Kim SH, and Hur DM. Semiconditional electrical stimulation of pudendal nerve afferents stimulation to manage neurogenic detrusor overactivity in patients with spinal cord injury. *Ann Rehabil Med.* 2011;35(5):605–12.

66. Fjorback MV, Rijkhoff N, Petersen T, Nohr M, and Sinkjaer T. Event driven electrical stimulation of the dorsal penile/clitoral nerve for management of neurogenic detrusor overactivity in multiple sclerosis. *Neurourol Urodyn.* 2006;25(4):349–55.

67. Lee Y, Creasey GH, Lim H, Song J, Song K, and Kim J. Detrusor and blood pressure responses to dorsal penile nerve stimulation during hyperreflexic contraction of the bladder in patients with cervical cord injury. *Arch Phys Med Rehabil.* 2003;84(1):136–40.

68. Reitz A, Schmid D, Curt A, Knapp PA, and Schurch B. Autonomic dysreflexia in response to pudendal nerve stimulation. *Spinal Cord.* 2003;41(10):539–42.

69. Sundin T, Carlsson C, and Kock NG. Detrusor inhibition induced from mechanical stimulation of the anal region and from electrical stimulation of pudendal nerve afferents. An experimental study in cats. *Invest Urol.* 1974;11(5):374–8.

70. Lindstrom S, Fall M, Carlsson CA, and Erlandson BE. The neurophysiological basis of bladder inhibition in response to intravaginal electrical stimulation. *J Urol.* 1983;129(2):405–10.

71. Lee YH and Creasey GH. Self-controlled dorsal penile nerve stimulation to inhibit bladder hyperreflexia in incomplete spinal cord injury: A case report. *Arch Phys Med Rehabil.* 2002;83(2):273–7.

72. Wheeler JS Jr, Walter J, and Sibley P. Management of incontinent SCI patients with penile stimulation: Preliminary results. *J Am Paraplegia Soc.* 1994;17(2):55–9.

73. Goldman H, Amundsen CL, Mangel J et al. Dorsal genital nerve stimulation for the treatment of overactive bladder symptoms. *Neurourol Urodyn.* 2008;27(6):499–50.

74. Lee YH, Kim S, Kim JM, Im HT, Choi IS, and Lee KW. The effect of semiconditional dorsal penile nerve electrical stimulation on capacity and compliance of the bladder with deformity in spinal cord injury patients: A pilot study. *Spinal Cord.* 2012;50(4):289–93.

75. Tanagho EA and Schmidt RA. Electrical stimulation in the clinical management of the neurogenic bladder. *J Urol.* 1998;140:1331–9.

76. Tanagho EA, Schmidt RA, and Orvis BR. Neural stimulation for control of voiding dysfunction: A preliminary report in 22 patients with serious neuropathic voiding disorders. *J Urol.* 1989;142:340–5.

77. Kessler TM, La Framboise D, Trelle S et al. Sacral neuromodulation for neurogenic lower urinary tract dysfunction: Systematic review and meta-analysis. *Eur Urol.* 2010;58(6):865–74.

78. Amend B, Matzel K, Abrams P, de Groat WC, and Sievert KD. How does neuromodulation work? *Neurourol Urodyn.* 2011;30(5):762–5.

79. Amend B, Bedke J, Khalil M, Stenzl A, and Sievert KD. Prolonged percutaneous SNM testing does not cause infection-related explanation. *BJU Int.* 2013;111(3):485–91.

80. De Wachter S, Vaganee D, Kessler TM. Sacral neuromodulation: Mechanism of action. *Eur Urol Focus.* 2020. doi: 10.1016/j.euf.2019.11.018. [Epub ahead of print]

81. Kurstjens M. Intraoperative recording of electroneurographic signals from cuff electrodes on the extradural sacral roots in humans. *Neururol Urodyn.* 2005;13(3):428–35.

82. Craggs M. SPARSI: An implant to empty the bladder and control incontinence without a posterior rhizotomy in spinal cord injury. *Br J Urol.* 2000;85(Suppl 2).

83. Chartier-Kastler EJ, Ruud Bosch JL, Perrigot M, Chancellor MB, Richard F, and Denys P. Long-term results of sacral nerve stimulation (S3) for the treatment of neurogenic refractory urge incontinence related to detrusor hyper-reflexia. *J Urol.* 2000;164:1476–80.

84. Yoo PB, Horvath E, Amundsen CL, Webster GD, and Grill WM. Multiple pudendal sensory pathways reflexly modulate bladder and urethral activity in patients with spinal cord injury. *J Urol.* 2011;185(2):737–43.

85. Schmidt RA, Bruschini H, and Tanagho EA. Urinary bladder and sphincter responses to stimulation of dorsal and ventral sacral roots. *Investigative Urol.* 1979;16:300–4.

86. Talalla A and Bloom JW. Sacral electrical stimulation for bladder control. In: Illis LS, ed. *Functional Stimulation (Spinal Cord Dysfunction, III).* Oxford, UK: Oxford University Press; 1992:206–18.

87. Sauerwein D. Surgical treatment of spastic bladder paralysis in paraplegic patients. Sacral deafferentation with implantation of a sacral anterior root stimulator. *Urologe A.* 1990;29:196–203.

88. Creasey GH. Electrical stimulation of sacral roots for micturition after spinal cord injury. *Urol Clin North Am.* 1993;20:505–15.

89. Sanders PMH, Ijzerman M, Roach MJ, and Gustafson KJ. Patient preferences for next generation neural prostheses to restore bladder function. *Spinal Cord.* 2010;49:113–9.

90. Sievert KD, Amend B, Gakis G et al. Early sacral neuromodulation prevents urinary incontinence after complete spinal cord injury. *Ann Neurol.* 2010;67(1):74–84.

91. Frodisch S, Frodisch Z, and Zimmermann S. A new technique for minimal invasive complete spinal cord injury in minipigs. *INUM Meeting*, Zurich, 2016.

92. Frodisch EE, Miclaus G, Patras I et al. A new technique for minimal invasive complete spinal cord injury in minipigs. *Acta Neurochir (Wien)*. 2018;160(3):459–65.

93. Redshaw JD, Lenherr S, Elliott SP et al. ; Neurogenic Bladder Research Group (Evaluation of the axonics modulation technologies sacral neuromodulation system for the treatment of urinary and fecal dysfunction. NBRG.org). Protocol for a randomized clinical trial investigating early sacral nerve stimulation as an adjunct to standard neurogenic bladder management following acute spinal cord injury. *BMC Urol*. 2018;18(1):72.

94. Cohn JA, Kowalik CG, Kaufman MR, Reynolds WS, Milam DF, and Dmochowski RR. Evaluation of the axonics modulation technologies sacral neuromodulation system for the treatment of urinary and fecal dysfunction. *Expert Rev Med Devices*. 2017;14(1):3–14.

95. Susan Heins. Axonics modulation tech receives CE mark for Its sacral neuromodulation system for the treatment of urinary and fecal dysfunction Jun 06,. 2016. https://www.biospace.com/article/releases/axonics-modulation-tech-receives-ce-mark-for-its-sacral-neuromodulation-system-for-the-treatment-of-urinary-and-fecal-dysfunction-/

96. https://www.fda.gov/medical-devices/recently-approved-devices/axonics-sacral-neuromodulation-snm-system-urinary-control-p180046

97. Blok B, Van Kerrebroeck P, deWachter S et al. A prospective, multicenter study of a novel, miniaturized rechargeable sacral neuromodulation system: 12-month results from the RELAX-OAB study. *Neurourol Urodyn*. 2019;38(2):689–95.

98. Siegel S, Noblett K, Mangel J et al. Results of a prospective, randomized, multicenter study evaluating sacral neuromodulation with InterStim therapy compared to standard medical therapy at 6-months in subjects with mild symptoms of overactive bladder. *Neurourol Urodyn*. 2015;34(3):224–30.

99. Siegel S, Noblett K, Mangel J et al. Five-year followup results of a prospective, multicenter study of patients with overactive bladder treated with sacral neuromodulation. *J Urol*. 2018;199(1):229–36.

100. Bycroft JA, Craggs M, Sheriff M, Knight S, and Shah PJ. Does magnetic stimulation of sacral nerve roots cause contraction or suppression of the bladder? *Neurourol Urodyn*. 2004;23(3):241–5.

101. Mendez A, Sawan M, Minagawa T, and Wyndaele JJ. Estimation of bladder volume from afferent neural activity. *IEEE Trans Neural Syst Rehabil Eng*. 2013;21(5):704–15.

102. Bourbeau D, Majerus S, Makovey I, Goldman HB, Damaser MS, and Bhunia S. Real-time classification of bladder events for effective diagnosis and treatment of urinary incontinence. *IEEE Trans Biomed Eng*. 2016;63(4):721–9.

103. Karam R, Majerus S, Bourbeau DJ, Damaser MS, and Bhunia S. Tunable and lightweight on-chip event detection for implantable bladder pressure monitoring devices. *IEEE Trans Biomed Circuits Syst*. 2017;11(6):1303–12.

104. Li P, Liao L, Chen G, Zhang F, and Tian Y. Early low-frequency stimulation of the pudendal nerve can inhibit detrusor overactivity and delay progress of bladder fibrosis in dogs with spinal cord injuries. *Neurorehabil Neural Repair*. 2009;23(6):615–26.

105. Gaunt RA and Prochazka A. Transcutaneously coupled, high-frequency electrical stimulation of the pudendal nerve blocks external urethral sphincter contractions. *Neurorehabil Neural Repair*. 2009;23(6):615–26.

106. Foditsch EE, Roider K, Patras I et al. Structural changes of the urinary bladder after chronic complete spinal cord injury in minipigs. *Int Neurourol J*. 2017;21(1):12–9.

107. De Groat WC. Nervous control of the urinary bladder of the cat. *Brain Res*. 1975;87:201–11.

108. Thor KB, Roppolo JR, Kawatani M, Erdman S, and deGroat WC. Plasticity in spinal opioid control of lower urinary tract function in paraplegic cats. *Neuroreport*. 1994;5(13):1673–8.

109. Brose SW, Bourbeau D, and Gustafson KJ. Genital nerve stimulation is tolerable and effective for bladder inhibition in sensate individuals with incomplete SCI. *J Spinal Cord Med*. 2018;41(2):174–81.

110. Knight SL, Edirisinghe N, Leaker B, Susser J, and Craggs MD. Conditional neuromodulation of neurogenic detrusor overactivity using transrectal stimulation in patients with spinal cord injury: A proof of principle study. *Neurourol Urodyn*. 2018;37(1):385–93.

111. Zheng M-X, Hua X-Y, Feng J-T et al. Trial of contralateral seventh cervical nerve transfer for spastic arm paralysis. *N Engl J Med*. 2018;378:22–34.

112. Li R, Li Y, Wu Y et al. Heparin-poloxamer thermosensitive hydrogel loaded with bFGF and NGF enhances peripheral nerve regeneration in diabetic rats. *Biomaterials*. 2018;168:24–37.

113. Darie R, Powell M, and Borton D. Delivering the sense of touch to the human brain. *Neuron*. 2017;93:728.

114. Capogrosso M, Milekovic T, Borton D et al. A brain-spinal interface alleviating gait deficits after spinal cord injury in primates. *Nature*. 2016;539:284–8.

115. Zheng H, Zhang Z, Jiang S et al. A shape-memory and spiral light-emitting device for precise multisite stimulation of nerve bundles. *Nature Commun*. 2019;10(1):2790.

116. Atala A, Bauer SB Soker S Yoo JJ Retik AB. Tissue-engineered autologous bladders for patients needing cystoplasty. *Lancet*. 2006;367(9518):1241–6.

117. De Wachter S, Knowles CH, Elterman DS, Kennelly MJ, Lehur PA, Matzel KE, Engelberg S, Van Kerrebroeck PEV. New technologies and applications in sacral neuromodulation: An Update. *Adv Ther*. 2020;37(2):637-643.

Chapter 31

SURGERY TO IMPROVE RESERVOIR FUNCTION

John P. Lavelle

THEORY

The actual storage volume of the normal human urinary bladder is quite variable and depends on a number of integrated factors under normal physiologic circumstances. The capacity of the bladder depends on intact storage reflexes,[1] which when the bladder is full, allow the voiding reflexes to take over, and at a socially appropriate time, enable voiding in a controlled coordinated manner. In women, normal bladder capacity ($n = 161$) ranges from 81 mL to 514 mL based on voiding diaries.[2] The urodynamic bladder capacity in normal subjects ($n = 28$ women 10 men) was on average 338 ± 242 mL (range 41–1281 mL) on free uroflow measurements and for men 541.3 ± 146.2 mL, range 317–926 mL and women 453 ± 146 mL range 321–822 mL on cystometry.[3] Large bladder capacity would be regarded as over 700 mL.[4] Children's bladder capacity is considered in two formulae: (1) $2 \times$ age (years) $+ 2 =$ capacity (ounces) up to 2 and (2) age (years) divided by $2 + 6 =$ capacity (ounces) for 2 years and older.[5]

Normal bladder compliance is considered to be greater than 30 mL in neurogenic bladders and greater than 40 mL per centimeter water.[6,3]

Urine storage should be at low pressures, and based on compliance measurements the end filling pressures should range between 10 and 15 cm water above baseline for normal capacities. Determination of small bladder capacity is up to the individual clinician. A reasonable volume to be considered small capacity would be less than 150 mL.[7] Poor compliance (less than 10 mL/cm water) unresponsive to treatment would also be considered an indication for bladder enlargement surgery.[8,9]

Neurologic injury leads to changes in muscle tension, and also in its reflexes, and the ability of the bladder to actively or passively accommodate and store urine. The chronic inflammatory changes also alter the matrix components of the bladder with an increased ratio of type III to type I collagen and suppression of elastin formation, which reduces compliance and thus shrinks the bladder capacity[7] with development

of potentially high storage pressures, and resultant leakage (incontinence), or reflux of urine, leading to renal damage by direct pressure or by recurrent episodes of pyelonephritis with scarring resulting in decreased renal function.

The primary principle of surgery to increase storage is to alter the bladder wall so that the storage pressures are decreased, and the storage volume expanded, in principle, with the law of LaPlace. The complications of reflux and renal damage may not be reversed; however, the aim is to stabilize these injuries, thus preventing further future damage. Importantly, if high-grade vesicoureteral reflux is present, this may not be reversible.

The primary outcomes are the reversal of the patient's symptoms and stabilization of conditions that may impair renal function or other complications. These include reduction in episodes of urinary tract infection, reduction in episodes of pyelonephritis, stabilization of renal function, reduced or cured urinary incontinence, and improvement in quality of life for the individual patient. By the same token, patient expectations on the outcomes should be carefully reviewed and understood by the patient, so that the patient's and surgeon's expectations are set to a reasonable outcome. The complications of metabolic upset, long-term complications to bone, vitamin B deficiency, bowel habit changes, augmentation failure, and potential of cancer need to be thoroughly discussed with and understood by the patient and caregivers prior to undertaking these surgeries, particularly in female patients, who may desire childbearing later.

SURGICAL PROCEDURES

DETRUSOR MYOMECTOMY
Indication: This procedure was originally described in children for patients with poor bladder capacity, decreased compliance, and intolerance or unresponsiveness to conservative measures to alter these parameters. Similarly, the procedure may be an option to be considered instead of augmentation

cystoplasty, as it avoids the metabolic side effects of enterocystoplasty. Stohrer et al. described its use in patients with spinal cord injury ($n = 11$)[8] (Figure 31.1).

Procedure: Originally described by Cartwright and Snow in 1989[9] (Figure 31.2), it primarily consists of carefully removing the muscle from the dome of the bladder, and thus creating a very large bladder diverticulum. Essentially, as an open procedure, an area around the dome is carefully circumscribed from posterior to anterior initially in the midline and then circumferentially, about three-quarters of the distance to the urothelium, with electrocautery and the rest of the way carefully separated using a hemostat; the bladder is then filled through a Foley catheter; and then Allis clamps are applied to one edge and the muscle of the dome of the bladder is carefully removed working laterally. This creates a very large diverticulum. Care is taken to not make holes in the urothelium. Bilateral psoas hitches are then performed with absorbable suture. It is generally considered that the extra capacity has to be maintained early after the operation, but how much volume or pressure has not been determined. Postoperatively, a cystogram should be performed to check for leakage, prior to restarting the intermittent catheterization, usually around 5–6 days, and also

a drain should be placed near the operative site to detect and control any urinary leaks and removed after confirmation of no leaks. The procedure seems to work well where the patients are younger, and also when the bladder capacity is about 75%–80% of expected capacity for age.[10]

Results: Cartwright initially reported on seven patients, aged 4–17 years with 4–24 months of follow-up. One was a technical failure, underwent enterocystoplasty, six were reported, all became continent, and except for one, all had improved bladder capacities. Two with decreased renal function improved, and one had improvement of hypertension. One who had six prior pelvic operations did not have resolution of symptoms and underwent enterocystoplasty 2.5 months postoperatively. One had vesicoureteral reflux (VUR), which was repaired at the time of autoaugmentation. Hansen et al. report that 19/25 children were continent on clean intermittent catheterization (CIC), with 4 undergoing enterocystoplasty. The follow-up was 0.1–15.6 years. They also recommended that the procedure is indicated for those with 50% of expected bladder capacity. Veenboer[11] reported in 47 adult myelodysplastic patients a similar success rate with only 4/25 requiring a enterocystoplasty, but the starting point was 80% of expected bladder capacity.

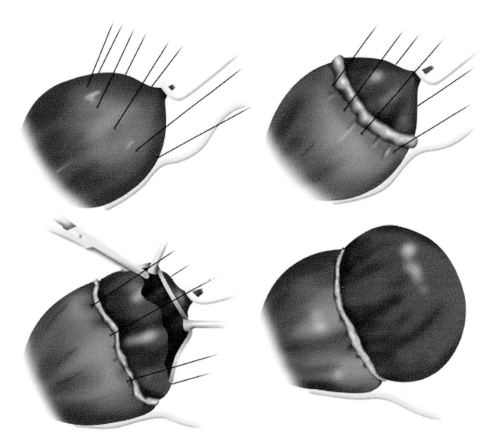

Figure 31.1   The auto-augmentation procedure (side view).

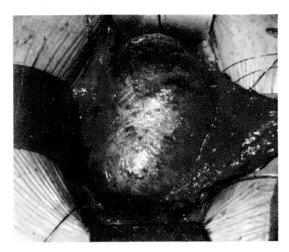

Figure 31.2 Surgical view during auto-augmentation procedure.

The results in both studies showed good increase in bladder capacity and compliance maintained over several years of follow-up.

However, MacNeily[12] reported that 15 of 17 patients failed with a 4–126 month follow-up period. A number of concomitant procedures were performed with this original myomectomy, and the authors did not introduce early bladder cycling. These may potentially be contributing factors in failure of the procedure. Eight of 17 patients failed to achieve continence, and 5 had hydronephrosis, of which 4 had enterocystoplasty.

Similarly, Marte[13] reported on 11 children with mean age 12.8 years with mean follow-up of 6.6 years. At 1 year, all had increased bladder capacities, with no reflux; however, over the follow-up period, four developed recurrent high-grade reflux, and one an hourglass deformity of the auto-augmentation; four patients had incontinence. The authors report that 7/11 failed the procedure. It should be noted that prior to the original auto-augmentation, four had vesicoureteral reflux treated by subtrigonal injections, of whom all but one had redeveloped the reflux at follow-up. It is also noted that Marte's and MacNeily's surgical techniques included suturing the bladder to the side wall of the pelvis in some fashion, which is not described in the original procedure.

Complications: The primary problem with this procedure is the ability to technically perform the operation without injuring the urothelium and causing perforations. Variously reported are fibrosis of the urothelium and also problems with formation of a narrow neck of the diverticulum leading to recurrent urinary tract infections (UTIs). It is also possible that the patients can perforate the diverticulum with the catheter during catheterization, which may require repair. Failure due to fibrosis may be addressed by enterocystoplasty.

Attempts to prevent fibrosis of the auto-augmented bladder included use of omental wrapping, dura patches, and demucosalized bowel or stomach, without success.

Conclusion: Like all other procedures for managing a neurogenic bladder, it is not ideal and does not pretend to provide a perfect solution. Auto-augmentation is and still remains a useful procedure, particularly when the bladder capacity is reasonable, compliance is poor, the patient is young, and there are reasons to augment with the urothelium, such as prevention of worsening acidosis, or concerns about long-term bone health. However, it is expected that the patient maintains the CIC regimen with care and attention to detail, as well as has constant follow-up on the part of the urologist to make sure the procedure remains successful.

BLADDER AUGMENTATION

Indication: The primary indication for augmentation cystoplasty is loss of bladder compliance, complicated by vesicoureteral reflux with or without recurrent pyelonephritis, urinary incontinence, due to the loss of bladder capacity, and failure of other noninvasive or invasive therapies.

Contraindications: Contraindications include short gut syndromes, inflammatory bowel disease, and potentially prior pelvic irradiation due to wound healing concerns. Patients with creatinine clearances below 40 mL/min may become more acidotic. However, controversy exists regarding use of bladder augmentation in renal insufficiency and also as a prelude to transplantation.[14-16] Also, all patients should be capable of performing CIC postoperatively to make sure that the bladder is adequately drained.

Procedure: Using a lower midline or Pfannenstiel incision, the bladder is exposed and the various segments of bowel for enterocystoplasty considered. The terminal ileum is the most commonly used segment; however, the augment segment may be made from sigmoid colon, or stomach depending on the characteristics of the bowel segment chosen. It is important that the mesentery of the chosen segment can easily reach the bladder (usually marked by reaching the pubic symphysis) and can lay on the posterior abdominal wall when routed to the bladder easily, to prevent tension and ischemia on the segment used. The augmented segment is composed of a detubularized segment of bowel, which in the case of the ileum, should be sewn together to create a larger patch. This in turn is then attached to a very widely opened bladder either transversely or in the anterior to posterior line or sometimes a U-shaped incision is used. This is important to maintain a wide-open augment and prevent an "hourglass" deformity that would render the augmentation useless. Also important is that the vascular pedicle is not on tension. Following attachment of the augment, the bladder volume is tested for leaks and then drained with a wide suprapubic (SP) tube, and Jackson-Pratt or similar drain on the outside. Bowel continuity is reestablished after isolation of the bowel segment. The wound is then closed, and the patient is allowed to recover. A cystogram is performed at about 2 weeks to check for leaks, and then the Foley is removed and SP capped. The patient may then be started on or resume CIC for bladder management; if problematic, the SP tube can be opened as a safety maneuver to drain the bladder. In the initial phases, there may be a lot of mucus production from the bowel, which may need to be irrigated out with a larger catheter.

Results: All studies report significant increases in bladder capacity with decreased storage pressures. Stabilization of hydronephrosis is also reported, or no subjects report developing postoperative hydronephrosis. Continence was reported from 67% to 100%. The complication rate is reported up to 40%–45%, and complications occur either early (within 3 years) or late (after 10 years). In one study, 41% of subjects had recurrent UTIs. Bowel problems were reported in 18%–22% of patients. In 86%–92%, improved quality of life parameters were reported. In one study, 3/79 patients died within 1 year of the procedure. The follow-up period was 6–10 years.[17-20]

Complications: Early complications include wound infections 5%–6.4%, small bowel obstruction 3%–5.7%, and bleeding with reoperation 0%–3%.[21] Revision surgery where the augmentation has failed is reported in 5%–42% of patients.[22] Subsequent augmentation or bladder malignancy occurs at a rate between 0 and 5%; however, controversy exists as to whether this truly represents an actual increased risk in malignancy, and also whether to screen for the malignancy. Approximately 90% of the malignancies are diagnosed at least 10 years after augmentation.[23-30] Screening for malignancies in bladder augmentations

and neurogenic bladder is controversial, as screening programs seem to have a low yield; however, if the patient presents with unexplained gross hematuria, the workup should be performed.

Up to 15% of patients postaugmentation may develop renal insufficiency progressing to renal failure. Also hyperchloremic acidosis requiring oral bicarbonate may be seen in up to 16% of patients. Some patients also may have, due to their neurologic disease, weak bladder necks, leading to nocturnal incontinence, requiring anticholinergic medication and potentially bladder neck reconstruction or diversion. Other short-term complications may include transient diarrhea due to the interruption of bowel continuity, which usually clears up at about 3–4 months but may be persistent. Mucus formation from the bowel mucosa can be troublesome as it can lead to mucus collections that require removal by irrigation by large-bore catheter as well as occasionally by cystoscopy. Due to the persistent bacteriuria due to the intermittent catheterization and also changes in the pH due to bowel secretions, there may also be increased urinary stone formation that will need to be treated as required. Also, due to the interruption of the terminal ileum (if used), the absorption of vitamin B12 may be altered, leading to the need for parenteral supplementation to prevent macrocytic anemia and neurologic sequalae. This may take 3–4 years to appear due to generally good reserves of B12 in most well-nourished individuals.

In the spina bifida population, many are being transitioned to adult care as longevity improves; however, the death rate in this population continues to be higher than in the able-bodied population.[31]

Conclusion: Enterocystoplasty is the final option in bladder expansion surgery. The results are generally good; however, there are a number of morbidities associated with the procedure. The primary objectives of the procedure, to improve bladder pressures and decrease complications for the patient, appear to be met, and the long-term quality of life outcomes are considerably improved. Care must be taken in patient selection and consideration made of the patients' comorbidities, especially hand and residual renal function.

FUTURE RESEARCH

Xiao and his colleagues innovatively studied bladder reinnervation and developed a way to establish a somatic-autonomic reflex pathway by ventral root micro-anastomosis between L7 and S2 or S3 roots experimentally in rats.[32] With this technique, they claimed to control detrusor overactivity and detrusor-sphincter dyssynergia in patients with suprasacral lesions. Encouraged by their preliminary results, they constructed artificial somatic-autonomic reflex pathways (skin–CNS–bladder reflex) in patients with overactive detrusor and acontractile bladders, and in patients with spina bifida in China.[33] Results of this interesting technique are discussed in detail in Chapter 32.

Another important problem in neurogenic bladder is the loss of bladder compliance. To date, the pathophysiologic mechanisms are poorly understood. Kanai has reported that relaxin-2 may reduce the production of extracellular matrix in inflammatory conditions and has shown following irradiation in mice that bladder muscle contractility and compliance are maintained by reduction in irradiation-induced fibrosis. These results provide early encouragement that it may have useful clinical application, if the findings can be translated to human bladders.[34,35]

Another interesting problem deserving more research is the "normality" of the bladder capacity in neurogenic bladder. There are little data on the appropriate treatment for patients with tetraplegia or high paraplegia (T1 through T6) who experience autonomic dysreflexia at low bladder volumes, and whether these patients should undergo enterocystoplasty or ileovesicostomy to prevent the long-term damaging sequalae from repeated episodes of autonomic dysreflexia, particularly in relatively young patients.

REFERENCES

1. de Groat WC, Griffiths D, and Yoshimura N. Neural control of the lower urinary tract. *Compr Physiol.* 2015;5(1):327–96.
2. Amundsen CL, Parsons M, Tissot B, Cardozo L, Diokno A, and Coats AC. Bladder diary measurements in asymptomatic females: Functional bladder capacity, frequency, and 24-hr volume. *Neurourol Urodyn.* 2007;26(3):341–9.
3. Wyndaele JJ. Normality in urodynamics studied in healthy adults. *J Urol.* 1999;161(3):899–902.
4. Purohit RS, Blaivas JG, Saleem KL et al. The pathophysiology of large capacity bladder. *J Urol.* 2008;179(3):1006–11.
5. Kaefer M, Zurakowski D, Bauer SB et al. Estimating normal bladder capacity in children. *J Urol.* 1997; 158(6):2261–4.
6. D'Ancona C, Haylen B, Oelke M et al. The International Continence Society (ICS) report on the terminology for adult male lower urinary tract and pelvic floor symptoms and dysfunction. *Neurourol Urodyn.* 2019;38(2):433–77.
7. Cantu H, Maarof SNM, and Hashim H. The inflammatory contracted bladder. *Curr Bladder Dysfunct Rep.* 2019;14(2):67–74.
8. Stohrer M, Kramer G, Goepel M, Lochner-Ernst D, Kruse D, and Rubben H. Bladder autoaugmentation

9. in adult patients with neurogenic voiding dysfunction. *Spinal Cord.* 1997;35(7):456–62.
9. Cartwright PC and Snow BW. Bladder autoaugmentation: Early clinical experience. *J Urol.* 1989;142(2 Pt 2):505–8; discussion 20-1.
10. Du K, Mulroy EE, Wallis MC, Zhang C, Presson AP, and Cartwright PC. Enterocystoplasty 30-day outcomes from National Surgical Quality Improvement Program Pediatric 2012. *J Pediatr Surg.* 2015;50(9):1535–9.
11. Veenboer PW, Nadorp S, de Jong TP et al. Enterocystoplasty vs detrusorectomy: Outcome in the adult with spina bifida. *J Urol.* 2013;189(3):1066–70.
12. MacNeily AE, Afshar K, Coleman GU, and Johnson HW. Autoaugmentation by detrusor myotomy: Its lack of effectiveness in the management of congenital neuropathic bladder. *J Urol.* 2003;170(4 Pt 2):1643–6; discussion 6.
13. Marte A, Di Meglio D, Cotrufo AM, Di Iorio G, De Pasquale M, and Vessella A. A long-term follow-up of autoaugmentation in myelodysplastic children. *BJU Int.* 2002;89(9):928–31.
14. Mehmood S, Seyam R, Firdous S, and Altaweel WM. Factors predicting renal function outcome after augmentation cystoplasty. *Int J Nephrol.* 2017;2017:3929352.
15. Budzyn J, Trinh H, Raffee S, and Atiemo H. Bladder augmentation (enterocystoplasty): The current state of a historic operation. *Curr Urol Rep.* 2019;20(9):50.
16. Taghizadeh AK, Desai D, Ledermann SE et al. Renal transplantation or bladder augmentation first? A comparison of complications and outcomes in children. *BJU Int.* 2007;100(6):1365–70.
17. Alfrey EJ, Salvatierra O Jr, Tanney DC et al. Bladder augmentation can be problematic with renal failure and transplantation. *Pediatr Nephrol (Berlin, Germany).* 1997;11(6):672–5.
18. Khastgir J, Hamid R, Arya M, Shah N, and Shah PJ. Surgical and patient reported outcomes of 'clam' augmentation ileocystoplasty in spinal cord injured patients. *Eur Urol.* 2003;43(3):263–9.
19. Herschorn S and Hewitt RJ. Patient perspective of long-term outcome of augmentation cystoplasty for neurogenic bladder. *Urology.* 1998;52(4):672–8.
20. Wu SY and Kuo HC. A real-world experience with augmentation enterocystoplasty—High patient satisfaction with high complication rates. *Neurourol Urodyn.* 2018;37(2):744–50.
21. Biers SM, Venn SN, and Greenwell TJ. The past, present and future of augmentation cystoplasty. *BJU Int.* 2012;109(9):1280–93.
22. Woodhams SD, Greenwell TJ, Smalley T, and Mundy AR. Factors causing variation in urinary N-nitrosamine levels in enterocystoplasties. *BJU Int.* 2001;88(3):187–91.
23. Cohen AJ, Pariser JJ, Anderson BB, Pearce SM, and Gundeti MS. The robotic appendicovesicostomy and bladder augmentation: The next frontier in robotics, are we there? *Urol Clin North Am.* 2015;42(1):121–30.
24. Cohen AJ, Brodie K, Murthy P, Wilcox DT, and Gundeti MS. Comparative outcomes and perioperative complications of robotic vs open cystoplasty and complex reconstructions. *Urology.* 2016;97:172–8.
25. Gill IS, Rackley RR, Meraney AM, Marcello PW, and Sung GT. Laparoscopic enterocystoplasty. *Urology.* 2000;55(2):178–81.
26. Docimo SG, Moore RG, Adams J, and Kavoussi LR. Laparoscopic bladder augmentation using stomach. *Urology.* 1995;46(4):565–9.

27. Smith P and Hardy GJ. Carcinoma occurring as a late complication of ileocystoplasty. *Br J Urol.* 1971;43(5):576–9.

28. Higuchi TT, Granberg CF, Fox JA, and Husmann DA. Augmentation cystoplasty and risk of neoplasia: Fact, fiction and controversy. *J Urol.* 2010;184(6): 2492–6.

29. Biardeau X, Chartier-Kastler E, Roupret M, and Phe V. Risk of malignancy after augmentation cystoplasty: A systematic review. *Neurourol Urodyn.* 2016;35(6):675–82.

30. Oakeshott P, Hunt GM, Poulton A, and Reid F. Expectation of life and unexpected death in open spina bifida: A 40-year complete, non-selective, longitudinal cohort study. *Dev Med Child Neurol.* 2010;52(8):749–53.

31. Xiao CG, Du MX, Li B et al. An artificial somatic-autonomic reflex pathway procedure for bladder control in children with spina bifida. *J Urol.* 2005;173(6):2112–6.

32. Xiao CG, Du MX, Dai C, Li B, Nitti VW, and de Groat WC. An artificial somatic-central nervous system-autonomic reflex pathway for controllable micturition after spinal cord injury: Preliminary results in 15 patients. *J Urol.* 2003;170(4 Pt 1):1237–41.

33. Peters KM, Girdler B, Turzewski C et al. Outcomes of lumbar to sacral nerve rerouting for spina bifida. *J Urol.* 2010;184(2):702–7.

34. Ikeda Y, Zabbarova IV, Birder LA et al. Relaxin-2 therapy reverses radiation-induced fibrosis and restores bladder function in mice. *Neurourol Urodyn.* 2018;37(8):2441–51.

35. Kanai AJ, Konieczko EM, Bennett RG, Samuel CS, and Royce SG. Relaxin and fibrosis: Emerging targets, challenges, and future directions. *Mol Cell Endocrinol.* 2019;487:66–74.

Chapter 32

SURGERY TO IMPROVE BLADDER OUTLET FUNCTION

Dayron Rodríguez and Philippe E. Zimmern

INTRODUCTION

The bladder outlet in patients with neurogenic voiding dysfunction is subject to two main abnormalities: (1) outlet underactivity, leading to urine leakage during increases in intra-abdominal pressure and (2) nonrelaxing urethral sphincter, resulting in reduced urine flow during voiding. This chapter is therefore divided into two sections: surgical treatment of the underactive or incompetent bladder outlet and surgical treatment of the nonrelaxing or hyperactive bladder outlet (detrusor-sphincter dyssynergia [DSD]).

SURGICAL MANAGEMENT OF THE INCOMPETENT BLADDER OUTLET

URETHRAL BULKING AGENTS (UBAS)
INTRODUCTION
UBAs work by augmenting or restoring the normal mucosal coaptation, increasing the urethral closure while having a minimal effect on voiding pressures.[1] Despite advances in biomedical engineering, the development of an ideal urethral bulking agent remains a persistent challenge due to concerns over long-term efficacy, cost-effectiveness, and patient safety.[2]

MACROPLASTIQUE
The main advantage of Macroplastique is its relatively large particle diameter (greater than 100 μm), which reduces the risk of particle migration, as well as its nonallergenic nature.[3] Due to its viscous nature, it is injected with a high-pressure injection gun under direct vision with a cystoscope under local anesthesia. A systematic review of Macroplastique treatment for stress urinary incontinence (SUI) showed improvement rates between 64% and 75% with dry rates of 36%–43%.[4]

COAPTITE
Coaptite (diameter: 75–125 μm) is nonantigenic, nonimmunogenic, and nontoxic and fared comparably with collagen (no longer available since 2011).[5] It can be easily injected using standard cystoscopic equipment available in most urology offices, and the material does not require refrigeration.

BULKAMID
First introduced in Europe in 1996, Bulkamid is composed of 2.5% polyacrylamide hydrogel and 97.5% water for injections. In a promising study on SUI or mixed urinary incontinence, 82% of 256 patients were cured or significantly improved with a high satisfaction rate at 3-years follow-up.[6]

STEM CELL THERAPY
While stem cell therapy has been tested in animal models with favorable results, there are only a few clinical trials available that demonstrate safety and potential efficacy in patients with SUI.[7-10] Most of these trials report that most subjects found transient benefit, while others achieved durable results. Ongoing studies will determine its role in the minimally invasive management of SUI. At present, and in most Western countries, it is recommended that outside of investigative protocols, physicians should not offer stem cell therapy to patients with stress incontinence.

INDICATIONS
The optimal candidate for UBA should have a stable, compliant, good capacity bladder with no urethral hypermobility and intrinsic sphincter deficiency typically diagnosed as low Valsalva leak point pressure (VLPP). Many investigators believe that concurrent detrusor overactivity or decreased compliance should be treated with anticholinergics and/or augmentation cystoplasty before attempting to treat an incompetent outlet with bulking agents.[11]

CONCLUSION
UBA offers minimal invasiveness, is easy to learn, and has low morbidity. Furthermore, UBA treatment does not jeopardize the performance and efficacy of other anti-incontinence procedures later on. The shortcomings of UBA include potential for repeat injections and at times a lesser degree of effectiveness compared to more invasive treatment modalities. Furthermore, the bulk of literature on UBAs focuses on nonneurogenic SUI. More research is necessary

in this neurogenic population, mainly the one using clean intermittent catheterization (CIC).

BLADDER NECK SLINGS AND WRAPS
INTRODUCTION
The fascial sling is commonly employed to treat urinary incontinence secondary to neurogenic outlet incompetence. Since those patients are already on CIC, there is no concern on tensioning the sling. Furthermore, the incidence of tension-induced erosion is low when autologous fascia is utilized as the sling material. Unfortunately, long-term experience with the bladder neck sling in the adult neurogenic bladder population rarely exceeds 4 years.

INDICATIONS
The ideal candidate is a female patient with bladder outlet incompetence, preserved urethral length, and a well-managed bladder on CIC. Its role in men is more disputed due to anatomic limitations resulting in variable functional outcomes. Whether or not to perform a concomitant enterocystoplasty is based on preoperative urodynamic findings consistent with elevated bladder storage pressures. In general, a cystogram/videourodynamics showing a wide-open bladder neck and a low VLPP will influence a decision to improve the bladder outlet concurrently.

RESULTS AND COMPLICATIONS
The literature on bladder neck slings to treat neurogenic SUI consists largely of case series, made up of mostly pediatric patients (Table 32.1), with continence rates greater than 70%.[12-15] Complications specific to the rectus fascia sling are relatively rare and include sling breakdown, angulated urethra, bladder neck contracture, urethral erosion, *de novo* detrusor overactivity (DO), retroperitoneal hematoma, and incisional hernia.[12] Because of the risk of exposure/erosion, there is very limited experience with synthetic slings. In one review, overall improved continence rates ranged from 29% to 80%.[16]

CONCLUSION
The bladder neck sling is a versatile addition to the armamentarium of the reconstructive surgeon. Its long-term durability is poorly described, which is an important consideration for young adults in whom the procedure may have to last decades.

ARTIFICIAL URINARY SPHINCTER
INTRODUCTION
Since 1973, the artificial urinary sphincter (AUS) (Figure 32.1) has provided high rates of efficacy and patient satisfaction, but also substantial revision

Table 32.1 Results of Fascial Slings and Wraps in Patients with Neurogenic Bladder Outlet Incompetence

Study	Year and Patient Population	Number and Type of Patients	Mean Follow-up (months)	Surgical Technique	Results	Other Surgical Procedures
Fontaine et al.[13]	1997, adult F	21: 9 MMC, 8 SCI, 3 SA, 1 sacral lipoma	28.6, range 6–60	RF sling done transabdominally, sutured to Cooper's	85.7% dry day and night, 95.2% dry day only	All had concomitant bladder augmentation
Mingin et al.[14]	2002, pediatric and adult M and F	37: 14 M, 23 F 36 neurogenic, 1 traumatic	48, range 6–120	Distally based rectus/pyramidalis myofascial flap wrapped around BN and sewn to contralateral RF	92% (34) dry 2 M failures, 1 F failure	33 concomitant augmentations, 9 mitrofanoft stomas, 5 reimplantations
Rutman et al.[15]	2005, adult F	Neurologic/congenital diseases, multiple prior anti-incontinence procedures	12 months, range 6–37	Soft polypropylene mesh wrap secured to anterior abdominal wall	20% failures, 80% improved or cured	91% concomitant urethrolysis, 20% concomitant prolapse repair
Athanasopoulos et al.[12]	2012, adult F	Mean age 37 years (range: 10–67) 21 MMC, 12 SCI	48 months	RF sling done	75.75% (25) totally dry, 5 15.15% (5) had markedly improved but still required one pad per day	14 concomitant augmentation cystoplasty and 3 myectomy

Abbreviations: BN, bladder neck; F, female; M, male; MMC, myelomeningocele; SA, sacral agenesis; SCI, spinal cord injury; RF, rectus fascia; SUI, stress urinary incontinence.

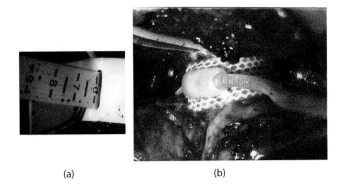

(a)   (b)

Figure 32.1   (a) Artificial urinary sphincter has been sized loosely and (b) placed around the proximal urethra.

rates secondary to mechanical failure, infection, and erosion resulting in sphincter removal.

INDICATIONS

The ideal candidate for an AUS should have a stable bladder with good compliance and capacity as well as adequate emptying. Elevated detrusor pressures can lead to upper tract deterioration once the outlet is occluded by the sphincter cuff. Many authors advocate an AUS as primary treatment for patients who void with weak or absent detrusor contraction, as those are the most likely to end up in lifelong retention should a fascial sling be performed.[17]

RESULTS

AUS continence rates range from 50% to 92%, with revision rates of 27%–57%, and removal rates of 19%–41% (Table 32.2).[18–22] In women, the procedure is less frequently performed due to technical challenges, including retropubic dissection of the whole urethra from the vaginal wall and proper sizing. More recently, robotic approaches have afforded good visualization and limited morbidity in expert hands.[23]

CONCLUSIONS

Despite many design modifications, AUS remains a time-tested procedure in this population for the well-selected patient aware of its risks and complications over time, including revisions. Newer sphincters and advances in robotics may further encourage its use.

BLADDER NECK CLOSURE

Bladder neck closure is a last-resort procedure[24] in patients with outlet incompetence who have failed multiple anti-incontinence procedures; those who are poor surgical candidates and cannot tolerate lengthy, complex reconstructive procedures; and cases of a destroyed urethra.[25] Closure of the bladder neck can be combined with a catheterizable cutaneous stoma or a chronic indwelling suprapubic tube depending on the constitutional and functional status of the

patient. In young males there are additional concerns regarding potency and ejaculation.[26] Bladder neck closure is highly effective with continence rates of 75%–100% at mean follow-up ranging from 1.5 to 3 years.[25,27–29] The main technical complication is bladder neck fistulization with continued leakage of urine, which has been reported to occur in 6%–25% of cases.[25,27–29]

SURGICAL TREATMENT OF HYPERACTIVE BLADDER OUTLET

INTRODUCTION

Detrusor external sphincter dyssynergia (DESD) is a common condition in patients with suprasacral spinal cord lesions, is associated with elevated intravesical pressures, and can result in substantial morbidity and mortality. By incising the external sphincter, sphincterotomy will result in continuous incontinence managed with a condom catheter. Botulinum toxin A (BTX-A), with its ability to induce a reversible chemical sphincterotomy, provides another option.

SPHINCTEROTOMY
INDICATIONS

Sphincterotomy is employed in the treatment of DESD in male patients with suprasacral spinal cord lesions and DO refractory to anticholinergics and CIC, or in those unable or unwilling to CIC. Sphincterotomy with condom catheter drainage may be preferable to a chronic indwelling catheter, which is still often used as the management of last resort in quadriplegic patients who do not have manual dexterity or caregiver support to perform CIC or change a condom catheter. Chronic indwelling catheters are associated with recurrent urosepsis, bladder calculi, and squamous cell carcinoma in this patient population.[30]

Table 32.2 Results of Artificial Urinary Sphincter Insertion for the Treatment of Incontinence in Patients with Neurogenic Bladder

Study	Year	Patient Population	Type and Location of Sphincter	Mean Follow-up Time	Results	Complications
Spiess et al.[22]	2002	Pediatric, 30 males with MMC	All AMS 800	6.5 years	63% dry, 20%, slightly wet	Only 8.3% lasted more than 100 months, mean lifetime 4.9 years
Pereira et al.[21]	2006	Adolescents: 35, 13 F, 22 M, MM 27, SA 4, 4 other	All AMS 800, BN, 13 also had augment	5.5 years (range 4–11)	91.4% dry	8.6% BN erosions, 20% mechanical failure, 7 with worsened bladder function
Bersch et al.[18]	2008	37 M + 14 F 37 SCI, 8 MMC, 2 others	Modified AMS 800, Peri-bladder neck	7.9 years (5–14.5)	90.2%	8% (4) infection, 27% (14) mechanical failure
Chartier et al.[19]	2011	Average age 35 years (18–58 years) MM16, SCI	All AMS 800, Junction between the bladder neck and the anterior face of the prostate	83 months (6–208 months)	74% had perfect or moderate continence	Complications noted in 19% (10/51), within 30 days after surgery: urinary infection (8), acute urinary retention (3), transient intracranial hypertension (1 myelomeningocele patient), and failure to perform IC (1)
Guillot-Tantay et al.[20]	2018	35 14 M patients, 4 SCI and 10 spina bifida	All AMS 800, Peribulbar ($n = 4$) and periprostatic position ($n = 10$)	18.3 years IQR (10.1–20.3 years)	50% continence rate	21.4% explanted due to erosion or infection.

Abbreviations: BN, bladder neck; BU, bulbar urethra; MMC, myelomeningocele; SA, sacral agenesis; SCI, spinal cord injury; UTI, urinary tract infection.

RESULTS AND COMPLICATIONS OF SPHINCTEROTOMY

Incising the external sphincter results in significant decreases in maximum detrusor pressure, postvoid residual, and the occurrence of autonomic dysreflexia. Bladder capacity is usually maintained. Sphincterotomy is irreversible and has been associated with intraoperative bleeding, clot retention, urosepsis, erectile dysfunction, and sphincterotomy failure secondary to urethral scarring. A reduction in long-term efficacy has also been observed, which may require repeat external sphincter or bladder neck incision.[31] Long-term use of a condom catheter can lead to skin ulceration, urethrocutaneous fistula, and penile retraction.[32] Treatment failure despite a technically perfect sphincterotomy occurs in 10%–50% of men treated for DESD. Reasons for failure include problems fitting the condom catheter as well as detrusor areflexia, which can result in poor bladder emptying despite an incompetent bladder outlet.[32]

BOTULINUM TOXIN A INJECTION INTO THE EXTERNAL URETHRAL SPHINCTER

INDICATIONS AND PATIENT SELECTION

BTX-A injection is a solution for patients with neurogenic hyperactive bladder outlet who have not decided to undergo surgical sphincterotomy. Dissatisfaction is mainly due to an increased incontinence grade that cannot be anticipated before the injection.[33]

RESULTS AND COMPLICATIONS

BTX-A injections effectively treat DESD symptoms with improvement rates 60%–88% at a mean follow-up ranging from 3 to 16 months.[34–37] Patient symptom improvements are related to decreased maximal voiding pressures leading to decreased postvoid residual volumes and lower CIC frequency, ultimately resulting in lower urinary tract infection rates. The effects last 3–9 months, with no significant adverse events reported.

CONCLUSION

Refractory DESD continues to be challenging. Sphincterotomy will undoubtedly continue to be considered in the management of these difficult cases, especially for patients who are unwilling or unable to perform CIC. For BTX-A injection, side effects such as incontinence and reinjection frequency have contributed to a low patient satisfaction rate and quality of life improvement. Long-term studies are lacking to firmly establish its role in DESD management.

CONCLUSIONS

The surgeon endeavoring to treat a patient with urinary incontinence secondary to neuropathic bladder outlet incompetence has a number of surgical options at his or her disposal. Injectable agents are often employed in female patients with mild degrees of incontinence, patients who leak small amounts after bladder neck sling or reconstruction, and patients who are not operative candidates or who are reluctant to undergo open surgery. The sling and AUS are commonly used when a more durable, long-term solution for incontinence is required. Because slings may be more successful in females than in males, some surgeons prefer to use slings as their first-line treatment in females and AUS as their primary treatment in males with neurogenic sphincteric incompetence. The fascial sling may be preferable to the AUS in patients who do not wish to have a foreign body implanted or who, because of their comorbidities or surgical history, are at high risk for cuff erosion or infection of the device. Bladder neck closure is a suitable option for select patients who have failed multiple surgical attempts to increase outlet resistance or who have poor functional and constitutional status. Sphincterotomy has been shown to be effective for DESD. Choice of treatment option is often guided by the irreversibility of sphincterotomy compared to BTX-A injection, but this most recent modality requires lifelong retreatments. Newer tools have emerged including new UBA agents and robotics for AUS placement, which may influence the long-term management of these patients.

REFERENCES

1. Hussain SM and Bray R. Urethral bulking agents for female stress urinary incontinence. *Neurourol Urodyn.* 2019;38(3):887–92.
2. Davis NF, Kheradmand F, and Creagh T. Injectable biomaterials for the treatment of stress urinary incontinence: Their potential and pitfalls as urethral bulking agents. *Int Urogynecol J.* 2013;24(6):913–9.
3. ter Meulen PH, Berghmans LC, Nieman FH, and van Kerrebroeck PE. Effects of Macroplastique implantation system for stress urinary incontinence and urethral hypermobility in women. *Int Urogynecol J Pelvic Floor Dysfunct.* 2009;20(2):177–83.
4. Ghoniem GM and Miller CJ. A systematic review and meta-analysis of Macroplastique for treating female stress urinary incontinence. *Int Urogynecol J.* 2013;24(1):27–36.
5. Mayer RD, Dmochowski RR, Appell RA et al. Multicenter prospective randomized 52-week trial of calcium hydroxylapatite versus bovine dermal collagen for treatment of stress urinary incontinence. *Urology.* 2007;69(5):876–80.
6. Pai A and Al-Singary W. Durability, safety and efficacy of polyacrylamide hydrogel (Bulkamid®) in the management of stress and mixed urinary incontinence: Three year follow up outcomes. *Cent European J Urol.* 2015;68(4):428–33.
7. Gras S, Klarskov N, and Lose G. Intraurethral injection of autologous minced skeletal muscle: A simple surgical treatment for stress urinary incontinence. *J Urol.* 2014;192(3):850–5.
8. Peters KM, Dmochowski RR, Carr LK et al. Autologous muscle derived cells for treatment of stress urinary incontinence in women. *J Urol.* 2014;192(2):469–76.
9. Sebe P, Doucet C, Cornu JN et al. Intrasphincteric injections of autologous muscular cells in women with refractory stress urinary incontinence: A prospective study. *Int Urogynecol J.* 2011;22(2):183–9.
10. Stangel-Wojcikiewicz K, Piwowar M, Jach R, Majka M, and Basta A. Quality of life assessment in female patients 2 and 4 years after muscle-derived cell transplants for stress urinary incontinence treatment. *Ginekol Pol.* 2016;87(3):183–9.
11. Kassouf W, Capolicchio G, Berardinucci G, and Corcos J. Collagen injection for treatment of urinary incontinence in children. *J Urol.* 2001;165(5):1666–8.
12. Athanasopoulos A, Gyftopoulos K, and McGuire EJ. Treating stress urinary incontinence in female patients with neuropathic bladder: The value of the autologous fascia rectus sling. *Int Urol Nephrol.* 2012;44(5):1363–7.
13. Fontaine E, Bendaya S, Desert JF, Fakacs C, Le Mouel MA, and Beurton D. Combined modified rectus fascial sling and augmentation ileocystoplasty for neurogenic incontinence in women. *J Urol.* 1997;157(1):109–12.
14. Mingin GC, Youngren K, Stock JA, and Hanna MK. The rectus myofascial wrap in the management of urethral sphincter incompetence. *BJU Int.* 2002;90(6):550–3.
15. Rutman MP, Deng DY, Shah SM, Raz S, and Rodriguez LV. Spiral sling salvage anti-incontinence surgery in female patients with a nonfunctional urethra: Technique and initial results. *J Urol.* 2006;175(5):1794–8; discussion 1798–9.
16. Myers JB, Mayer EN, and Lenherr S; Neurogenic Bladder Research Group. Management options for sphincteric deficiency in adults with neurogenic bladder. *Transl Androl Urol.* 2016;5(1):145–57.
17. Kryger JV, Leverson G, and Gonzalez R. Long-term results of artificial urinary sphincters in children are independent of age at implantation. *J Urol.* 2001;165(6 Pt 2):2377–9.
18. Bersch U, Gocking K, and Pannek J. The artificial urinary sphincter in patients with spinal cord lesion: Description of a modified technique and clinical results. *Eur Urol.* 2009;55(3):687–93.

19. Chartier Kastler E, Genevois S, Game X et al. Treatment of neurogenic male urinary incontinence related to intrinsic sphincter insufficiency with an artificial urinary sphincter: A French retrospective multicentre study. *BJU Int.* 2011;107(3):426–32.

20. Guillot-Tantay C, Chartier-Kastler E, Mozer P et al. [Male neurogenic stress urinary incontinence treated by artificial urinary sphincter AMS 800 (Boston Scientific, Boston, USA): Very long-term results (>25 years)]. *Prog Urol.* 2018;28(1):39–47.

21. Lopez Pereira P, Somoza Ariba I, Martinez Urrutia MJ, Lobato Romero R, and Jaureguizar Monroe E. Artificial urinary sphincter: 11-year experience in adolescents with congenital neuropathic bladder. *Eur Urol.* 2006;50(5):1096–101; discussion 1101.

22. Spiess PE, Capolicchio JP, Kiruluta G, Salle JP, Berardinucci G, and Corcos J. Is an artificial sphincter the best choice for incontinent boys with Spina Bifida? Review of our long term experience with the AS-800 artificial sphincter. *Can J Urol.* 2002;9(2):1486–91.

23. Yates DR, Phe V, Roupret M et al. Robot-assisted laparoscopic artificial urinary sphincter insertion in men with neurogenic stress urinary incontinence. *BJU Int.* 2013;111(7):1175–9.

24. Zimmern P, Hou J, and Lemack G. Transvaginal Bladder Neck Closure. Vol Video 18.2: *Native Tissue Repair for Incontinence and Prolapse. Springer;* 2017.

25. Zimmern PE, Hadley HR, Leach GE, and Raz S. Transvaginal closure of the bladder neck and placement of a suprapubic catheter for destroyed urethra after long-term indwelling catheterization. *J Urol.* 1985;134(3):554–7.

26. Hoebeke P, De Kuyper P, Goeminne H, Van Laecke E, and Everaert K. Bladder neck closure for treating pediatric incontinence. *Eur Urol.* 2000;38(4):453–6.

27. Bergman J, Lerman SE, Kristo B, Chen A, Boechat MI, and Churchill BM. Outcomes of bladder neck closure for intractable urinary incontinence in patients with neurogenic bladders. *J Pediatr Urol.* 2006;2(6):528–33.

28. Hensle TW, Kirsch AJ, Kennedy WA2nd , and Reiley EA. Bladder neck closure in association with continent urinary diversion. *J Urol.* 1995;154(2 Pt 2):883–5.

29. Jayanthi VR, Churchill BM, McLorie GA, and Khoury AE. Concomitant bladder neck closure and Mitrofanoff diversion for the management of intractable urinary incontinence. *J Urol.* 1995;154(2 Pt 2):886–888.

30. Watanabe T, Rivas DA, Smith R, Staas WE, Jr, and Chancellor MB. The effect of urinary tract reconstruction on neurologically impaired women previously treated with an indwelling urethral catheter. *J Urol.* 1996;156(6):1926–8.

31. Pan D, Troy A, Rogerson J, Bolton D, Brown D, and Lawrentschuk N. Long-term outcomes of external sphincterotomy in a spinal injured population. *J Urol.* 2009;181(2):705–9.

32. Reynard JM, Vass J, Sullivan ME, and Mamas M. Sphincterotomy and the treatment of detrusor-sphincter dyssynergia: Current status, future prospects. *Spinal Cord.* 2003;41(1):1–11.

33. Kuo HC. Satisfaction with urethral injection of botulinum toxin A for detrusor sphincter dyssynergia in patients with spinal cord lesion. *Neurourol Urodyn.* 2008;27(8):793–6.

34. de Seze M, Petit H, Gallien P et al. Botulinum A toxin and detrusor sphincter dyssynergia: A double-blind lidocaine-controlled study in 13 patients with spinal cord disease. *Eur Urol.* 2002;42(1):56–62.

35. Phelan MW, Franks M, Somogyi GT et al. Botulinum toxin urethral sphincter injection to restore bladder emptying in men and women with voiding dysfunction. *J Urol.* 2001;165(4):1107–10.

36. Schurch B, Hauri D, Rodic B, Curt A, Meyer M, and Rossier AB. Botulinum-A toxin as a treatment of detrusor-sphincter dyssynergia: A prospective study in 24 spinal cord injury patients. *J Urol.* 1996;155(3):1023–9.

37. Smith CP, Nishiguchi J, O'Leary M, Yoshimura N, and Chancellor MB. Single-institution experience in 110 patients with botulinum toxin A injection into bladder or urethra. *Urology.* 2005;65(1):37–41.

Chapter 33

URINARY DIVERSION

Véronique Phé and Gilles Karsenty

INTRODUCTION

Management of neurogenic bladder aims

- To maintain low-pressure urinary storage and complete voiding thus preserving the upper urinary tract
- To achieve urinary continence thus improving patient quality of life and self-esteem

When all conservative treatments fail, urinary diversion (UD) can be offered rather than resorting to indwelling catheters. Although there have been no randomized prospective long-term trials, patients with indwelling catheters have more morbidity, such as infectious complications, lithiasis, and radiographic abnormalities, than those managed with intermittent self-catheterization (ISC).[1,2] Though a long-term Foley catheter or suprapubic tube may be convenient for some patients, UD may be a reasonable option.

An outline of management of neurogenic bladder in relation to UD is shown in Figure 33.1.

SELECTION OF URINARY DIVERSION TYPE

Noncontinent urinary diversion (NCUD) can be offered to patients in whom ISC cannot be performed due to anatomic barriers, cognitive impairment, or limited dexterity.[3] Ultimately, NCUD can be considered in patients who are wheelchair bound or bedridden with untreatable incontinence, in devastated lower urinary tract (including skin ulcers with urinary fistula), when the upper urinary tract is severely compromised, and in patients who refuse other therapy.

Continent urinary diversion (CUD) is proposed to patients who are willing to perform ISC but who are unable to use the native urethra because of upper limb disability, difficulties in reaching or finding the urethra, or urethral destruction. Although CUD is considered appropriate in highly selected patients, these procedures are technically more challenging and are associated with higher short-term and long-term complication rates than the NCUD technique.[4]

The choice of UD procedure must be based on a multidisciplinary evaluation involving primarily the urologist and the neurorehabilitation physician with the patient and family/caregivers.

In addition to clear information on potential risks and benefits of each UD type given by the physicians, speaking to other patients with various forms of diversions often helps the patient to better realize the reality of a UD and to avoid inappropriate or unrealistic expectations.

Ability and willingness to perform ISC life long, motivation to comply with self-care and follow-up, progressivity of the neurologic disease, medical comorbidities, and age are some of the main criteria to be taken into account to end up in a concerted choice.

GENERAL SURGICAL PRINCIPLES

BOWEL PREPARATION

Enhanced recovery after surgery (ERAS) programs have demonstrated a 50% reduction in postoperative complications and a 30%–50% reduction in hospital stay in almost all major surgeries specialties.[5] Key points of ERAS gastrointestinal measures include overnight fasting of carbohydrate drinks 2 hours before surgery, avoidance of bowel preparation and nasogastric tube, pharmacologic prophylaxis of postoperative vomiting, early (day 1) postoperative oral feeding, liberal use of laxative, and Alvimopan. Although ERAS has not been evaluated specifically in neuro-urologic patients, similar results have been reported after cystectomy and UD for bladder cancer with the same advantages.

INTESTINAL ANASTOMOSIS

Much of the early morbidity and mortality associated with UD relates to intestinal complications.[6] The fundamental principles of intestinal anastomoses include adequate mobilization, maintenance of blood supply, apposition of mucosa-to-mucosa of the two bowel segments, and creation of a watertight and tensionless anastomotic line. Sutures or staples can be used, both having similar complication rates.[7]

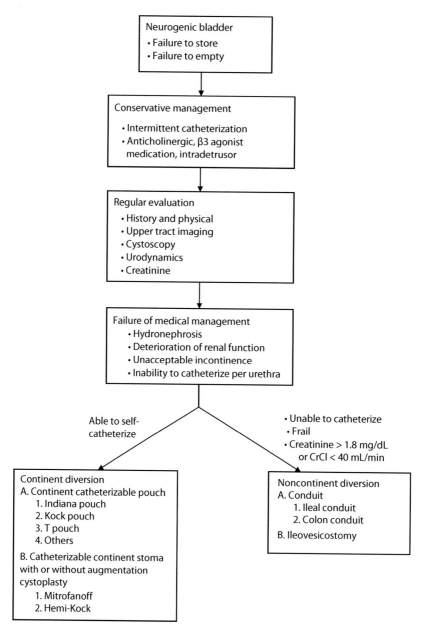

Figure 33.1 Surgical management of patients with neurogenic bladders requiring urinary diversion.

URETEROINTESTINAL ANASTOMOSES

Basic surgical principles of ureterointestinal anastomoses are as follows:

- Minimal ureter mobilization to allow a tensionless anastomosis
- Periadventitial tissue sparing to ensure adequate blood supply
- Creation of a watertight mucosa-to-mucosa apposition with fine (4–0 or 5–0) delayed absorbable sutures
- Refluxing anastomoses (Bricker or Wallace technique) for ileal conduits (Figures 33.2 and 33.3)

STOMA

The stoma is a very important aspect of the surgery. Much of the success of a UD can be dependent on an appropriate stomal site and aspect.

In NCUD, stomal site and technique should accommodate a collection device that does not leak in any position (supine, sitting, or standing), while maintaining patient comfort when wearing clothes (Figure 33.5). The position is commonly located in the right lower quadrant (Figure 33.4) but should be chosen and marked preoperatively to fit each patient specification, like a stoma above the umbilicus in a quadriplegic wheelchair-bound patient.

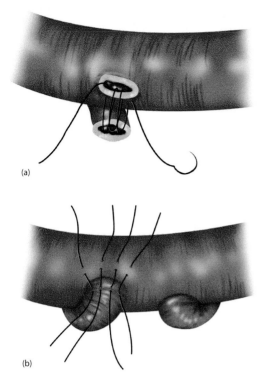

(a)

(b)

Figure 33.2 Bricker ureterointestinal anastomosis. (a) A full-thickness serosa and mucosal plug are removed from the bowel. Interrupted 5-0 delayed absorbable suture approximates the ureter to the full thickness of the bowel mucosa and serosa. (b) A supportive suture layer can be added from the adventitia of the ureter to the serosa of the bowel. (From McDougal W, and McDougal WS, In: *Campbell's Urology*, WB Saunders, Philadelphia, PA, 2002, p. 3766.)

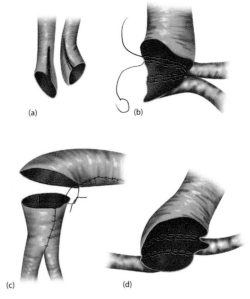

(a) (b)

(c) (d)

Figure 33.3 Wallace ureterointestinal anastomosis. (a) Both ureters are spatulated and are laid adjacent to each other. (b) The apex of one ureter is sutured to the apex of the other ureter. The medial walls of both ureters are then sutured together with interrupted or running 5-0 delayed absorbable suture. The lateral walls are then sutured to the bowel. (c) A Y-type variant. (d) The head-to-tail variant. (From McDougal W and McDougal WS, In: *Campbell's Urology*, WB Saunders, Philadelphia, PA, 2002, p. 3766.)

In CUD, although the umbilicus is often the preferred location because of easier access and cosmetic reasons, the actual site would ideally be chosen preoperatively with an occupational therapist, especially if the patient has upper limb impairment.[8]

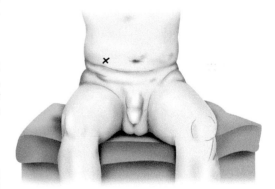

Figure 33.4 The stoma site is selected and marked on the surface of the abdomen where the skin is not rolled into folds while the patient is either sitting or standing. (From Hinman F Jr, *Atlas of Urologic Surgery*, WB Saunders, Philadelphia, PA, 1998, p. 647.)

NONCONTINENT URINARY DIVERSIONS

CONDUITS

Since 1950, the Bricker ileal conduit has been the standard for NCUD.[9] In a few cases, colon conduit may be chosen when there are functional or anatomic factors that preclude the use of the ileum (as extensive irradiation). Concomitant to the creation of an ileal conduit, a cystectomy is usually performed since retained bladder exposes the patient to the risk of pyocystis bladder cancer, pain, and hematuria.[10]

TECHNIQUE

Blood supply is based on the superior mesenteric artery (jejunal and ileal branches). After transection, the left ureter is brought under the sigmoid colon through the sigmoid mesentery to the right side.

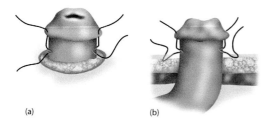

(a)   (b)

Figure 33.5 (a,b) Rosebud stoma. Five to 6 cm of intestine is brought through the abdominal wall. The open bowel is sutured to the skin with four quadrant sutures of 3-0 delayed absorbable sutures that pass through the skin edge, then catch the adventitia of the bowel well below the level of the skin, and finally go through the mucosal edge, thus everting the stoma. Additional sutures are placed through the skin and bowel edge between the quadrant sutures to close the gap. (From McDougal W, and McDougal WS, *Campbell's Urology*, WB Saunders, Philadelphia, PA, 2002, p. 3760.)

About 20 cm from the ileocecal valve, a 10 cm segment of ileum is selected and transected. The disconnected ileal segment is placed inferior to the remaining bowel segments. The bowel is reanastomosed, then ureteroileal anastomoses are performed either separately (Bricker) or co-joined (Wallace technique) at the proximal end of the loop. The final step is the creation of the stoma (Figure 33.6).

ILEAL VESICOSTOMY

The ileal vesicostomy is an alternative to ileal conduit in some patients. It avoids the complications of ureterointestinal anastomosis, while maintaining the native ureteral antireflux mechanism. The addition of a small segment of ileum from the bladder to the abdominal wall acts to maintain low pressure in the bladder. Theoretically, this results in a low-pressure reservoir that, if indicated at a later date, can be converted back to normal anatomy (Figure 33.7).

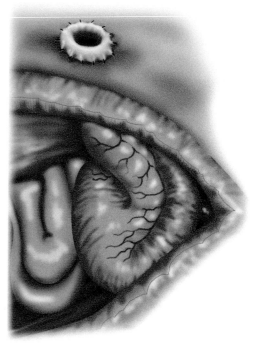

Figure 33.7 The ileovesicostomy. (From Hinman F Jr, *Atlas of Urologic Surgery*, WB Saunders, Philadelphia, PA, 1998, p. 641.)

CONTINENT URINARY DIVERSION

CUD includes any reservoir subserved by a catheterizable efferent mechanism other than the native urethra and bladder neck.[11]

In the most complex situation, a surgical reanimation program of hand function could even improve tetraplegic patient eligibility for a CUD.[8,12]

If possible, it is preferable to preserve the bladder, thus maintaining the ureteral antireflux mechanism. If needed, the bladder capacity can be increased and the pressure lessened with an intestinal augmentation combined. When this cannot be achieved due to significant bladder disease, a continent catheterizable supravesical reservoir (pouch) may be a better option.

CONTINENCE MECHANISMS

The most demanding technical aspect of a CUD is the construction of the continence mechanism.

Three general principles have been described[7]:

- Intussuscepted nipple valve (Kock, Benchekroun, Mainz III without appendix pouch) bearing a risk of nipple destabilization despite the most experienced surgeons.[13,14]

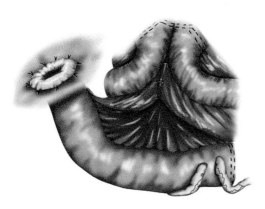

Figure 33.6 The ileal conduit at completion. (From Hinman F Jr, *Atlas of Urologic Surgery*, WB Saunders, Philadelphia, PA, 1998, p. 654.)

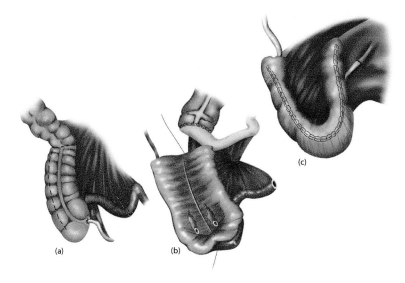

Figure 33.8 Indiana pouch. (a) A 25–30 cm segment of cecum, ascending colon, and hepatic flexure, in addition to 8–10 cm terminal ileum, is selected. The ascending colon is split down the antimesenteric border to within 2 cm of the caudal tip. (b) Perform an ileocolostomy using a suture technique or by a stapled method. Insert the ureters by a submucosal technique. (c) Place a Malecot catheter through the wall of the lowest part of the complex, in a position to allow direct exit through the abdominal wall. Close the U-shaped defect by folding the distal portion of the colon into the proximal end, and suture it in place with a running 3-0 absorbable suture. Add a serosal Lembert stitch with occasional lock stitches. Leave the ileum to form the cutaneous conduit with tapering. (From Hinman F Jr, *Atlas of Urologic Surgery*, WB Saunders, Philadelphia, PA, 1998, p. 698.)

- Tapered or imbricated, or both, terminal ileum used in right colon pouches (Indiana [Figure 33.8], Florida Mainz II) with the ileocecal valve as a ready-made continence mechanism.[13,15–17].

- Efferent appendicular or pseudo-appendicular tubes are based on a technical principle described by Mitrofanoff in 1980 (Figures 33.10 through 33.12), using the appendix or ureter to create a flap valve, and at the same time a neourethral conduit to the bladder[18,19] (Figure 33.9) (see details in Chapter 34). When appendix is not available, a detubularized and remodeled ileal segment (Monti, Casale) can be built. The Mitrofanoff principle can be used as well in the native bladder (augmented or not) as in any type of intestinal pouch.[13] The Mitrofanoff principle is the most commonly used CUD technique in neuro-urology.[20]

brought out through the abdominal wall as a stoma (Figures 33.8 and 33.9).

ILEAL CONTINENT RESERVOIR

Ileal reservoirs maintain the ileocecal valve and use only the small bowel to create a low-pressure reservoir.[21] The Kock pouch was the first described (Figures 33.13 and 33.14). It has been criticized for being technically difficult and is associated with a high complication rate (including failure due to eversion and effacement of the intussusception, ischemic atrophy requiring a new nipple be constructed, stone formation on eroded or exposed staples). As such, it has been abandoned by many urologists. Other types of ileal pouches that combine an ileal reservoir with a T-valve or the Mitrofanoff principle without an intussuscepted segment have been described.[22,23]

TYPES OF CONTINENT SUPRAVESICAL RESERVOIRS
ILEOCECAL CONTINENT RESERVOIR

The Indiana,[15] Florida,[16] University of Miami, or Mainz III pouch[17] use the detubularized right colon as a reservoir while using reinforcement of the ileocecal valve for continence. The remaining ileal limb acts as the neourethra, which can be tapered and

OUTCOMES OF URINARY DIVERSION

NCUD, especially ileal conduit, allows preservation of the renal function and autonomy related to urinary function in patients with spinal cord injury.[24] In patients with advanced multiple sclerosis,[25] improvement of the urinary quality of life has been reported.[25,27]

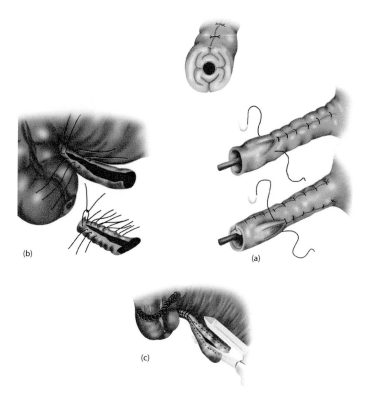

Figure 33.9 Tapering of ileal cutaneous conduit for Indiana pouch. (a) Apply apposing Lembert sutures on each side of the terminal ileum. Excess ileum can also be tapered (b) by suturing or (c) by a stapling technique. (From Benson, MC, Olsson, CA, *Campbell's Urology*, WB Saunders, Philadelphia, PA, 2002, p. 3821.)

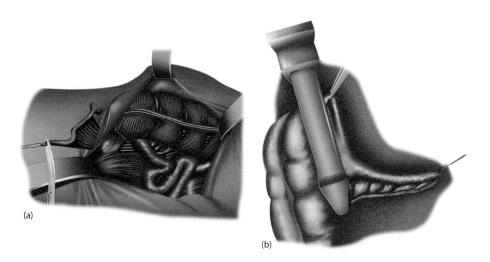

Figure 33.10 Mitrofanoff (appendicovesicostomy). (a) Stay sutures are placed at the base of the appendix, and the wall of the cecum is incised circumferentially to take a small cuff of cecum with the appendix. The appendiceal mesentery is separated a short distance from that of the cecum, preserving all of the appendiceal blood supply. The cecal defect is closed. The appendix is extraperitonealized behind the ileocecal junction. For umbilical placement of the stoma, it is not necessary to extraperitonealize the appendix. (b) For a short appendix or an obese patient, the appendix can be made longer by incorporating some of the cecal wall. (From Hinman F Jr, *Atlas of Urologic Surgery*, WB Saunders, Philadelphia, PA, 1998, p. 709.)

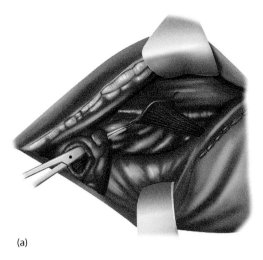
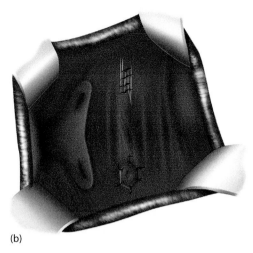

(a)   (b)

Figure 33.11   (a,b) Through a cystotomy, a submucosal tunnel is made in the posterolateral wall of the bladder, beginning well above the right ureteral orifice. The appendix tip is implanted. A bladder augmentation is usually done next. (From Hinman F Jr, *Atlas of Urologic* Surgery, WB Saunders, Philadelphia, PA, 1998, p. 710.)

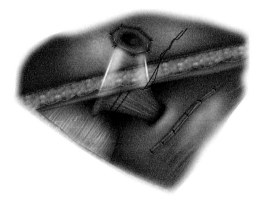

Figure 33.12   The appendiceal base is passed through an opening in the abdominal wall muscles large enough to accommodate a finger. The appendiceal opening is sutured to the skin (sometimes at the umbilicus). The bladder should be hitched to the anterior abdominal wall, and a catheter left in the appendix. (From Hinman F Jr, *Atlas of Urologic Surgery*, WB Saunders, Philadelphia, PA, 1998, p. 710.)

Regarding CUD, the European Association of Urology guideline on neuro-urology has reported in a systematic review an ability to catheterize rate of 84% or greater and the continence rate at stoma greater than 75%.[20]

Perceived global satisfaction has been found to be high with both conduit and CUD; it has also been noted that most patients would choose the same procedure again.[28] Moreover, the creation of a CUD results in an improved body image, a better quality of life, and even a better sex life when compared to patients' prior management.[29,30]

Ileal conduit is offered to neuro-urological patients after failure of conservative therapies or as a salvage therapy, as a last resort procedure. However, high perioperative morbidity and late complication rates have been reported.[24]

The complications are displayed in Table 33.1. The most common early postoperative complication is wound infection, followed by ureteroileal anastomotic leakage (prevalence 3%–9%),[31,32] intestinal obstruction, intestinal fistulas, and acute pyelonephritis. Long-term complications include stomal stenosis, ureteroileal stenosis favored by previous anastomotic leakage (prevalence 1%–14%),[33] subsequent failure of the loop to propel urine adequately, and deterioration of the upper urinary tract[34].

The specific complication rate of CUD is meaningful. Tube stenosis occurred in 4%–32% of the cases. The difference between CUD techniques regarding the stenosis rate has never been assessed in the literature. In order to decrease morbidity and instead of being an end-stage treatment, CUD should probably be considered earlier in the management of neuro-urological patients.

Since complications can occur as late as 20 years and later after both NCUD and CUD, a regular (yearly) and lifelong follow-up with upper tract imaging and kidney function test can be suggested.

Metabolic alterations have been described and are dependent on many variables including the segment of bowel used, the surface area of the

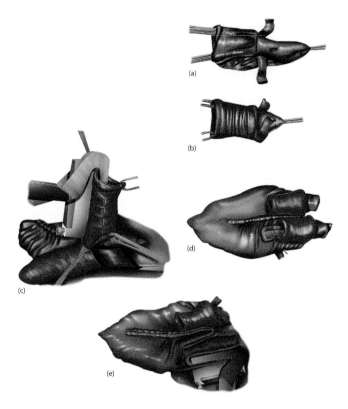

(a)

(b)

(c)

(d)

(e)

Figure 33.13 Construction of a nipple valve for the Kock pouch. (a) A 15 cm segment of terminal ileum is isolated and opened along its antimesenteric wall. The proximal 10 cm serves as the continent intussusception and the distal 5–10 cm as the patch. The size of the patch varies according to the size of the excised segment. (b) A Babcock clamp is advanced into the terminal ileum, the full thickness of the intussuscipiens is grasped, and it is prolapsed into the pouch. (c) Three rows of 4.8 mm staples are applied to the intussuscepted nipple valve using the TA-55 stapler. (d) A small buttonhole is made in the back wall of the ileal plate to allow the anvil of the TA-55 stapler to be passed through and advanced into the nipple valve. A fourth row of staples is applied. The figure shows two valve mechanisms. In this instance, there would be only one. (e) The anvil of the stapler can be directed between the two leaves of the intussuscipiens and the fourth row of staples applied in this manner. The figure shows two valve mechanisms. In this instance, there would be only one. ([a] From Ghoneim MA et al. *J. Urol.* 138, 1150–1154, 1987. [b–e] From Hinman F Jr, *Atlas of Urologic Surgery*, WB Saunders, Philadelphia, PA, 1998, pp. 688–9; Benson MC, and Olsson CA, *Campbell's Urology*, WB Saunders, Philadelphia, PA, 2002, p. 3808.)

bowel, the duration the urine is exposed to the bowel, the concentration of the solutes in the urine, the renal function, and the pH (see Table 33.2). Ionogram and alkali reserve can be included in the follow-up in the case of acid-based imbalance symptoms. When an ileocecal intestinal segment has been used, vitamin B12 can be verified every second year.

About three-quarters of those with conduits and patients with catheterizable pouches have bacteriuria at any time, yet many of them are asymptomatic and do not require treatment for their colonization.[26]

To conclude, such patients may be better referred to expert centers that can counsel the patient, offer all types of UD procedures, and provide adapted perioperative care and long-term follow-up by a multidisciplinary team.

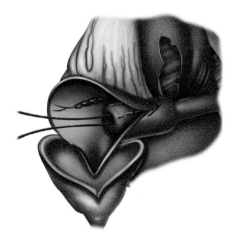

Figure 33.14 Hemi-Kock augmentation cystoplasty. (From Hinman F Jr, *Atlas of Urologic Surgery*, WB Saunders, Philadelphia, PA, 1998, p. 732.)

Table 33.1   Complications of Urinary Intestinal Diversion

Complications	Type of Diversion	Patients (complications/N)	Incidence (%)
Bowel obstruction	Ileal conduit	124/1289	10
	Colon conduit	9/230	5
	Gastric conduit	2/21	10
	Continent diversion	2/250	4
Ureteral intestinal obstruction	Ileal conduit	90/1142	8
	Antireflux colon conduit	25/122	20
	Colon conduit	8/92	9
	Continent diversion	16/461	4
Urine leak	Ileal conduit	23/886	3
	Colon conduit	6/130	5
	Continent diversion	104/629	17
	Ileum colon	5/123	4
Stomal stenosis or hernia	Ileal conduit	196/806	24
	Colon conduit	45/227	20
	Continent diversion	28/310	9
Renal calculi	Ileal conduit	70/964	7
	Antireflux colon conduit	5/94	5
Pouch calculi	Continent diversion	42/317	13
Acidosis requiring treatment	Ileal conduit	46/296	16
	Antireflux colon conduit	5/94	5
	Gastric conduit	0/21	0
	Continent diversion		
	Ileum	21/263	8
	Colon or colon-ileum	17/63	27
Pyelonephritis	Ileal conduit	132/1142	12
	Antireflux colon conduit	13/96	13
	Continent diversion	15/296	5
Renal deterioration	Ileal conduit	146/808	18
	Antireflux colon conduit	15/103	15

Source: Dahl DM, and McDougal WS, *Campbell-Walsh Urology*, WB Saunders, Philadelphia, PA, 2012, pp. 2411–49.

Table 33.2   Metabolic Changes According to Intestinal Segment used to Build Continent Urinary Diversion

Digestive Tract Segment	Complications of Loss of a Digestive Segment	Complications Related to the Contact of Urine with the Digestive Tract
Gastric	Intrinsic factor and vitamin B12 deficiency Gastric ulceration Bone demineralization In patients with normal renal function, this is usually not clinically significant.	Hypochloremic alkalosis, hypokalemic metabolic acidosis. In patients with normal renal function, this is usually not clinically significant.
Jejunal	Few complications	Water loss syndrome (dehydration, hyponatremia, hypochloremia, hyperkalemia, metabolic acidosis), lethargy, nausea, vomiting, dehydration, weakness, and hyperthermia.
Ileal	Loss of bile salt Altered lipid metabolism Kidney lithiasis Vitamin B12 deficit Diarrhea and malabsorption	Water loss syndrome Hyperchloremic acidosis, fatigability, anorexia, weight loss, polydipsia, and lethargy. Regardless of the type of diversion, patients require regular screening of their electrolytes.[33]
Colic	Diarrhea	Hyperchloremic acidosis

REFERENCES

1. Jamil F, Williamson M, Ahmed YS, and Harrison SC. Natural-fill urodynamics in chronically catheterized patients with spinal-cord injury. *BJU Int.* 1999;83:396–9. doi:10.1046/j.1464-410x.1999.00933.x

2. Weld KJ and Dmochowski RR. Association of level of injury and bladder behavior in patients with post-traumatic spinal cord injury. *Urology.* 2000;55:490–4. doi:10.1016/s0090-4295(99)00553-1

3. Legrand G, Roupret M, Comperat E, Even-Schneider A, Denys P, and Chartier-Kastler E. Functional outcomes after management of end-stage neurological bladder dysfunction with ileal conduit in a multiple sclerosis population: A monocentric experience. *Urology.* 2011;78:937–41. doi:10.1016/j.urology.2011.06.015

4. McKiernan J, DeCastro G, and Benson M. Cutaneous continent diversion. In: Wein A, Kavoussi LR, Novick AC, Partin AW, Peters CA, eds. *Campbell-Walsh Urology.* Vol 3. Philadelphia, PA: Elsevier, WB Saunders; 2012:2450–78.

5. Ljungqvist O, Scott M, and Fearon KC. Enhanced recovery after surgery: A review. *JAMA Surg.* 2017;152:292–8. doi:10.1001/jamasurg.2016.4952

6. Månsson W, Colleen S, and Stigsson L. Four methods of uretero-intestinal anastomosis in urinary conduit diversion. A comparative study of early and late complications and the influence of radiotherapy. *Scand J Urol Nephrol.* 1979;13:191–9. doi:10.3109/00365597909181176

7. Dahl D and McDougal W. Use of intestinal segments in urinary diversion. In: Wein A, Kavoussi LR, Novick AC, Partin AW, and Peters CA, eds. *Campbell-Walsh Urology,* 10th ed. Vol 3. Philadelphia, PA: Elsevier, WB Saunders; 2012:2411–49.

8. Bernuz B, Guinet A, Rech C et al. Self-catheterization acquisition after hand reanimation protocols in C5-C7 tetraplegic patients. *Spinal Cord.* 2011;49:313–7. doi:10.1038/sc.2010.120

9. Bricker EM. Bladder substitution after pelvic evisceration. *Surg Clin North Am.* 1950;30:1511–21. doi:10.1016/s0039-6109(16)33147-4

10. Chartier-Kastler EJ, Mozer P, Denys P, Bitker M-O, Haertig A, and Richard F. Neurogenic bladder management and cutaneous non-continent ileal conduit. *Spinal Cord.* 2002;40:443–8. doi:10.1038/sj.sc.3101346

11. Kaefer M and Retik AB. The Mitrofanoff principle in continent urinary reconstruction. *Urol Clin North Am.* 1997;24:795–811.

12. Perrouin-Verbe M-A, Chartier-Kastler E, Even A, Denys P, Roupret M, and Phé V. Long-term complications of continent cutaneous urinary diversion in adult spinal cord injured patients. *Neurourol Urodyn.* 2016;35:1046–50. doi:10.1002/nau.22879

13. Benson M and Olsson C. Cutaneous continent urinary diversion. In: Walsh PC, Retik AB, Vaughan EDJ, and Wein AJ, eds. *Campbell's Urology.* Philadelphia, PA: WB Saunders; 2002:3789–834.

14. Benchekroun A. Hydraulic valve for continence and antireflux. A 17–year experience of 210 cases. *Scand J Urol Nephrol Suppl.* 1992;142:66–70.

15. Rowland RG, Mitchell ME, Bihrle R, Kahnoski RJ, and Piser JE. Indiana continent urinary reservoir. *J Urol.* 1987;137:1136–9. doi:10.1016/s0022-5347(17)44428-4

16. Lockhart JL. Remodeled right colon: An alternative urinary reservoir. *J Urol.* 1987;138:730–4. doi:10.1016/s0022-5347(17)43355-6

17. Bejany DE and Politano VA. Stapled and nonstapled tapered distal ileum for construction of a continent colonic urinary reservoir. *J Urol.* 1988;140:491–4. doi:10.1016/s0022-5347(17)41699-5

18. Mitrofanoff P. [Trans-appendicular continent cystostomy in the management of the neurogenic bladder]. *Chir Pediatr.* 1980;21:297–305.

19. Keating MA, Rink RC, and Adams MC. Appendicovesicostomy: A useful adjunct to continent reconstruction of the bladder. *J Urol.* 1993;149:1091–4. doi:10.1016/s0022-5347(17)36305-x

20. Phé V, Boissier R, Blok BFM et al. Continent catheterizable tubes/stomas in adult neuro-urological patients: A systematic review. *Neurourol Urodyn.* 2017;36:1711–22. doi:10.1002/nau.23213

21. Kock NG, Nilson AE, Nilsson LO, Norlén LJ, and Philipson BM. Urinary diversion via a continent ileal reservoir: Clinical results in 12 patients. *J Urol.* 1982;128:469–75. doi:10.1016/s0022-5347(17)53001-3

22. Marino G and Laudi M. Ileal T-pouch as a urinary continent cutaneous diversion: Clinical and urodynamic evaluation. *BJU Int.* 2002;90:47–50. doi:10.1046/j.1464-410x.2002.02784.x

23. Vuichoud C, Perrouin-Verbe M-A, Phe V, Bitker M-O, Parra J, and Chartier-Kastler E. [Continent cutaneous urinary diversion after cystectomy for cancer: A reliable alternative? A monocentric retrospective study]. *Progres En Urol J Assoc Francaise Urol Soc Francaise Urol.* 2016;26:642–50. doi:10.1016/j.purol.2016.09.061

24. Guillot-Tantay C, Chartier-Kastler E, Perrouin-Verbe M-A, Denys P, and Léon P, Phé V. Complications of non-continent cutaneous urinary diversion in adults with spinal cord injury: A retrospective study. *Spinal Cord.* 2018;56:856–62. doi:10.1038/s41393-018-0083-1

25. Guillotreau J, Castel-Lacanal E, Roumiguié M et al. Prospective study of the impact on quality of life of cystectomy with ileal conduit urinary diversion for neurogenic bladder dysfunction. *Neurourol Urodyn.* 2011;30:1503–6. doi:10.1002/nau.21121

26. Skinner DG, Lieskovsky G, Skinner EC, and Boyd SD. Urinary diversion. *Curr Probl Surg.* 1987;24:399–471.

27. Guillotreau J, Panicker JN, Castel-Lacanal E et al. Prospective evaluation of laparoscopic assisted cystectomy and ileal conduit in advanced multiple sclerosis. *Urology.* 2012;80:852–7. doi:10.1016/j.urology.2012.06.039

28. Hardt J, Petrak F, Filipas D, and Egle UT. Adaptation to life after surgical removal of the bladder-an application of graphical Markov models for analysing longitudinal data. *Stat Med.* 2004;23:649–66. doi:10.1002/sim.1596

29. Moreno JG, Chancellor MB, Karasick S, King S, Abdill CK, and Rivas DA. Improved quality of life and sexuality with continent urinary diversion in quadriplegic women with umbilical stoma. *Arch Phys Med Rehabil.* 1995;76:758–62. doi:10.1016/s0003-9993(95)80531-1

30. Watanabe T, Rivas DA, Smith R, Staas WJ, and Chancellor M. The effect of urinary tract reconstruction on neurologically impaired women previously treated with an indwelling urethral catheter. *J Urol.* 1988;140(5 Pt 2):1152–6.

31. Beckley S, Wajsman Z, Pontes JE, and Murphy G. Transverse colon conduit: A method of urinary diversion after pelvic irradiation. *J Urol.* 1982;128:464–8. doi:10.1016/s0022-5347(17)52999-7

32. Loening SA, Navarre RJ, Narayana AS, and Culp DA. Transverse colon conduit urinary diversion. *J Urol.* 1982;127:37–9. doi:10.1016/s0022-5347(17)53593-4

33. McDougal W and McDougal WS. Use of intestinal segments and urinary diversion. In: Walsh PC, Retik AB, Vaughan EDJ, and Wein AJ, eds. *Campbell's Urology*, 8th ed. Philadelphia, PA: WB Saunders; 2002:3745–88.

34. Nurmi M, Puntala P, and Alanen A. Evaluation of 144 cases of ileal conduits in adults. *Eur Urol.* 1988;15(1–2):89–93.

35. Hinman F Jr, *Atlas of Urologic Surgery*, WB Saunders, Philadelphia, PA, 1998, p. 647. ISBN 10 : 0721664040 ISBN 13 : 9780721664040.

TRANSAPPENDICULAR CONTINENT CYSTOSTOMY TECHNIQUE (MITROFANOFF PRINCIPLE)

Ali Alsulihem and Jacques Corcos

BACKGROUND

Mitrofanoff first described the use of the appendix as a continent catheterizable channel in 1980 for pediatric patients with neurogenic bladder.[1] Shortly after, it became a popular procedure and has expanded to various indications and the adult population.[2] The continence mechanism of this procedure is the tunneled flap valve. In this chapter, we review the technical details of this procedure.

INDICATIONS

It is indicated in patients who desire an alternative route to reach the bladder (native or augmented) by clean intermittent catheterization because of damaged urethra, impaired upper limb function, or urethral meatus inaccessibility (obesity, lower limb spasticity, female gender, etc.).[3-7]

PREOPERATIVE EVALUATION AND PREPARATION

Careful evaluation of patients' history and physical examination is essential. Prior abdominal surgeries should be reviewed. The patient's mental and physical ability to perform clean intermittent catheterization should be thoroughly evaluated. The presence of the appendix should be checked and preparation of possible alternative procedures done if a patient has a previous appendectomy. The position of stoma should be marked preoperatively. The usual location is the umbilicus, but it can be shifted to the right lower quadrant if a patient is obese or if umbilical implantation is not appropriate, in case of girls or young women who might consider future pregnancy.[8] See Table 34.1.

Table 34.1   Patient Selection

Patient capable of personal control
Good knowledge of self-catheterization via the urethra
The bladder can be emptied via two continence orifices
Early and long-term treatment
Associated Malone cecostomy
A commitment of the surgeon to treat possible residual incontinence

Preoperative mechanical bowel preparation is usually performed, along with appropriate antimicrobial prophylaxis coverage.[9]

OPERATIVE TECHNIQUE

The general surgical principle is summarized in Table 34.2.

SKIN INCISION AND UMBILICUS PREPARATION

The skin incision is usually done by lower midline with periumbilical paramedian incision (Figure 34.1). The skin incision is made at least 10 mm away from the umbilicus, with the subcutaneous incision made

Table 34.2   Broad Principles of Cystostomy Performance

Give preference to an appendix that is usable
Keep the appendix for the bladder
Implant in the bladder (and not in an intestinal patch)
"Parietalize" the bladder and fix it to the anterior abdominal wall
Follow a rectilinear and downward trajectory to the bladder neck
Give preference to the umbilicus, except in women who could be pregnant

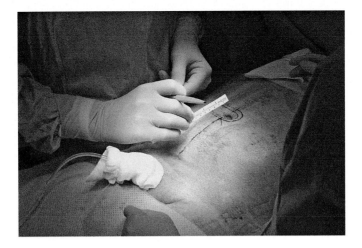

Figure 34.1   Median sub- and periumbilical laparotomy.

medial until the release of the umbilical attachments. It is important not to traumatize the umbilical skin to reduce the risk of stomal stenosis. The bottom of the umbilicus is resected to allow a 20F catheter to pass through.[8]

APPENDIX PREPARATION

After opening the peritoneum, mobilizing the bowel, and releasing possible adhesions, if present, the appendix should be easily found and palpated. Then, the release of mesoappendix is done by freeing its medial attachments to the cecum and tying it with 4-0 absorbable sutures (Figure 34.2a). The appendix should be released until it reaches the bladder implantation site. Then, the ascending colon should be clamped, and the appendix tip should be cut to allow passage of a 14F catheter. If it does not pass a 14F catheter, then re-cutting the edge is done until the 14F catheter can pass.

Then, evaluation of the appendix length is made. If the appendix is long enough to reach the skin stoma

site, the transection of the appendix proximal end with the cecum is made with a cold knife, and closure of the cecum is similarly done with absorbable suture to appendectomy.[8,9]

If the appendix is short, a cecal cuff can be taken over 14F catheter (Figure 34.2b) to add a length of 4–8 cm.[8] If the appendix cannot be used, a reconfigured ileal segment (Yang-Monti or Casale) can be used similar to the appendix.[7–9]

Then, the distal 2 cm tip is cleared from its mesoappendix by bipolar cautery, and the mucosa is exteriorized by absorbable sutures (Figure 34.3a,b).[8] The distal tip will be implanted into the bladder. The appendix is then washed with saline until clear efflux is obtained and then intubated with a 14F catheter.

At the end of the appendix preparation phase, the appendix should be:

1. Mobile and able to reach the bladder and the stoma site

(a)   (b)

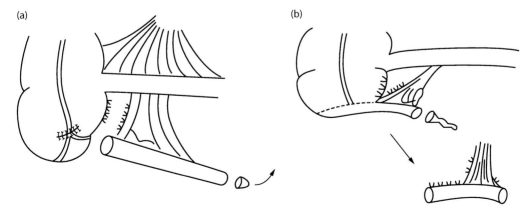

Figure 34.2   (a) The appendix tip is resected for insertion of a 14F catheter. The appendix is then mobilized with selective ligatures of the mesoappendix vessels, and a cecal collar is sectioned. (b) If the appendix is too short, and if the mesoappendix is favorable, we perform a cecoplasty to enlarge the appendix 4–8 cm.

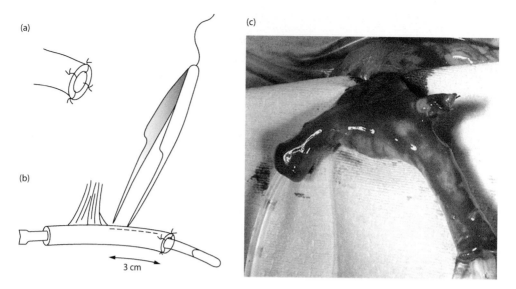

Figure 34.3 (a) After resection of the appendix tip, the mucosa is fixed to the appendix wall by four stitches of rapidly absorbable 5-0 sutures. (b) At the end of preparation, the appendix conduit must be freed from the mesoappendix up to 2 cm to allow its implantation in the bladder. (c) An operative view of the same step.

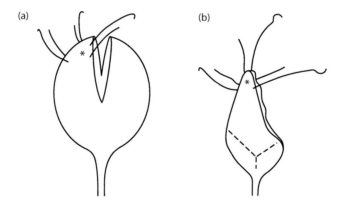

Figure 34.4 If the bladder is large, it is opened along the median line, and the implantation zone is marked off with three absorbable Mon 2-0 sutures. (b) If the bladder is small, an inverted Y- or V-shaped incision is made in such a way that a long anterior tip reaches the area chosen for the continent stoma.

2. In straight alignment to avoid kinking of the stoma
3. Wide caliber that can adapt at least 14F catheter without resistance
4. Has well-vascularized mucosal ends of the appendix to prevent stenosis of both tips (Figure 34.3c)[8]

CYSTOSTOMY, BLADDER FLAP, AND ANTIREFLUX APPENDIX IMPLANTATION

The bladder should be filled, and a bladder incision is made at midline if large bladder capacity (Figure 34.4a), or an inverted V or Y incision is made in case of low

bladder capacity (Figure 34.4b) to create a sizable anterior wall flap (Figure 34.5).[8] Another description of bladder flap creation in small bladders is to create it in a similar fashion to a Boari bladder flap.[9]

Then, the bladder flap edges are fixed with three stay sutures at 4, 6, and 12 o'clock positions (triangulating sutures) (Figure 34.6a). Then the cystostomy opening is made, at least 15 mm away from each flap edge, 20F wide, and the distal tip of the appendix is passed through that opening. Then a second mucosal incision is made 2 cm proximal to the cystostomy incision toward the bladder base (Figure 34.6b). Then, a wide submucosal tunnel is created, and the appendix is implanted in Glen-Anderson fashion with a 2 cm tunnel. The external part of the appendix is then fixed to the external bladder wall with three interrupted

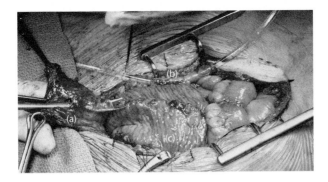

Figure 34.5 The interest of creating an anterior bladder flap (a) with an inverted V-shaped incision: creation of submucosal channel becomes easy, appendix (b) will have straight implantation, and starting bladder augmentation (c) is easier to perform.

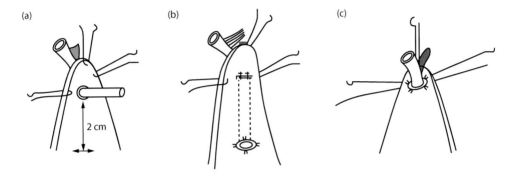

Figure 34.6 (a) The distal part of the appendix, relieved of its mesoappendix up to 2 cm, is passed through the opening situated 1 cm from the tip. (b) The appendix is positioned in the bladder submucosa for a length of at least 2 cm. (c) The appendix is lightly fixed to the bladder exterior by three stitches with absorbable 3-0 sutures.

sutures (Figure 34.6c). The mucosal end is then attached to the bladder mucosa with five absorbable sutures in interrupted fashion.[8] The trajectory of the catheterization should be aligned toward the bladder base. Then, the bladder flap with the appendix is attached to the anterior abdominal wall with three to five slowly absorbable sutures. The mesoappendix should be oriented between the bladder flap and the abdominal wall. It is essential to have a straight path and avoid kinking of the channel, and if necessary, the surgeon should shorten the appendix to achieve straight alignment. Then, the bladder flap in which the appendix has been fixed should be fixed to the abdominal wall by three to five absorbable sutures. The 14F catheter should serve as a guide for sutures (Figure 34.7a).

APPENDIX TO SKIN ANASTOMOSIS (STOMA CREATION)

The appendix should be anastomosed to the skin at this point. The stoma can be created at the umbilicus

or alternatively done at the right lower quadrant if it cannot be attached to the umbilicus.

If the umbilicus is chosen as the stoma site, six to eight monofilament 5-0 sutures should be used to perform the appendix to umbilical skin anastomosis, over a 14F Foley catheter. The surgeon must make sure to have wide and equal skin and appendix diameters, and if needed, spatulation of the appendix or skin should be performed to have uniform alignment between the two edges of the anastomosis.[8] Then, the previously mentioned three triangulating sutures of the bladder flap should be fixed to the abdominal wall (Figure 34.7b,c). The positioning of these three fixating sutures should orient the appendix into a straight direction without kinking. The appendix should cross the midline 1–3 cm from the umbilical skin anastomosis to the right side, and there is no excess appendix tube.

If the desired stoma site is on the right lower quadrant, the appendix should be passed through the rectus fascia[9] and anastomosed to the skin flap. A wide V or U flap can be used with a spatulated appendix in thin patients.[8,9] In the case of obesity, the VR flap or VQZ flap can be used to adapt according to the

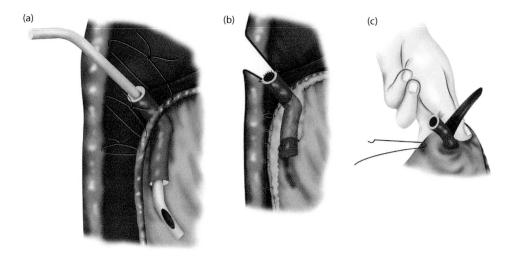

Figure 34.7 (a) The bladder and appendix are brought toward the opening under slight tension. (b) The three sutures for the presentation of the bladder are fixed to the abdominal wall. The 14F catheter, which is calibrated to the suture scars, serves as a guide to assemble the appendix-bladder. (c) The three stitches are tightened and then knotted for perfect positioning of the appendix and the mesoappendix.

abdomen shape.[8] The skin-appendix anastomosis should be done in a similar fashion to the umbilical anastomosis, and the bladder should be attached to the abdominal wall in the same manner. Usually, implantation of the appendix to the right lower quadrant is generally easier than the umbilical site.[8] Table 34.3 summarizes specific troubleshooting and solutions to avoid complications intraoperatively.

BLADDER DRAINAGE AND CLOSURE

After completion of the appendix attachment to the bladder and skin with a 14F catheter in the channel, the surgeon then should address the closure of the bladder or augmentation with the bowel if planned. The bladder should be drained with a suprapubic, large-caliber (20–24F Malecot) catheter through the native bladder. A urethral catheter can be used, but

this has been discouraged.[8] The perivesical space should be drained using a drain, such as Jackson-Pratt drain.[8] Then, any mesenteric defect should be closed to avoid the risk of ileus. Finally, closure of the abdominal wall should be done carefully with slowly absorbable suture. The surgeon should be careful to avoid involving the channel and/or the mesoappendix.[8] It has been suggested to use interrupted 1 PDS sutures to prevent the risk of compressing the appendix or mesoappendix.[8]

POSTOPERATIVE CARE

The drains are removed once no leakage is confirmed a few days postoperatively. The large-caliber suprapubic tube is kept for 3 weeks, along with closed 14F catheter on the appendicovesicostomy tract as a stent. Some have advocated a cystogram after 3 weeks

Table 34.3 Specific Problems and Solutions during Implantation

Appendix Part	Specific Problems	Prevention and Solutions
External part	Stenosis	1. Large interrupted suture with a big cecal collar 2. Interposition of a cutaneous flap in an appendicular incision
Middle part	Mesoappendix constriction	Always inspect the mesoappendix and color of the appendix
		• At bladder fixation points • During closure of the median incision
	Nonrectilinear trajectory (kink) because of excessive length	Reposition the parietal mooring, shorten the appendix
Terminal part	Submucosal trajectory is too short (incontinence)	Re-do the assembly

to rule out leakage from the vesicoappendiceal anastomosis.[9]

At 3 weeks, the suprapubic tube should be clamped, the 14F appendiceal catheter is removed, and the surgeon should assess the ease of catheterization and its direction toward the bladder neck.[8] The patient then should try to catheterize every 4 hours, and if no problems, the suprapubic catheter then should be removed.[9]

OUTCOMES AND LONG-TERM RESULT

Major reported complications are stomal incontinence and stenosis. The reported stomal continence rate in adult series ranges between 100% and 66%, and the reported total continence rate is between 96% and 66%. The reported stenosis rate varies between case series from 6.8% to 54%. The stenosis level is reported as being at skin or more proximal at fascia level or on bladder level. The overall revision rate for complications varied between 20% and 67%.[10-14] The recently reported and largest case series have shown that the appendix channel has fewer complications that reconfigured ileal channels,[15] with channel stenosis of 17.2% versus 22.2% ($P = 0.3$), and incontinence rate of 19.5% versus 36% ($P = 0.03$) for the appendix and reconfigured ileal channels, respectively. Of those patients, 75% were still using the channel at a mean follow-up of 78.6 months. And there was a 90% continence rate.

A recent systematic review of continent catheterizable channels in neuro-urological patients has shown that the Mitrofanoff procedure was the most reported procedure done for neuro-urological adult patients with a stenosis rate of 32.3% for the Mitrofanoff or Casale procedure.[16] They have found no statistically significant difference in the surgical revision rate between appendix or reconfigured ileum.[16]

MANAGEMENT OF COMPLICATIONS

Stomal prolapse is a less common complication, which has been reported to be 2%–5%, which might require revision if not amiable to silver nitrite treatment.[17-19]

A short tunnel usually causes stomal incontinence. Evaluation should be done thoroughly to exclude other causes, such as high reservoir pressure. Using a bulking agent can be tried with some success in the short term,[20] but long-term data are lacking. The reported agent used is dextranomer/hyaluronic acid.[20-23] If failed, surgical revision can be undertaken by either complete take-down and use

of ileal segment, or alternatively leaving the existing channel and wrapping an additional detrusor muscle over the channel.[24]

Difficult catheterization can be caused by stomal stenosis, channel angulation, channel redundancy, and/or channel diverticulum or false passage, which can be managed by conservative management; if failed, formal revision should be carried out.[24]

Types of revision for stomal stenosis have been divided into suprafascial revision and subfascial revision. Suprafascial revision includes excising all scar tissue and reanastomosing the channel to skin flap in YV or VQZ plasty fashion.[24] Subfascial revision should be addressed by removing adherent tissue to the channel and excising the stenotic part, then either reanastomosing to another position or replacing the whole channel if the remaining segment is too short.[24]

CONCLUSION

The Mitrofanoff procedure is the most performed continent catheterizable channel procedure, with acceptable long-term outcomes. The surgeon should be familiar with indications, technical aspects, possible alternative procedures, long-term results, and management of its complications. Strict adherence to the technical details should minimize the risk of future complications.

REFERENCES

1. Mitrofanoff P. Cystostostornie continente trans-appendiculaire dans le traiterent des vessie neuro-logiques. *Chir Pediatr.* 1980;21:297–305.
2. Woodhouse CR and MacNeily AE. The Mitrofanoff principle: Expanding upon a versatile technique. *Br J Urol.* 1994;74(4):447–53.
3. Redshaw JD, Elliott SP, Rosenstein DI et al. Procedures needed to maintain functionality of adult continent catheterizable channels: A comparison of continent cutaneous ileal cecocystoplasty with tunneled catheterizable channels. *J Urol.* 2014;192(3):821–6.
4. Lapides J, Diokno AC, Silber SM et al. Clean, intermittent self-catheterization in the treatment of urinary tract disease. 1972. *J Urol.* 2002;167:1584.
5. Bakke A, Irgens LM, Malt UF et al. Clean intermittent catheterization-performing abilities, aversive experiences and distress. *Spinal Cord.* 1993;31:288.
6. Touma NJ, Horovitz D, Shetty A et al. Outcomes and quality of life of adults undergoing continent catheterizable vesicostomy for neurogenic bladder. *Urology.* 2007;70:454.
7. Levi ME and Elliott SP. Reconstructive techniques for creation of catheterizable channels: Tunneled and nipple valve channels. *Transl Androl Urol.* 2016;5(1):136–44.

8. Boillot B, Corcos J, and Mitrofanoff P. The trans-appendicular continent cystostomy technique (Mitrofanoff principle). In: Jacques Corcos DG, and Gilles K, eds. *Textbook of the Neurogenic Bladder.* 1. 3rd ed. Boca Raton, FL: CRC Press, Taylor & Francis Group; 2016:563–70.

9. Thomas JC. Appendicovesicostomy. In: Joseph A, Smith J, Howards SS, Preminger GM, and Dmochowski RR, eds. *Hinman's Atlas of Urologic Surgery,* 4th ed. Philadelphia, PA: Elsevier; 2018:410–2.

10. Perrouin-Verbe MA, Chartier-Kastler E, Even A, Denys P, Rouprêt M, and Phé V. Long-term complications of continent cutaneous urinary diversion in adult spinal cord injured patients. *Neurourol Urodyn.* 2016;35(8):1046–50.

11. Van der Aa F, Joniau S, De Baets K, and De Ridder D. Continent catheterizable vesicostomy in an adult population: Success at high costs. *Neurourol Urodyn.* 2009;28(6):487–91.

12. Hadley D, Anderson K, Knopick CR, Shah K, and Flynn BJ. Creation of a continent urinary channel in adults with neurogenic bladder: Long-term results with the Monti and Casale (Spiral Monti) procedures. *Urology.* 2014;83(5):1176–80.

13. De Ganck J, Everaert K, Van Laecke E, Oosterlinck W, and Hoebeke P. A high easy-to-treat complication rate is the price for a continent stoma. *BJU Int.* 2002;90(3):240–3.

14. Sahadevan K, Pickard RS, Neal DE, and Hasan TS. Is continent diversion using the Mitofanoff principle a viable long-term term option for adults requiring bladder replacement? *BJU Int.* 2008;102(2):236–40.

15. O'Connor EM, Foley C, Taylor C et al. Appendix or ileum—Which is the best material for Mitrofanoff channel formation in adults? *J Urol.* 2019;202(4):757–62.

16. Phé V, Boissier R, Blok BFM et al. Continent catheterizable tubes/stomas in adult neuro-urological patients: A systematic review. *Neurourol Urodyn.* 2017;36(7):1711–22.

17. Süzer O, Vates TS, Freedman AL et al. Results of the Mitrofanoff procedure in urinary tract reconstruction in children. *Br J Urol.* 1997;79: 279–82.

18. Leslie B, Lorenzo AJ, Moore K et al. Long-term followup and time to event outcome analysis of continent catheterizable channels. *J Urol.* 2011;185:2298–302.

19. Welk BK, Afshar K, Rapoport D et al. Complications of the catheterizable channel following continent urinary diversion: Their nature and timing. *J Urol.* 2008;180:1856–60.

20. Prieto JC, Perez-Brayfield M, Kirsch AJ et al. The treatment of catheterizable stomal incontinence with endoscopic implantation of dextranomer/hyaluronic acid. *J Urol.* 2006;175:709–11.

21. Guys JM, Fakhro A, Haddad M et al. Endoscopic cure of stomal leaks in continent diversion. *BJU Int.* 2002;89:628–9.

22. Halachmi S, Farhat W, Metcalfe P et al. Efficacy of polydimethylsiloxane injection to the bladder neck and leaking diverting stoma for urinary continence. *J Urol.* 2004;171:1287–90.

23. Roth CC, Donovan BO, Tonkin JB et al. Endoscopic injection of submucosal bulking agents for the management of incontinent catheterizable channels. *J Pediatr Urol* 2009;5:265–8.

24. Hampson LA, Baradaran N, and Elliott SP. Long term complications of continent catheterizable channels: A problem for transitional urologists. *Transl Androl Urol.* 2018;7(4):558–66.

Chapter 35

TISSUE ENGINEERING AND CELL THERAPIES FOR NEUROGENIC BLADDER AUGMENTATION AND URINARY CONTINENCE RESTORATION

René Yiou

INTRODUCTION

Research in the field of cell-based therapy and tissue engineering for functional urologic disorders has advanced considerably over the past decade, allowing several recent clinical trials. Here, we review these new technologies applied to neuro-urologic disorders, namely, bladder-tissue engineering for neurogenic bladder and cell therapy for urethral rhabdosphincter insufficiency.

PART 1: BLADDER REPLACEMENT FOR PATIENTS WITH NEUROGENIC BLADDER

Hypertonic low-compliant bladder responsible for urinary incontinence or reflux in the upper urinary tract can develop during the course of several neurologic disorders.[1,2] Bladder augmentation performed to treat neurogenic bladder traditionally involves the use of intestinal segments, which can lead to complications such as urolithiasis, and metabolic disturbances.[3]

In recent years, attention has turned to tissue engineering as an alternative to free tissue grafts for bladder augmentation.[4–12] Promising results were obtained in various animal models of cystectomy. Acellular matrices or scaffolds made of various materials have been tested, either alone or after seeding with viable cells.

BIOMATERIALS

The ideal biomaterial for tissue engineering should be biocompatible, promote cellular interactions, and enhance tissue development, thus replicating the functions of the normal ECM. The biomaterial should degrade slowly after implantation while undergoing colonization by host cells, so that it is eventually replaced by ECM components produced by the seeded or ingrowing cells. Biomaterials that

have been evaluated for engineering genitourinary tissues include naturally derived materials, such as collagen and alginate; decellularized tissue matrix such as bladder submucosa and small intestinal submucosa (SIS); and synthetic polymers such as polyglycolic acid (PGA), polylactic acid (PLA), and polylactic-coglycolic acid (PLGA) (Figure 35.1). The degradation products of PGA, PLA, and PLGA are nontoxic and slowly eliminated from the body in the form of carbon dioxide and water.

Because these polymers are thermoplastics, they can easily be formed into a three-dimensional scaffold with a desired microstructure, gross shape, and dimension by various techniques.

CLINICAL REPORTS OF BLADDER AUGMENTATION USING TISSUE ENGINEERING

In 2006, Atala and colleagues reported the first clinical trial of tissue-engineered bladders in seven patients who had myelomeningocele with poorly compliant bladders and frequent urinary leakage as often as every 30 minutes despite maximal pharmacotherapy.[12] For the scaffolds, collagen matrix derived from decellularized bladder submucosa was used in the first four patients and a composite of collagen and PGA in the next three patients. The scaffolds were seeded with autologous smooth muscle and urothelial cells. A bladder biopsy of 1–2 cm^2 was obtained from the bladder dome through a small suprapubic incision. Smooth muscle cells and urothelial cells were cultured separately for 7 weeks. Then, the smooth muscle cells were seeded on the outer surface and the urothelial cells on the inner surface of the scaffold. The scaffold was covered with omentum in four patients (including the three patients with composite scaffolds) (Figure 35.2). Compared to preoperative values, mean maximum bladder capacity decreased by 30% in the three patients treated with collagen scaffolds and no omental wrap. A 1.22-fold increase (from 438 mL to a mean of 535 mL) was noted in the patient treated with collagen and omental wrap, suggesting a major role of the omentum in the development of an adequate vascular bed in the neobladder. In the

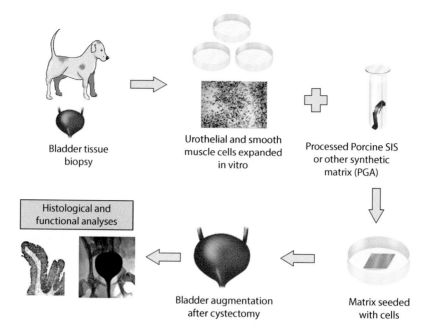

Figure 35.1 Design of bladder tissue engineering protocols. PGA, polyglycolic acid; SIS, small intestinal submucosa.

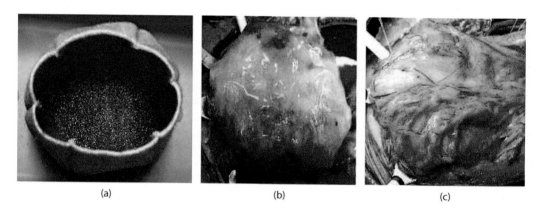

(a)   (b)   (c)

Figure 35.2 Scaffold seeded with cells (a) and engineered bladder anastomosed to native bladder with running 4-0 polyglycolic sutures (b). Implant covered with fibrin glue and omentum (c). (Reproduced with permission from Atala A et al. Tissue-engineered autologous bladders for patients needing cystoplasty. *Lancet*. 2006;367(9518):1241–6.)

three patients treated with the composite scaffold and omental wrap, mean maximum bladder capacity increased 1.58-fold (Figure 35.3), and the maximum mean dry intervals during the day increased from 3 to 7 hours. This pioneering study shows that tissue engineering can be used to generate bladders for patients who require cystoplasty. The beneficial effects of omental wrap emphasize the crucial role played by the vascular supply in the development of the seeded scaffold. Several questions remain, such as the long-term fate of cultivated cells and the risk of premature senescence. In addition, recurrence of the urinary symptoms is theoretically possible, since the underlying neurologic disease remains present.

3D Printing

3D printing has recently emerged as one of the most promising technologies in the field of tissue engineering.[31] It relies on a methodology known as additive manufacturing, which uses digital data of a 3D structure and converts it into an actual object. In contrast to the classical tissue engineering process that involves scaffolds, 3D printing creates complex structures from the bottom-up.

The main approaches for 3D bioprinting are inkjet printing, stereolithography, and extrusion printing. Inkjet bioprinters can deliver biomaterials and cells in controlled volumes like ink in a cartridge delivers droplets to paper to create documents.

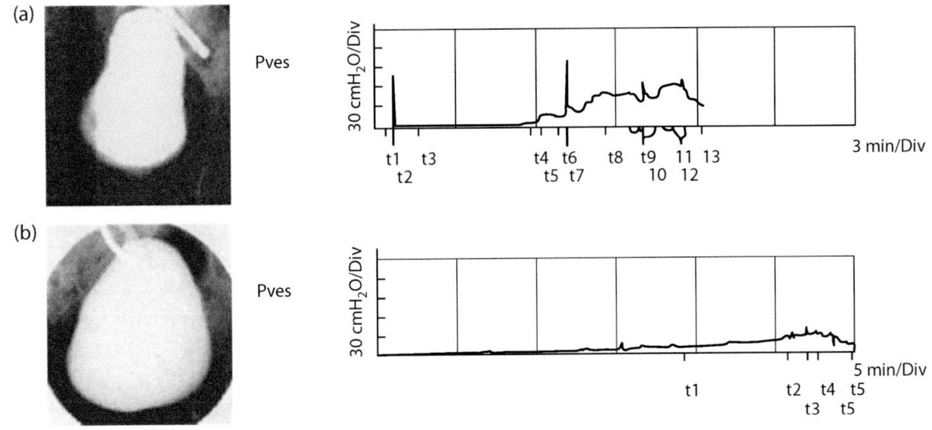

Figure 35.3 Preoperative (a) and 10-month postoperative (b) cystograms and urodynamic findings in patient with a collagen-polyglycolic acid scaffold engineered bladder. Note irregular bladder on cystogram, abnormal bladder pressures on urodynamic study preoperatively, and improved findings postoperatively. (Reproduced with permission from Atala A et al. Tissue-engineered autologous bladders for patients needing cystoplasty. *Lancet*. 2006;367(9518):1241–6.)

One of the main challenges of 3D bioprinting is to avoid thermal or mechanical cell damage associated with droplet production. Further studies are required to define the role of this technology for bladder reconstruction.

PART 2: CELL THERAPY FOR URETHRAL RHABDOSPHINCTER INSUFFICIENCY

Urinary incontinence due to intrinsic urethral sphincter insufficiency develops in many central or peripheral neurologic disorders affecting the nerves that supply the urethral rhabdosphincter.

Cell therapy holds promise for restoring urethral tonicity and sphincter function in patients with urinary sphincter insufficiency, since it represents the first therapeutic option aimed at repairing the cellular damages at the origin of urinary incontinence. Several types of precursor or stem cells have been tested to improve the tone exerted by the smooth or striated components of the urethral musculature; these are mainly stem cells derived from bone marrow,[44–46] adipose tissue,[4,47] or skeletal muscle. At present, urethral injection of striated muscle precursor cells (MPCs) remains the most extensively studied cell therapy approach to urinary incontinence.[48–53] In rodents, improved contractility of the urethral rhabdosphincter was noted after the injection of autologous MPCs.[48,50] Results of several clinical trials conducted with MPCs are now available.[49,52–57] Here, we provide an overview of MPC-based cell therapy for skeletal muscle diseases, and we discuss the biological basis for MPC transfer into the urethra to treat urinary incontinence.

ORIGIN AND FUNCTION OF SKELETAL MUSCLE PRECURSOR CELLS

Satellite cells constitute the main population of MPCs. In the event of muscle injury, the satellite cells proliferate and differentiate into secondary myoblasts, which fuse into new myotubes or repair the parental myofibers.

Importantly, resident satellite cells can fully reconstitute the myofiber mass lost after a muscle injury, although they initially contribute less than 1% of all myonuclei.[58] The considerable myogenic potential of MPCs was recently emphasized by Collins et al.,[20] who found that as few as seven satellite cells could generated more than 100 new myofibers, each of which contained thousands of myonuclei.

The main challenge faced by autologous MPC transfer resides in the high sensitivity of these cells to ischemia, which may impair their survival after implantation. Several solutions to this problem have been investigated. Beauchamps et al. showed that the majority of MPCs died after injection into muscle, despite *in vitro* evidence of vitality, and that the tiny minority that survived exhibited stem cell characteristics.[19] These findings were confirmed by several other groups, prompting researchers to investigate new preparation methods that select MPC exhibiting the stem-cell phenotype.[60,61] However, no clinical studies of such selected MPCs are available.

Other groups investigated the impact of the cell preparation process on myoblast survival.[18,20–24] The few animal studies comparing injections of myoblasts with or without prior culturing consistently showed deleterious effects of culture conditions. Enzymatic disaggregation of muscle biopsies was a major cause of MPC death following implantation.[20] MPC exposure to culture conditions may also contribute to loss of myogenic potential.[23] Montarras et al. found that culturing prior to transplantation markedly reduced the regenerative efficiency of MPCs, so that culture expansion seemed to constitute an "empty" process yielding the same amount of muscle as the number of cells from which the culture was initiated.[18] Thus, there is evidence that the myogenic potential of injected MPCs can be impaired by the cell preparation process, most notably the enzyme digestion step, and by cell culture conditions. It remained to be determined whether injecting small numbers of cells without previous cultivation is more effective than injecting large numbers of MPCs previously expanded *in vitro*.

CHALLENGES FACED BY USING MUSCLE PRECURSOR CELLS TO TREAT INTRINSIC URETHRAL RHABDOSPHINCTER INSUFFICIENCY

Paracrine and Neurotrophic Effects of Muscle Precursor Cell Injections

Whether the host tissue can innervate MPC-derived myotubes is of special concern when seeking to treat intrinsic sphincter insufficiency, since this condition is often associated with chronic muscle denervation.[70] Several groups found that activated MPCs and the myofiber regeneration process promoted motoneuron sprouting.[50,71,72] For instance, following experimental muscle denervation via afferent nerve transection, myofibers and the surrounding ECM released potent neurotrophic factors, such as neuroleukin, insulin-like growth factor, and neural cell adhesion molecules, which can stimulate the sprouting of nearby nerve endings, ultimately leading to myofiber reinnervation.[72] These cytokines and growth factors represent the main mechanism for self-repair of the neuromuscular junction.

Consequently, the injection of MPC or myofibers with attached satellite cells may improve neurogenic intrinsic sphincter insufficiency by activating the sprouting of urethral nerves thought a paracrine effect.

We recently described a new method of MPC transfer into the urethra, in which myofibers and their attached satellite cells, without prior tissue processing, were implanted near the bladder neck at a distance from the rhabdosphincter.[73] The satellite cells underwent activation and fusion, replacing the parent myofibers, which degenerated rapidly after implantation. A large number of myotubes exerting tonic contraction developed. Importantly, these myotubes had cholinergic receptors connected to nerve endings after 1 month, demonstrating connection with urethral nerves. Thus, it can be assumed that the myogenic process allows self-innervation of the new muscle in an ectopic position through a potent paracrine and neurotrophic effect on the environment.

RESULTS OF CLINICAL TRIALS USING MUSCLE PRECURSOR CELLS

Several clinical trials have been conducted with different methods of MPC preparation.

Gräs et al.[82] investigated intraurethral injection of autologous minced skeletal muscle as a means to deliver MPC without expansion *in vitro* in 35 women with stress urinary incontinence. After 1 year, significant reductions in mean number of leakages ($p < .01$) and in ICIQ-SF scores ($p < .001$) were observed: in patients with uncomplicated incontinence, cure (defined as zero leaks in 3 days and an ICIQ-SF score of 5 or less) and improvement were observed in 25% and 63% of patients, and in the complicated group they were noted in 7% and 57%, respectively.

The authors concluded that intraurethral injection of minced autologous muscle tissue is a simple surgical procedure that yields similar results to previous reports of *in vitro* expanded MPCs.

We assessed the safety of periurethral myofiber implantation in 10 patients (5 men after radical prostatectomy and 5 women) with severe urinary incontinence due to intrinsic sphincter deficiency.[57] The objective was to assess the myogenic process resulting from direct implantation of myofiber with their satellite cells—the main MPCs—without cell culture expansion. The maximum urethral closure pressure (MUCP) and concomitant periurethral electromyographic (EMG) activity were recorded before surgery and 1 and 3 months after surgery. Continence was assessed using the 24-hour pad test and self-completed questionnaires, for 12 months. No serious side effect was detected. Continence improved significantly during the 12-month follow-up in 4/5 women, including 2 who recovered normal continence. In the women, MUCP increased twofold and *de novo* EMG periurethral activity was recorded. In the men, MUCP and EMG recordings showed similar improvements, but the effect on continence was moderate. The small number of patients enrolled could affect these results; however, this is the first report of a one-step procedure for transferring autologous MPCs via myofiber implantation that showed improvement of periurethral muscular activity.

Peters et al. tested for urinary incontinence the stem cell–like population of MPC called muscle-derived stem cells (MDSCs) isolated from biopsies of patient's quadriceps femoris and expanded *in vitro* before injection. They included 80 females who were divided in four dose groups (10×106; 50×106; 100×106; 200×106) of MDSCs that were injected via transurethral (56 of 80 patients) or periurethral (24 of 80) approach. All dose groups showed a significant reduction in the diary reported stress leaks, IIQ-7 and UDI-6 at 12 months; and a dose response was suggested by the authors. However, it is not clear how many patients were considered as cured in this study. Seven of the 22 patients of the high-dose group reported zero stress leaks during 3 days after 1 year, but this ratio seemed to differ from other groups.

Gerullis et al.[55] reported the results of transurethral injections of autologous muscle-derived cells into the urinary sphincter in 222 male patients with stress urinary incontinence after prostate surgery. The transplanted cells were characterized after culture using different markers of myogenic differentiation. Overall, 120 patients responded to therapy, of whom 26 patients (12%) were continent, and 94 patients (42%) showed improvement. In 102 (46%) patients, the therapy was ineffective. Clinical improvement was observed on average 4.7 months after transplantation and continued in all improved patients. The authors conclude that transurethral injection of muscle-derived cells into the damaged urethral sphincter of a male patient is a safe procedure and improves continence.

Overall, initial clinical results are encouraging in the setting of intrinsic sphincter deficiency in women and in the men after radical prostatectomy. No clinical trials are available in the context of neurogenic incontinence. However, basic science and research in animal models suggest that the neurotrophic effects mediated by MPC injection may find application in neurogenic incontinence. The most appropriate procedure of cell preparation and transfer into the urethra remains to be determined.

OTHER PROMISING SOURCES OF STEM CELLS TO TREAT URINARY INCONTINENCE

Bone marrow and adipose tissue contain mesenchymal stem cells that were investigated in several animal models of sphincter damage,[4,45–47,84–90] and clinical cases of patients treated with such cells have been reported.[91,92] The rationale behind the use of mesenchymal stem cells for urinary incontinence is in their (1) capacity to transdifferentiate into muscle cells, (2) antiapoptotic effects, (3) releasing of angiogenic and neurotrophic growth factors, (4) ability to recruit local stem cells to participate to the regeneration process, and (5) ability to fuse with preexisting cells.

Mesenchymal stem cells may be harvested from adipose tissue after enzymatical digestion or from bone marrow by simple centrifugation in a Ficoll gradient. Cell culture is required to select mesenchymal stem cells, but protocols of cell injection avoiding this step are now available. In the absence of culture selection, the population of cells obtained is more heterogeneous and also contains endothelial progenitors or endothelial cells that may also have a therapeutic implication.

REFERENCES

1. Kiddoo DA, Carr MC, Dulczak S, and Canning DA. Initial management of complex urological disorders: Bladder exstrophy. Urol Clin North Am. 2004;31:417–26, vii–viii.
2. Snodgrass WT and Adams R. Initial urologic management of myelomeningocele. Urol Clin North Am. 2004;31:427–34, viii.
3. McDougal WS. Metabolic complications of urinary intestinal diversion. J Urol. 1992;147:1199–208.
4. Jack GS, Almeida FG, Zhang R, Alfonso ZC, Zuk PA, and Rodriguez LV. Processed lipoaspirate cells for tissue engineering of the lower urinary tract: Implications for the treatment of stress urinary incontinence and bladder reconstruction. J Urol. 2005;174:2041–5.
5. Zhang Y, Kropp BP, Moore P et al. Coculture of bladder urothelial and smooth muscle cells on small intestinal submucosa: Potential applications for tissue engineering technology. J Urol. 2000;164:928–34; discussion 34–5.
6. Zhang Y, Kropp BP, Lin HK, Cowan R, and Cheng EY. Bladder regeneration with cell-seeded small intestinal submucosa. Tissue Eng. 2004;10:181–7.
7. Yoo JJ, Meng J, Oberpenning F, and Atala A. Bladder augmentation using allogenic bladder submucosa seeded with cells. Urology. 1998;51:221–5.
8. Vaught JD, Kropp BP, Sawyer BD et al. Detrusor regeneration in the rat using porcine small intestinal submucosal grafts: Functional innervation and receptor expression. J Urol. 1996;155:374–8.
9. Schultheiss D, Gabouev AI, Cebotari S et al. Biological vascularized matrix for bladder tissue engineering: Matrix preparation, reseeding technique and short-term implantation in a porcine model. J Urol. 2005;173:276–80.
10. Kropp BP, Rippy MK, Badylak SF et al. Regenerative urinary bladder augmentation using small intestinal submucosa: Urodynamic and histopathologic assessment in long-term canine bladder augmentations. J Urol. 1996;155:2098–104.
11. Kropp BP, Cheng EY, Lin HK, and Zhang Y. Reliable and reproducible bladder regeneration using unseeded distal small intestinal submucosa. J Urol. 2004;172:1710–3.
12. Atala A, Bauer SB, Soker S, Yoo JJ, and Retik AB. Tissue-engineered autologous bladders for patients needing cystoplasty. Lancet. 2006;367:1241–6.
13. Badylak SF, Kropp B, McPherson T, Liang H, and Snyder PW. Small intestinal submucosa: A rapidly resorbed bioscaffold for augmentation cystoplasty in a dog model. Tissue Eng. 1998;4:379–87.
14. de Boer WI, Rebel JM, Vermey M, de Jong AA, and van der Kwast TH. Characterization of distinct functions for growth factors in murine transitional epithelial cells in primary organotypic culture. Exp Cell Res. 1994;214:510–8.
15. Oberpenning F, Meng J, Yoo JJ, and Atala A. De novo reconstitution of a functional mammalian urinary bladder by tissue engineering. Nat Biotechnol. 1999;17:149–55.
16. Lin HK, Cowan R, Moore P et al. Characterization of neuropathic bladder smooth muscle cells in culture. J Urol. 2004;171:1348–52.
17. Dozmorov MG, Kropp BP, Hurst RE, Cheng EY, and Lin HK. Differentially expressed gene networks in cultured smooth muscle cells from normal and neuropathic bladder. J Smooth Muscle Res. 2007;43:55–72.

18. Montarras D, Morgan J, Collins C et al. Direct isolation of satellite cells for skeletal muscle regeneration. *Science.* 2005;309:2064–7.

19. Beauchamp JR, Morgan JE, Pagel CN, and Partridge TA. Dynamics of myoblast transplantation reveal a discrete minority of precursors with stem cell-like properties as the myogenic source. *J Cell Biol.* 1999;144:1113–22.

20. Collins CA, Olsen I, Zammit PS et al. Stem cell function, self-renewal, and behavioral heterogeneity of cells from the adult muscle satellite cell niche. *Cell.* 2005;122:289–301.

21. Fan Y, Beilharz MW, and Grounds MD. A potential alternative strategy for myoblast transfer therapy: The use of sliced muscle grafts. *Cell Transplant.* 1996;5:421–9.

22. Fan Y, Maley M, Beilharz M, and Grounds M. Rapid death of injected myoblasts in myoblast transfer therapy. *Muscle Nerve.* 1996;19:853–60.

23. Smythe GM and Grounds MD. Exposure to tissue culture conditions can adversely affect myoblast behavior *in vivo* in whole muscle grafts: Implications for myoblast transfer therapy. *Cell Transplant.* 2000;9:379–93.

24. Smythe GM, Hodgetts SI, and Grounds MD. Problems and solutions in myoblast transfer therapy. *J Cell Mol Med.* 2001;5:33–47.

25. Bartsch G, Yoo JJ, De Coppi P et al. Propagation, expansion, and multilineage differentiation of human somatic stem cells from dermal progenitors. *Stem Cells Dev.* 2005;14:337–48.

26. De Coppi P, Bartsch G Jr, Siddiqui MM et al. Isolation of amniotic stem cell lines with potential for therapy. *Nat Biotechnol.* 2007;25:100–6.

27. Walles T, Herden T, Haverich A, and Mertsching H. Influence of scaffold thickness and scaffold composition on bioartificial graft survival. *Biomaterials.* 2003;24:1233–9.

28. Nomi M, Atala A, Coppi PD, and Soker S. Principals of neovascularization for tissue engineering. *Mol Aspects Med.* 2002;23:463–83.

29. Shea LD, Smiley E, Bonadio J, and Mooney DJ. DNA delivery from polymer matrices for tissue engineering. *Nat Biotechnol.* 1999;17:551–4.

30. Kinnaird T, Stabile E, Epstein SE, and Fuchs S. Current perspectives in therapeutic myocardial angiogenesis. *J Interv Cardiol.* 2003;16:289–97.

31. Kaushik G, Leijten J, and Khademhosseini A. Concise review: Organ engineering: Design, technology, and integration. *Stem Cells.* 2017;35:51–60.

32. Haab F, Zimmern PE, and Leach GE. Female stress urinary incontinence due to intrinsic sphincteric deficiency: Recognition and management. *J Urol.* 1996;156:3–17.

33. Thuroff JW, Abrams P, Andersson KE et al. EAU Guidelines on Urinary Incontinence. *Actas Urol Esp.* 2011;35:373–88.

34. Mottet N, Boyer C, Chartier-Kastler E, Ben Naoum K, Richard F, and Costa P. Artificial urinary sphincter AMS 800 for urinary incontinence after radical prostatectomy: The French experience. *Urol Int.* 1998;60(Suppl 2):25–9; discussion 35.

35. Costa P, Poinas G, Ben Naoum K et al. Long-term results of artificial urinary sphincter for women with type III stress urinary incontinence. *Eur Urol.* 2013;63:753–8.

36. Abrams P, Andersson KE, Birder L et al. Fourth International Consultation on Incontinence Recommendations of the International Scientific Committee: Evaluation and treatment of urinary incontinence, pelvic organ prolapse, and fecal incontinence. *Neurourol Urodyn.* 2010;29:213–40.

37. Hubner WA, Gallistl H, Rutkowski M, and Huber ER. Adjustable bulbourethral male sling: Experience after 101 cases of moderate-to-severe male stress urinary incontinence. *BJU Int.* 2011;107:777–82.

38. Hubner WA and Schlarp OM. Treatment of incontinence after prostatectomy using a new minimally invasive device: Adjustable continence therapy. *BJU Int.* 2005;96:587–94.

39. Kjaer L, Fode M, Norgaard N, Sonksen J, and Nordling J. Adjustable continence balloons: Clinical results of a new minimally invasive treatment for male urinary incontinence. *Scand J Urol Nephrol.* 2012;46:196–200.

40. Lebret T, Cour F, Benchetrit J et al. Treatment of postprostatectomy stress urinary incontinence using a minimally invasive adjustable continence balloon device, ProACT: Results of a preliminary, multicenter, pilot study. *Urology.* 2008;71:256–60.

41. Keegan PE, Atiemo K, Cody J, McClinton S, and Pickard R. Periurethral injection therapy for urinary incontinence in women. *Cochrane Database Syst Rev.* 2007:CD003881.

42. Haab F, Zimmern PE, and Leach GE. Urinary stress incontinence due to intrinsic sphincteric deficiency: Experience with fat and collagen periurethral injections. *J Urol.* 1997;157:1283–6.

43. Wilson TS, Lemack GE, and Zimmern PE. Management of intrinsic sphincteric deficiency in women. *J Urol.* 2003;169:1662–9.

44. Adamiak A and Rechberger T. Potential application of stem cells in urogynecology. *Endokrynol Pol.* 2005;56:994–7.

45. Stangel-Wojcikiewicz K, Majka M, Basta A et al. Adult stem cells therapy for urine incontinence in women. *Ginekol Pol.* 2010;81:378–81.

46. Smaldone MC, Chen ML, and Chancellor MB. Stem cell therapy for urethral sphincter regeneration. *Minerva Urol Nefrol.* 2009;61:27–40.

47. Zhao W, Zhang C, Jin C et al. Periurethral injection of autologous adipose-derived stem cells with controlled-release nerve growth factor for the treatment of stress urinary incontinence in a rat model. *Eur Urol.* 2011;59:155–63.

48. Cannon TW, Lee JY, Somogyi G et al. Improved sphincter contractility after allogenic muscle-derived progenitor cell injection into the denervated rat urethra. *Urology.* 2003;62:958–63.

49. Strasser H, Marksteiner R, Margreiter E et al. Stem cell therapy for urinary incontinence. *Urol A.* 2004;43:1237–41.

50. Yiou R, Yoo JJ, and Atala A. Restoration of functional motor units in a rat model of sphincter injury by muscle precursor cell autografts. *Transplantation.* 2003;76:1053–60.

51. Peyromaure M, Sebe P, Praud C et al. Fate of implanted syngenic muscle precursor cells in striated urethral sphincter of female rats: Perspectives for treatment of urinary incontinence. *Urology.* 2004;64:1037–41.

52. Sebe P, Doucet C, Cornu JN et al. Intrasphincteric injections of autologous muscular cells in women with refractory stress urinary incontinence: A prospective study. *Int Urogynecol J.* 2011;22:183–9.

53. Cornu JN, Doucet C, Sebe P et al. Prospective evaluation of intrasphincteric injections of autologous muscular cells in patients with stress urinary incontinence following radical prostatectomy. *Prog Urol.* 2011;21:859–65.

54. Strasser H, Marksteiner R, Margreiter E et al. Autologous myoblasts and fibroblasts versus collagen for treatment of stress urinary incontinence in women: A randomised controlled trial. *Lancet.* 2007;369:2179–86.

55. Gerullis H, Eimer C, Georgas E et al. Muscle-derived cells for treatment of iatrogenic sphincter damage and urinary incontinence in men. *Sci World J.* 2012;2012:898535.

56. Carr LK, Steele D, Steele S et al. 1-year follow-up of autologous muscle-derived stem cell injection pilot study to treat stress urinary incontinence. *Int Urogynecol J Pelvic Floor Dysfunct.* 2008;19:881–3.

57. Yiou R, Hogrel JY, Loche CM et al. Periurethral skeletal myofibre implantation in patients with urinary incontinence and intrinsic sphincter deficiency: A phase I clinical trial. *BJU Int.* 2013;111:1105–16.

58. Zammit PS, Heslop L, Hudon V et al. Kinetics of myoblast proliferation show that resident satellite cells are competent to fully regenerate skeletal muscle fibers. *Exp Cell Res.* 2002;281:39–49.

59. Beauchamp JR, Heslop L, Yu DS et al. Expression of CD34 and Myf5 defines the majority of quiescent adult skeletal muscle satellite cells. *J Cell Biol.* 2000;151:1221–34.

60. Gussoni E, Soneoka Y, Strickland CD et al. Dystrophin expression in the mdx mouse restored by stem cell transplantation. *Nature.* 1999;401:390–4.

61. Qu-Petersen Z, Deasy B, Jankowski R et al. Identification of a novel population of muscle stem cells in mice: Potential for muscle regeneration. *J Cell Biol.* 2002;157:851–64.

62. Tavian M, Zheng B, Oberlin E et al. The vascular wall as a source of stem cells. *Ann N Y Acad Sci.* 2005;1044:41–50.

63. Dreyfus PA, Chretien F, Chazaud B et al. Adult bone marrow-derived stem cells in muscle connective tissue and satellite cell niches. *Am J Pathol.* 2004;164:773–9.

64. Partridge TA, Morgan JE, Coulton GR, Hoffman EP, and Kunkel LM. Conversion of mdx myofibres from dystrophin-negative to -positive by injection of normal myoblasts. *Nature.* 1989;337:176–9.

65. Mendell JR, Kissel JT, Amato AA et al. Myoblast transfer in the treatment of Duchenne's muscular dystrophy. *N Engl J Med.* 1995;333:832–8.

66. Menasche P, Hagege AA, Scorsin M et al. Myoblast transplantation for heart failure. *Lancet.* 2001;357:279–80.

67. Tremblay JP, Malouin F, Roy R et al. Results of a triple blind clinical study of myoblast transplantations without immunosuppressive treatment in young boys with Duchenne muscular dystrophy. *Cell Transplant.* 1993;2:99–112.

68. Urish K, Kanda Y, and Huard J. Initial failure in myoblast transplantation therapy has led the way toward the isolation of muscle stem cells: Potential for tissue regeneration. *Curr Top Dev Biol.* 2005;68:263–80.

69. Qu Z, Balkir L, van Deutekom JC, Robbins PD, Pruchnic R, and Huard J. Development of approaches to improve cell survival in myoblast transfer therapy. *J Cell Biol.* 1998;142:1257–67.

70. Hale DS, Benson JT, Brubaker L, Heidkamp MC, and Russell B. Histologic analysis of needle biopsy of urethral sphincter from women with normal and stress incontinence with comparison of electromyographic findings. *Am J Obstet Gynecol.* 1999;180:342–8.

71. van Mier P and Lichtman JW. Regenerating muscle fibers induce directional sprouting from nearby nerve terminals: Studies in living mice. *J Neurosci.* 1994;14:5672–86.

72. English AW. Cytokines, growth factors and sprouting at the neuromuscular junction. *J Neurocytol.* 2003;32:943–60.

73. Lecoeur C, Swieb S, Zini L et al. Intraurethral transfer of satellite cells by myofiber implants results in the formation of innervated myotubes exerting tonic contractions. *J Urol.* 2007;178:332–7.

74. Gosling JA, Dixon JS, Critchley HO, and Thompson SA. A comparative study of the human external sphincter and periurethral levator ani muscles. *Br J Urol.* 1981;53:35–41.

75. Yiou R, Delmas V, Carmeliet P et al. The pathophysiology of pelvic floor disorders: Evidence from a histomorphologic study of the perineum and a mouse model of rectal prolapse. *J Anat.* 2001;199:599–607.

76. Badra S, Andersson KE, Dean A, Mourad S, and Williams JK. Long-term structural and functional effects of autologous muscle precursor cell therapy in a nonhuman primate model of urinary sphincter deficiency. *J Urol.* 2013;190(5):1938–45.

77. Eberli D, Aboushwareb T, Soker S, Yoo JJ, and Atala A. Muscle precursor cells for the restoration of irreversibly damaged sphincter function. *Cell Transplant.* 2012;21:2089–98.

78. Zini L, Lecoeur C, Swieb S et al. The striated urethral sphincter of the pig shows morphological and functional characteristics essential for the evaluation of treatments for sphincter insufficiency. *J Urol.* 2006;176:2729–35.

79. Bacou F, Rouanet P, Barjot C, Janmot C, Vigneron P, and d'Albis A. Expression of myosin isoforms in denervated, cross-reinnervated, and electrically stimulated rabbit muscles. *Eur J Biochem.* 1996;236:539–47.

80. Mitterberger M, Pinggera GM, Marksteiner R et al. Functional and histological changes after myoblast injections in the porcine rhabdosphincter. *Eur Urol.* 2007;52:1736–43.

81. Morgan DM, Umek W, Guire K, Morgan HK, Garabrant A, and DeLancey JO. Urethral sphincter morphology and function with and without stress incontinence. *J Urol.* 2009;182:203–9.

82. Gras S, Klarskov N, and Lose G. Intraurethral injection of autologous minced skeletal muscle: A simple surgical treatment for stress urinary incontinence. *J Urol.* 2014;192:850–5.

83. Peters KM, Dmochowski RR, Carr LK et al. Autologous muscle derived cells for treatment of stress urinary incontinence in women. *J Urol.* 2014;192:469–76.

84. Zou XH, Zhi YL, Chen X et al. Mesenchymal stem cell seeded knitted silk sling for the treatment of stress urinary incontinence. *Biomaterials.* 2010;31:4872–9.

85. Smaldone MC and Chancellor MB. Muscle derived stem cell therapy for stress urinary incontinence. *World J Urol.* 2008;26:327–32.

86. Lin CS and Lue TF. Stem cell therapy for stress urinary incontinence: A critical review. *Stem Cells Dev.* 2012;21:834–43.

87. Kinebuchi Y, Aizawa N, Imamura T, Ishizuka O, Igawa Y, and Nishizawa O. Autologous bone-marrow-derived mesenchymal stem cell transplantation into injured rat urethral sphincter. *Int J Urol.* 2010;17:359–68.

88. Furuta A, Jankowski RJ, Pruchnic R, Yoshimura N, and Chancellor MB. The promise of stem cell therapy to restore urethral sphincter function. *Curr Urol Rep.* 2007;8:373–8.

89. Furuta A, Carr LK, Yoshimura N, and Chancellor MB. Advances in the understanding of stress urinary incontinence and the promise of stem-cell therapy. *Rev Urol.* 2007;9:106–12.

90. Corcos J, Loutochin O, Campeau L et al. Bone marrow mesenchymal stromal cell therapy for external urethral sphincter restoration in a rat model of stress urinary incontinence. *Neurourol Urodyn.* 2011;30:447–55.

91. Yamamoto T, Gotoh M, Kato M et al. Periurethral injection of autologous adipose-derived regenerative cells for the treatment of male stress urinary

incontinence: Report of three initial cases. *Int J Urol.* 2012;19:652–9.

92. Gotoh M, Yamamoto T, Kato M et al. Regenerative treatment of male stress urinary incontinence by periurethral injection of autologous adipose-derived regenerative cells: 1-year outcomes in 11 patients. *Int J Urol.* 2014;21(3):294–300.

Chapter 36

NEUROPROTECTION AND REPAIR AFTER SPINAL CORD INJURY

Jehane H. Dagher

INTRODUCTION

The pathophysiology of spinal cord injury (SCI) has generated significant research interest, and many attempts to limit injury (neuroprotection), improve regeneration, or augment the function of surviving tissue (neuroaugmentation) have met success in animal models. This chapter is an overview of the predominant mechanisms of SCI and therapeutic approaches identified in preclinical and human studies.

PRIMARY AND SECONDARY SPINAL CORD INJURY

Primary SCI is the result of physical forces of the initial traumatic event and is often the most important determinant of injury severity; physical forces include compression, shearing, laceration, and acute stretch/distraction.[1] Secondary injury mechanisms include ischemia, sodium- and calcium-mediated cell injury, glutamatergic excitotoxicity, hemorrhage, and inflammation. The secondary injury amplifies the primary damage and promotes cystic degeneration and glial scar formation, thereby preventing functional recovery.[2]

INJURY MECHANISMS AND NEUROPROTECTION

ISCHEMIA

Vascular alterations after SCI include vasospasm due to mechanical vascular and endothelial injury as well as the release of vasoactive amines; thrombosis; edema due to increased vascular permeability and cytotoxicity; impaired vascular autoregulation; impaired venous outflow; and systemic hypotension.[3]

Aggressive hemodynamic and respiratory management in an intensive care setting reduces morbidity, mortality, and length of stay. In light of consistently observed improvement in morbidity and mortality associated with blood pressure augmentation, the 2012 Guidelines for the Management of Acute Cervical Spine and Spinal Cord Injury recommend the maintenance of mean arterial pressure (MAP) between 85 and 90 mm Hg in the first 7 days following acute SCI (level 3 recommendation).[4]

IONIC MECHANISMS AND EXCITOTOXICITY

Disruptions of homeostasis of Na^+ and Ca^{2+} appear pivotal in the pathophysiology of SCI.[5] Following SCI, several factors, most prominently ischemia, lead to energy depletion and decreased intracellular adenosine triphosphate. This leads to a breakdown of the normal membrane electrochemical gradients and membrane depolarization. These pathologic changes in turn trigger the opening of voltage-gated Na^+ channels, further exacerbating the dissipation of the normal membrane electrochemical gradient. Increased intracellular Na^+ causes cell swelling and cytotoxic edema; activation of phospholipases; intracellular acidification; increased intracellular Ca^{2+}; and reverse operation of Na^+-dependent glutamate transporters, exacerbating rises in extracellular glutamate and excitotoxicity.[6]

SODIUM CHANNEL BLOCKER

The results of recently completed early phase trials have provided the rationale for further study through randomized controlled human studies.[7-9] Riluzole, a sodium channel blocker currently used in the treatment of amyotrophic lateral sclerosis, is thought to reduce both aberrant sodium channel activation and glutamate release following SCI.[10] Clinical trial showed efficacy and safety of riluzole, particularly in patients with incomplete cervical injury.[7,11,12]

CALCIUM CHANNEL BLOCKERS

Animal SCI models have confirmed both the neuroprotective benefits of calcium channel blockade[13-15] and an associated increase in post traumatic spinal blood flow.[16,17] Pointillart et al. investigated the calcium channel blocker nimodipine as well as methylprednisolone in 106 patients with acute SCI; however, no benefits were significant in humans.[18]

APOPTOSIS

Early neuronal apoptosis in SCI is followed by a delayed wave of predominantly oligodendroglial programmed cell death in degenerating white matter tracts.[19-28] These observations point to a longer therapeutic window for antiapoptotic strategies in SCI than that of therapies aimed at other secondary mechanisms.[19] Glial apoptosis occurs, at least in part, as a consequence of axonal degeneration[29-31] and activation of programmed cell death,[32,33] including activation of cell death programs in the oligodendrocyte.[28,34]

GRANULOCYTE COLONY-STIMULATING FACTOR

In response to ischemia and central nervous system (CNS) injury, granulocyte colony-stimulating factor (G-CSF) and its receptor (CD114; G-CSFR) are upregulated in neurons and endogenous stem cells, initiating a compensatory neuroprotective mechanism. By binding to its cognate receptor, G-CSF counteracts programmed cell death in mature neurons, induces neurogenesis, and promotes neuronal differentiation of adult neural stem cells. Improvements in motor and sensory scores were significant; However, all studies were open-label and non-randomized, and double-blinded randomized controlled clinical trials for G-CSF are needed.[35-41]

GLIAL SCAR

In SCI, glial scars are thought to act as a barrier to regeneration and recovery. A glial scar's cellular component is composed predominantly of reactive astrocytes with the surrounding matrix rich in proteoglycans.[42] This structure is thought to provide a physical barrier to axonal extension as well as to express proteins such as chondroitin sulfate proteoglycans that inhibit axonal growth.[42] Chondroitinase ABC, which removes glycosaminoglycan side chains from these molecules, promotes axonal extension and functional recovery after SCI.[43] In addition to being a potentially useful primary treatment in SCI, in limiting the glial scar and in reducing its inhibitory effects, chondroitinase ABC may be key in strategies involving cell transplant. Following cell transplantation, axons that traverse a cell transplant may be inhibited from reentering the CNS distally in part by glial scar.[44]

Recent evidence may indicate that the glial scar also provides some important beneficial functions after injury. Targeted depletion of reactive astrocytes that undergo mitosis indicated that after injury, this component of the glial scar serves to repair the blood-brain barrier, prevent an overwhelming inflammatory response, and limit cellular degeneration.[45,46] The role of the glial scar may also be to seclude the injury site from healthy tissue, preventing spreading tissue damage.[46]

MYELIN-ASSOCIATED INHIBITORY PROTEINS

It has long been recognized that CNS myelin is a nonpermissive substrate for neurite extension.[47] Attempts to identify the molecular components responsible for that inhibition have identified three proteins of key interest: Nogo,[48] MAG, and oligodendrocyte myelin glycoprotein.[49,50] These ligands and their shared receptors, therefore, provide targets that may disinhibit neurite extension in a myelin environment. Inhibition of Nogo using a portion of its receptor or neutralizing antiserum has shown evidence of improved axonal extension and improved functional recovery.[51,52] Anti-Nogo-A antibody has been shown to promote axonal sprouting and improve functional recovery following injury.[53] A non-randomized, open-label phase I clinical trial of humanized anti-Nogo-A antibody was initiated to assess the feasibility, tolerability, and safety of either repeated intrathecal bolus injections or continuous intrathecal delivery in acute SCI (4–14 days after injury); results are pending (ATI-355; Novartis Pharmaceuticals).

HYPOTHERMIA

The safety of systemic hypothermia as a means to ameliorate secondary injury has also been demonstrated.[54]

METHYLPREDNISOLONE

Three National Acute Spinal Cord Injury Studies (NASCIS) evaluated the clinical safety and efficacy of varying methylprednisolone sodium succinate (MPSS) dose and timing. NASCIS results have been retrospectively analyzed on numerous occasions to derive meaningful conclusions: MPSS does not increase the risk of infections and confers significant short term effects when given within the first 8 hours of injury.[55] Patients with cervical SCI and reduced baseline injury severity seem to benefit most from this treatment.[56] These improvements have tremendous impact on patients' quality of life; hence, the most recent AOSpine guideline currently recommends a 24-hour treatment of intravenous MPSS when initiated within the first 8 hours of SCI, independent of injury level.[57]

GANGLIOSIDES

Gangliosides are found in high concentration in the outer cell membranes of CNS cells, especially in the vicinity of synapses. The proposed mechanisms of action of exogenously administered gangliosides include antiexcitotoxic activities, prevention of apoptosis, augmentation of neurite outgrowth, and induction of neuronal sprouting and regeneration.[58-61] The proposed neuroregenerative benefits of GM-1 ganglioside provided the impetus for clinical trials in humans with acute SCI, but results had no statistically significant improvement with treatment.[62,63]

MINOCYCLINE

The neuroprotective benefits of minocycline, a synthetic tetracycline antibiotic, are thought to include the inhibition of microglial activation and proliferation, reduction of excitotoxicity, limitation of neuronal and oligodendroglial apoptosis through mitochondrial stabilization, removal of oxygen free radicals, attenuation of inflammation, and Ca^{2+} chelation. Improved neurologic recovery following administration of minocycline has been demonstrated in animal models of ischemic stroke, Parkinson's disease, multiple sclerosis, Huntington's disease, as well as SCI.[64-66]

Although results of an early phase clinical trial are encouraging,[67] the efficacy of minocycline in the treatment of human SCI has yet to be definitively established.

CELLULAR TRANSPLANTATION

The transplantation of various cellular subtypes including stems cells, bone marrow stromal cells, autologous macrophages, Schwann cells, and olfactory ensheathing glia, the controversial fetal cells, induced pluripotent stem cells (iPSCs) following SCI has been the subject of extensive preclinical studies.[68] Their proposed mechanisms of promoting neurologic recovery include the release of growth stimulating trophic factors, reduction of glial scar, removal of inhibitory myelin debris, amelioration of inflammation, and cellular replacement.[69] They may allow the creation of a permissive environment for axonal extension (e.g., Schwann cells and olfactory ensheathing glia), although to be successful, regenerative strategies require extension into distal spinal tissue from the transplanted environment.[70] They may elaborate growth factors that can influence local neurons and axonal elements (e.g., by *ex vivo* genetic modification).[71] They also may have the potential of differentiating into neurons or glia providing the cellular elements for true regeneration (e.g., stem cells).[69] Many of these therapies are first cultured, perhaps modified, and then introduced into the spinal cord. Predominantly done in the subacute and chronic phases of injury, only a few cell transplantation strategies are thought to have neuroprotective potential for the acutely injured spinal cord. Although serious adverse events associated with cellular transplantation have been rare among early phase uncontrolled human studies,[72-80] their efficacy is difficult to determine given the natural history of modest recovery that frequently occurs following acute SCI.

Several randomized controlled trials investigating cellular transplantation following SCI have been successfully performed to date.[81-85]

Despite little evidence of efficacy to date, interest remains in cellular transplantation strategies.

CONCLUSIONS

Neuroprotection has the potential to improve recovery of motor, sensory, and autonomic function following SCI. Further research is necessary to delineate the efficacy of treatment on recovery.

REFERENCES

1. Ackery A, Tator C, and Krassioukov A. A global perspective on spinal cord injury epidemiology. *J Neurotrauma.* 2004;21(10):1355–70.
2. Ulndreaj A, Badner A, and Fehlings MG. Promising neuroprotective strategies for traumatic spinal cord injury with a focus on the differential effects among anatomical levels of injury. *F1000 Res.* 2017;6.
3. Tator CH and Fehlings MG. Review of the secondary injury theory of acute spinal cord trauma with emphasis on vascular mechanisms. *J Neurosurg.* 1991;75(1):15–26.
4. Ryken TC, Hurlbert RJ, Hadley MN et al. The acute cardiopulmonary management of patients with cervical spinal cord injuries. *Neurosurgery.* 2013;72(Suppl 2):84–92.
5. Agrawal S, Nashmi R, and Fehlings M. Role of L- and N-type calcium channels in the pathophysiology of traumatic spinal cord white matter injury. *Neuroscience.* 2000;99(1):179–88.
6. Xu G-Y Hughes MG, Ye Z, Hulsebosch CE, McAdoo DJ. Concentrations of glutamate released following spinal cord injury kill oligodendrocytes in the spinal cord. *Exp Neurol.* 2004;187(2):329–36.
7. Grossman RG, Fehlings MG, Frankowski RF et al. A prospective, multicenter, phase I matched-comparison group trial of safety, pharmacokinetics, and preliminary efficacy of riluzole in patients with traumatic spinal cord injury. *J Neurotrauma.* 2014;31(3):239–55.
8. Fehlings MG, Theodore N, Harrop J et al. A phase I/IIa clinical trial of a recombinant Rho protein antagonist in acute spinal cord injury. *J Neurotrauma.* 2011;28(5):787–96.
9. McKerracher L, and Anderson KD. Analysis of recruitment and outcomes in the phase I/IIa Cethrin clinical trial for acute spinal cord injury. *J Neurotrauma.* 2013;30(21):1795–804.
10. Schwartz G, and Fehlings MG. Secondary injury mechanisms of spinal cord trauma: A novel therapeutic approach for the management of secondary pathophysiology with the sodium channel blocker riluzole. In: Mara D (ed.). *Progress in Brain Research.* New York, NY: Elsevier; 2002:177–90.
11. Fehlings MG, Nakashima H, Nagoshi N, Chow DS, Grossman RG, Kopjar B. Rationale, design and critical end points for the Riluzole in Acute Spinal Cord Injury Study (RISCIS): A randomized, double-blinded, placebo-controlled parallel multi-center trial. *Spinal Cord.* 2016;54(1):8-15.
12. Fehlings MG, Wilson JR, Frankowski RF et al. Riluzole for the treatment of acute traumatic

spinal cord injury: Rationale for and design of the NACTN Phase I clinical trial. *J Neurosurg Spine*. 2012;17(Suppl 1):151–6.

13. De Ley G and Leybaert L. Effect of flunarizine and methylprednisolone on functional recovery after experimental spinal injury. *J Neurotrauma*. 1993;10(1):25–35.

14. Pointillart V, Gense D, Gross C et al. Effects of nimodipine on posttraumatic spinal cord ischemia in baboons. *J Neurotrauma*. 1993;10(2):201–13.

15. Ross IB, Tator CH, and Theriault E. Effect of nimodipine or methylprednisolone on recovery from acute experimental spinal cord injury in rats. *Surg Neurol*. 1993;40(6):461–70.

16. Guha A, Tator CH, and Piper I. Effect of a calcium channel blocker on posttraumatic spinal cord blood flow. *J Neurosurg*. 1987;66(3):423–30.

17. Ross IB and Tator CH. Spinal cord blood flow and evoked potential responses after treatment with nimodipine or methylprednisolone in spinal cord-injured rats. *Neurosurgery*. 1993;33(3):470–7.

18. Pointillart V, Petitjean ME, Wiart L et al. Pharmacological therapy of spinal cord injury during the acute phase. *Spinal Cord*. 2000;38(2):71–6.

19. Casha S, Yu W, and Fehlings M. Oligodendroglial apoptosis occurs along degenerating axons and is associated with FAS and p75 expression following spinal cord injury in the rat. *Neuroscience*. 2001;103(1):203–18.

20. Li GL, Brodin G, Farooque M et al. Apoptosis and expression of Bcl-2 after compression trauma to rat spinal cord. *J Neuropathol Exp Neurol*. 1996;55(3):280–9.

21. Li GL, Farooque M, Holtz A, Olsson Y et al. Apoptosis of oligodendrocytes occurs for long distances away from the primary injury after compression trauma to rat spinal cord. *Acta Neuropathol*. 1999;98(5):473–80.

22. Katoh K, Ikata T, Katoh S et al. Induction and its spread of apoptosis in rat spinal cord after mechanical trauma. *Neurosci Lett*. 1996;216(1):9–12.

23. Lou J, Lenke LG, Ludwig FJ, O'Brien MF et al. Apoptosis as a mechanism of neuronal cell death following acute experimental spinal cord injury. *Spinal Cord*. 1998;36(10):683–90.

24. Crowe MJ, Bresnahan JC, Shuman SL et al. Apoptosis and delayed degeneration after spinal cord injury in rats and monkeys. *Nat Med*. 1997;3(1):73–6.

25. Liu XZ, Xu XM, Hu R et al. Neuronal and glial apoptosis after traumatic spinal cord injury. *J Neurosci*. 1997;17(14):5395–406.

26. Yong C, Arnold PM, Zoubine MN et al. Apoptosis in cellular compartments of rat spinal cord after severe contusion injury. *J Neurotrauma*.1998;15(7):459–72.

27. Emery E, Aldana P, Bunge MB et al. Apoptosis after traumatic human spinal cord injury. *J Neurosurg*. 1998;89(6):911–20.

28. Shuman SL, Bresnahan JC, and Beattie MS. Apoptosis of microglia and oligodendrocytes after spinal cord contusion in rats. *J Neurosci Res*. 1997;50(5):798–808.

29. Warden P et al. Delayed glial cell death following wallerian degeneration in white matter tracts after spinal cord dorsal column cordotomy in adult rats. *Exp Neurol*. 2001;168(2):213–24.

30. Abe Y, Bamber NI, Li H et al. Apoptotic cells associated with Wallerian degeneration after experimental spinal cord injury: A possible mechanism of oligodendroglial death. *J Neurotrauma*. 1999;16(10):945–52.

31. Bjartmar C, Yin X, and Trapp BD. Axonal pathology in myelin disorders. *J Neurocytol*. 1999;28(4–5):383–95.

32. Fernandez P-A, Tang DG, Cheng L, Prochiantz A, Mudge AW, Raff MC et al. Evidence that axon-derived neuregulin promotes oligodendrocyte survival in the developing rat optic nerve. *Neuron*. 2000;28(1):81–90.

33. Flores AI, Mallon S, Matsui T et al. Akt-mediated survival of oligodendrocytes induced by neuregulins. *J Neurosci*. 2000;20(20):7622–30.

34. Yin X, Crawford TO, Griffin JW et al. Myelin-associated glycoprotein is a myelin signal that modulates the caliber of myelinated axons. *J Neurosci*. 1998;18(6):1953–62.

35. Chung J, Kim MH, Yoon YJ, Kim KH, Park SR, Choi BH. Effects of granulocyte colony–stimulating factor and granulocyte-macrophage colony–stimulating factor on glial scar formation after spinal cord injury in rats. *J Neurosurg Spine*. 2014;21(6):966–73.

36. Schneider A, Krüger C, Steigleder T et al. The hematopoietic factor G-CSF is a neuronal ligand that counteracts programmed cell death and drives neurogenesis. *J Clin Invest*. 2005;115(8):2083–98.

37. Kawabe J, Koda M, Hashimoto M et al. Neuroprotective effects of granulocyte colony-stimulating factor and relationship to promotion of angiogenesis after spinal cord injury in rats. *J Neurosurg Spine*. 2011;15(4):414–21.

38. Hartung T. Anti-inflammatory effects of granulocyte colony-stimulating factor. *Curr Opin Hematol*. 1998;5(3):221–5.

39. Kamiya K, Koda M, Furuya T et al. Neuroprotective therapy with granulocyte colony-stimulating factor in acute spinal cord injury: A comparison with high-dose methylprednisolone as a historical control. *Eur Spine J*. 2015;24(5):963–7.

40. Inada T, Takahashi H, Yamazaki M et al. Multicenter prospective nonrandomized controlled clinical trial to prove neurotherapeutic effects of granulocyte colony-stimulating factor for acute spinal cord injury: Analyses of follow-up cases after at least 1 year. *Spine*. 2014;39(3):213–9.

41. Saberi H, Derakhshanrad N, and Yekaninejad MS. Comparison of neurological and functional outcomes after administration of granulocyte-colony-stimulating factor in motor-complete versus motor-incomplete postrehabilitated, chronic spinal cord injuries: A phase I/II study. *Cell Transplant*. 2014;23(1 Suppl):19–23.

42. Silver J and Miller JH. Regeneration beyond the glial scar. *Nat Rev Neurosci*. 2004;5(2):146.

43. Bradbury EJ, Moon LD, Popat RJ et al. Chondroitinase ABC promotes functional recovery after spinal cord injury. *Nature*. 2002;416(6881):636.

44. Chau C, Shum DK, Li H et al. Chondroitinase ABC enhances axonal regrowth through Schwann cell-seeded guidance channels after spinal cord injury. *FASEB J*. 2004;18(1):194–6.

45. Bush TG, Puvanachandra N, Horner CH et al. Leukocyte infiltration, neuronal degeneration, and neurite outgrowth after ablation of scar-forming, reactive astrocytes in adult transgenic mice. *Neuron*. 1999;23(2):297–308.

46. Faulkner JR, Herrmann JE, Woo MJ, Tansey KE, Doan NB, Sofroniew MV. Reactive astrocytes protect tissue and preserve function after spinal cord injury. *J Neurosci*. 2004;24(9):2143–55.

47. Ramón y Cajal S. Degeneration and regeneration of the nervous system. Javier DeFelipe and Edward G. Jones. editors. Translated by R. M. May. Oxford University Press, 1995.

48. Chen MS, Huber AB, van der Haar ME et al. Nogo-A is a myelin-associated neurite outgrowth inhibitor

and an antigen for monoclonal antibody IN-1. *Nature.* 2000;403(6768):434-9.

49. Wang KC, Koprivica V, Kim JA et al. Oligodendrocyte-myelin glycoprotein is a Nogo receptor ligand that inhibits neurite outgrowth. *Nature.* 2002;417(6892):941.

50. Cafferty WB, Duffy P, Huebner E, Strittmatter SM. MAG and OMgp synergize with Nogo-A to restrict axonal growth and neurological recovery after spinal cord trauma. *J Neurosci.* 2010;30(20):6825-37.

51. Fouad K, Klusman I, and Schwab M. Regenerating corticospinal fibers in the Marmoset (*Callitrix jacchus*) after spinal cord lesion and treatment with the anti-Nogo-A antibody IN-1. *Eur J Neurosci.* 2004;20(9):2479-82.

52. Li S, Liu BP, Budel S et al. Blockade of Nogo-66, myelin-associated glycoprotein, and oligodendrocyte myelin glycoprotein by soluble Nogo-66 receptor promotes axonal sprouting and recovery after spinal injury. *J Neurosci.* 2004;24(46):10511-20.

53. Freund P, Wannier T, Schmidlin E et al. Anti-Nogo-A antibody treatment enhances sprouting of corticospinal axons rostral to a unilateral cervical spinal cord lesion in adult macaque monkey. *J Comparative Neurol.* 2007;502(4):644-59.

54. Martirosyan NL, Patel AA, Carotenuto A et al. The role of therapeutic hypothermia in the management of acute spinal cord injury. *Clin Neurol Neurosurg.* 2017;154:79-88.

55. Evaniew N, Belley-Côté EP, Fallah N, Noonan VK, Rivers CS, Dvorak MF. Methylprednisolone for the treatment of patients with acute spinal cord injuries: A systematic review and meta-analysis. *J Neurotrauma.* 2016;33(5):468-81.

56. Evaniew N, Noonan VK, Fallah N et al. Methylprednisolone for the treatment of patients with acute spinal cord injuries: A propensity score-matched cohort study from a Canadian multi-center spinal cord injury registry. *J Neurotrauma.* 2015;32(21):1674-83.

57. Fehlings MG, Wilson JR, Tetreault LA et al. A clinical practice guideline for the management of patients with acute spinal cord injury: Recommendations on the use of methylprednisolone sodium succinate. *Global Spine J.* 2017;7(3 Suppl):203S-11S.

58. Zeller CB, and Marchase RB. Gangliosides as modulators of cell function. *Am J Physiol Cell Physiol.* 1992;262(6):C1341-55.

59. Rahmann H. Brain gangliosides and memory formation. *Behavioural Brain Res.* 1995;66(1-2):105-16.

60. Sabel BA, and Stein DG. Neurology: Pharmacological treatment of central nervous system injury. *Nature.* 1986;323(6088):493.

61. Gorio A. Gangliosides as a possible treatment affecting neuronal repair processes. *Adv Neurol.* 1988;47:523.

62. Geisler FH, Dorsey FC, and Coleman WP. Recovery of motor function after spinal-cord injury—A randomized, placebo-controlled trial with GM-1 ganglioside. *N Engl J Med.* 1991;324(26):1829-38.

63. Geisler FH, Coleman WP, Grieco G et al. The Sygen® multicenter acute spinal cord injury study. *Spine.* 2001;26(24S):S87-98.

64. Ahmad M, Zakaria A, and Almutairi KM. Effectiveness of minocycline and FK506 alone and in combination on enhanced behavioral and biochemical recovery from spinal cord injury in rats. *Pharmacol Biochem Behav.* 2016;145:45-54.

65. Aras M, Altas M, Motor S et al. Protective effects of minocycline on experimental spinal cord injury in rats. *Injury.* 2015;46(8):1471-4.

66. Sonmez E, Kabatas S, Ozen O et al. Minocycline treatment inhibits lipid peroxidation, preserves spinal cord ultrastructure, and improves functional outcome after traumatic spinal cord injury in the rat. *Spine.* 2013;38(15):1253-9.

67. Casha S, Zygun D, McGowan MD, Bains I, Yong VW, Hurlbert RJ et al. Results of a phase II placebo-controlled randomized trial of minocycline in acute spinal cord injury. *Brain.* 2012;135(4):1224-36.

68. Sahni V, and Kessler JA. Stem cell therapies for spinal cord injury. *Nat Rev Neurol.* 2010;6(7):363.

69. Kwon BK, Liu J, Oschipok L, Teh J, Liu ZW, Tetzlaff W. Rubrospinal neurons fail to respond to brain-derived neurotrophic factor applied to the spinal cord injury site 2 months after cervical axotomy. *Exp Neurol.* 2004;189(1):45-57.

70. Xu XM, Chen A, Guénard V, Kleitman N, Bunge MB. Bridging Schwann cell transplants promote axonal regeneration from both the rostral and caudal stumps of transected adult rat spinal cord. *J Neurocytol.* 1997;26(1):1-16.

71. Murray M, Kim D, Liu Y, Tobias C, Tessler A, Fischer I. Transplantation of genetically modified cells contributes to repair and recovery from spinal injury. *Brain Res Rev.* 2002;40(1-3):292-300.

72. Geffner L, Santacruz P, Izurieta M et al. Administration of autologous bone marrow stem cells into spinal cord injury patients via multiple routes is safe and improves their quality of life: Comprehensive case studies. *Cell Transplant.* 2008;17(12):1277-93.

73. Yoon SH, Shim YS, Park YH et al. Complete spinal cord injury treatment using autologous bone marrow cell transplantation and bone marrow stimulation with granulocyte macrophage-colony stimulating factor: Phase I/II clinical trial. *Stem Cells.* 2007;25(8):2066-73.

74. Syková E, Homola A, Mazanec R et al. Autologous bone marrow transplantation in patients with subacute and chronic spinal cord injury. *Cell Transplant.* 2006;15(8-9):675-87.

75. Deda H, Inci MC, Kürekçi AE et al. Treatment of chronic spinal cord injured patients with autologous bone marrow-derived hematopoietic stem cell transplantation: 1-year follow-up. *Cytotherapy.* 2008;10(6):565-74.

76. Mackay-Sim A, Féron F, Cochrane J et al. Autologous olfactory ensheathing cell transplantation in human paraplegia: A 3-year clinical trial. *Brain.* 2008;131(9):2376-86.

77. Lima C, Escada P, Pratas-Vital J et al. Olfactory mucosal autografts and rehabilitation for chronic traumatic spinal cord injury. *Neurorehabil Neural Repair.* 2010;24(1):10-22.

78. Saberi H, Firouzi M, Habibi Z et al. Safety of intramedullary Schwann cell transplantation for postrehabilitation spinal cord injuries: 2-year follow-up of 33 cases. *J Neurosurg Spine.* 2011;15(5):515-25.

79. Knoller N, Auerbach G, Fulga V et al. Clinical experience using incubated autologous macrophages as a treatment for complete spinal cord injury: Phase I study results. *J Neurosurg Spine.* 2005;3(3):173-81.

80. Squillaro T, Peluso G, and Galderisi U. Clinical trials with mesenchymal stem cells: An update. *Cell Transplant.* 2016;25(5):829-48.

81. Lammertse D, Jones LA, Charlifue SB et al. Autologous incubated macrophage therapy in acute, complete spinal cord injury: Results of the phase 2 randomized controlled multicenter trial. *Spinal Cord.* 2012;50(9):661.

82. Ahuja CS, Nori S, Tetreault L et al. Traumatic spinal cord injury—Repair and regeneration. *Neurosurgery.* 2017;80(3S):S9–22.

83. Xu P, and Yang X. The efficacy and safety of mesenchymal stem cell transplantation for spinal cord injury patients: A meta-analysis and systematic review. *Cell Transplant.* 2019;28(1):36–46.

84. Deng J, Zhang Y, Xie Y, Zhang L, Tang P. Cell transplantation for spinal cord injury: Tumorigenicity of induced pluripotent stem cell-derived neural stem/progenitor cells. *Stem Cells Int.* 2018:5653787.

85. Jin MC, Jin MC, Medress ZA, Azad TD, Doulames VM, Veeravagu A. Stem cell therapies for acute spinal cord injury in humans: A review. *Neurosurg Focus.* 2019;46(3):E10.

Chapter 37

NEURAL REROUTING IN PATIENTS WITH SPINAL CORD INJURY

Chuan-Guo Xiao and Kenneth I. Glassberg

INTRODUCTION

Neurogenic bladder can be caused by a spinal cord injury (SCI), diseases such as myelomeningocele, and radical surgery of pelvic organs. Clean intermittent catheterization (CIC), antimuscarinics, and other pharmacologic agents have improved the daily management of these bladders often with improving compliance and sometimes salvaging a threatened upper tract but without having an effect on volitional voiding.

Bladder reinnervation resurfaced with a new concept and procedure with promising results in patients who have sustained a SCI and in patients born with myelomeningocele. The procedure, as reported by Xiao and coauthors, involves a somatic-autonomic neural rerouting procedure and subsequently has often been referred to as the Xiao procedure[1,2] (Figure 37.1). Since this book focuses on adult neurogenic bladder, the Xiao procedure for patients with SCI is the focus of this chapter. Its use in patients with myelomeningocele is most often performed in childhood and adolescence and is, therefore, only briefly discussed.

BACKGROUND TO XIAO PROCEDURE

A few investigators have tried to reinnervate the bladder using a whole lumbar or costal nerve to sacral nerve anastomosis, without satisfactory results.[8] The Xiao procedure differs from previous attempts in that only the motor axons of a somatic reflex arc are used to regenerate into autonomic preganglionic nerves; thus, reinnervating bladder parasympathetic ganglion cells and, thereby, transferring somatic reflex activity initiated by sensory dermatome stimulation to bladder smooth muscle. Xiao's attempts using his somatic-autonomic reflex pathway procedure were developed in animals and then employed in animals (rats, cats, and canines) who had a neurogenic bladder created beforehand with

spinal cord transection. Following surgery, these animals successfully regained bladder function as demonstrated by postoperative neural tracings, electrophysiologic studies, and urodynamics.[1–3] Once the technique was shown to be effective in animals, the procedure was then performed with Institutional Review Board (IRB) approval in human adults with SCI and, subsequently, in children with spinal bifida.

XIAO PROCEDURE FOR SPINAL CORD INJURY (INCLUDING OUTCOMES)

The Xiao procedure is in fact a microneurosurgical procedure including laminectomy and ventral root (VR) microanastomosis, usually between the L5/S1 and S2/3 VRs. The L5/S1 dorsal root (DR) is left intact as the trigger for micturition once axonal regeneration has taken place. In 1995, the first clinical trial of the artificial somatic-CNS (central nervous system)-autonomic reflex pathway procedure was instituted.[4] Fifteen male volunteers with overactive neurogenic bladder and DESD secondary to complete suprasacral SCI underwent the Xiao procedure. The mean follow-up period was 3 years. All patients underwent urodynamic evaluation before surgery and during follow-up. Among the 15 patients, 10 (67%) regained satisfactory bladder control within 12–18 months. The average postvoid residual urine decreased from 332 to 31 mL. Issues with recurrent urinary infection and overflow incontinence resolved. Urodynamic studies revealed a change from detrusor hyperreflexia with DESD and high detrusor pressure to normalized compliance and synergistic voiding, but the 18 months' postoperation mean max P_{det} 62.83 cm H_2O was still higher than normal, though reduced significantly from 82.33 preoperatively ($p < 0.0025$). Impaired renal function returned to normal. Two patients (13%) who required a skin stimulator instead of just scratching to evoke voiding following the VR anastomosis exhibited a partial recovery but had over 100 mL of residual urine. One patient was lost to follow-up and two failed. In short, it is possible

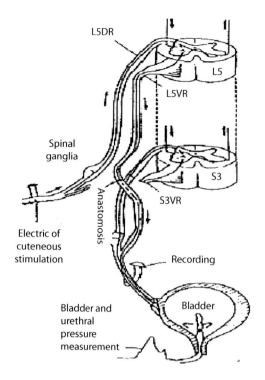

L5

L5VR

Spinal ganglia

S3

Anastomosis

S3VR

Electric of cuteneous stimulation

Recording

Bladder and urethral pressure measurement

Bladder

Figure 37.1 Skin-CNS-bladder (somatic-CNS-autonomic) reflex pathway. (From Xiao et al. *J Urol.* 2003;170:1237, with permission.)

with this novel concept to surgically establish an artificial somatic-CNS-autonomic reflex arc for controlling bladder emptying and improving bladder function for patients with complete suprasacral SCI and a neurogenic overactive bladder in association with DESD.[4] Since then, we (CGX) have been using the Xiao procedure for both neurogenic overactive bladder secondary to complete suprasacral SCI, and noncontractile neurogenic bladder secondary to conus medullaris injury or cauda equina injury.[6]

Two other major centers in China have been working on bladder reinnervation. Hou's team in the Second Army Medical University of China has been working on somatic-autonomic reinnervation for neurogenic bladder caused by SCI since 2008.[9] They chose only the S1 nerve root to enable initiation of the somatic-CNS-autonomic reflex by tapping on the Achilles tendon in addition to skin stimulation, creating an Achilles-tendon-to-bladder reflex pathway. Nine of 12 paraplegic patients (75%) with overactive neurogenic bladder and detrusor external urethral sphincter (EUS) dyssynergia caused by complete suprasacral SCI regained bladder control within 6–12 months after surgery. Urodynamic studies 1 year after the surgery demonstrated elimination of detrusor-sphincter dyssynergy as well as increased bladder capacity. They also tried T11 ventral root to S3 ventral root for atonic bladder after conus

medullaris injury and reported similar success except for a longer regenerating time, i.e., 2 years. Hou's team has performed the somatic-autonomic reinnervation procedure in about 400 patients with SCI, with an effective rate of about 70% by questionnaires.[10,11] Cao's team in Nanjing Medical University modified the Xiao procedure by extradural S1 to S2 ventral root anastomosis with shorter operating room (OR) time, shorter regeneration distance, and fewer complications such as spinal fluid leaking and headache.[12,13]

There were similar reports of success in the United States. A National Institutes of Health (NIH) supported clinical trial was carried out at New York University Medical Center using the Xiao procedure for neurogenic bladder caused by complete SCI. The positive results confirmed the principle of somatic-autonomic reinnervation.[14] At Louisiana State University, Patwardhan reported a 6-year-old girl with SCI secondary to a gunshot. Five months postsurgery, she had already regained voluntary voiding.[15]

Tuite et al. performed the Xiao procedure in a 10-year-old boy with chronic T10-T11 paraplegia, but it failed to produce effective results due to neuroma formation. The only way to correct the situation is to remove the neuroma surgically and redo the anastomosis.[16]

In Denmark, one group reported lack of success in 10 patients with SCI. These failures were possibly due to not following some of the guidelines that had been recommended in the past and are discussed in the section on "What We Have Learned Over Time."[23]

XIAO PROCEDURE FOR SPINA BIFIDA

Encouraged by the success of the Xiao procedure in patients with SCI with restoration of bladder storage and emptying, we initiated an investigation in 2000 on the value of the Xiao procedure for 20 children with neurogenic bladder secondary to spina bifida and reported the results in 2005.[5] All children were incontinent. Seventeen of the 20 patients gained satisfactory bladder control and continence with demonstrable improvement on postoperative urodynamic studies in 8–12 months after Xiao procedure. Overall, three cases failed to exhibit any improvement. As with patients with SCI, those patients with spina bifida who gained bladder control after the Xiao procedure also gained bowel control.

Peters and his colleagues at Beaumont Hospital reported the U.S. pilot study of the Xiao procedure for children with spina bifida with neurogenic bladder. The results were similar to those from

Xiao. In the 10 of 13 children who returned at 3 years, renal function remained stable, and mean maximum cystometric capacity (MCC) increased ($p = 0.0135$), 8 were treatment responders with voiding efficiency greater than 50%, and 9 had discontinued antimuscarinics. Only 2/8 with baseline neurogenic detrusor overactivity (NDO) still had NDO, all 3 with compliance less than 10 mL/cm H_2O had normalized, 7/10 considered their bowels normal, 5/10 were continent of stool, and 8/10 would undergo the procedure again.[17–19]

On the other hand, Tuite et al recruited 20 children with spina bifida in a "double-blind" study: 10 had a cord detethering surgery, 10 had cord detethering plus Xiao procedure,. While the initial report showed no improvement postoperatively, 4 months later, Tuite et al. published an updated article about the same trial with more positive outcomes.[20,22,23]

WHAT WE HAVE LEARNED OVER TIME

From our own experience, reports in the literature by other researchers, and our conversations with other surgeons regarding their experience with this rerouting technique, we have identified certain criteria that need to be met before considering a candidate for the procedure and certain adjustments that need to be made in caring for patients following the surgery.[21]

In China, most patients with SCI use a condom catheter for keeping them dry, whether the incontinence is secondary to detrusor overactivity or overflow incontinence.[9] When the New York University Medical Center trial was instituted, it was realized, in preparing the protocol for the NIH and IRB, that there was a conflict between routine antimuscarinic usage and achieving neural reinnervation of the bladder after the Xiao procedure. Antimuscarinics are used to block the neural connection between postganglionic nerves and the detrusor, and thereby inhibit detrusor contractions and make the bladder a low-pressure storage tank for CIC. In other words, antimuscarinics, in a way, paralyze the bladder. The Xiao procedure, however, reestablishes neural control of the lower urinary tract via the somatic-autonomic reinnervation. The postganglionic nerve to detrusor connection is the last and most important leg of the somatic-CNS-autonomic reflex arc; if this leg is blocked by continuous antimuscarinics, the newly established reflex pathway created by the surgery would be unable to be activated, and the patient would be unable to initiate a detrusor contraction in order to void. As a result, the New York University study did not allow patients to take antimuscarinics or stay on CIC, and patients with a bladder capacity

of greater than 700cc were excluded from the study.[7] Most of the patients with disappointing results in the Denmark study were maintained on antimuscarinics and also had volumes well above 700 cc, volumes we believe are too large and too chronically distended to allow for a successful response to reinnervation.[23]

In order to have a good outcome for the Xiao procedure, it is most important to make sure the donor VR is alive with good quality axons, which should be confirmed by preoperative neurophysiology study and intraoperative neural physiological monitoring. Since the intradural neural roots are very fragile and cannot hold the suture to make notes, the dura should be used as the "bed" to fix the anastomosis between L5 or S1 VR and S2/S3 VR. This technique also can avoid the anastomosis floating in the spinal fluid. Children with spina bifida with complete S1 and L5 damage need neural graft between higher lumbar VR and S2-S3 VR. Grafting will increase the regeneration time and may reduce the effective rate.

The most fascinating and unexpected result of the 2005 trial in patients with spina bifida was that the children who gained bladder storage and emptying function also gained bladder sensory function. A preexisting sensory infrastructure may have been activated by stretch as the detrusor tone and bladder storage function improved. Since spinal cord continuity was not interrupted as in SCI, the CNS at both spinal and supraspinal levels may have plasticity to accommodate the artificial somatic-autonomic reflex pathway for micturition (Figure 37.2).

GUIDELINE TO OPTIMIZE EFFICACY OF XIAO PROCEDURE

Our current guidelines in regard to patients being evaluated for the Xiao procedure for neurogenic bladder secondary to SCI include the following: (1) Presurgery urodynamic testing must be done, and in all cases, antimuscarinics should be discontinued 2 weeks prior to the urodynamics. (2) Presurgery bladder capacity should not be larger than 700 mL. (3) Antimuscarinics and CIC should be avoided after the initial 3 months after surgery or when bowel function starts to improve, a signal that a new somatic-autonomic reflex arc is developing, and volitional voiding can start to take place. (4) Suprapubic urinary diversion or very punctual CIC should be maintained after the Xiao procedure for neurogenic overactive bladders with DESD and hydronephrosis, until the new voiding mechanism becomes functional. (5) For patients who can walk, patients may use only one side—one-half S1 VR or one-third of L5 VR—to avoid or minimize the negative impact on the motor function of the foot. (6) For spina bifida, it is best

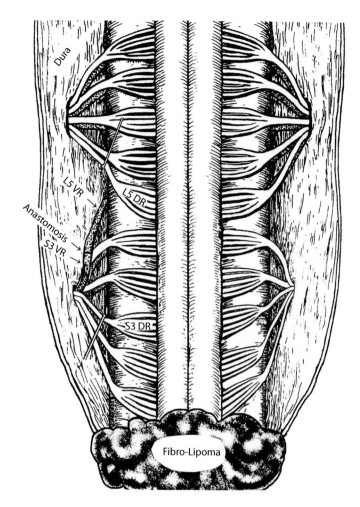

Figure 37.2 The somatic-autonomic reflex pathway procedure.

to select the first 10 children who can walk on their own for fastest and best results, then move on to more difficult cases.

CONCLUSION

In conclusion, the Xiao procedure in carefully selected patients is usually effective, reliable, and associated with infrequent side effects in the treatment of neurogenic bladder in patients with SCI and spina bifida. Understanding and following the guidelines of the Xiao procedure are critical for satisfactory results.

REFERENCES

1. Xiao CG and Godec CJ. A possible new reflex pathway for micturition after spinal cord injury. *Paraplegia*. 1994;32(5):300–7.

2. Xiao CG, de Groat WC, Godec CJ, Dai C, and Xiao Q. "Skin-CNS-bladder" reflex pathway for micturition after spinal cord injury and its underlying mechanisms. *J Urol*. 1999;162(3 Pt 1):936–42.

3. Wang HZ, Li SR, Wen C, Xiao CG, and Su BY. Morphological changes of cholinergic nerve fibers in the urinary bladder after establishment of artificial somatic-autonomic reflex arc in rats. *Neurosci Bull*. 2007;23(5):277–81.

4. Xiao CG, Du MX, Dai C, Li B, Nitti VW, and de Groat WC. An artificial somatic-central nervous system-autonomic reflex pathway for controllable micturition after spinal cord injury: Preliminary results in 15 patients. *J Urol*. 2003;170(4 Pt 1):1237–41.

5. Xiao CG, Du MX, Li B et al. An artificial somatic-autonomic reflex pathway procedure for bladder control in children with spina bifida. *J Urol*. 2005;173(6):2112–6.

6. Xiao CG. Re-innervation for neurogenic bladder: Historic review and introduction of a somatic-autonomic reflex pathway procedure for patients with spinal cord injury or spina bifida. *Eur Urol*. 2006;49(1):22–8; discussion 8–9.

7. Xiao CG. Xiao procedure for neurogenic bladder in spinal cord injury and spina bifida. *Curr Bladder Dysfunct Rep*. 2012;7(2):83–7.

8. Gomez-Amaya SM, Barbe MF, de Groat WC et al. Neural reconstruction methods of restoring bladder function. *Nat Rev Urol*. 2015;12(2):100–18.

9. Lin H, Hou C, Zhen X, and Xu Z. Clinical study of reconstructed bladder innervation below the level of spinal cord injury to produce urination by Achilles tendon-to-bladder reflex contractions. *J Neurosurg Spine*. 2009;10(5):452–7.

10. Lin H and Hou C. Transfer of normal S1 nerve root to reinnervate atonic bladder due to conus medullaris injury. *Muscle Nerve*. 2013;47(2):241–5.

11. Lin H, Hou CL, Zhong G, Xie Q, and Wang S. Reconstruction of reflex pathways to the atonic bladder after conus medullaris injury: Preliminary clinical results. *Microsurgery*. 2008;28(6):429–35.

12. Ma J, Sui T, Zhu Y, Zhu A, Wei Z, and Cao XJ. Micturition reflex arc reconstruction including sensory and motor nerves after spinal cord injury: Urodynamic and electrophysiological responses. *J Spinal Cord Med*. 2011;34(5):510–7.

13. Zhou X, Liu Y, Ma J, Sui T, Ge Y, and Cao X. Extradural nerve anastomosis technique for bladder re-innervation in spinal cord injury: Anatomical feasibility study in human cadavers. *Spine*. 2014;39(8):635–41.

14. Kelley C, Xiao CG, and Weiner H. Xiao procedure for neurogenic bladder in patients with spinal cord injury: Preliminary results of first 2 USA patients. *J Urol*. 2005;173:1132A.

15. Patwardhan R and Mata J. Case report on Xiao procedure for a 6 year old SCI girl to gain bladder control. *Supplement of First International Neural Regeneration Conference*, 2009.

16. Tuite GF, Storrs BB, Homsy YL et al. Attempted bladder re-innervation and creation of a scratch reflex for bladder emptying through a somatic-to-autonomic intradural anastomosis. *J Neurosurg Pediatr*. 2013;12(1):80–6.

17. Peters KM, Girdler B, Turzewski C et al. Outcomes of lumbar to sacral nerve rerouting for spina bifida. *J Urol*. 2010;184(2):702–7.

18. Peters K, Feber K, and Girdler B. Three-year clinical outcomes with lumbar to sacral nerve rerouting in spina bifida. *J Urol*. 2011;185:e602.

19. Peters KM, Gilmer H, Feber K et al. US pilot study of lumbar to sacral nerve rerouting to restore voiding and bowel function in spina bifida: 3-Year experience. *Adv Urol*. 2014;2014:863209.

20. Tuite GF, Polsky EG, Homsy Y et al. Lack of efficacy of an intradural somatic-to-autonomic nerve anastomosis (Xiao procedure) for bladder control in children with myelomeningocele and lipomyelomeningocele: Results of a prospective, randomized, double-blind study. *J Neurosurg Pediatr*. 2016; 18(2):150–63.

21. Xiao CG. Xiao procedure: Problems with ethics, methodology, and results from the double-blind trial of Tuite et al. *J Neurosurg Pediatr*. 2017;19(2):265–9.

22. Tuite GF, Homsy Y, Polsky EG et al. Urological outcome of the Xiao procedure in children with myelomeningocele and lipomyelomeningocele undergoing spinal cord detethering. *J Urol*. 2016;196(6):1735–40.

23. Rasmussen MM, Rawashdeh YF, Clemmensen D et al. The artificial somato-autonomic reflex arch does not improve lower urinary tract function in patients with spinal cord lesions. *J Urol*. 2015;193(2): 598–604.

24. Xiao C-G, Du M-X, Dai C, Li B, Nitti V W and de Groat WC. An artificial somatic-central nervous system-autonomic reflex pathway for controllable micturition after spinal cord injury: Preliminary results in 15 patients. *J Urol*. 2003;170:1237.

Part VI

SYNTHESIS OF TREATMENT

AN OVERVIEW OF TREATMENT ALTERNATIVES FOR DIFFERENT TYPES OF NEUROGENIC BLADDER DYSFUNCTION IN ADULTS

Jacques Corcos

INTRODUCTION

This chapter is intended for readers who may want to have an integrated overview of the different existing treatments detailed in Chapters 28 to 39. We inspired ourselves from these chapters to summarize, in the most comprehensive way, alternatives offered to physicians for the treatment of neurogenic bladder (NB) overactivity or hypoactivity and/or outlet overactivity or insufficiency. We avoided discussing treatments not yet widely approved by lack of strong evidence or abandoned by lack of efficacy or because of their adverse effects. Details and references are available in the different quoted chapters.

MANAGEMENT OF ALTERED RESERVOIR FUNCTION

Neurologic diseases can modify bladder reservoir function with two possible end results: underactive or acontractile bladder and overactive bladder.

EMPTYING UNDERACTIVE OR ACONTRACTILE BLADDERS

In this situation, the bladder cannot empty, or partially empty, leaving a high postvoid residual volume. Complete bladder emptying, which is necessary to maintain a low bladder pressure and control urinary infections, can be achieved by the following techniques:

1. *Credé's maneuver*: This maneuver is more efficacious, especially in females, where the pelvic floor muscles are paralyzed. The increased abdominal pressure is dissipated in part by the flaccid pelvic floor, and lesser pressure will be exerted simultaneously on the proximal urethra. Bladder evacuation, however, is rarely complete with this technique. Very little literature exists

on this widely used emptying technique, and no comparative studies with clean intermittent catheterization (CIC) or indwelling catheters have ever been done.[1,2]

2. *Catheterization*: Whenever the clinical situation permits, CIC is the best way to ensure adequate bladder emptying. The credit for this revolutionary technique goes to Guttman and Lapides, who demonstrated that self-catheterization does not need to be sterile and is safe and harmless if the catheter is simply clean.[3-5] Their observations, which revolutionized the management of patient bladder evacuation problems, are based on the premise that one of the mechanisms for the bladder to resist bacterial colonization is its periodic and complete emptying. This is still considered the safest way to empty a poorly contractile bladder.[6]

As detailed in Chapter 28 use of an indwelling catheter, either per the urethra or the suprapubic catheter, remains an acceptable option for bladder drainage depending on different characteristics of the patient and/or the disease.

MANAGEMENT OF DETRUSOR OVERACTIVITY

The most frequent consequences of an overactive detrusor are incontinence, frequency, and recurrent urinary tract infections. Treatment of neurogenic detrusor overactivity is based on several techniques used alone or in combination.

PHARMACOLOGIC MANIPULATION

1. *Oral administration*: In the last decade, a large number of pharmacologic substances have been developed to control bladder overactivity. Most of these substances have antimuscarinic properties, interfering with M3-type receptors. Their overall efficacy in neurogenic overactivity is about 50%.[7-18] The recently approved β_3 agonists appear to have, in overactive bladder (OAB), similar efficacy compared to anticholinergics

but with a much better tolerability profile with regard to dry mouth and constipation. They have not yet been studied in NBs. Combination therapy with antimuscarinics and β_3 agonist is another option for patients refractory to single-drug therapy.[17]

2. *Transcutaneous administration*: Davila et al.[14] reported the results of a multicenter trial with transcutaneous oxybutynin. Compared with oral administration, the transdermal route had equal efficacy and a significantly improved side-effect profile in adults with urge urinary incontinence. No data have been seen in NBs.

3. *Intravesical drug instillations*: This option is exceptionally used in adult NBs. It could at times, in patients using intermittent catheterization, help achieve good control of the overactivity with minimal side effects.[16-22]

4. *Intravesical drug injections*: Multisite intradetrusor botulinum toxin A injection in the bladder is frequently used for detrusor overactivity refractory to oral therapy. Since the initial study by Schurch et al.[23] numerous trials have been performed. Treatment of neurogenic detrusor overactivity with onabotulinumtoxinA has shown to significantly improve urodynamics, including maximal cystometric bladder capacity, detrusor pressures, compliance, as well as clinical parameters such as urinary incontinence. The main duration of response is approximately 9 months.[23,24] This treatment, which has completely revolutionized the management of NBs, is further discussed in Chapter 29.

NEUROSTIMULATION

Neurostimulation (when electrical stimulation is applied directly to a nerve fiber to achieve a sphincter contraction or detrusor relaxation) and neuromodulation (when electrical stimulation is applied indirectly to modify sensory and/or motor functions of the lower urinary tract) are widely used in NB.

Neurostimulation is applied mainly in patients with complete SCI and preserved detrusor function, excluding patients with noncontractile bladder. Introduced by Tanagho and Schmidt[25], then by Brindley et al.[26], this technique is associated with bilateral sacral posterior rhizotomies to reduce overactivity and autonomic dysreflexia. The success rate is high for bladder function but less for rectal and erectile function.[25-28] The techniques and expertise required for this procedure are rare, and only a few specialized centers perform them, mainly in Europe.

The role of electrical stimulation of the lower urinary tract is extensively covered in Chapter 31.

SURGERY

Two main surgical procedures have been proposed in the literature to decrease detrusor overactivity and/or to manage low-compliant bladders: partial detrusorectomy (autoaugmentation) and enterocystoplasty. The ultimate goal of each procedure is to increase reservoir capacity and reduce the amplitude of detrusor contractions. According to what we know, autoaugmentation is not performed anymore due to its inconsistent results and complications.

Enterocystoplasty is contemplated in patients with small bladder capacity. Most commonly, a detubularized segment of the distal ileum is used for this purpose, but a detubularized colic segment or part of the gastric wall can also be used. Excellent long-term results were reported in about 75% of patients, with improvement in another 20%.[29,30] In the future, the use of tissue engineering techniques may create a new interest for this augmentation technique (see also Chapter 32).

SUMMARY: MANAGEMENT OF NEUROGENIC OVERACTIVE DETRUSOR

Medication remains the first-line treatment for bladder activity, followed in case of bad tolerance or inefficacy by intradetrusor botulinum toxin A injections. Electrical stimulation/modulation and bladder augmentation techniques are used in rare cases.

ALTERED OUTLET FUNCTION

The outlet can be in neurologically impaired patients, either overactive (dyssynergic) or hypoactive.

INTRAVESICAL FUNCTIONAL OBSTRUCTION PHARMACOLOGIC APPROACH

Theoretically, α-blocking agents and medications that relax the striated sphincter/pelvic floor (i.e., Lioresal) should decrease urethral resistance during micturition. The use of alpha-blockers in the neurologic patient is less effective than their use in Benign prostatic hypertrophy (BPH).[31]

Phelan et al.[34] reported on the efficacy of botulinum toxin injections in the urethral sphincter of men and women with acontractile bladder. All but 1 of the 21 patients treated voided without catheterization, postvoid residual decreased by 71%, and voiding pressure decreased by 38%. Transient incontinence was sometimes observed.[32–40] Indications and practicality of botulinum toxin A injections in the urethral striated sphincter are discussed in Chapter 29.

Steers et al.[53] showed that intrathecal infusion of baclofen not only abolished bladder hyperreflexia in all patients but also eliminated vesicosphincteric dyssynergia in 40% of them.[41]

SURGICAL PROCEDURES
Sphincterotomy
In case of external sphincter dyssynergia in patients unable to perform CIC or for patients able to reflex void into a condom catheter, external sphincterotomy is an acceptable option. Optimally, this will result in decreased voiding pressures, decreased postvoid residuals, and a lessened chance to experience issues such as urinary tract infection and autonomic dysreflexia. Long-term success rates appear to be 40%–60%. Many neuro-urologists and patients prefer a suprapubic catheter to this definitive surgery.[42]

HYPOTONIC OUTLET INCONTINENCE
Sphincteric insufficiency is commonly seen in NBs especially in Cauda equina syndrome. Many options to increase urethral resistance exist but it should be pointed out that the prerequisite to augment outlet resistance is a low-pressure bladder reservoir.

URETHROPEXY AND SLINGS
Compared to nonneurologic patients, very limited literature exists regarding the use of slings in neurogenic sphincteric deficiency in males and females.[43–50]

Suburethral sling operations are reported mainly in children with spina bifida; however, a few cases in adult males with puboprostatic slings have also been described.[49,50] No long-term results are available for the recently developed devices that provide a fixed urethral compression to ensure continence in males. However, one should be cautious when considering a sling with polypropylene if the goal is to place the sling *tight* and cause the patient, using CIC, urinary retention.

PERIURETHRAL BULKING AGENTS
These interesting techniques that offer minimal invasiveness with a fast learning curve and low morbidity are detailed in Chapter 33. However, this treatment modality has not been widely studied in the neurogenic adult population.[51–58] Only a few reports reviewing the experience in patients with NB dysfunction exist in literature.[56,58]

Periurethral bulking agent (UBA) treatment does not jeopardize the performance and efficacy of other anti-incontinence procedures later on. The shortcomings of UBA include potential for repeat injections and at times a lesser degree of effectiveness compared to more invasive treatment modalities.

ARTIFICIAL URINARY SPHINCTER
Artificial urinary sphincter remains the gold standard, especially in males, for the treatment of urinary incontinence secondary to sphincter weakness. Fulford et al.[59] reported on 68 patients, all of them followed for more than 10 years: 75% had satisfactory continence, but only 13% still retained their original device. This suggests that the lifetime of the artificial sphincter is around 10–15 years, confirmed by Spiess et al.[60] who studied 30 children with meningomyelocele in whom an artificial sphincter was implanted at the bladder neck or the bulbar urethra. Survival analysis of the sphincter device revealed a sharp drop after 100 months, with only 8.3% of the sphincters still functioning beyond this point. A recent long-term follow-up (13 years) suggests that artificial urinary sphincter implantation remains a durable treatment also for the NB patient population.[61]

URETHRAL REPLACEMENT
When the urethra is judged nonsalvageable from the functional point of view, it can be replaced by a muscular tube obtained from the detrusor. The Young-Dees-Leadbetter technique creates a muscular tube from the trigone. This necessitates reimplantation of both ureters in an extratrigonal site. Long-term results showed perfect continence in 57% of adults and 70% of children.[62]

Tanagho[63] proposed the creation of the tube from the anterior bladder wall. This leaves the ureterovesical junction undisturbed. Good-to-excellent results were obtained in 71.5% of the 56 patients operated (for more techniques and their results see also Chapter 33).

SUPRAURETHRAL DIVERSION
When the clinical situation is such that neither the Young-Dees-Leadbetter operation nor the Tanagho technique is feasible, supraurethral diversion might become necessary. This creates an abdominal stoma that can be continent or incontinent. It may require, especially in females, the simultaneous closure of the bladder neck (see Chapter 32).

REFERENCES

1. Küss R and Grégoire W. *Histoire illustrée de l'Urologie de l'Antiquité à nos Jours*. Paris, France: R Dacosta, 1988.
2. Kitahara S, Iwatsubo E, Yasuda K et al. Practice patterns of Japanese physicians in urologic surveillance and management of spinal cord injury patients. *Spinal Cord.* 2006;44(6):362–8.
3. Lapides J, Diokno AC, Silber SJ, and Lowe BS. Clean, intermittent self-catheterization in the treatment of urinary tract disease. *J Urol.* 1972;107:458–61.
4. Lapides J, Diokno AC, Lowe BS, and Kalish MD. Follow-up on unsterile, intermittent self-catheterization. *J Urol.* 1974;111:184–7.

5. Diokno AC, Sonda P, Hollander JB, and Lapides J. Fate of patients started on clean intermittent self-catheterization therapy 10 years ago. *J Urol.* 1983;129:1120–2.

6. Weld KJ and Dmochowski RR. Effect of bladder management on urological complications in spinal cord injured patients. *J Urol.* 2000;163:768–72.

7. Appel RA. Pharmacotherapy for overactive bladder: An evidence-based approach to selecting an antimuscarinic agent. *Drugs.* 2006;66:1361–70.

8. Appel RA. Treatment of overactive bladder with once-daily extended release tolterodine or oxybutynin: The antimuscarinic clinical effectiveness trial (ACET). *Curr Urol Rep.* 2002;3:343–4.

9. Elliott DS and Barrett DM. Surgical and medical management of the neurogenic bladder. *AUA Update Series.* 2002;21:138–43.

10. Rovner E. Tropsium chloride in the management of overactive bladder. *Drugs.* 2004;64:2433–46.

11. Khullar V, Chapple C, Gabriel Z, and Dooley JA. The effects of antimuscarinics on health-related quality of life in overactive bladder: A systemic review and meta-analysis. *Urology.* 2006;68(Suppl 2):38–48.

12. Horstmann M, Schaefer T, Aguilar Y, Stenzl A, and Sievert KD. Neurogenic bladder treatment by doubling the recommended antimuscarinic dosage. *Neurourol Urodyn.* 2006;25:441–5.

13. Abrams P, Kelleher C, Staskin D et al. Combination treatment with mirabegron and solifenacin in patients with overactive bladder: Efficacy and safety results from a randomised, double-blind, dose-ranging, phase 2 study (symphony). *Eur Urol.* 2015;67(3):577–88.

14. Davila GW, Daugherty CA, and Sanders SW. Transdermal Oxybutynin Study Group. A short-term, multicenter, randomized double-blind dose titration study of the efficacy and anticholinergic side effects of transdermal compared to immediate release oxybutynin treatment of patients with urge urinary incontinence. *J Urol.* 2001;166:140–5.

15. Brandler CB, Radebaugh LC, and Mohler JL. Topical oxybutynin chloride for relaxation of dysfunctional bladders. *J Urol.* 1989;141:1350–2.

16. Madersbacher H and Jilg G. Control of detrusor hyperreflexia by the intravesical installation of oxybutynin chloride. *Paraplegia.* 1991;29:84–90.

17. Massad CA, Kogan BA, and Trigo-Rocha FE. Pharmacokinetics of intravesical and oral oxybutynin chloride. *J Urol.* 1992;148:595–7.

18. Di Stasi SM, Giannantoni A, Navarra P et al. Intravesical oxybutynin: Mode of action assessed by passive diffusion and electromotive administration with pharmacokinetics of oxybutynin and N-desethyl-oxybutynin. *J Urol.* 2001;166:2232–6.

19. de Sèze M, Wiart L, Joseph PA et al. Capsaicin and neurogenic detrusor hyperreflexia: A double-blind placebo-controlled study in 20 patients with spinal cord lesions. *Neurourol Urodyn.* 1998;17:513–23.

20. Maggi CA, Patacchini R, Tramontana M et al. Similarities and differences in the action of resiniferatoxin and capsaicin on central and peripheral endings of primary sensory neurons. *Neuroscience.* 1990;37:531–9.

21. de Ridder D and Baert L. Vanilloids and the overactive bladder. *BJU Int.* 2000;86:172–80.

22. Ekström B. Intravesical instillation of drugs in patients with detrusor hyperactivity. *Scand J Urol Nephrol.* 1992;149(Suppl):1–67.

23. Schurch B, Stöhrer M, Kramer G et al. Botulinum-A toxin for treating detrusor hyperreflexia in spinal cord-injured patients: A new alternative to anticholinergic drugs? Preliminary results. *J Urol.* 2000;164:692–7.

24. Fowler CJ. Bladder afferents and their role in overactive bladder. *Urology.* 2002;59(Suppl 5A):37–42.

25. Tanagho EA and Schmidt RA. Electrical stimulation in the clinical management of the neurogenic bladder. *J Urol.* 1988;140:1331–9.

26. Brindley GS, Pulkey CE, Rushton DN, and Cardozo L. Sacral anterior root stimulators for bladder control in paraplegia: The first 50 cases. *J Neurol Neurosurg Psychiatry.* 1986;49:1104–14.

27. Chartier-Katler EJ, Denys P, Chancellor MB et al. Urodynamic monitoring during percutaneous sacral nerve neurostimulation in patients with neurogenic detrusor hyperreflexia. *Neurourol Urodyn.* 2001;20:61–71.

28. Van Kerrebroeck PE, Koldewijn EL, and Debruyne FM. Worldwide experience with the Finetech-Brindley sacral anterior root stimulator. *Neurourol Urodyn.* 1993;12:497–503.

29. Flood HD, Malhotra SJ, O'Connell HE et al. Long-term results and complications using augmentation cystoplasty in reconstructive urology. *Neurourol Urodyn.* 1995;14:297–309.

30. Leng WW, Blalock HJ, Frederiksson WH et al. Enterocystoplasty or myomectomy? Comparison of indications and outcomes for bladder augmentation. *J Urol.* 1999;161:758–63.

31. Kim DK. Current pharmacological and surgical treatment of underactive bladder. *Investig Clin Urol.* 2017;58(Suppl 2):S90–8.

32. Dykstra DD and Sidi AA. Treatment of detrusor sphincter dyssynergia with botulinum A toxin: A double blind study. *Arch Phys Med Rehab.* 1990:71:24–6

33. Fowler CJ, Betts CD, Christmas TJ et al. Botulinum toxin in the treatment of chronic urinary retention in women. *Br J Urol.* 1992;70:387–9.

34. Phelan MW, Franks M, Somogyi GT et al. Botulinum toxin urethral sphincter injection to restore bladder emptying in men and women with voiding dysfunction. *J Urol.* 2001;164:1107–10.

35. Boyd RN, Britton TC, Robinson RO, and Borzyskowski M. Transient urinary incontinence after botulinum A toxin. *Lancet.* 1996;348(9025):481–2. Letter.

36. Kuo HC. Effect of botulinum toxin A in the treatment of voiding dysfunction due to detrusor underactivity. *Urology.* 2003;61:550–4.

37. Karsenty G, Baazeem A, Elzayat E, and Corcos J. Injection of botulinum toxin type A in the urethral sphincter to treat lower urinary tract dysfunction: A review of indications, techniques and results. *Can J Urol.* 2006;13:3027–33.

38. Mamas MA, Reynard JM, and Brading AF. Augmentation of nitric oxide to treat detrusor-external sphincter dyssynergia in spinal cord injury. *Lancet.* 2001;357(9272):1964–7.

39. Reitz A, Bretscher S, Knapp PA et al. The effect of nitric oxide on the resting tone and the contractile behaviour of the external urethral sphincter: A functional urodynamic study in healthy humans. *Eur Urol.* 2004;45:367–73.

40. Reitz A, Knapp PA, Muntener M, and Schurch B. Oral nitric oxide donors: A new pharmacological approach to detrusor-sphincter dyssynergia in spinal cord injured patients. *Eur Urol.* 2004; 45:516–20.

41. Steers WD, Meythaller JM, and Haworth C. Effects of acute bolus and continuous intrathecal Baclofen

on genito-urinary dysfunction due to spinal cord pathology. *J Urol.* 1992;148:1849–55.

42. Rivas DA and Chancellor MB. Sphincterotomy and sphincter stent prosthesis placement. In: Corcos J, Schick E, eds. *The Urinary Sphincter.* New York, NY: Marcel Dekker, 2001:565–82.

43. Bezerra CA, Bruschini H, and Cody DJ. Traditional suburethral sling operations for urinary incontinence in women. *Cochrane Database Syst Rev.* 2005;3:CD001754.

44. Daneshmand S, Ginsberg DA, Bennet JK et al. Puboprostatic sling repair for treatment of urethral incompetence in adult neurogenic incontinence. *J Urol.* 2003;169:199–202.

45. Athanasopoulos A, Gyftopoulos K, and McGuire EJ. Treating stress urinary incontinence in female patients with neuropathic bladder: The value of the autologous fascia rectus sling. *Int Urol Nephrol.* 2012;44(5):1363–7. doi:10.1007/s11255-012-0247-4

46. Abdul-Rahman A, Attar KH, Hamid R, and Shah PJ. Long-term outcome of tension-free vaginal tape for treating stress incontinence in women with neuropathic bladders. *BJU Int.* 2010;106(6):827–30. doi:10.1111/j.1464–4

47. Castellan M, Gosalbez R, Labbie A, Ibrahim E, and Disandro M. Bladder neck sling for treatment of neurogenic incontinence in children with augmentation cystoplasty: Long-term followup. *J Urol.* 2005;173:2128–31.

48. Dik P, Klijn AJ, van Gool JD, and de Jong TP. Transvaginal sling suspension of bladder neck in female patients with neurogenic sphincter incontinence. *J Urol.* 2003;170(2 Pt 1):580–1.

49. Triaca V, Twiss CO, and Raz S. Urethral compression for the treatment of postprostatectomy urinary incontinence: Is history repeating itself? *Eur Urol.* 2007;51:304–5. Editorial.

50. Groen LA, Spinoit AF, Hoebeke P et al. The AdVance male sling as a minimally invasive treatment for intrinsic sphincter deficiency in patients with neurogenic bladder sphincter dysfunction: A pilot study. *Neurourol Urodyn.* 2012;31(8):1284–7.

51. Berg S. Polytef augmentation urethroplasty. *Arch Surg.* 1973;107:379–81.

52. Malizia AA, Reiman HM, Myers RP et al. Migration and granulomatous reaction after periurethral injection of polytef (Teflon). *JAMA.* 1984;251:3277–81.

53. Corcos J and Fournier C. Periurethral collagen injection for the treatment of female stress urinary incontinence:4-Year follow-up results. *Urology.* 1999;54:815–18.

54. Santarosa RP and Blaivas JG. Periurethral injection of autologous fat for the treatment of sphincteric incontinence. *J Urol.* 1994;151:607–11.

55. Barrett DM, Ghoniem G, Bruskewitz R et al. The Genisphere: A new percutaneously placed anti-incontinence device. *J Urol.* 1990;141:224A.

56. Pineda EB, Hadley HR. Urethral injection treatment for stress urinary incontinence. In: Corcos J, Schick E, eds. *The Urinary Sphincter.* New York, NY: Marcel Dekker, 2001:497–515.

57. Ghoniem G, Corcos J, Comiter C, Westney OL, and Herschorn S. Durability of urethral bulking agent injection for female stress urinary incontinence: 2-Year multicenter study results. *J Urol.* 2010; 183(4):1444–9.

58. Kassouf W, Capolechio J, Bernardinucci G, and Corcos J. Collagen injection for treatment of urinary incontinence in children. *J Urol.* 2001;165:1666–8.

59. Fulford SC, Sutton C, Bales G et al. The fate of the "modern" artificial urinary sphincter with a follow-up of more than 15 years. *Br J Urol.* 1997;79:713–6.

60. Spiess PE, Capolicchio JP, Kiruluta G et al. Is an artificial sphincter the best choice for incontinent boys with spina bifida? Review of our long term experience with the AS800 artificial sphincter. *Can J Urol.* 2002;9:1486–91.

61. Lai HH, Hsu EI, Teh BS, Butler EB, and Boone TB. 13 Years of experience with artificial urinary sphincter implantation at Baylor College of Medicine. *J Urol.* 2007;177:1021–5.

62. Leadbetter GW Jr. Surgical reconstruction for complete urinary incontinence: A 10 to 22 year follow-up. *J Urol.* 1985;113:205–6.

63. Tanagho EA. Bladder neck reconstruction for total urinary incontinence: 10 Years of experience. *J Urol.* 1981;125:321–6.

Part VII

COMPLICATIONS

Chapter 39

COMPLICATIONS RELATED TO NEUROGENIC BLADDER DYSFUNCTION I
Infection, Lithiasis, and Neoplasia

Gamal Ghoniem

INFECTION

INCIDENCE

Urinary tract infections (UTIs) are among the most common urologic complications of neurogenic bladder (NGB). It has been estimated that approximately 33% of patients with spinal cord injury (SCI) have bacteriuria at any time.[1] One prospective study on patients on intermittent catheterization or condom catheterization reported an incidence of febrile UTIs of 1.8 per person per year.[2] UTI is the most common cause of fever in the patient with SCI[3] and can be acute or chronic, relapsing, or recurrent. The term "relapse" implies infection by the same organism, while "recurrent" implies infection with a different strain of bacteria.[4]

SPECIMEN COLLECTION FOR CULTURE

In patients with SCI who have an indwelling catheter (urethral or suprapubic), the urine specimen should be obtained from a new, freshly inserted catheter and not from the old catheter and cultured as soon as possible.[5]

RISK FACTORS

The 1992 National Institute on Disability and Rehabilitation Research Consensus Conference examined the problems associated with UTIs in patients with SCI. Among the risk factors identified were overdistension of the bladder, elevated intravesical pressure, increased risk of urinary obstruction, vesicoureteral reflux (VUR), presence of bladder diverticula, impaired voiding, instrumentation, and increased incidence of stones (Figure 39.1). Other factors that have been implicated are decreased fluid intake, poor hygiene perineal colonization, decubiti and other evidence of local tissue trauma, and reduced host defense associated with chronic illness.[2]

The method of bladder management has a profound impact on UTI. Suprapubic catheters and indwelling urethral catheters eventually have an equivalent infection rate.[8] Since its introduction by Lapides et al.[7] in 1972, clean (but not sterile) intermittent catheterization (CIC) has been shown to decrease lower tract infections by maintaining low intravesical pressure and reducing the incidence of stones.[6,8]

A recent study showed male gender, severe bladder deformity, ASIA impairment scale of AIS C or more, the number of CICs, and use of quinolones were significantly associated with febrile UTI occurrence in neurogenic bladder patients employing routine CIC.[9]

BACTERIOLOGY AND LABORATORY FINDINGS

Urinalysis will show bacteriuria and pyuria. The National Institute on Disability and Rehabilitation Research Consensus Statement recommended the following criteria for the diagnosis of significant bacteriuria in SCI patients. Any detectable bacteria from indwelling or suprapubic catheter aspirates was considered significant because the majority of patients show an increase greater than 105 cfu (colony forming unit/mL) within a short period. For patients on CIC, greater than 102 cfu/mL was considered significant. For catheter-free males, a clean voided specimen showing greater than or equal to 104 cfu/mL is considered significant.[10,11]

Escherichia coli is isolated in approximately 20% of patients. *Enterococci, Proteus mirabilis,* and *Pseudomonas* are more common among patients with SCI than patients with intact spinal cords. Other organisms that are quite often cultured include *Klebsiella, Proteus, Serratia, Providencia, Staphylococcus,* and *Candida* species.

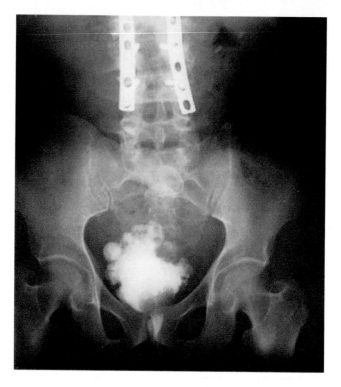

Figure 39.1 Cystogram of an 18-year-old patient with posttraumatic spinal cord injury. Classic "Christmas tree" bladder can be seen with an indwelling urethral catheter inside it. Ogawa Classification Grade III bladder deformity.

The bacteria that produce urease are particularly harmful because of significant alkalinization of urine, which promotes the precipitation of struvite stone (magnesium-ammonium-phosphate and calcium carbonate). The most common organism associated with struvite calculi is *Proteus mirabilis*. Other organisms include *Ureaplasma urealyticum*, *Providencia stuartii*, *Yersinia enterocolitica*, and *Bacteroides* corrodens.[12,13]

Most bacteriuria in short-term catheterization are of a single organism, whereas patients catheterized for longer than a month will usually show a polymicrobial flora caused by a wide range of gram-negative and gram-positive bacterial species.[14] Such specimens commonly have two to four bacterial species.[15]

Two of the most persistent species are *Escherichia coli* and *Providencia stuartii*. *Providencia stuartii* is rarely found outside the long-term catheterized urinary tract and may use the catheter itself as a niche.[16,17]

PREVENTION

Although the efficacy of prophylactic antibiotic therapy has been demonstrated, the possibility of bacterial resistance is a real concern. In recurrent UTIs, alternating antibiotics or use of methenamine for 2 months alternating with nitrofurantoin can be effective. Use of a catheter should be minimized according to the guidelines developed by the Centers for Disease Control and Prevention (CDC). The strategies developed by Infectious Diseases Society of America (IDSA) are effective and proven to decrease catheter-associated urinary tract infections (CAUTIs).[18]

LOWER URINARY TRACT INFECTIONS
CYSTITIS

Cystitis is the most common complication of neurogenic bladder. Because of partial or complete loss of sensation, patients do not usually experience frequency, urgency, or dysuria. More often, they complain of fever, back or abdominal discomfort, leakage between catheterizations, increased spasticity, malaise, lethargy, and/or cloudy, malodorous urine.[3] Urinalysis usually shows bacteriuria, pyuria, and hematuria.

Treatment is by giving the specific antibiotics. The duration of therapy is not established, but 4–5 days is recommended for the mild symptomatic patient and 10–14 days for sicker patients. Recurrent UTIs may be associated with high storage pressures, and intervention to decrease storage pressure may decrease the incidence of symptomatic UTIs.[10]

URETHRITIS AND EPIDIDYMITIS

This usually occurs in patients with indwelling urethral catheters, and less commonly with CIC. Occasionally, blockage of the periurethral gland by the catheter occurs; with secondary infection, this

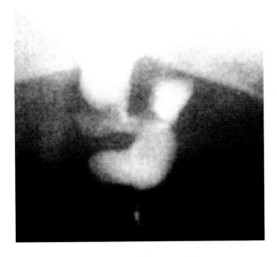

Figure 39.2 Voiding cystourethrogram (VCUG) of a 28-year-old female with urethral diverticulum developing after history of chronic indwelling catheterization. Note the saddle configuration of the diverticulum.

will lead to the formation of a periurethral abscess.[18] It may drain inside the urethral lumen, creating a diverticulum that needs surgical excision, otherwise recurrent periurethral abscess may develop (Figure 39.2). Quinolones can be given until the result of culture appears.

PROSTATITIS

In patients with NGB, high voiding pressure may increase intraprostatic ductal reflux in susceptible individuals (Figure 39.3).

The most common cause of prostatitis is the Enterobacteriaceae family of gram-negative bacteria, commonly strains of *Escherichia coli*, identified in 65% to 80% infections. *Pseudomonas aeruginosa*, *Serratia* species, *Klebsiella* species, and *Enterobacter aerogenes* are identified in a further 10%–15%.[19]

The most important clue in the diagnosis is a history of documented recurrent UTIs.[20] Urinalysis is usually free of pus cells. Segmented lower urinary tract cultures should be done to localize the infection in the prostate.[21] Treatment consists mainly of antibiotics that have good diffusion power into the prostatic tissues, such as trimethoprim and fluoroquinolones. Other agents such as alpha-blockers and anti-inflammatory drugs may also be used.

UPPER URINARY TRACT INFECTION (PYELONEPHRITIS)

Acute pyelonephritis in NBD patients is considered a complicated infection and requires hospitalization. At first, the patient should be adequately hydrated, blood culture and urine culture should be done, and broad-spectrum intravenous antibiotics (ampicillin-gentamicin) should be started until the results of cultures appear. On day 3, appropriate oral antibiotic should be started, and the duration of therapy should be 14 days.[22]

If symptoms persist beyond 72 hours, however, the possibility of perinephric or intrarenal abscesses, urinary tract abnormalities, or obstruction should be considered, and radiologic investigation with ultrasonography or computed tomography (CT) should be performed.[23]

LITHIASIS

INCIDENCE

It is estimated that 10%–20% of patients with SCI will have struvite stones within 10 years of injury; of these, 7% will have renal stones.[24] Once a kidney

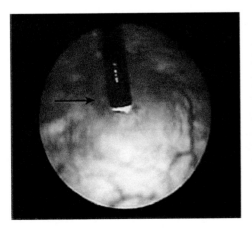 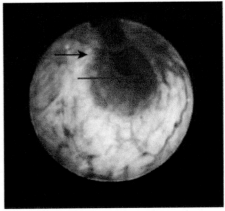

Figure 39.3 Cystoscopy of the same patient showing closed bladder neck with bladder filling (left side, black arrow). On bladder contraction, the bladder neck opens (right side, black arrow), but the external sphincter contracts at the same time (right side, blue arrow) leaving only the prostatic urethra opened.

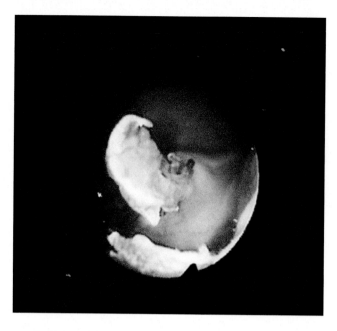

Figure 39.4 Cystoscopy of a 22-year-old male patient with a history of chronic indwelling catheter. Multiple typical eggshell-shaped stones could be seen, which were formed around the balloon of the Foley's catheter.

stone develops, there is a 34% chance of a second stone developing within the next 5 years.[25]

RISK FACTORS

The main risk factors for stone development are recurrent UTIs, especially due to urea-splitting organisms, infravesical obstruction producing stasis, indwelling catheters, VUR, hypercalciuria resulting from immobilization, demineralization of bone, and high specific gravity of urine.[26]

The risk of patients with SCI developing a stone is six times greater than in the general population.

STONE COMPOSITION

For the last few decades, most studies have reported that patients with NBD exclusively develop struvite stones composed of magnesium ammonium phosphate. This was attributed to UTI with urea-splitting organisms that render the urine pH greater than 7.24.[27] Recent studies, however, reported that many patients with NBD harboring calculi have been found to have metabolic stones.[28,29] The importance of this observation is that once a metabolically derived stone is identified, the patient should be offered further metabolic evaluation and medical and dietary therapy.[30]

DIAGNOSIS

Patients with renal stones usually have nonspecific symptoms including feeling unwell, abdominal discomfort, increased spasms, and autonomic dysreflexia (AD). A CT urogram becomes essential for diagnosis.[31]

Bladder stones usually start as small pieces of thin struvite calculi formed around the balloon of the Foley's

catheter. These calculi may grow but retain the typical eggshell shape that appears in cystoscopy (Figure 39.4).

TREATMENT

Successful treatment of renal stones depends on complete elimination of the calculus, eradication of infection, and removal of the obstruction. Selection of the best method of treatment should be individualized and adapted to every patient.

In paraplegic and quadriplegic patients, typical extracorporeal shock wave lithotripsy (ESWL) alone is not recommended because of the difficulty in eliminating the stone fragments, and ESWL may predispose to the development of AD.[32,33] The recommended technique for treatment is percutaneous nephrolithotripsy (PCNL). It is considered the "gold standard," specially for stone size above 2 cm. Nephrectomy should be performed when the kidney is nonfunctioning, or if there is pyonephrosis (Figure 39.5).

Ureteric stones can be managed through ureteroscopic fragmentation and extraction. Access can be limited by lower limb contractures.

Treatment of bladder stones is straightforward because of easy access to the bladder, both endoscopically and surgically, however, it could be complicated in augmented neurogenic bladder (Figure 39.6).

PREVENTION

Successful prevention of urinary stones in NBD patients depends on regular positioning of the paralyzed patients, high fluid intake, early mobilization, proper treatment of UTI, prevention of subsequent infection, and the use of urinary acidifiers.[34]

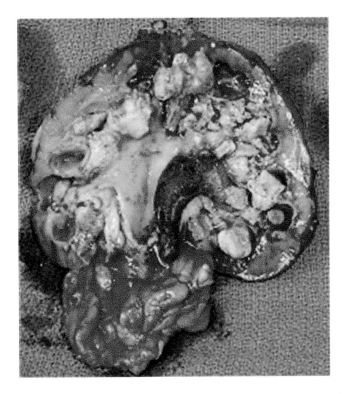

Figure 39.5   A surgical specimen from a 31-year-old patient who underwent nephrectomy for a nonfunctioning kidney harboring a staghorn stone.

NEOPLASM

INCIDENCE AND TYPES

It is estimated that patients with NBD are 16–28 times more susceptible to develop bladder cancer than the normal population.[35] Recent studies reported a bladder cancer incidence of 0.1%–2.4%. Patients with SCI tend to present with bladder cancer at an earlier age and a more advanced stage, on average 18–24 years after the onset of SCI.[36] The most common histologic type occurring in these patients is squamous cell carcinoma.[38]

RISK FACTORS

The most important risk factor for the development of bladder carcinoma is irritation of the bladder mucosa. This includes chronic bladder infection, prolonged indwelling catheterization, and bladder stone disease. Other risk factors include smoking and altered immunologic function.

SCREENING

The screening of NBD patients with chronic indwelling catheterization is controversial. Some advocate the use of screening cystoscopy after 5–7 years of using chronic catheterization.[37,38]

Screening cytology may be of benefit. Stonehill et al. recommended yearly cytology in all patients with chronic indwelling catheters, followed by biopsy if it was positive.[39]

A new onset of gross hematuria should be investigated in the same way as in the neurologically normal population.

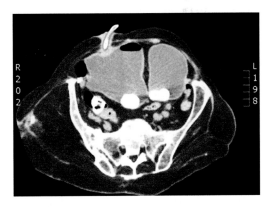

Figure 39.6   Computed tomography scan of an augmented bladder in a patient with spinal cord injury with bladder and augment stones. The augmentation scarred down and formed an hourglass appearance with poor drainage into native bladder. Patient presented 7 years after augmentation with sepsis, retention, and renal failure. (Courtesy of Dr. Ghoniem.)

REFERENCES

1. Stover SL, Lioyd LK, Waites KB, and Jackson AB. Urinary tract infection in spinal cord injury. *Arch Phys Med Rehab.* 1989;70:47–54.
2. Waites KB, Canupp CK, and Devivo MJ. Epidemiology and risk factors for urinary tract infection following spinal cord injury. *Arch Phys Med Rehab.* 1993;74:691.
3. Beraldo PSS, Neves EGC, Alves CMF et al. Pyrexia in hospitalized spinal cord injury patients. *Paraplegia.* 1993;31:186.
4. Ward TT, Jones SR. Genitourinary tract infections. In: Reese RE, and Betts RF, eds. *A Logical Approach to Infectious Diseases,* 3rd ed. Boston, MA: Little, Brown and Company; 1991:357–89.
5. Horton JA 3rd, Kirshblum SC, Lisenmeyer TA, Johnston M, and Rustagi A. Does refrigeration of urine alter culture results in hospitalized patients with neurogenic bladder? *J Spinal Cord Med.* 1998;21:342–7.
6. Gilmore DS, Schick DJ, Young MN, and Montgomerie JZ. Effect of external urinary collection system on colonization and urinary tract infections with *Pseudomonas* and *Klebsiella* in men with spinal cord injury. *J Am Paraplegia Soc.* 1992;15:155.
7. Lapides J, Diokno AC, Silber SJ et al. Clean intermittent self-catheterization in the treatment of urinary tract disease. *J Urol.* 1972;107(3):458–61.
8. Tambyah PA and Maki DG. Catheter-associated urinary tract infection is rarely symptomatic: A prospective study of 1,497 catheterized patients. *Arch Intern Med.* 2000;160:678.
9. Shigemura K, Kitagawa K, Nomi M et al. Risk factors for febrile genito-urinary infection in the catheterized patients by with spinal cord injury-associated chronic neurogenic lower urinary tract dysfunction evaluated by urodynamic study and cystography: A retrospective study. *World J Urol.* 2020;38(3):733–40.
10. Cardenas DD and Hooton TM. Urinary tract infection in persons with spinal cord injury. *Arch Phys Med Rehab.* 1995;76:272.
11. National Institute on Disability and Rehabilitation Research Consensus Statement. The prevention and management of urinary tract infections among people with spinal cord injury. *SCI Nurs.* 1993;10:49–61.
12. Babayan RK. Urinary calculi and endourology. In: Siroky MB, Krane RJ, eds. *Manual of Urology.* Boston, MA: Little, Brown and Company; 1990:123–31.
13. Silverman DE and Stamey TA. Management of infection stones: The Stanford experience. *Medicine (Baltim).* 1983;62:44–51.
14. Edwards LE, Lock R, Powell C, and Jones P. Post-catheterization urethral strictures: A clinical and experimental study. *Br J Urol.* 1983;55:53.
15. Nickel JC, Olson ME, and Costerton JW. *In vivo* coefficient of kinetic friction: Study of urinary catheter biocompatibility. *Urology.* 1987;14:501.
16. Hockstra D. Hyaluronan-modified surfaces for medical devices. *Med Device Diagn Ind.* 1999:48–56.
17. Liedberg H and Lundeberg T. Silver alloy-coated catheters reduce catheter-associated bacteriuria. *Br J Urol.* 1990;65:379.
18. Hooton TM, Bradley SF, Cardenas DD et al. Diagnosis, prevention, and treatment of catheter associated urinary tract infection in adults: 2009 International Clinical Guidelines from the Infectious Disease Society of America. *Clin Infect Dis.* 2010;50(5):625–63.
19. Kaplan SA, Te AE, and Jacobs BZ. Urodynamic evidence of vesical neck obstruction in men with misdiagnosed chronic nonbacterial prostatitis and the therapeutic role of endoscopic incision of the bladder neck. *J Urol.* 1994;152:2063–5.
20. Weidner W and Ludwig M. Diagnostic management of chronic prostatitis. In: Weidner W, Madsen PO, and Schiefer HG, eds. *Prostatitis – Etiopathology, Diagnosis and Therapy.* Berlin, Germany: SpringerVerlag; 1994:158–74.
21. Stamey TA, Meares EMJ, and Winningham DG. Chronic bacterial prostatitis and the diffusion of drugs into prostatic fluid. *J Urol.* 1970;103:187–94.
22. Talan DA, Stamm WE, Hooton TM et al. Comparison of ciprofloxacin (7 days) and trimethoprim-sulfamethoxazole (14 days) for acute uncomplicated pyelonephritis in women. *JAMA.* 2000;12:1583.
23. Soulen MC, Fishman EK, Goldman SM et al. Bacterial renal infection: Role of CT. *Radiology.* 1989;171:703.
24. Chen Y, DeVivo MJ, and Roseman JM. Current trend and risk factors for kidney stones in persons with spinal cord injury: A longitudinal study. *Spinal Cord.* 2000;38:346–53.
25. Chen Y, DeVivo MJ, Stover SL, and Lioyd LK. Recurrent kidney stone: A 25 year follow up study in persons with spinal cord injury. *Urology.* 2002;60:228–32.
26. Ost MC and Lee BR. Urolithiasis in patients with spinal cord injuries: Risk factors, management, and outcomes. *Curr Opin Urol.* 2006;16(2):93–109.
27. Burr RG. Urinary calculi composition in patients with spinal cord lesions. *Arch Phys Med Rehab.* 1978;59:84–9.
28. Nikakhter B, Vaziri ND, Khonsary F, Gordon S, and Mirahmadi MD. Urolithiasis in patients with spinal cord injury. *Paraplegia.* 1981;19:363–9.
29. Matlaga BR, Kim SC, Watkins SL et al. Changing composition of renal calculi in patients with neurogenic bladder. *J Urol.* 2006;175(5):1716–9.
30. Donnellan SM and Bolton DM. The impact of contemporary bladder management techniques on struvite calculi associated with spinal cord injury. *BJU Int.* 1999;84:280–7.
31. Mardis HK, Parks JH, Muller G, Ganzel K, and Coe FL. Outcome of metabolic evaluation and medical treatment for calcium nephrolithiasis in a private urological practice. *J Urol.* 2004;171:85–93.
32. Niedrach WL, Davis RS, Tonetti FW, and Cockett AT. Extracorporeal shock-wave lithotripsy in patients with spinal cord dysfunction. *Urology.* 1991, 38:152–6.
33. Stow DF, Bernstein JS, Madson KE, McDonald DJ, and Ebert TJ. Autonomic hyperreflexia in spinal cord injured patients during extracorporeal shock wave lithotripsy. *Anath Analg.* 1989;68:788–91.
34. Jeantet A, Thea A, Fernando U et al. Infectious nephrolithiasis: Results of treatment with methenamine mandelate. *Contrib Nephrol.* 1987;58:233–5.
35. Hess MJ, Zhan Eh, Foo DK, and Yalla SV. Bladder cancer in patients with spinal cord injury. *J Spinal Cord Med.* 2003;26(4):335–8.

36. Welk B, McIntyre A, Teasell R, Potter P, and Loh E. Bladder cancer in individuals with spinal cord injuries. *Spinal Cord.* 2013;51:516–21.

37. van Velzen D, Kirshnan KR, Parsons KF et al. Comparative pathology of dome and trigone of urinary bladder mucosa in paraplegics and tetraplegics. *Paraplegia.* 1995;33:565–72.

38. Navon JD, Soliman H, Khonsari F, and Ahlering T. Screening cystoscopy and survival of SCI patients with squamous cell carcinoma of the bladder. *J Urol.* 1997;157:2109–11.

39. Stonehill WH, Goldman HB, and Dmochowski RR. The use of urine cytology for diagnosing bladder cancer in spinal cord injured patients. *J Urol.* 1997;157:2112–14.

COMPLICATIONS RELATED TO NEUROGENIC BLADDER DYSFUNCTION II
Upper Urinary Tract

Claire C. Yang

INTRODUCTION

The function of the bladder and sphincters depends on an intact nervous system. Neurogenic bladder (NGB) dysfunction results from lesions or derangements in the nervous system and can result in a number of bladder problems, such as urinary tract infections (UTIs), urinary incontinence, and retention. Lower urinary tract dysfunction can also affect the upper urinary tract (i.e., the kidneys and ureters), with complications such as vesicoureteral reflux (VUR), hydronephrosis, and loss of renal function. Thus, minimizing the complications of NGB dysfunction—particularly the health- and life-threatening upper tract changes—remains the goal of treatment.

Historically, patients with significant NGB dysfunction had poor survival after the development of bladder failure. However, in the 1960s and 1970s, the medical community recognized that, in large part, renal failure resulted from inadequate bladder management. Improved bladder emptying, along with more widespread antibiotic use, improved both renal function and, ultimately, survival rates in persons with NGB dysfunction. Consequently, upper tract sequelae have decreased dramatically in the last 50 years for patients with access to adequate medical care. These complications still occur, and healthcare providers of patients with NGB dysfunction must continuously remember the possibility of upper tract deterioration as they treat their patients.

This chapter discusses the clinical conditions that contribute to upper tract deterioration, the pathophysiology of upper tract deterioration in patients with NGB dysfunction, and the incidence of upper tract damage in common neurologic conditions that results in NGB dysfunction. Other chapters in this textbook discuss the evaluation, diagnosis, and management of upper tract complications.

CLINICAL CONDITIONS CONTRIBUTING TO UPPER TRACT DETERIORATION IN NEUROGENIC BLADDER DYSFUNCTION

Renal and ureteral injury in NGB dysfunction can result from both acute and chronic conditions. Acute causes include infection and sudden obstruction. Pyelonephritis occurs due to ascending bacteriuria from the lower urinary tract, as a result of catheterization or poor bladder emptying. Acute obstruction of a renal unit is typically caused by nephrolithiasis, which is a risk factor for developing both temporary and permanent renal insufficiency. In patients with NGB dysfunction, stones are frequently composed of struvite ("infection stone"), due to the high urinary pH typical in persons with chronic bacteriuria, although metabolic stones can be present as well.[1] In acute nephrolithiasis, the degree of obstruction, duration of obstruction, and presence of bacteriuria all affect the severity of the renal injury and the likelihood of functional recovery. It is likely that the high incidence of nephrolithiasis in some groups of patients with NGB dysfunction (e.g., reported as 7%–30% in patients with spinal cord injury [SCI][2,3]) contributes to the higher risk of renal insufficiency compared to the general population.

Chronic infections and obstruction compound the likelihood of upper tract damage. For example, repeated episodes of pyelonephritis or chronic pyelonephritis result in cortical and medullary scarring[4] and loss of renal function. However, repeated episodes of pyelonephritis uncomplicated by obstruction, structural alterations of the urinary tract, or NGB dysfunction, do *not* result in end-stage renal disease.[4,5] Compared to chronic infections, chronic obstruction has worse outcomes for patients with NGB dysfunction. On a structural level, repeated episodes of acute obstruction or chronic, untreated obstruction eventually result in permanent nephron loss and a decrease in glomerular filtration rate (GFR).

A more insidious—oftentimes silent—etiology for the loss of renal function in NGB dysfunction is the presence of chronically high pressures within the bladder in the absence of acute obstruction. These pressures result from a poorly compliant bladder, high contraction pressures, or a poorly emptying bladder, all obstructing urine drainage from the kidney. In the first case, the fibrotic, noncompliant bladder becomes the point of obstruction for ureteral drainage, and hydronephrosis develops. In fact, several studies have shown that urodynamic parameters such as persistent poor compliance and high detrusor pressures predict upper tract decompensation.[6–8]

Elevated detrusor storage or voiding pressures may also contribute to the development of VUR, which further increases the risk of upper tract deterioration. This was nicely demonstrated in a study of 170 patients with SCI with NGB dysfunction, followed for 5 years following injury. These patients were injured in the mid-20th century, without the aggressive antibiotic and bladder management currently available. In this series, the incidence of renal dysfunction temporally tracks with the development of VUR.[9]

In healthy bladders, the valvular function of the ureterovesical junction (UVJ) protects the low-pressure upper urinary tract from urine refluxing from the bladder. When an individual has NGB dysfunction, chronically high detrusor pressures compromise this protective function and are believed to alter the anatomy of the bladder trigone, distorting the angle of ureteral entry into the trigone and shortening the tunneled portion of the intramural ureter.[10] This altered intramural obliquity triggers urinary reflux from the bladder back into the ureter (Figure 40.1). With VUR, the low-pressure upper tracts are then exposed to higher pressures and result in a loss of GFR (see later). VUR also facilitates ascending bacteriuria and predisposes the renal unit to struvite stone growth.[3]

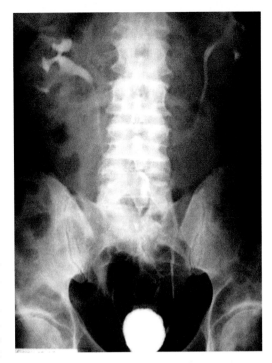

Figure 40.1 Bilateral vesicoureteral reflux. Retrograde cystogram demonstrating bilateral vesicoureteral reflux in a 48-year-old male patient with spinal cord injury.

the lower urinary tract is generated. Whether the bladder pressure results in loss of integrity of the UVJ (causing VUR) or compromises efficient renal drainage, the elevated pressures are eventually transmitted to the upper tracts. Intrarenal pressure increases, hydronephrosis develops, GFR decreases, and ultimately, nephron loss results. The most important goal of managing NGB is to preserve renal function, and this is primarily achieved through treatment aimed at minimizing the generation of elevated pressure in the lower urinary tract.

INCIDENCE OF UPPER TRACT DAMAGE RELATED TO NEUROGENIC BLADDER DYSFUNCTION IN PATIENTS WITH NEUROLOGIC CONDITIONS

PATHOPHYSIOLOGY OF RENAL DETERIORATION

A healthy bladder remains compliant during the filling phase and empties without excessive detrusor contraction pressures, thus maintaining an environment without resultant high bladder pressures. However, NGB dysfunction can result in poor bladder compliance, high detrusor contraction pressures, and incomplete bladder emptying. In all three conditions, excessively high pressure in

Individuals with neurologic injury or disease resulting in NGB dysfunction, particularly injury or disease affecting the spinal cord, experience higher risks of bladder dysfunction and related renal insufficiency compared to the general population. The increased risk is in part due to the lack of coordination between detrusor contractions and sphincter relaxation, a pathophysiology common to spinal conditions. These conditions include SCI, neural tube defects (e.g., spina bifida), and multiple sclerosis (MS).

SPINAL CORD INJURY

As noted earlier, SCI has historically been associated with frequent urologic sequelae. Hydronephrosis, VUR, pyelonephritis, and renal insufficiency in patients with minimally treated NGB were commonplace, with incidence increasing with time from injury.[9,11] Compared to historic levels, contemporary incidence of upper tract complications in SCI has dropped significantly. In 2005, Ku and colleagues retrospectively reported on 179 patients with traumatic SCI for a minimum of 10 years to identify the risk of complication of the upper urinary tract in relation to bladder management.[12] In this series, 32.4% of patients developed some degree of renal deterioration. In 2001, Lawrenson and colleagues used a large, community-based data set, comparing patients with SCI with the general population. Patients with SCI were found to have a fivefold increased risk of renal failure compared with the general population.[13] But overall, genitourinary causes of death (primarily renal failure) in patients with SCI have become significantly less common. In a large database of 29,000 patients with SCI in the United States, genitourinary causes of death ranked eleventh, behind pneumonia, septicemia, cancer, heart disease, and other etiologies.[14] Other parts of the world have also documented the same findings.[15]

NEURAL TUBE DEFECTS

Historically, children born with neural tube defects and significant NGB dysfunction did not typically live to adulthood, often as a result of renal failure.[16] In 2005, only 60% of children with spina bifida in the United Kingdom reached the age of 21 years,[17] with renal failure still one of the leading causes of death, presumably a sequela of NGB dysfunction. In two UK series, renal failure was the most common cause of death (18%), especially in those with sensory levels above T11.[18] In the United Kingdom, Singhal and Mathew examined an unselected group of adult patients with spina bifida, and in their series of 30 patients with identifiable causes of death, 10 died as a result of renal failure.[19] Moreover, the aforementioned Lawrenson study estimated that the risk of renal failure for patients with neural tube defects was eight times that of the general population.[13] Recent studies show that with early evaluation, follow-up examinations, and adequate therapy, a reduction in renal function was noticed in only 1.2%–2.1% of children with spina bifida.[20,21] However, the low incidence of renal deterioration may not be maintained as these children transition through puberty and progress through adulthood.[17] As demonstrated in patients with SCI, patients with neural tube defects have also benefitted from improved urinary tract management, but upper tract complications of NGB dysfunction are still cause for concern.

MULTIPLE SCLEROSIS

Bladder dysfunction, resulting in abnormalities in both storage and emptying, affects up to 90% of patients with MS.[22] It has long been recognized that detrusor overactivity and external sphincter dyssynergia are the most common forms of bladder and sphincter dysfunction.[23] Furthermore, the greater the impairment with MS, the greater the risk of urinary tract abnormalities.[24] Despite these findings, renal insufficiency secondary to NGB in patients with MS is not particularly common. A meta-analysis of 14 studies comprising 2076 patients by Koldewijn and colleagues in 1995 found a 0.34% incidence of hydronephrosis or renal complications.[25] In addition, Lawrenson and colleagues reported no increased risk in persons with MS for the development of renal insufficiency when compared to the general population.[13]

SUMMARY

NGB dysfunction affects many individuals with compromised nervous systems, particularly persons with SCI and neural tube disorders. Healthcare providers must remain vigilant in evaluating and treating patients with NGB dysfunction to prevent long-term kidney damage.

REFERENCES

1. Matlaga BR, Kim SC, Watkins SL, Kuo RL, Munch LC, and Lingeman JE. Changing composition of renal calculi in patients with neurogenic bladder. *J Urol.* 2006;175(5):1716–9.
2. Comarr AE, Kawaichi GK, and Bors E. Renal calculosis of patients with traumatic cord lesions. *J Urol.* 1962;87:647–56.
3. Hall MK, Hackler RH, Zampieri TA, and Zampieri JB. Renal calculi in spinal cord-injured patient: Association with reflux, bladder stones, and foley catheter drainage. *Urology.* 1989;34(3):126–8.
4. Freedman LR. Natural history of urinary infection in adults. *Kidney Int Suppl.* 1975;4:S96–100.
5. Asscher AW, McLachlan MS, Jones RV et al. Screening for asymptomatic urinary-tract infection in schoolgirls. A two-centre feasibility study. *Lancet.* 1973;2(7819):1–4.
6. Styles RA, Ramsden PD, and Neal DE. Chronic retention of urine. The relationship between upper tract dilatation and bladder pressure. *Br J Urol.* 1986;58(6):647–51.
7. Ghoniem GM, Bloom DA, McGuire EJ, and Stewart KL. Bladder compliance in meningomyelocele children. *J Urol.* 1989;141(6):1404–6.

8. Ghoniem GM, Roach MB, Lewis VH, and Harmon EP. The value of leak pressure and bladder compliance in the urodynamic evaluation of meningomyelocele patients. *J Urol*. 1990;144(6):1440–2.

9. Hutch JA and Bunts RC. The present urologic status of the war-time paraplegic. *J Urol*. 1951;66(2): 218–28.

10. Morales PA. Renal complications of the neurogenic bladder. In: Boyarsky S, ed. *The Neurogenic Bladder*. Baltimore, MD: Williams and Wilkins; 1967.

11. Bors E. Neurogenic bladder. *Urol Surv*. 1957;7(3):177–250.

12. Ku JH, Choi WJ, Lee KY et al. Complications of the upper urinary tract in patients with spinal cord injury: A long-term follow-up study. *Urol Res*. 2005;33(6):435–9.

13. Lawrenson R, Wyndaele JJ, Vlachonikolis I, Farmer C, and Glickman S. Renal failure in patients with neurogenic lower urinary tract dysfunction. *Neuroepidemiology*. 2001;20(2):138–43.

14. The 2012 Annual Statistical Report for the Spinal Cord Injury Model Systems. Table 10: Cause of Death. 2012:8. https://www.nscisc.uab. edu/PublicDocuments/reports/pdf/2012%20 NSCISC%20Annual%20Statistical%20Report%20 Complete%20Public%20Version.pdf

15. Soden RJ, Walsh J, Middleton JW, Craven ML, Rutkowski SB, and Yeo JD. Causes of death after spinal cord injury. *Spinal Cord*. 2000;38(10):604–10.

16. Doran PA and Guthkelch AN. Studies in spina bifida cystica. I. General survey and reassessment of the problem. *J Neurol Neurosurg Psychiatry*. 1961;24:331–45.

17. Woodhouse CR. Myelomeningocele in young adults. *BJU Int*. 2005;95(2):223–30.

18. Hunt G, Lewin W, Gleave J, and Gairdner D. Predictive factors in open myelomeningocele with special reference to sensory level. *Br Med J*. 1973;4(5886):197–201.

19. Singhal B and Mathew KM. Factors affecting mortality and morbidity in adult spina bifida. *Eur J Pediatr Surg*. 1999;9(Suppl 1):31–2.

20. Hopps CV and Kropp KA. Preservation of renal function in children with myelomeningocele managed with basic newborn evaluation and close followup. *J Urol*. 2003;169(1):305–8.

21. Dik P, Klijn AJ, van Gool JD, de Jong-de Vos van Steenwijk CC, and de Jong TP. Early start to therapy preserves kidney function in spina bifida patients. *Eur Urol*. 2006;49(5):908–13.

22. McGuire EJ and Savastano JA. Urodynamic findings and long-term outcome management of patients with multiple sclerosis-induced lower urinary tract dysfunction. *J Urol*. 1984;132(4):713–5.

23. Bradley WE. Urinary bladder dysfunction in multiple sclerosis. *Neurology*. 1978;28(9 Pt 2):52–8.

24. Betts CD, D'Mellow MT, and Fowler CJ. Urinary symptoms and the neurological features of bladder dysfunction in multiple sclerosis. *J Neurol Neurosurg Psychiatry*. 1993;56(3):245–50.

25. Koldewijn EL, Hommes OR, Lemmens WA, Debruyne FM, and van Kerrebroeck PE. Relationship between lower urinary tract abnormalities and disease-related parameters in multiple sclerosis. *J Urol*. 1995;154(1):169–73.

BENIGN PROSTATIC HYPERPLASIA AND LOWER URINARY TRACT SYMPTOMS IN MEN WITH NEUROGENIC BLADDER

Jeffrey Thavaseelan and Akhlil Hamid

INTRODUCTION

Diagnosis and management of benign prostatic hyperplasia (BPH) in neurologically impaired patients is challenging. The assumption that lower urinary tract symptoms (LUTS) in these patients are invariably due to the underlying neuropathology may result in inadequate treatment of BPH. However, ignoring the underlying neurologic condition can exacerbate symptoms and dramatically worsen quality of life.

With increasing age, we not only see an increase in BPH but also an increase in age-related detrusor dysfunction and an increase in the incidence of neurologic disease, in particular, neurodegenerative disease (Figure 41.1).

ASSESSMENT

Figure 41.2 illustrates a diagnostic workup of LUTS in men over the age of 40 years.[1] It is important to note that the presence of neurologic disease automatically necessitates further evaluation.

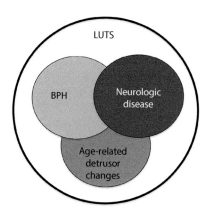

Figure 41.1 Illustration of the multiple factors contributing to luts with increasing age.

It is important to note that LUTS due to neurologic diseases may precede the diagnosis and may not be related to BPH. For example, in multiple system atrophy (MSA), LUTS may be the first manifestation, seen significantly before the diagnosis is made.[2]

Physical examination should include a focused urologic assessment with examination of the prostate and neurologic system. The latter should include perianal sensation, anal tone, and bulbocavernosus reflex. This is particularly relevant in sacral neurologic pathology.

Tests that further contribute to assessment include a 3-day bladder diary, urinalysis, and assessment of flow rate and residual volume.[3]

As per Figure 41.2, patients with or suspected of having neurologic disease require further evaluation, and this includes renal ultrasound, serum creatinine, and urodynamics.[4]

Important to identify are risk factors for renal tract deterioration, including detrusor–external sphincter dyssynergia (DESD), poor bladder compliance, urethral obstruction, and increased postvoid residual (PVR).[4]

URODYNAMIC TESTING

There are primarily five questions that need to be answered when performing urodynamic assessment:

1. Is there detrusor overactivity (DO) during fill phase?
2. Is there DESD?
3. Is the bladder compliant?
4. Is there obstruction during voiding and, if so, at which level?
5. What is the contractility of the bladder during voiding?

DO may be neurogenic or nonneurogenic, as is the case in BPH.[5] Between 46% and 66% of men with prostatic obstruction may have concurrent DO.[6] In

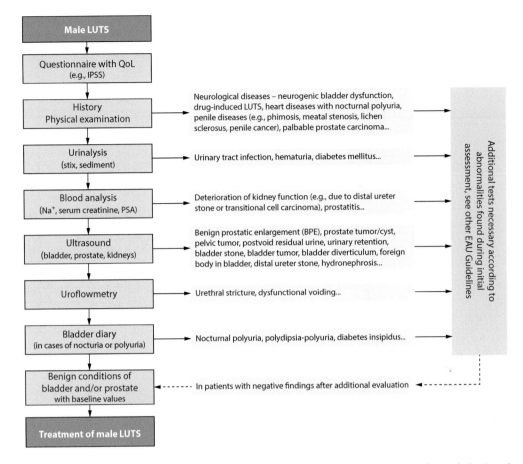

Figure 41.2 Algorithm showing recommended assessment for patients with benign prostatic hyperplasia. Note that additional tests are necessary for patients with neurologic diseases. (https://uroweb.org/wp-content/uploads/EAU-Guidelines-Male_LUTS-2013.pdf.) (Reproduced with permission from Oelke, M et al., Guidelines on the Management of Male Lower Urinary Tract Symptoms [LUTS], incl. Benign Prostatic Obstruction [BPO].)

men with BPH and underlying neurologic disease, it can be difficult to determine the true cause of DO.

Several publications have attempted to classify DO characteristics into clinical groups.[7,8] Kageyama et al.[8] published a classification of DO and likelihood of persisting problems after transurethral resection of the prostate (TURP).[8] DO occurring at low volume, high pressure, and phasic were more suggestive of underlying neurogenic disease. However, one cannot always rely on this, and assessment requires an individualized holistic clinical approach.

DESD is defined by the International Continence Society (ICS) as a "detrusor contraction concurrent with an involuntary contraction of the urethral and/or periurethral striated muscle.[5]" Occasionally flow can be prevented altogether and can only be diagnosed with urodynamic studies (Figure 41.3). It only arises in the patient with pathology between the pontine micturition center (PMC) and the sacral micturition center (S2 through S4).[9] Examples include spinal cord injury, multiple sclerosis, spinal dysraphism, and transverse myelitis.

In a patient who does not have spinal cord pathology as described, a similar discrepancy can be seen between detrusor and sphincter activity but is referred to as dysfunctional voiding.

In the absence of DESD, diagnosis of LUTS due to BPH requires urodynamic demonstration of obstruction at the level of the posterior urethra. The most widely used parameter is detrusor pressure at maximum flow (P_{det} at Q_{max}).[10]

Voiding cystourethrogram (VCUG) is helpful in demonstrating narrowing of the posterior urethra during voiding.

UNDERLYING DISEASE

The following discussion concentrates on special circumstances that must be considered in patients with certain underlying diseases.

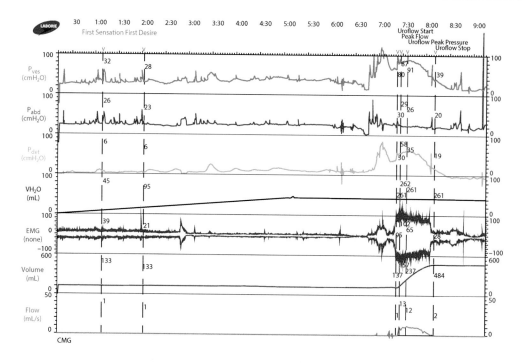

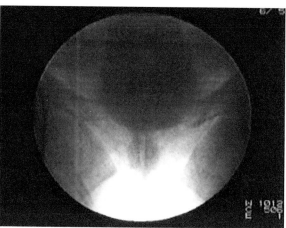

Figure 41.3 Voiding cystourethrogram showing the classical dilated bladder neck and posterior urethra with narrowing at the external sphincter with voiding.

PARKINSON'S DISEASE

LUTS associated with Parkinson's disease (PD) is primarily a disorder of bladder storage rather than voiding; however, the severity of the symptoms tends to be exacerbated by the immobility, cognitive impairment, and poor manual dexterity that are typically seen in this condition.[11] The most common symptoms described are nocturia (77.5%), urgency (36.7%), and increased urinary frequency (32.6%), which reflect DO commonly seen in urodynamic testing.[11,12] There may also be voiding symptoms including hesitancy,

straining to void, and diminished flow. Historically, this was thought to be due to pseudodyssynergia, where the patient voluntarily contracts their pelvic floor to prevent leakage or sphincter bradykinesia.[13] However, it is not as common as previously thought and in the older patient with PD, BPH may be the cause of voiding symptoms. There is also evidence to suggest higher resting urethral pressures secondary to levodopa or its metabolites, a common treatment for PD, which leads to increased bladder neck tone via the α_1-adrenoceptor.[14]

Urodynamic studies are mandatory in patients with PD to determine treatment. The key question is, if outflow obstruction can be demonstrated and there is clinical evidence of an enlarged prostate, is it safe to perform surgery if conservative therapy fails? Roth et al.[15] published a series of patients with PD who underwent TURP with prior urodynamic assessment. At 3 years, success following TURP was 70%. Of the ten patients with urge urinary incontinence, five resolved, and three improved; no patients experienced *de novo* incontinence.[15]

Historically there has been a hesitancy to perform outflow surgery in patients with PD due to a high incidence of incontinence that had been reported.[16] However, in those studies, it was noted that some of these patients were likely to have had MSA.[2] Distinguishing between PD and MSA is critical before surgical intervention for BPH is considered. The reason for this is outlined in the following section.

MULTIPLE SYSTEM ATROPHY

MSA is a progressive degenerative neurologic disorder, which shares symptoms with PD and is considered a form of atypical parkinsonism.

Although sometimes misdiagnosed as PD, its underlying neuropathology is more extensive, involving not only the substantia nigra, but other areas such as the cerebellar hemisphere, inferior olivary nucleus, locus coeruleus (PMC), intermediolateral cell column, and Onuf's nucleus.[17]

Consistent with the sites of abnormal pathology, urinary symptoms are seen in a significant proportion (greater than 80%) of MSA patients, tend to occur earlier in the disease process than with PD, and may be the first presenting symptom.[18]

Most important, however, is the recognition that in MSA there is denervation of the external urethral sphincter (EUS) as a consequence of the involvement of Onuf's nucleus.[14,15] This is best diagnosed using electromyography (EMG). Clearly, therefore, surgical treatment of BPH in patients with MSA could result in genuine stress incontinence.

Patients diagnosed as having PD but with early onset and marked urinary incontinence, more extensive pyramidal or cerebellar signs, erectile dysfunction, and severe postural hypotension, may need to be reassessed for possibility of MSA prior to considering outflow surgery.

STROKE

The prevalence of urinary incontinence following stroke has been reported to range between 28% and 79%.[19] The most common cause of incontinence was traditionally thought to be DO; however, urodynamic testing in these patients has shown that DO, acontractility, and also normal bladder function can be evident.[19,20] In this cohort, the symptoms described as most bothersome by patients include nocturia (53%), urgency (48%), and daytime frequency (40%).[21]

Lum and Marshall[22] published a series of 39 patients who had a history of stroke and underwent endoscopic prostatectomy. Better outcomes were achieved in patients under the age of 70 years and those who had their operation more than 1 year after the stroke.[22] In addition, patients with left cerebral hemisphere lesions did better than those with right or bilateral lesions.[22]

DIABETES MELLITUS

Bladder dysfunction is a common sequela to diabetes and usually secondary to peripheral neuropathy. Symptoms include decreased sensation, increased bladder capacity, DO, urinary incontinence, poor urinary flow rate, and incomplete bladder emptying with high PVRs. The prevalence of urodynamically diagnosed bladder DO varies between 25% and 90% and can exist either with or without impaired detrusor contractility.[23] The pathophysiology behind this may not only be due to peripheral neuropathy but also central neuropathy, with up to 76% of diabetic patients with DO having multiple cerebral infarctions on MRI.[24] Indeed, urinary incontinence is a greater complication than neuropathy and nephropathy in diabetes.[25] In addition, there are other ways in which diabetes may give rise to LUTS. These include diabetic polyuria, neurogenic dysfunction of detrusor smooth muscle cells, and a greater risk of symptomatic urinary tract infections. Certainly, the modern understanding of diabetic cystopathy is a combination of impaired detrusor contractility leading to incomplete emptying but also elements of DO and increased sensation.[26] Therefore, the use of urodynamic testing is useful in the management of patients with diabetes and LUTS. In a study by Kaplan et al., of 182 patients, 55% had DO, 23% had impaired detrusor contractility, and 10% had bladder atonia. Significantly, 36% of patients were also found to have bladder outflow obstruction.[26]

MULTIPLE SCLEROSIS

Multiple sclerosis (MS) is a chronic inflammatory disease of the central nervous system (CNS) leading to multiple physical disabilities. Patients with MS can

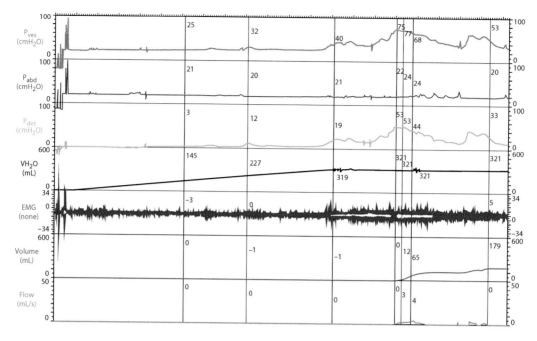

Figure 41.4 Urodynamic test in male with multiple sclerosis with lower urinary tract symptoms (LUTS) and benign prostatic hyperplasia (BPH). Trace shows high pressure and poor flow, but increased electromyographic activity during void indicative of detrusor external sphincter dyssynergia rather than BPH being the cause of LUTS.

present with abnormalities to the detrusor, EUS, or both, and therefore may have failure to store or failure to empty or a combination of both. Indeed, 60%–80% of patients show neurogenic DO, which results in a functionally small capacity bladder and may present with urgency, frequency, and urge incontinence. Approximately 20% suffer from impaired detrusor contractility and atonic bladder presenting with overflow incontinence, poor flow, and incomplete emptying.[27] Furthermore, 25% of patients have a degree of DESD from spinal cord involvement. DESD can lead to incomplete emptying and urinary retention, or present with urgency, frequency, and incontinence.[28] Less commonly, MS in the sacral cord can produce a hypotonic bladder that empties poorly.

As MS is primarily a disease that occurs in the younger age group and more so in women, the issue of bladder dysfunction in relation to BPH is rare. In these rare cases, differentiating LUTS associated with BPH from that which is caused by MS becomes a very difficult task. Urodynamic testing is crucial to delineate the pathophysiologic cause but is likely to be more useful in ensuring the absence of DESD as the cause of obstruction (Figure 41.4).

CONCLUSION

Diagnosis and management of LUTS and BPH in the older man with underlying neurologic disease

is complex. The potential for an adverse outcome following surgical intervention in these patients with BPH reinforces the importance of a detailed clinical history and knowledge of how neurologic conditions present themselves with respect to LUTSs. VCUG with/without EMG is an essential part of the diagnostic process, but it must be recognized that it is not always possible to discriminate between LUTS secondary to BPH and LUTS secondary to neurologic disease. As a consequence, in many circumstances, conservative treatment is preferable to irreversible surgical intervention.

REFERENCES

1. Oelke M, Bachmann A, Descazeaud A et al. Guidelines on the management of male lower urinary tract symptoms (LUTS), incl. benign prostatic obstruction (BPO). 2012. https://uroweb.org/wp-content/uploads/EAU-Guidelines-Male_LUTS-2013.pdf
2. Fowler CJ, Dalton C, and Panicker JN. Review of neurologic diseases for the urologist. *Urol Clin North Am.* 2010;37:517–26.
3. American Urological Association. Guidelines on the management of benign prostatic hyperplasia. 2010. http://www.auanet.org/education/guidelines/benign-prostatic-hyperplasia.cfm
4. Blaivas J. Benign prostatic hyperplasia and lower urinary tract symptoms in men with neurogenic bladder. In: Corcos ES, and Schik E, eds. *Textbook of Neurogenic Bladder: Adults and Children.* Boca Raton, FL: CRC Press; 2008:860–78.

5. Abrams P, Cardozo L, Fall M et al. The standardisation of terminology of lower urinary tract function: Report from the Standardisation Sub-committee of the International Continence Society. *Neurourol Urodyn.* 2002;21:167–78.

6. Blaivas JG, Marks BK, Weiss JP, Panagopoulos G, and Somaroo C. Differential diagnosis of overactive bladder in men. *J Urol.* 2009;182:2814–7.

7. Flisser AJ, Walmsley K, and Blaivas JG. Urodynamic classification of patients with symptoms of overactive bladder. *J Urol.* 2003;169:529–33; discussion 33–4.

8. Kageyama S, Watanabe T, Kurita Y et al. Can persisting detrusor hyperreflexia be predicted after transurethral prostatectomy for benign prostatic hypertrophy? *Neurourol Urodyn.* 2000;19:233–40.

9. Sadananda P, Vahabi B, and Drake MJ. Bladder outlet physiology in the context of lower urinary tract dysfunction. *Neurourol Urodyn.* 2011;30:708–13.

10. Eri LM, Wessel N, Tysland O, and Berge V. Comparative study of pressure-flow parameters. *Neurourol Urodyn.* 2002;21:186–93.

11. Ragab MM and Mohammed ES. Idiopathic Parkinson's disease patients at the urologic clinic. *Neurourol Urodyn.* 2011;30:1258–61.

12. Vaughan CP, Juncos JL, Trotti LM, Johnson TM 2nd, and Bliwise DL. Nocturia and overnight polysomnography in Parkinson's disease. *Neurourol Urodyn.* 2013;32:1080–5.

13. Galloway NT. Urethral sphincter abnormalities in Parkinsonism. *Br J Urol.* 1983;55:691–3.

14. Sakakibara R, Hattori T, Uchiyama T, and Yamanishi T. Videourodynamic and sphincter motor unit potential analyses in Parkinson's disease and multiple system atrophy. *J Neurol Neurosurg Psychiatry.* 2001;71:600–6.

15. Roth B, Studer UE, Fowler CJ, and Kessler TM. Benign prostatic obstruction and Parkinson's disease—Should transurethral resection of the prostate be avoided? *J Urol.* 2009;181:2209–13.

16. Staskin DS, Vardi Y, and Siroky MB. Post-prostatectomy continence in the parkinsonian patient: The significance of poor voluntary sphincter control. *J Urol.* 1988;140:117–8.

17. Ahmed Z, Asi YT, Sailer A et al. The neuropathology, pathophysiology and genetics of multiple system atrophy. *Neuropathol Appl Neurobiol.* 2012;38:4–24.

18. Stefanova N, Bucke P, Duerr S, and Wenning GK. Multiple system atrophy: An update. *Lancet Neurol.* 2009;8:1172–8.

19. McKenzie P and Badlani GH. The incidence and etiology of overactive bladder in patients after cerebrovascular accident. *Curr Urol Rep.* 2012;13:402–6.

20. Linsenmeyer TA. Post-CVA voiding dysfunctions: Clinical insights and literature review. *Neuro Rehabilitation.* 2012;30:1–7.

21. Tibaek S, Gard G, Klarskov P et al. Prevalence of lower urinary tract symptoms (LUTS) in stroke patients: A cross-sectional, clinical survey. *Neurourol Urodyn.* 2008;27:763–71.

22. Lum SK and Marshall VR. Results of prostatectomy in patients following a cerebrovascular accident. *Br J Urol.* 1982;54:186–9.

23. Kirschner-Hermanns R, Daneshgari F, Vahabi B et al. Does diabetes mellitus-induced bladder remodeling affect lower urinary tract function? ICI-RS 2011. *Neurourol Urodyn.* 2012;31:359–64.

24. Yamaguchi C, Sakakibara R, Uchiyama T et al. Overactive bladder in diabetes: A peripheral or central mechanism? *Neurourol Urodyn.* 2007;26:807–13.

25. Daneshgari F, Liu G, Birder L, Hanna-Mitchell AT, and Chacko S. Diabetic bladder dysfunction: Current translational knowledge. *J Urol.* 2009;182:S18–26.

26. Kaplan SA, Te AE, and Blaivas JG. Urodynamic findings in patients with diabetic cystopathy. *J Urol.* 1995;153:342–4.

27. Tubaro A, Puccini F, de Nunzio C et al. The treatment of lower urinary tract symptoms in patients with multiple sclerosis: A systematic review. *Curr Urol Rep.* 2012;13:335–42.

28. Mahfouz W and Corcos J. Management of detrusor external sphincter dyssynergia in neurogenic bladder. *Eur J Phys Rehabil Med.* 2011;47:639–50.

Part VIII

SEXUAL DYSFUNCTION AND REPRODUCTION IN NEUROLOGIC DISORDERS

Chapter 42

PATHOPHYSIOLOGY OF MALE SEXUAL DYSFUNCTION AFTER SPINAL CORD INJURY

Pierre Denys and Charles Joussain

INTRODUCTION

After spinal cord injury (SCI), the impairment of neural command and its consequences on reproductive organs have been extensively described in humans. Overall, sexual activity and satisfaction decrease,[1] but sexuality remains a major concern before locomotion for paraplegics,[2,3] often male and young at the time of injury.[4,5] The quality of life satisfaction with respect to sexuality after spinal cord lesion has a significant correlation with the quality of relationship with a sexual partner, with sexual desire, and with the mental well-being of the subject, but not to preserved sexual abilities.[2,6] Moreover, the type and enjoyment of sexual activities engaged substantially change after SCI.[1]

IMPACT OF SPINAL CORD INJURY ON SEXUAL BEHAVIOR

Sexual behavior is controlled by supraspinal structure and spinal centers.[7] Impairment in sexual behavior can be due to lesion of the spinal centers per se and/or by lesion of descending and/or ascending pathways from and to the brain, respectively. The impact of SCI on self-esteem and body image can also have a deleterious effect on sexual behavior.[2] Except for desire and central arousal, the other components of sexual response, i.e., erection, ejaculation, and general physiologic events during sexual climax, can occur in case of complete SCI, independently from any brain control. In clinical practice, it is well known that patients with SCI have specific problems such as dissociation between desire, erection, ejaculation, and orgasm.[8,9] As for the able-bodied general population, the sexual concerns, activities, satisfaction, and responsiveness to treatments in men with SCI evolve with age, and this is a concern for physicians in charge of sexual counseling and management.[10,11]

DESIRE AND AROUSAL

After injury, about 20% of men with SCI describe their sexual desire to be weak and decreased as compared to before injury. Moreover, areas specified by men with SCI to induce sexual arousal when stimulated change as compared to before injury; some men develop new areas of arousal above the level of injury, for instance, the head, neck, and torso. This "arousal neuroplasticity" is unsurprisingly more frequently reported by men with complete SCI.[1,12-14]

Underdiagnosed traumatic brain injuries in SCI patients[15] may lead to cognitive, behavioral, and neuroendocrine impairment that might affect sexual behavior.[16] Besides traumatic brain injury (TBI), total testosterone serum levels can be low after isolated SCI.[13,17,18] But correlation between testosterone level and sexual function has not been evidenced in patients with SCI.[13,19]

ERECTION

Erection is often impaired after SCI. In response to penile glans and perineal stimulation, reflexogenic erection requires at least partial preservation of the sacral parasympathetic centers (S2 through S4).[20] In response to psychogenic stimulation, i.e., thoughts, dreams, and visual, auditory, or olfactory stimuli, psychogenic erection can occur if the sympathetic centers are located above the injury (Figure 42.1).[20,21] The decrease of vasoconstrictor tone (sympathetic brake) on erection may induce a soft swelling but not a rigid enough erection.[9,20] If the upper limit of lesion is below T12, sparing at least part of the erection spinal sympathetic centers, and the lower limit is above S2, mixed, i.e., psychogenic, and reflex erection can occur.[20] Overall, before development, proerectile drug erection was reported to occur in 54%–95% of patients with SCI and intromission followed by sexual

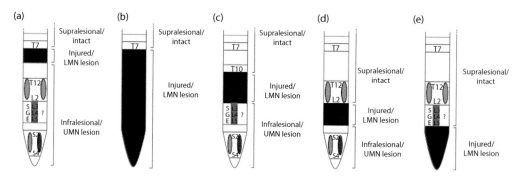

Figure 42.1 Prototypical type of complete spinal cord injuries and related sexual functions are (a) lesion above thoracolumbar and sacral spinal cord: reflex erection +, psychogenic erection −, reflex rhythmic forceful ejaculation +, psychogenic ejaculation −; (b) thoracolumbar and sacral lesion: erection and ejaculation are unlikely to occur; (c) thoracolumbar lesion: reflex erection +, psychogenic erection −, reflex and psychogenic ejaculation −; (d) mid- and lower lumbar lesion: reflex and psychogenic erection +, psychogenic and reflex ejaculation unlikely −; (e) sacral lesion: reflex erection −, psychogenic erection +, reflex ejaculation −, psychogenic ejaculation (emission without involvement of somatic centers, possibly premature) +. LMN, lower motor neuron; UMN, upper motor neuron.

intercourse achieved by 5%–75% of patients with SCI.[1,22,23] Without medication, erection is reported as not reliable because of not lasting long enough and/or not being firm enough by the vast majority of patients with SCI.[14]

EJACULATION

Ejaculation is severely impaired after SCI. Only 12% of patients with complete SCI and 33% of patients with incomplete SCI can ejaculate during masturbation or sexual intercourse without the aid of medication or devices.[24] Penile vibratory stimulation (PVS) represents the first line of treatment for sperm retrieval.[25] PVS is a high-intensity stimulation. Overall, about 50% of patients with SCI can ejaculate in response to PVS.[24] As for erection, the ability to ejaculate depends on the lesion characteristics. Secretion, the first phase of emission, is under the control of spinal parasympathetic centers (segments S2 through S4). Lesion of the parasympathetic centers impairs reflective erection, secretion, and transmission of the genital stimuli to the spinal cord. The sympathetic centers (segments T12 through L2) induce sexual glands and seminal tract smooth muscle cell contraction and bladder neck closure. Lesion of these centers severely impairs ejaculation. In particular, lesion of two or three spinal segments (T12, L1, L2) usually precludes ejaculation occurrence. Once seminal fluid reaches the prostatic urethra, the expulsion phase occurs under the control of the somatic centers. Lesion of the sacral spinal cord impairs, but less severely, ejaculation, and if ejaculation occurs, semen expulsion throughout the urethral meatus is not rhythmically forceful but dribbling (Figure 42.2).[24,26]

ORGASM

The impairment of orgasm by SCI is difficult to assess; more than 20 definitions of orgasm have been proposed.[27] Overall, orgasm tends to be defined as a psychologic, transient peak sensation of pleasure with altered state of consciousness, and a physiologic experience including sex flush; sweating; myotonia; rhythmic pelvic muscle contractions; and increased heart rate, respiration, and blood pressure.[28,29] Contrarily to erection or ejaculation, orgasm monitoring is difficult and requires compilation of self-reported perceptions and blood pressure, heart, and respiratory rates.[30] Following SCI, depending on reports, up to 50% of men with SCI can achieve orgasm.[1,13] In laboratory conditions, Sipski et al. reported that orgasm was achieved by 64.4% of patients with SCI without a lesion of the sacral parasympathetic and somatic centers and 50% with a lesion as compared to 100% of able-bodied men. Men with incomplete SCI are more likely to experience orgasm (82%) than men with complete SCI (50%). Of interest is that patients with SCI may experience orgasm without ejaculation or ejaculate without achieving orgasm.[31] Overall, one should keep in mind that, if experienced by men with SCI, feelings perceived during sexual climax are usually reported as weakened, sometimes unpleasant, and even painful.[30,32]

Some studies reported cardiovascular, respiratory, muscular, and autonomic events during sexual climax in men with SCI to be similar to those in able-bodied men.[33,34] Patients with SCI with lesion cranial to T6[36] can experience autonomic dysreflexia (AD) during sexual climax, defined by an increase in

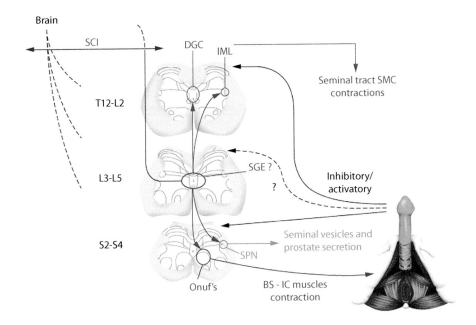

Figure 42.2   Impact of a complete spinal cord injury, with lower limit above T12, on ascending and descending projections from/to the spinal centers controlling sexual behavior. Disruption of the brain projections to the autonomic and somatic centers and to the spinal generator of ejaculation (SGE). Disruption of the lumbar spinothalamic pathway to the subparafascicular nucleus (purple). Preservation of the genito-spino-genital reflex pathway. Black, afferents; green, orange, red, and purple, efferents; BS, bulbospongiosus; DGC, dorsal gray commissure; IC, ischiocavernosus; IML, intermediolateralis column; SMC, smooth muscle cells; SPN, sacral parasympathetic nucleus.

systolic blood pressure (SBP) of at least 20 mm Hg and often accompanied by pulsatile headaches, tightness of the chest, hot flushes, goosebumps, tachycardia or bradycardia, sweating, and skeletal muscle spasms.[35,37] Cardiovascular events associated with sexual climax in able-bodied men satisfy the definition of AD, as an SBP increase of 40–60 mm Hg can occur associated with signs of autonomic arousal. The main differences with men with SCI are the intensity, especially SBP increase, and the duration of autonomic arousal signs with a return to baseline within 2 minutes after ejaculation.[28,37,38] A questionnaire has been developed and validated by Courtois et al. Men with an upper limit of SCI below T6 usually do not experience AD and describe that muscular, including pelviperineal, and/or autonomic and/or cardiovascular, events lack climactic characteristics in opposition to men with more cranial SCI.[30]

Although beyond the scope of this review, it is of interest that in women with SCI, sensory information from the genitals and hypogastric area can bypass the spinal cord and reach the brainstem via the vagus nerve to finally be integrated by the encephalon.[39] Such an accessory pathway may explain why, even in the case of complete SCI, some women with SCI report experiencing orgasms "as before the injury."[40]

Few therapeutic options exist to induce or enhance orgasm after SCI. PVS is an efficient and simple tool to elicit ejaculation and thus sexual climax. Associated with PVS, midodrine, an α_1 agonist prescribed to prevent orthostatic hypotension,[41,42] increases ejaculation rate[43] and orgasm occurrence.[44] Some results about midodrine and orgasm are conflicting[30,44]

ANIMAL MODELS TO STUDY SEXUAL BEHAVIOR AFTER SPINAL CORD INJURY

The rat is the animal model most extensively used to investigate sexual behavior after SCI.[45–47] Sexual function studies in SCI rats require a lesion above autonomic centers, usually midthoracic, and 15 days of follow-up to restore stable reflex activity.[47] Early behavioral studies on rats with transections at the midthoracic level showed an enhanced erectile and depressed ejaculatory reflex.[47–49] Nout et al. used telemetric monitoring of corpus spongiosum penis pressure and reported that the number of full erectile episodes decreased significantly 24 days after T10 standardized lesions, but the level of pressure registered in the bulb increased during erection.[50] Johnson and colleagues developed rodent models with chronic midthoracic incomplete SCI to assess the function of descending pathways involved in ejaculation. Spinal ejaculatory pathways are dependent on bilateral pathways from the brainstem which modulate pudendal motor reflex and pudendal nerve autonomic fiber activities. Sensory input from the dorsal nerve of the penis required to trigger ejaculation is no longer inhibited from the nucleus paragigantocellularis (nPGi) after unilateral incomplete lesion. This inhibition is important in the organization of rhythmic contractions of the perineal muscles during the expulsion phase of ejaculation. Chronic incomplete unilateral lesion of the descending pathways from the brain to the spinal cord results in new connections of the pudendal reflex inhibitory and pudendal sympathetic activatory pathways across the midline below the lesion, which contributes to poor coordination of the perineal muscles during the contractions that are mandatory for ejaculation.[51] After spinal transection, when ejaculation is elicited by electrical[52] or pharmacologic stimulation,[53] the specific pattern of urogenital smooth and striated muscle cell contractions comparable to the one described in intact animals[54,55] occurs involving the vas deferens, seminal vesicles, and prostate during emission, followed by bulbospongiosus muscle during expulsion associated with ischiocavernosus and bulbospongiosus muscle contraction responsible for phasic penile erection.[45] In both sexes, rhythmic firing of the hypogastric, pelvic, and pudendal motor nerves is recorded.[56] This pattern of reflex contractions is relatively insensitive to the effects of gonadal hormones.[57,58] Because of the similarities of this reflex pattern of contractions in lower mammals to the physiology of sexual climax in humans, it is thought that a similar pattern of neural activity generated and coordinated at the spinal level may occur at sexual climax in men and women with SCIs.[59-61]

SPINAL GENERATOR OF EJACULATION

The description of a spinal generator of ejaculation (SGE) has changed the way of thinking about modifications induced by spinal lesions. A group of lumbar spinothalamic (LSt) neurons projects to the parvocellular subparafascicular thalamic nucleus.[62] Another subset of neurons expresses gastrin-releasing peptide (GRP).[63] Altogether, these neurons form an SGE connected with motor neurons of the dorsomedial nucleus and both sympathetic and parasympathetic preganglionic neurons innervating the bulbospongiosus muscle and the prostate, respectively.[52,64-66] The impact of spinal lesions on ejaculation and orgasm should be considered in terms of the existence of a putative SGE in the lumbar spinal cord.

EVIDENCE FOR THE EXISTENCE OF SPINAL GENERATOR OF EJACULATION IN MAN

How could normal ejaculation as well as somatic and autonomic events occur during sexual climax despite the loss of supraspinal control? Even though normal ejaculation, i.e., rhythmic forceful ejaculation, is often not possible, ejaculation can still occur in response to peripheral stimulation in patients with complete SCI. The autonomic and somatic spinal centers that control emission and expulsion can be activated in a coordinated manner without any supraspinal input. This leads to the hypothesis that an SGE might also exist in humans. Some physiologic data support the existence of an SGE in man. In men with an upper limit of complete SCI above T12, Sonksen recorded the intraurethral pressures at the level of the internal and external urinary sphincter during PVS or electroejaculation procedures. A specific and reproducible pattern of pressure variations occurred during ejaculation. Moreover, the discontinuation of vibratory or electrical stimulation, once this pattern began, did not prevent the specific series of contractions from occurring.[61]

The historical approach consists of characterizing sexual response to the level and extent of the injury in men and women.[67] This provided a lot of information on the respective roles of the spinal segments (i.e., sacral, thoracolumbar) for reflexogenic, psychogenic erection and ejaculation, orgasm, and sexual response in both men and women.[9,20,68-70] The ejaculation rate is significantly reduced when the spinal segments controlling ejaculation, i.e., sympathetic (T12 through L2) and parasympathetic and somatic (S2 through S4) are lesioned.[9] Unsurprisingly, the lesion of the somatic centers precludes ejaculation being rhythmic and forceful. Numerous studies highlight the crucial role of the T12 through L2 segments in the control of ejaculation insomuch that it is supposed to be "the ejaculation center."[26,71] Other authors assessed the importance of an intersegmental pathway between L2 and S1 to be uninjured for ejaculation to occur.[72-75] More than a pathway to connect autonomic and somatic spinal centers, these segments probably harbor an SGE. In light of the description of an SGE in the rat, studies that assessed the occurrence of ejaculation as a function of the status of the spinal segments have been reviewed and meta-analyses have been conducted. The results strengthen the role of the spinal ejaculation centers at the level of T12 through L2 and S2 through S4 but also point out a key role for segments L3 through L5 (Figure 42.2). The ejaculation rate drops sharply when the injury extends to segments L3 and below. Apart from the limits inherent to the variable methods used to elicit ejaculation and the heterogeneity of the studies, this analysis provides only indirect evidence for the existence of an SGE in man.[24]

In the rodent model, within the dorsal horn after SCI, the dendritic arborization of calcitonin gene-related peptide (CGRP), immunoreactive, small-diameter, primary afferent neurons enlarge significantly,[76] and the extent of this immunoreactivity correlates with the magnitude of AD.[77] This modification of afferent arbors seems to be dependent on nerve growth factor (NGF) action. Furthermore, treatment with high-affinity NGF antibody of trk A-IgG fusion protein delivered intraspinally can limit the development of afferent sprouting and the magnitude of AD.[78,79] This strongly suggests an ongoing process after SCI led by neuroplasticity. Sexual stimulation during masturbation, coitus, or PVS can induce AD even in the absence of ejaculation. In other patients, AD only occurs at ejaculation.[80-82] Complete SCI disrupts the pathways that convey pleasurable sensation to the brain, especially putative LSt neuronal axons that could convey orgasm-specific information to the thalamus (Figure 42.2). The perception of "autonomic arousal" or AD signs during sexual climax concurrent with, and possibly induced by, the activation of the SGE might be one of the mechanisms whereby men with complete SCI experience orgasm at sexual climax.[30]

SUMMARY

Spinal cord lesions dramatically impair sexual behavior in animals and humans. Sexual behavior after SCI depends on the location and extent of the SCI and on the dynamic process of reorganization within the spinal cord of pathways and centers involved in sexual function. Desire is often decreased after SCI, even in the absence of associated TBI. Erectile dysfunction and efficacy of medical treatments depend on the status of the sympathetic and somatic but mostly the parasympathetic centers. Ejaculation and orgasm are more severely impaired, and the functional prognosis depends on the status of the lumbosacral spinal cord, especially the putative location of an SGE in segments L3 through L5. An ongoing process of reorganization occurs after SCI, which can be correlated with a difficulty in inducing ejaculation via stimulation of perineal afferents and with the development of AD after SCI.

REFERENCES

1. Alexander CJ, Sipski ML, and Findley TW. Sexual activities, desire, and satisfaction in males pre- and post-spinal cord injury. *Arch Sex Behav.* 1993;22(3):217–28.
2. Reitz A, Tobe V, Knapp PA, and Schurch B. Impact of spinal cord injury on sexual health and quality of life. *Int J Impot Res.* 2004;16(2):167–74.
3. Anderson KD. Targeting recovery: Priorities of the spinal cord-injured population. *J Neurotrauma.* 2004;21(10):1371–83.
4. Jackson AB, Dijkers M, Devivo MJ, and Poczatek RB. A demographic profile of new traumatic spinal cord injuries: Change and stability over 30 years. *Arch Phys Med Rehabil.* 2004;85(11):1740–8.
5. Devivo MJ. Epidemiology of traumatic spinal cord injury: Trends and future implications. *Spinal Cord.* 2012;50(5):365–72.
6. Phelps J, Albo M, Dunn K, and Joseph A. Spinal cord injury and sexuality in married or partnered men: Activities, function, needs, and predictors of sexual adjustment. *Arch Sex Behav.* 2001;30(6):591–602.
7. Sakamoto H. Brain-spinal cord neural circuits controlling male sexual function and behavior. *Neurosci Res.* 2012;72(2):103–16.
8. Everaert K, de Waard WI, Van Hoof T et al. Neuroanatomy and neurophysiology related to sexual dysfunction in male neurogenic patients with lesions to the spinal cord or peripheral nerves. *Spinal Cord.* 2010;48(3):182–91.
9. Grossiord A, Chapelle PA, Lacert P, Pannier S, and Durand J. The affected medullary segment in paraplegics. Relation to sexual function in men [author's transl.]. *Rev Neurol (Paris)* 1978;134(12):729–40.
10. Lombardi G, Macchiarella A, Cecconi F, Aito S, and Del Popolo G. Sexual life of males over 50 years of age with spinal-cord lesions of at least 20 years. *Spinal Cord.* 2008;46(10):679–83.
11. Larsen E and Hejgaard N. Sexual dysfunction after spinal cord or cauda equina lesions. *Paraplegia.* 1984;22(2):66–74.
12. Cardoso FL, Savall AC, and Mendes AK. Self-awareness of the male sexual response after spinal cord injury. *Int J Rehabil Res.* 2009;32(4):294–300.
13. Phelps G, Brown M, Chen J et al. Sexual experience and plasma testosterone levels in male veterans after spinal cord injury. *Arch Phys Med Rehabil.* 1983;64(2):47–52.
14. Anderson KD, Borisoff JF, Johnson RD, Stiens SA, and Elliott SL. Long-term effects of spinal cord injury on sexual function in men: Implications for neuroplasticity. *Spinal Cord.* 2007;45(5):338–48.
15. Tolonen A, Turkka J, Salonen O, Ahoniemi E, and Alaranta H. Traumatic brain injury is under-diagnosed in patients with spinal cord injury. *J Rehabil Med.* 2007;39(8):622–6.
16. Sander AM, Maestas KL, Pappadis MR et al. Sexual functioning 1 year after traumatic brain injury: Findings from a prospective traumatic brain injury model systems collaborative study. *Arch Phys Med Rehabil.* 2012;93(8):1331–7.
17. Durga A, Sepahpanah F, Regozzi M, Hastings J, and Crane DA. Prevalence of testosterone deficiency after spinal cord injury. *PM&R* 2011;3(10):929–32.

18. Safarinejad MR. Level of injury and hormone profiles in spinal cord-injured men. *Urology.* 2001;58(5):671–6.

19. Celik B, Sahin A, Caglar N et al. Sex hormone levels and functional outcomes: A controlled study of patients with spinal cord injury compared with healthy subjects. *Am J Phys Med Rehabil.* 2007;86(10):784–90.

20. Chapelle PA, Durand J, and Lacert P. Penile erection following complete spinal cord injury in man. *Br J Urol* 1980;52(3):216–9.

21. Sipski M, Alexander C, Gómez-Marín O, and Spalding J. The effects of spinal cord injury on psychogenic sexual arousal in males. *J Urol.* 2007;177(1):247–51.

22. Biering-Sorensen F and Sonksen J. Penile erection in men with spinal cord or cauda equina lesions. *Semin Neurol.* 1992;12(2):98–105.

23. Courtois FJ, Goulet MC, Charvier KF, and Leriche A. Posttraumatic erectile potential of spinal cord injured men: How physiologic recordings supplement subjective reports. *Arch Phys Med Rehabil.* 1999;80(10):1268–72.

24. Chéhensse C, Bahrami S, Denys P et al. The spinal control of ejaculation revisited: A systematic review and meta-analysis of anejaculation in spinal cord injured patients. *Hum Reprod Update.* 2013;19(5):507–26.

25. Brackett NL, Lynne CM, Ibrahim E, Ohl DA, and Sonksen J. Treatment of infertility in men with spinal cord injury. *Nat Rev Urol.* 2010;7(3):162–72.

26. Chapelle PA, Colbeau-Justin P, Durand J, and Richard F. [Ejaculation problems in traumatic paraplegia]. *Sem Hop,* 1982;58(28–29):1691–7.

27. Mah K and Binik YM. The nature of human orgasm: A critical review of major trends. *Clin Psychol Rev.* 2001;21(6):823–56.

28. Masters WH and Johnson VE. *Human Sexual Response.* San Rafael, CA: Ishi Press International; 2010.

29. Bohlen JG, Held JP, Sanderson MO, and Patterson RP. Heart rate, rate-pressure product, and oxygen uptake during four sexual activities. *Arch Intern Med.* 1984;144(9):1745–8.

30. Courtois F, Charvier K, Vézina JG et al. Assessing and conceptualizing orgasm after a spinal cord injury. *BJU Int.* 2011;108(10):1624–33.

31. Sipski M, Alexander CJ, and Gomez-Marin O. Effects of level and degree of spinal cord injury on male orgasm. *Spinal Cord.* 2006;44(12):798–804.

32. Dahlberg A, Alaranta HT, Kautiainen H, and Kotila M. Sexual activity and satisfaction in men with traumatic spinal cord lesion. *J Rehabil Med.* 2007;39(2):152–5.

33. Courtois F, Charvier K, Leriche A, Vézina J-G, and Jacquemin G. Sexual and climactic responses in men with traumatic spinal cord injury: A model for rehabilitation. *Sexologies.* 2009;18:79–82.

34. Szasz G and Carpenter C. Clinical observations in vibratory stimulation of the penis of men with spinal cord injury. *Arch Sex Behav.* 1989;18(6):461–74.

35. Karlsson AK. Autonomic dysreflexia. *Spinal Cord.* 1999;37(6):383–91.

36. Lindan R, Joiner E, Freehafer AA, and Hazel C. Incidence and clinical features of autonomic dysreflexia in patients with spinal cord injury. *Paraplegia.* 1980;18(5):285–92.

37. Courtois F, Geoffrion R, Landry E, and Bélanger M. H-reflex and physiologic measures of ejaculation in men with spinal cord injury. *Arch Phys Med Rehabil.* 2004;85(6):910–8.

38. Pollock ML and Schmidt DH. *Heart Disease and Rehabilitation,* 3rd ed. Champaign, IL: Human Kinetics; 1995:243–76.

39. Komisaruk BR, Gerdes CA, and Whipple B. 'Complete' spinal cord injury does not block perceptual responses to genital self-stimulation in women. *Arch Neurol.* 1997;54(12):1513–20.

40. Sipski ML, Alexander CJ, and Rosen R. Sexual arousal and orgasm in women: Effects of spinal cord injury. *Ann Neurol.* 2001;49(1):35–44.

41. Lossnitzer K and Letzel H. Efficacy of midodrin in orthostatic circulatory disorders. Results of a 2D multicentric field study of 942 patients. *Med Welt.* 1983;34(42):1190–3.

42. Wright RA, Kaufmann HC, Perera R et al. A double-blind, dose-response study of midodrine in neurogenic orthostatic hypotension. *Neurology.* 1998;51(1):120–4.

43. Soler JM, Previnaire JG, Plante P, Denys P, and Chartier-Kastler E. Midodrine improves ejaculation in spinal cord injured men. *J Urol.* 2007;178(5):2082–6.

44. Soler JM, Previnaire JG, Plante P, Denys P, and Chartier-Kastler E. Midodrine improves orgasm in spinal cord-injured men: The effects of autonomic stimulation. *J Sex Med.* 2008;5(12):2935–41.

45. McKenna KE, Chung SK, and McVary KT. A model for the study of sexual function in anesthetized male and female rats. *Am J Physiol.* 1991;261(5 Pt 2):R1276–85.

46. Hart BL. Sexual reflexes and mating behavior in the male rat. *J Comp Physiol Psychol.* 1968;65(3):453–60.

47. Sachs BD and Garinello LD. Spinal pacemaker controlling sexual reflexes in male rats. *Brain Res.* 1979;171(1):152–6.

48. Hart BL and Odell V. Elicitation of ejaculation and penile reflexes in spinal male rats by peripheral electric shock. *Physiol Behav.* 1981;26(4):623–6.

49. Hart BL and Odell V. Effects of intermittent electric shock on penile reflexes of male rats. *Behav Neural Biol* 1980;29(3):394–8.

50. Nout YS, Schmidt MH, Tovar CA, Culp E, Beattie MS, and Bresnahan JC. Telemetric monitoring of corpus spongiosum penis pressure in conscious rats for assessment of micturition and sexual function following spinal cord contusion injury. *J Neurotrauma.* 2005;22(4):429–41.

51. Johnson RD. Descending pathways modulating the spinal circuitry for ejaculation: Effects of chronic spinal cord injury. *Prog Brain Res.* 2006;152:415–26.

52. Borgdorff AJ, Bernabé J, Denys P, Alexandre L, and Giuliano F. Ejaculation elicited by microstimulation of lumbar spinothalamic neurons. *Eur Urol.* 2008;54(2):449–56.

53. Clément P, Bernabé J, Denys P, Alexandre L, and Giuliano F. Ejaculation induced by i.c.v. injection of the preferential dopamine D³ receptor agonist 7-hydroxy-2-(di-N-pro-pylamino)tetralin in anesthetized rats. *Neuroscience.* 2007;145(2):605–10.

54. Beyer C, Contreras JL, Larsson K, Olmedo M, and Morali G. Patterns of motor and seminal vesicle activities during copulation in the male rat. *Physiol Behav.* 1982;29(3):495–500.

55. Holmes GM, Chapple WD, Leipheimer RE, and Sachs BD. Electromyographic analysis of male rat perineal muscles during copulation and reflexive erections. *Physiol Behav.* 1991;49(6):1235–46.

56. Cai RS, Alexander MS, and Marson L. Activation of somatosensory afferents elicit changes in vaginal blood flow and the urethrogenital reflex via autonomic efferents. *J Urol.* 2008;180(3):1167–72.

57. Park JH, Bonthuis P, Ding A, Rais S, and Rissman EF. Androgen- and estrogen-independent regulation of copulatory behavior following castration in male B6D2F1 mice. *Horm Behav.* 2009;56(2):254–63.

58. Holmes GM and Sachs BD. Erectile function and bulbospongiosus EMG activity in estrogen-maintained castrated rats vary with behavioral context. *Horm Behav.* 1992;26(3):406–19.

59. Bohlen JG, Held JP, Sanderson MO, and Ahlgren A. The female orgasm: Pelvic contractions. *Arch Sex Behav.* 1982;11(5):367–86.

60. Bohlen JG, Held JP, and Sanderson MO. The male orgasm: Pelvic contractions measured by anal probe. *Arch Sex Behav.* 1980;9(6):503–21.

61. Sonksen J, Ohl DA, and Wedemeyer G. Sphincteric events during penile vibratory ejaculation and electroejaculation in men with spinal cord injuries. *J Urol.* 2001;165(2):426–9.

62. Ju G, Melander T, Ceccatelli S, Hökfelt T, and Frey P. Immunohistochemical evidence for a spinothalamic pathway co-containing cholecystokinin- and galanin-like immunoreactivities in the rat. *Neuroscience.* 1987;20(2):439–56.

63. Sakamoto H, Matsuda K, Zuloaga DG et al. Sexually dimorphic gastrin releasing peptide system in the spinal cord controls male reproductive functions. *Nat Neurosci.* 2008;11(6):634–6.

64. Truitt WA and Coolen LM. Identification of a potential ejaculation generator in the spinal cord. *Science.* 2002;297(5586):1566–9.

65. Xu C, Giuliano F, Yaici ED et al. Identification of lumbar spinal neurons controlling simultaneously the prostate and the bulbospongiosus muscles in the rat. *Neuroscience.* 2006;138(2):561–73.

66. Xu C, Yaici ED, Conrath M et al. Galanin and neurokinin-1 receptor immunoreactive [corrected] spinal neurons controlling the prostate and the bulbo- spongiosus muscle identified by transsynaptic labeling in the rat. *Neuroscience.* 2005;134(4):1325–41.

67. Grossiord A, Buzacoux J, Maury M, and Barthes G. Studies on motor metamerisation of the upper and lower limbs. *Paraplegia* 1963;1:81–97.

68. Berard EJ. The sexuality of spinal cord injured women: Physiology and pathophysiology. A review. *Paraplegia.* 1989;27(2):99–112.

69. Bors EC. Neurological disturbances of sexual function with special reference to 529 patients with spinal cord injury. *Urol Surv.* 1960;10:191–221.

70. Munro D, Horne HW Jr, and Paull DP. The effect of injury to the spinal cord and cauda equina on the sexual potency of men. *N Engl J Med.* 1948;239(24):903–11.

71. Nehra A, Werner MA, Bastuba M, Title C, and Oates RD. Vibratory stimulation and rectal probe electroejaculation as therapy for patients with spinal cord injury: Semen parameters and pregnancy rates. *J Urol.* 1996;155(2):554–9.

72. Brindley GS. Reflex ejaculation under vibratory stimulation in paraplegic men. *Paraplegia.* 1981;19(5):299–302.

73. Bird VG, Brackett NL, Lynne CM, Aballa TC, and Ferrell SM. Reflexes and somatic responses as predictors of ejaculation by penile vibratory stimulation in men with spinal cord injury. *Spinal Cord.* 2001;39(10):514–9.

74. Sonksen J. Assisted ejaculation and semen characteristics in spinal cord injured males. *Scand J Urol Nephrol Suppl.* 2003;213(213):1–31.

75. Ohl DA, Menge AC, and Sonksen J. Penile vibratory stimulation in spinal cord injured men: Optimized vibration parameters and prognostic factors. *Arch Phys Med Rehabil.* 1996;77(9):903–5.

76. Wong ST, Atkinson BA, and Weaver LC. Confocal microscopic analysis reveals sprouting of primary afferent fibres in rat dorsal horn after spinal cord injury. *Neurosci Lett.* 2000;296(2–3):65–8.

77. Krenz NR and Weaver LC. Changes in the morphology of sympathetic preganglionic neurons parallel the development of autonomic dysreflexia after spinal cord injury in rats. *Neurosci Lett.* 1998;243(1–3):61–4.

78. Krenz NR, Meakin SO, Krassioukov AV, and Weaver LC. Neutralizing intraspinal nerve growth factor blocks autonomic dysreflexia caused by spinal cord injury. *J Neurosci.* 1999;19(17):7405–14.

79. Marsh DR, Wong ST, Meakin SO, MacDonald JI, Hamilton EF, and Weaver LC. Neutralizing intraspinal nerve growth factor with a trkA-IgG fusion protein blocks the development of autonomic dysreflexia in a clip-compression model of spinal cord injury. *J Neurotrauma.* 2002;19(12):1531–41.

80. McBride F, Quah SP, Scott ME, and Dinsmore WW. Tripling of blood pressure by sexual stimulation in a man with spinal cord injury. *J R Soc Med.* 2003;96(7):349–50.

81. Sheel AW, Krassioukov AV, Inglis JT, and Elliott SL. Autonomic dysreflexia during sperm retrieval in spinal cord injury: Influence of lesion level and sildenafil citrate. *J Appl Physiol.* 2005;99(1):53–8.

82. Courtois FJ, Charvier KF, Leriche A, Vézina JG, Côté M, and Bélanger M. Blood pressure changes during sexual stimulation, ejaculation and midodrine treatment in men with spinal cord injury. *BJU Int.* 2008;101(3):331–7.

Chapter 43

TREATMENT MODALITIES FOR ERECTILE DYSFUNCTION IN NEUROLOGIC PATIENTS

Jean-Jacques Wyndaele

INTRODUCTION

Erectile dysfunction (ED) in neurologic patients (NED) is one of the consequences of disturbance/disruption of the innervation related to the function of the sexual organs. Prevalence can differ between causes.[1,2] Neurogenic pathology accounts for 10%–19% of all causes of ED.[3] ED has been reported in up to 70% in multiple sclerosis,[4] 80% after spinal cord injury (SCI),[5] 17%–48% after cerebrovascular accident,[6] 3%–58% in epilepsy,[7] 50%–69% in Parkinson's disease,[8] and 75% in spina bifida.[9] It is an early prominent sign in 40% of men with multiple system atrophy[10] and will develop in the majority.[11] Neurologic problems are a risk factor for ED in patients with human T-cell lymphotropic virus type 1 (HTLV-1) infection.[12]

There is a tendency to approach NED mainly from a neuropathophysiologic angle, but erection as part of sexuality is much more than that. Age, other health problems, attitude, psychological, sociocultural, educational, sociological, cognitive, and iatrogenic factors, and much more should also be taken into account to permit a proper individual approach. Disease-related factors such as depression, decreased physical and mental function, the burden of chronic illness, and loss of independence may preclude sexual intimacy and lead to ED as well.[2]

The clinical approach follows the traditional steps of patient history, physical examination, investigation of erectile function, investigation of the neurologic lesion, and laboratory tests. The results should lead to an accurate idea of what causes ED and how the dysfunction negatively influences the patient's and the partner's life.

As etiologies are seldom curable, initial treatment is largely empirical and the approach stepwise: lifestyle modification, drugs, vacuum devices, intraurethral suppositories, and intracavernosal injection of vasoactive substances. Prosthesis implantation is the end-of-the-line treatment.

THE BEGINNING OF MANAGEMENT

Even today it is not easy for a patient to talk about sexuality to a third person, even to his physician. There are different ways to approach this. If the patient puts trust in a paramedic, they can be advised to go and talk to the physician. Specialized SCI rehabilitation centers around the world organize group information sessions, including a session on sexuality. These are usually followed with great interest by patients. Most want to have an individual consultation afterward. If the physician introduces questions about sexuality during a general consultation, this is often positively received. The patient has the right to decline sexual consultation, but such refusal happens rarely.

It is of great importance to be open and rather direct in the questioning: when sexual life started, how it developed further, which habits existed, and if there have ever been problems before. Several will have tried some sexual activity after the neurologic lesion occurred, and to discuss problems that were encountered is very useful. If no sexual activity has taken place, a short explanation about how sexual function may have been altered is a good introduction. Patients can then be invited to try it out and report on what they observe. It is theoretically possible to give statistical data on what incidences in the particular lesion have been described. But this has limited value, as a patient is not interested in what happens in 100 men with a similar lesion; he wants to know what his case will be. Trial is the most direct approach: send them to properly experience and come back to report. Models to use in talking about sexuality are the PLISSIT model[13] and the OSEC model.[14]

To include the partner from the start of the counseling, if agreed by the patient, is helpful.

Most questions from many couples will be about fertility, but this will not be developed further in this chapter.

When a problem of erection is reported at a consecutive consultation, details are necessary: can erection be elicited by stimulation of the penis or does it occur spontaneously during sexual thoughts/ dreams/fantasies, when watching erotic movies, reading erotic publications, or by a combination of genital and psychologic arousal? Erection may occur but stay for a very short time, not get rigid enough, show a bended shaft, or other concerns.

If the need for treatment is obvious, different possibilities can be discussed.

Sexual rehabilitation techniques: Daily practicing of the bulbocavernosus reflex may increase muscular strength in the perineal area and improve penile erection.[15,16]

PDE5i

Oral PDE5 inhibitors (PDE5i), unless contraindicated, are often used first.[17] Sildenafil, introduced in 1998, had a large impact due to its easy applicability, effectiveness, and safety. Its formats, delay of action, and half-life are given in Table 43.1.[18] Its efficacy has been repeatedly demonstrated, mostly in men with SCI. The presence of an upper motor neuron lesion was significantly associated with therapeutic success, while patients with lower motor neuron lesions and cauda equina syndrome were poorer responders.[19] Other PDE5i have become commercialized: vardenafil, tadalafil, and more recently avanafil, udenafil, and miradenafil, are available in some countries. The pharmacokinetics behind the drug's activity have been described before.[20,21] The medications differ in time of onset, duration of action, and side effects (Table 43.1). How to use the drug must be clearly explained. It can be taken daily (e.g., tadalafil 5 mg) or on demand.[22] It is not always the patient's first choice due to its restricted duration. Discontinuation of the intake is not rare and can be due to unawareness that sexual excitement is needed. There is a learning curve, and four to five trials with one drug are suggested before switching to another.[21] The contraindication is the use of nitrate because of the risk of hypotension, including nitrogen paste used in rehabilitation centers for autonomic hyperreflexia. Caution is also needed in men with multiple system atrophy.[10,20] Other limitations are uncontrolled hypertension, unstable angina, and the intake of alpha-blockers. Vardenafil should not be taken by men on type 1A or type 3 antiarrhythmics or in the presence of a prolonged QT syndrome.[22]

Tadalafil has the advantage of its longer duration of action. Daily use may be considered. In patients with conus or cauda lesions, a dose of 20 mg may be insufficient.

PDE5i have few side effects. Dyspepsia, headache, and more rarely myalgia, flushing, low back pain, and rhinitis have been reported. The most common side effect is headache or dizziness, seen in nearly 10%. Due to these side effects, 5% stopped the treatment.[24]

Lombardi et al. reported good evidence of benefit in men with SCI, especially with incomplete lesion above T12, and some residual erection.[25] Other publications gave good results, especially when psychogenic and/ or reflexive erections are present.[24]

In Parkinson's disease good results have been published,[23] as well as in multiple sclerosis and spina bifida.[20] Few data are available in other neurologic disorders.[19] No deaths, priapism, or autonomic dysreflexia have been associated with this treatment. Matos et al. warned that PDE5i are potentially proconvulsant; thus, caution is needed for use in men with epilepsy.[26] Apomorphine subcutaneous or sublingual may be an alternative to sildenafil, though lower efficacy has been described.[27]

INTRACAVERNOSAL INJECTIONS OF VASOACTIVE DRUGS

If insufficient neuronal and/or endothelial nitric oxide prevent proper activity of PDE5i, direct generation of cAMP and vasodilatation can be obtained by injection of vasoactive drugs in the corpora cavernosa.[28] Several products have been used: phentolamine, papaverine, prostaglandin, and vasoactive intestinal peptide. Their application alone or in combination has been reported as very efficacious in up to 90%[28–30] of patients with SCI, especially those with thoracic and cervical lesions, who will often respond to a lower dosage, which can minimize the risk for prolonged erection.[31]

The most used is prostaglandin E1, U.S. Food and Drug Administration approved (edex or Caverject), available in 10 and 20 μg. The resulting erection is independent of sexual arousal and comes quick. If prostaglandin E1 is not or insufficiently successful, combination with another vasoactive drug can improve the results. The risk of priapism and penile fibrosis can be lowered by careful titration, proper patient education, and monitoring: first self-injections under medical surveillance, permitting to observe

Table 43.1 PDE5i Summary of Action

	Format	Half-Life	Delay of Action
Sildenafil	25 mg, 50 mg, 100 mg	3–5 hours	30–60 min
Tadalafil	10 mg, 20 mg	17–24 hours	45–60 min
Vardenafil	5 mg, 10 mg, 20 mg	4–5 hours	15–60 min

the time before erection occurs, rigidity, and the time before the erection disappears. Incremental dosage adjustment will help determine the right dose for home use. If self-injection is impossible, the assistance of a properly trained partner may be mandatory. In a young patient with SCI, a few micrograms may be sufficient, while up to 40 micrograms can be required if endothelial dysfunction is present.[31]

An adverse event may be penile pain, which is mostly self-limited in chronic use. Other side effects may be facial flushing and headache.[29-31]

The risk of priapism is low with proper application and dosage.[29] When a patient is admitted for a prolonged erection, initial treatment consists of a simple puncture of the corpora cavernosa to aspirate blood to decompress the corpora. If need be, the corpora cavernosa are irrigated using normal saline and a diluted solution of phenylephrine or other similar α-adrenergic agents under careful cardiovascular monitoring, especially in patients with a previous history of cardiovascular disease. A surgical procedure (surgical shunt) is rarely needed.

INTRAURETHRAL DELIVERY OF ALPROSTADIL (MUSE, VITAROS)
This application was seen as promising as many patients were accustomed to catheterization. The results were rather disappointing.[32] A dosage of 1000 μg may be needed,[33,34] with a dosage of only 300–500 μg in the commercially available medications (Vitaros or Muse), and the use of a constriction ring has been advocated to prevent hypotension.

VACUUM CONSTRICTION DEVICES AND PENILE RING
A vacuum constriction device (VCD) consists of a cylinder with a vacuum pump and a constrictive tension ring. After inserting the penis, a negative pressure is created in the cylinder. Blood is drawn into the penis and mechanically blocked by a tension ring applied at the base of the penis. VCDs have been reported to be effective in up to 90% in certain ED populations, but it is not well accepted in patients with SCI.[35] Patients with preserved sensation may experience bruising, sensation of cold penis, and pain. Limited hand function, cost, the artificial nature, a buried penis, and use of anticoagulants may limit its use.

A penile ring can also be used separately if erection can be achieved but not sustained. It exists in different diameters. A band can remain in place for a maximum of 20–30 minutes. There are few contraindications and the method is cheap but can provoke local allergies or cutaneous lesions.

PENILE PROSTHESIS IMPLANT SURGERY
The implants are considered a last alternative as the implantation destroys the internal penile tissue.

The prosthesis comes in various formats. Semirigid prostheses are not recommended for men with SCI with lack of sensation because of their sitting position and spasticity, which with infection can cause perforation. Inflatable prostheses are preferable but may be difficult to manage for tetraplegic men with limited hand function. Zerman et al. found 82% satisfaction reported by the patient and 67% by their partner.[36] Complications are infection (3%–5%), corporal and urethral perforation (especially with placement of a malleable device implanted through a subcoronal incision), erosion, bowing of the glans, and technical dysfunction.

Besides the sexual indication, malleable prostheses have been used in incontinent patients using a urine-collecting device, as it can facilitate application and maintenance.

RECENT EVOLUTION
Melanotan-II (MT-II) applied dermatologically can give an erection but is suspected to possibly induce melanoma.[37] Gene therapy and stem cell research need further investigation in humans.

CONCLUSION

There are different therapeutic means to treat erectile dysfunction in neurologic patients. It is important to have proper sexual counseling before proposing and implementing a treatment. The partner should be closely involved. The application has to be properly explained and application controlled. The overall results are satisfactory. The complications and side effects are not very frequent.

REFERENCES

1. Yafi FA, Jenkins L, Albersen M et al. Erectile dysfunction. *Nat Rev Dis Primers*. 2016;4(2):16003.
2. Shridharani AN, Brant WO. The treatment of erectile dysfunction in patients with neurogenic disease. *Transl Androl Urol*. 2016;5(1):88–101.
3. Abicht JH. Testing the autonomic system. In: Jonas U, Thon WF, and Stief CG, eds. *Erectile Dysfunction*. Berlin, Germany: Springer Verlag; 1991:187–94.
4. Zorzon M, Zivadinov R, Monti Bragadin L et al. Sexual dysfunction in multiple sclerosis: A 2-year follow-up study. *J Neurol Sci*. 2001;187(1–2):1–5.
5. Courtois FJ, Charvier KF, Leriche A, and Raymond DP. Sexual function in spinal cord injury men. I. Assessing sexual capability. *Paraplegia*. 1993;31(12):771–84.
6. Bener A, Al-Hamaq AO, Kamran S, and Al-Ansari A. Prevalence of erectile dysfunction in male stroke patients, and associated co-morbidities and risk factors. *Int Urol Nephrol*. 2008;40(3):701–8.

7. Smaldone M, Sukkarieh T, Reda A, and Khan A. Epilepsy and erectile dysfunction: A review. *Seizure.* 2004;13(7):453–9.

8. Bronner G, Royter V, Korczyn AD, and Giladi N. Sexual dysfunction in Parkinson's disease. *J Sex Marital Ther.* 2004;30(2):95–105.

9. Gamé X, Moscovici J, Gamé L, Sarramon JP, Rischmann P, and Malavaud B. Evaluation of sexual function in young men with spina bifida and myelomeningocele using the International Index of Erectile Function. *Urology.* 2006;67(3):566–70.

10. Kirchhof K, Apostolidis AN, Mathias CJ, and Fowler CJ. Erectile and urinary dysfunction may be the presenting features in patients with multiple system atrophy: A retrospective study. *Int J Impot Res.* 2003;15(4):293–8.

11. Papatsoris AG, Papapetropoulos S, Singer C, and Deliveliotis C. Urinary and erectile dysfunction in multiple system atrophy (MSA). *Neurourol Urodyn.* 2008;27(1):22–7.

12. de Oliveira CJV, Neto JAC, Andrade RCP, Rocha PN, and de Carvalho Filho EM. Risk factors for erectile dysfunction in men with HTLV-1. *J Sex Med.* 2017;14(10):1195–200.

13. Annon JS. The PLISSIT model: A proposed conceptual scheme for behavioural treatment of sexual problems. *J Sex Ed Ther.* 1976;2(2):1–15.

14. Bronner G. Practical strategies for the management of sexual problems in Parkinson's disease. *Parkinsonism Relat Disord.* 2009;15(Suppl 3):s96–s100.

15. Courtois FJ, Mathieu C, Charvier K, and Bélanger M. Sexual rehabilitation for men with spinal cord injury: Preliminary report on a behavioral strategy. *Sex Disabil.* 2001;19(2):149–57.

16. Courtois FJ, Charvier KF, Leriche A, Côté M, and Lemieux AA. L'évaluation et le traitement des troubles des réactions sexuelles chez l'homme et la femme blessés médullaires. [Assessment and treatment of sexual dysfunctions in men and women with spinal cord injury.] *Sexologies.* 2009; 18(1):51–9.

17. Montague DK, Jarow JP, Broderick GA et al. Erectile Dysfunction Guideline Update Panel. Chapter 1: The management of erectile dysfunction: An AUA update. *J Urol.* 2005;174(1):230–9.

18. Boolell M, Gepi-Attee S, Gingell JC, and Allen MJ. Sildenafil, a novel effective oral therapy for male erectile dysfunction. *BR J Urol.* 1996;78(2):257–61.

19. Lombardi G, Nelli F, Celso M, Mencarini M, and Del Popolo G. Treating erectile dysfunction and central neurological diseases with oral phosphodiesterase type 5 inhibitors. Review of the literature. *J Sex Med.* 2012;9(4):970–85.

20. Basson R and Bronner G. Management and rehabilitation of neurologic patients with sexual and bladder dysfunction. In: Vodusek D, and Boller F, eds. *Handbook of Clinical Neurology 130. Neurology of Sexual and Bladder Disorders.* Amsterdam: Elsevier; 2015. Chapter Section 5: 415–34.

21. Kendirci M, Tanriverdi O, Trost, L, and Helstrom WJ. Management of sildenafil treatment failures. *Curr Opin Urol.* 2006;16(6):449–59.

22. Morganroth J, Ilson BE, Shaddinger BC et al. Evaluation of vardenafil and sildenafil on cardiac repolarisation. *Am J Cardiol.* 2004;93(11):1378–83.

23. Raffaele R, Vecchio I, Giammusso B, Morgia G, Brunetto MB, and Rampello L. Efficacy and safety of fixed-dose oral sildenafil in the treatment of sexual dysfunction in depressed patients with idiopathic Parkinson's disease. *Eur Urol.* 2002;41(4):382–6.

24. Schmid DM, Schurch B, and Hauri D. Sildenafil in the treatment of sexual dysfunction in spinal cord-injured male patients. *Eur Urol.* 2000;38(2):184–93.

25. Lombardi G, Musco S, Wyndaele JJ, and Del Popolo G. Treatments for erectile dysfunction in spinal cord patients: Alternatives to phosphodiesterase type 5 inhibitors? A review study. *Spinal Cord.* 2015;853(12):849–54.

26. Matos G, Scorza FA, Cavalheiro EA, Tufik S, and Andersen ML. PDEI-5 for erectile dysfunction: A potential role in seizure susceptibility. *J Sex Med.* 2012;9(8):2111–21.

27. Perimenis P, Gyftopoulos K, Giannitsas K et al. A comparative, crossover study of the efficacy and safety of sildenafil and apomorphine in men with evidence of arteriogenic erectile dysfunction. *Int J Impot Res.* 2004;16(1):2–7.

28. Dinsmore WW and Wyllie MG. Vasoactive intestinal polypeptide/phentolamine for intracavernosal injection in erectile dysfunction. *BJU Int.* 2008;102(8):933–7.

29. Vidal J, Curcoll, L, Roig T, and Bagunya J. Intracavernous pharmacotherapy for management of erectile dysfunction in multiple sclerosis patients. *Rev Neurol.* 1995;24(12):269–71.

30. Rabini-Movaghar V and Vaccaro AR. Management of sexual disorders in spinal cord injured patients. *Acta Med Iran.* 2012;50(5):295–9.

31. Lakin MM, Montague DK, VanderBrug Medendorp S, Tesar L, and Schover LR. Intracavernous injection therapy: Analysis of results and complications. *J Urol.* 1990;143(6):1138–41.

32. Costa P and Potempa AJ. Intraurethral alprostadil for erectile dysfunction: A review of the literature. *Drugs.* 2012;72(17):2243–54.

33. Mulhall JP, Jahoda AE, Ahmed A, and Parker M. Analysis of the consistency of intraurethral prostaglandin E(1) (MUSE) during at-home use. *Urology.* 2001;58(2):262–6.

34. Bodner DR, Haas CA, Krueger B, and Seftel AD. Intraurethral alprostadil for treatment of erectile dysfunction in patients with spinal cord injury. *Urology.* 1999;53(1):199–202.

35. Biering-Sørensen I, Hansen RB, and Biering-Sørensen F. Sexual function in a traumatic spinal cord injured population 10–45 years after injury. *J Rehabil Med.* 2012;44(11):926–31.

36. Zermann DH, Kutzenberger J, Sauerwein D, Schubert J, and Loeffler U. Penile prosthetic surgery in neurologically impaired patients: Long-term followup. *J Urol.* 2006;175(3Pt1):1041–4; discussion 1044.

37. Paurobally D, Jason F, Dezfoulian B, and Nikkels AF. Melanotan-associated melanoma. *Br J Dermatol.* 2011;164(6):1403–5.

Chapter 44

FERTILITY ISSUES IN MEN WITH SPINAL CORD INJURY

Jeanne Perrin

INTRODUCTION

Spinal cord injury (SCI) most often affects young men of reproductive age: several million men between 16 and 45 years of age face quadriplegia or paraplegia worldwide.[1] A recent study evaluated that in male patients with SCI, the prevalence of biological parenthood was statistically lowered compared to the general population.[2] Indeed, only 10% of them can father children without medical assistance, due to three main factors impairing the fertility of patients with SCI:

- Ejaculatory dysfunction, addressed in Chapter 42
- Erectile dysfunction, addressed in Chapters 42 and 43
- Semen parameters' impairment[3]

SEMEN PARAMETERS ARE USUALLY IMPAIRED IN PATIENTS WITH SPINAL CORD INJURY

Numerous studies have demonstrated that more than 90% of patients with SCI show altered semen parameters, characterized by asthenozoospermia, necrozoospermia, and leukocytospermia.[4-8] Ejaculate volume is usually normal but may be reduced in cases of partially retrograde ejaculation.[9] Leukocytospermia is often observed in the absence of an associated infection of the urinary tract and/or seminal ducts. There are two clinical factors that are associated with better semen characteristics: (1) the ability to obtain ejaculation by masturbation (which occurs in one out of ten patients with SCI)[10] and (2) incomplete lesion of the spinal cord (i.e., ASIA impairment scale grades B, C, and D).[11] When semen can be obtained by ejaculation, the total number of motile sperm in the ejaculate is usually greater than 5 millions; this result generally allows for intravaginal insemination (IVI) or the use of simple assisted reproductive techniques (ARTs) like intrauterine insemination (IUI).[8]

The main abnormalities related to semen impairment in patients with SCI can be divided into issues seen in the acute and chronic phases of their SCI. In the acute phase there is alteration of the testis environment (hormonal and neural regulations of Sertoli and Leydig cells),[12-14] impairment of the blood-testis barrier (leading to systemic autoimmunity),[15] and early alteration of cyclic adenosine monophosphate signaling and caspase-1 expression (leading to the disruption of germ cell differentiation and to increased apoptosis).[16] In the chronic phase the autoimmunity and oxidative stress impair sperm motility (by seminal fluid alteration and prostate gland dysfunction),[17] and the chronic testicular hyperthermia induces meiosis impairment, germ cell apoptosis, and oxidative damage (leading to increased sperm DNA fragmentation and aneuploidy).[18-20]

BIOLOGICAL FATHERHOOD AFTER SPINAL CORD INJURY

HAVING CHILDREN: AN IMPORTANT PART OF THE REHABILITATION PROGRAM

SCI mainly affects young men of parenting age, who are expected to live many decades after injury. For most of them, biological fatherhood and family foundation are of utmost importance as a way to rebuild a life after the spinal injury.[21] Consequently, male SCI fertility should be considered as an important item of the rehabilitation program.[22] As the great majority of patients with SCI cannot achieve antegrade ejaculation by masturbation and/or sexual intercourse and present impaired semen parameters,[23] medical care is generally required to obtain a pregnancy.[6]

STRATEGY TO OBTAIN BIOLOGICAL FATHERHOOD

The management of the male patient with SCI to obtain fatherhood involves a multidisciplinary trained and well-coordinated staff.

COUPLE EVALUATION

The ART technique mainly depends on the sperm collection method and semen quality; ART treatments should allow as much privacy as possible for the couple.[24] First, the ability of the patient to retrieve ejaculated semen, the semen parameters, and the feminine characteristics are analyzed in order to choose the ART leading to the best pregnancy chances in the couple. After male and female evaluation, ART using fresh semen is usually proposed. Anterograde ejaculation is not always obtained by masturbation, penile vibratory stimulation (PVS) with midodrine adjunction, or electroejaculation (EEJ), but these techniques often allow for retrograde ejaculation and sperm collection from the bladder.[25,26] If sperm cannot be harvested in an antegrade or retrograde fashion, then surgical sperm retrieval from the seminal tract/testis is proposed.[24,27,28] Surgical sperm extraction is also used in cases of azoospermia or severe necrozoospermia.

In case of worsening of semen and/or patient's ability to retrieve sperm by ejaculation, ART can use cryopreserved sperm when semen has been previously banked[22] (Figure 44.1).

When the patient is able to retrieve semen by antegrade ejaculation, the ART is chosen according to the results of semen parameters' analysis[6,29]:

- When a sufficient count of progressive motile sperm is present in the ejaculate and when feminine characteristics are favorable, self-inseminations at home and/or intrauterine insemination (IUI) should be proposed.

- When a sufficient count of progressive motile sperm is present in the ejaculate and when feminine characteristics are not optimal, *in vitro* fertilization (IVF) should be proposed.
- When a low count of motile sperm is present in the ejaculate, and when feminine characteristics allow it, intracytoplasmic sperm injection (ICSI) should be proposed.

SPERM RETRIEVAL BY EJACULATION

A meta-analysis concluded that 16% of patients with SCI (12% complete SCI and 33% incomplete SCI) can obtain antegrade ejaculation by masturbation and/or sexual intercourse[10] (Table 44.1). In other patients with SCI, PVS is a simple and efficient technique to induce antegrade ejaculation.[30,31] As a first-line treatment, PVS allows 52% of patients with SCI to obtain antegrade ejaculation[10] (Table 44.1). The ejaculation success rate is also related to the patients' injury level and extent. Ejaculation is obtained by PVS in more than 80% of patients with complete and incomplete SCI at a level above T10 and in 21% with an injury level T11 or below.[10,23] In patients with complete SCI, ejaculation success depends on the integrity of spinal ejaculation centers (Table 44.2). For emission, the T12 through L2 segments have to be infralesional, and for expulsion the S2 through S4 segments have to be infralesional.[10] Ejaculation "dyssynergia" may induce a lack of expulsion; after PVS, if no anterograde ejaculation is obtained, sperm

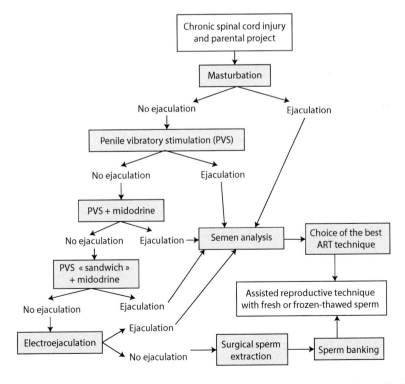

Figure 44.1 Protocol of semen retrieval for assisted reproductive techniques in male patients with chronic spinal cord injury. (ART, assisted reproductive technique; PVS, penile vibratory stimulation.)

Table 44.1 Ejaculation Rates in Patients with Complete and Incomplete Spinal Cord Injuries, According to the Stimulation Technique

Stimulation Technique	SCI Type: Complete/ Incomplete (n)	Ejaculation Rate (%, CI)
Masturbation/ coitus	C+I	16 (2.5–19.5)
PVS	C (1161)	11.8 (10.1–13.8)
	I (343)	33.2 (28.5–38.4)
	C+I	52.1 (45.3–58.9)
	C (597)	47.4 (43.4–51.4)
	I (305)	52.8 (47.2–58.3)

Source: Adapted from Chéhensse et al. *Hum Reprod Update.* 2013;19(5):507–26.
Abbreviations: C, complete; CI, confidence interval; I, incomplete; PVS, penile vibratory stimulation; SCI, spinal cord injury.

Table 44.2 Ejaculation Rates in Patients with Complete Spinal Cord Injury after Penile Vibratory Stimulation, According to the Status of Spinal Ejaculation Centers

SEC Status in Patients with Complete SCI	Technique	Ejaculation Rate (%, CI)
Complete lesion of T12-S5 segment (n=21)	PVS	0 (0–13.5)
T12-S5 segment infralesional (n=53)	PVS	73.6 (60.3–83.7)
Lesion encompassing T12-L2 segment (n=5)	PVS	0 (0–48.9)
T12-L2 segment infralesional (n=30)	PVS	90 (73.6–97.3)
Lesion encompassing S2-S4 segment (n=4)	PVS	0 (0–54.6)
S2-S4 segment infralesional (n=47)	PVS	76.6 (62.6–86.6)

Source: Adapted from Chéhensse et al. *Hum Reprod Update.* 2013;19(5):507–26.
Abbreviations: PVS, penile vibratory stimulation; SCI, spinal cord injury; SEC, spinal ejaculation center.

from the prostatic urethra should by collected by careful catheterization.[32]

For patients not responding to PVS, the adjunction of midodrine is safe and efficient to improve ejaculation rates.[27] As a second-line treatment, EEJ induces an ejaculation in more than 91% of patients.[23,29,33]

When only retrograde ejaculation can be obtained, it is possible to retrieve spermatozoa in the bladder for ART.[24] The oral adjustment of urinary pH and osmolarity by various methods (NaHCO$_3$ tablets, carbonated beverages, "Liverpool solution") is simple and inexpensive. However, there is no consensus for a validated method, and osmolarity is not always

corrected, leading to failures to retrieve motile sperm in the bladder.[34,35] Alternatively, the instillation of sterile medium (such as FertiCult, JCD) in the empty bladder before ejaculation is simple, efficient, and may allow sperm cryopreservation for subsequent use in ART.[25,26,36] Semen parameters in bladder samples show normal sperm concentration (25–34 M/mL) but low progressive motility (4%–40%).[37–39]

SPERM RETRIEVAL BY SURGICAL EXTRACTION

Kafetsoulis et al. highlighted that in the United States, 28% of fertility centers proposed surgical sperm retrieval as first-line treatment for patients with SCI because they lacked equipment and training to obtain ejaculated semen by PVS and/or EEJ.[6] Surgery should be restricted to rigorous indications in SCI.[40] Surgical sperm retrieval yields smaller quantities of poorer quality sperm than ejaculation and involves the use of more invasive and expensive ART.[41]

Nevertheless, in a minority of patients with SCI, ejaculated sperm cannot be obtained and/or azoospermia or severe necrozoospermia is found. In patients with SCI, the motility and viability of sperm extracted from the vas deferens are statistically higher than ejaculated sperm.[42] When surgical sperm extraction is needed, it is successful for more than 85% of patients.[43,44]

FERTILITY SUCCESS RATES OF ASSISTED REPRODUCTIVE TECHNIQUES IN COUPLES WITH MALE PARTNER WITH SPINAL CORD INJURY

Couples who are able to manage PVS and the risk of autonomic dysreflexia and who meet the clinical and biological eligibility criteria for semen self-insemination at home show a pregnancy rate of 29% per couple and a live birth rate of 22% per couple.[6,29] The results of IUI in couples with a male partner with SCI are comparable to those in infertile couples with no SCI: 9%–18% pregnancy per cycle and 30%–60% cumulative pregnancy rate per couple.[6,45]

Similarly, the results of IVF and ICSI in couples with male partners with SCI are comparable to those in infertile couples with no SCI.[45,46] Fertilization rates obtained by ICSI of sperm retrieved from the bladder and from surgical extraction are comparable to those obtained by ICSI of ejaculated sperm.[25,26,45,47] In total, ICSI constitutes a cumulative pregnancy rate of 57% per couple and a cumulative live birth rate of 50% per couple.[29]

SHOULD PATIENTS BANK SPERM AFTER SPINAL CORD INJURY?

As previously stated, two retrospective studies suggested that semen parameters are stable during the chronic phase of SCI except for a mild but significant decrease in sperm concentration. However, most authors consider that preventative sperm banking is not useful for the fertility management of male patients with SCI.[29,48,49]

Nevertheless, some authors also suggest that the fertility of patients with SCI during the chronic phase is at higher risk than in infertile patients without SCI.

In patients with SCI, impairment of basic semen parameters is frequent; higher levels of oxidative stress and sperm DNA damage are widely described.[11,20,48–50] Though no clinically significant decrease in basic semen parameters has been assessed by retrospective studies,[48,49] there is no scientific evidence that sperm DNA damage remains stable during the chronic phase of SCI. Sperm DNA damage in patients with SCI is at least in part related to oxidative stress; as the incidence of seminal tract and accessory gland infections is higher in patients with chronic SCI (28%–38%) than in infertile patients without SCI (10%),[51–53] the question of the evolution of DNA damage during the chronic phase of SCI is raised. Orchitis and epididymitis also induce a higher risk of semen impairment and obstructive sequelae, leading to possible oligo-/azoospermia.[53–55]

Moreover, the increasing use of intradetrusor injection of botulinum toxin for the treatment of neurogenic bladder could lead to retrograde ejaculation in many patients. A prior report noted toxin diffusion to the bladder neck and sexual accessory tract, resulting in an increased incidence of retrograde ejaculation and a significant decrease of ejaculate volume.[56]

All these factors may induce the use of bladder- or surgically retrieved sperm for ART and commit couples to ICSI.[22] From the patients' perspective, this scenario should be avoided because ICSI treatments are very expensive and more invasive for the female partner than IUI and self-inseminations at home.

As the fertility of patients with SCI is at higher risk compared to patients without SCI, sperm banking has been proposed in order to ensure patient-centered care of these patients.[22] The protocol proposes early sperm banking to all patients with SCI after the phase of spinal shock, while they are in the rehabilitation center postinjury. When ejaculated sperm are retrieved, they are frozen and stored. EEJ and surgical sperm extraction are only proposed to patients with SCI who desire biological parenthood. When the patient with SCI starts infertility treatment, fresh or frozen-thawed sperm may be used, according to the ability of patient to ejaculate and the quality of the sperm and semen parameters (Figure 44.2). Sperm banking is

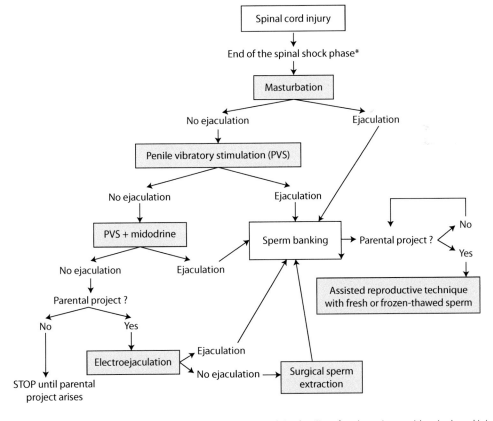

Figure 44.2 Proposition of a patient-centered management of the fertility of male patients with spinal cord injury (SCI) by early sperm banking. (*Patient should be informed that SCI increases the risk of impaired fertility.)

simple and affordable and could benefit patients with SCI by avoiding the need for future sperm surgical extraction and ICSI,[22] which is more invasive and not affordable for many patients with SCI.

CONCLUSION

Semen parameters are rapidly impaired by SCI. During the acute phase, spermatogenesis, blood-testis barrier, and seminal vesicle function are impacted. During the chronic phase, patients face a markedly decreased sperm motility and viability, due to various testicular and seminal factors including autoimmune, oxidative, and heat stresses.

The management of the fertility of patients with SCI involves a multidisciplinary staff and should be patient-centered care. As robust scientific data are lacking about the evolution of semen parameters and sperm DNA damage during the chronic phase, early sperm banking may be proposed. The ART management of male patients with SCI should use the better-quality sperm available (fresh or frozen-thawed), and the technique should be carefully adapted to feminine characteristics. Patient-centered care gives the best pregnancy chances to the couple and avoids preventable surgical sperm extractions. The results of ART treatments in couples with male partners with SCI are expected to be comparable to those of couples without SCI.

REFERENCES

1. National Spinal Cord Injury Statistical Center. 2018 Annual Statistical Report for the Spinal Cord Injury Model Systems. University of Alabama at Birmingham: Birmingham, Alabama. https://www.nscisc.uab.edu/Public_Pages/ReportsStats December 2018.
2. van den Borne K, Brands I, Spijkerman D, Adriaansen JJE, Postma K, and van den Berg-Emons HJG. Prevalence of parenthood in wheelchair-dependent persons with long-term spinal cord injury in the Netherlands. *Spinal Cord.* 2018;56(6):607–13.
3. Elliott SP. Sexual dysfunction and infertility in men with spinal cord disorders. In: Lin V, ed. *Spinal Cord Medicine: Principles and Practice.* New York, NY: Demos Medical; 2003:349–65.
4. Brindley GS. The Ferrier lecture, 1986. The actions of parasympathetic and sympathetic nerves in human micturition, erection and seminal emission, and their restoration in paraplegic patients by implanted electrical stimulators. *Proc R Soc Lond Ser B.* 1988;235(1279):111–20.
5. Momen MN, Fahmy I, Amer M, Arafa M, Zohdy W, and Naser TA. Semen parameters in men with spinal cord injury: Changes and aetiology. *Asian J Androl.* 2007;9(5):684–9.
6. Kafetsoulis A, Brackett NL, Ibrahim E, Attia GR, and Lynne CM. Current trends in the treatment

7. Dimitriadis F, Karakitsios K, Tsounapi P et al. Erectile function and male reproduction in men with spinal cord injury: A review. *Andrologia.* 2010;42(3):139–65.
8. Brackett NL, Lynne CM, Ibrahim E, Ohl DA, and Sønksen J. Treatment of infertility in men with spinal cord injury. *Nat Rev Urol.* 2010;7(3):162–72.
9. da Silva BF, Borrelli M Jr, Fariello RM et al. Is sperm cryopreservation an option for fertility preservation in patients with spinal cord injury-induced anejaculation? *Fertil Steril.* 2010;94(2):564–73.
10. Chéhensse C, Bahrami S, Denys P, Clément P, Bernabé J, and Giuliano F. The spinal control of ejaculation revisited: A systematic review and meta-analysis of anejaculation in spinal cord injured patients. *Hum Reprod Update.* 2013;19(5):507–26.
11. Iremashvili VV, Brackett NL, Ibrahim E, Aballa TC, and Lynne CM. A minority of men with spinal cord injury have normal semen quality—Can we learn from them? A case-control study. *Urology.* 2010;76(2):347–51.
12. Lee S, Miselis R, and Rivier C. Anatomical and functional evidence for a neural hypothalamic-testicular pathway that is independent of the pituitary. *Endocrinology.* 2002;143(11):4447–54.
13. Ottenweller JE, Li MT, Giglio W, Anesetti R, Pogach LM, and Huang HF. Alteration of follicle-stimulating hormone and testosterone regulation of messenger ribonucleic acid for Sertoli cell proteins in the rat during the acute phase of spinal cord injury. *Biol Reprod.* 2000;63(3):730–5.
14. Huang HF, Linsenmeyer TA, Li MT et al. Acute effects of spinal cord injury on the pituitary-testicular hormone axis and Sertoli cell functions: A time course study. *J Androl.* 1995;16(2):148–57.
15. Dulin JN, Moore ML, Gates KW, Queen JH, and Grill RJ. Spinal cord injury causes sustained disruption of the blood-testis barrier in the rat. *PLOS ONE.* 2011;6(1):e16456.
16. Nikmehr B, Bazrafkan M, Hassanzadeh G et al. The correlation of gene expression of inflammasome indicators and impaired fertility in rat model of spinal cord injury: A time course study. *Urol J.* 2017;14(6):5057–63.
17. Camargo M, Intasqui P, and Bertolla RP. Understanding the seminal plasma proteome and its role in male fertility. *Basic Clin Androl.* 2018;28(6).
18. Paul C, Teng S, and Saunders PTK. A single, mild, transient scrotal heat stress causes hypoxia and oxidative stress in mouse testes, which induces germ cell death. *Biol Reprod.* 2009;80(5):913–9.
19. Restelli AE, Bertolla RP, Spaine DM, Miotto A Jr, Borrelli M Jr, and Cedenho AP. Quality and functional aspects of sperm retrieved through assisted ejaculation in men with spinal cord injury. *Fertil Steril.* 2009;91(3):819–25.
20. Qiu Y, Wang L-G, Zhang L-H, Li J, Zhang A-D, and Zhang M-H. Sperm chromosomal aneuploidy and DNA integrity of infertile men with anejaculation. *J Assist Reprod Genet.* 2012;29(2):185–94.
21. Anderson KD. Targeting recovery: Priorities of the spinal cord-injured population. *J Neurotrauma.* 2004;21(10):1371–83.
22. Karsenty G, Bernuz B, Metzler-Guillemain C et al. Should sperm be cryopreserved after spinal cord injury? *Basic Clin Androl.* 2013;23(6).
23. Brackett NL, Ibrahim E, Iremashvili V, Aballa TC, and Lynne CM. Treatment for ejaculatory dysfunction in men with spinal cord injury: An 18-year single center experience. *J Urol.* 2010;183(6):2304–8.

24. Perrin J, Saïas-Magnan J, Thiry-Escudié I et al. [The spinal cord injured patient: Semen quality and management by assisted reproductive technology]. *Gynécologie Obstétrique Fertil*. 2010;38(9):532–5.

25. Perrin J, Saïas-Magnan J, Lanteaume A et al. [Initial results of a novel technique for sperm retrieval in male infertility due to refractory retrograde ejaculation]. *Prog En Urol J Assoc Fr Urol Société Fr Urol*. 2011;21(2):134–8.

26. Philippon M, Karsenty G, Bernuz B et al. Successful pregnancies and healthy live births using frozen-thawed sperm retrieved by a new modified Hotchkiss procedure in males with retrograde ejaculation: First case series. *Basic Clin Androl*. 2015;25:5.

27. Soler JM, Previnaire JG, Plante P, Denys P, and Chartier-Kastler E. Midodrine improves ejaculation in spinal cord injured men. *J Urol*. 2007;178(5):2082–6.

28. Soler JM and Previnaire JG. Ejaculatory dysfunction in spinal cord injury men is suggestive of dyssynergic ejaculation. *Eur J Phys Rehabil Med*. 2011;47(4):677–81.

29. DeForge D, Blackmer J, Garritty C et al. Fertility following spinal cord injury: A systematic review. *Spinal Cord*. 2005;43(12):693–703.

30. Sønksen J, Biering-Sørensen F, and Kristensen JK. Ejaculation induced by penile vibratory stimulation in men with spinal cord injuries. The importance of the vibratory amplitude. *Paraplegia*. 1994;32(10):651–60.

31. Fode M, Ohl DA, and Sønksen J. A step-wise approach to sperm retrieval in men with neurogenic anejaculation. *Nat Rev Urol*. 2015;12(11):607–16.

32. Soler J-M, Previnaire JG, and Mieusset R. Evidence of a new pattern of ejaculation in men with spinal cord injury: Ejaculation dyssynergia and implications for fertility. *Spinal Cord*. 2016;54(12):1210–4.

33. Soeterik TF, Veenboer PW, Oude-Ophuis RJ, and Lock TM. Electroejaculation in patients with spinal cord injuries: A 21-year, single-center experience. *Int J Urol Off J Jpn Urol Assoc*. 2017;24(2):157–61.

34. Aust TR, Brookes S, Troup SA, Fraser WD, and Lewis-Jones DI. Development and *in vitro* testing of a new method of urine preparation for retrograde ejaculation; the Liverpool solution. *Fertil Steril*. 2008;89(4):885–91.

35. Scammell GE, Stedronska-Clark J, Edmonds DK, and Hendry WF. Retrograde ejaculation: Successful treatment with artificial insemination. *Br J Urol*. 1989;63(2):198–201.

36. Jefferys A, Siassakos D, and Wardle P. The management of retrograde ejaculation: A systematic review and update. *Fertil Steril*. 2012;97(2):306–12.

37. Glezerman M, Lunenfeld B, Potashnik G, Oelsner G, and Beer R. Retrograde ejaculation: Pathophysiologic aspects and report of two successfully treated cases. *Fertil Steril*. 1976;27(7):796–800.

38. Jimenez C, Grizard G, Pouly JL, and Boucher D. Birth after combination of cryopreservation of sperm recovered from urine and intracytoplasmic sperm injection in a case of complete retrograde ejaculation. *Fertil Steril*. 1997;68(3):542–4.

39. Ranieri DM, Simonetti S, Vicino M, Cormio L, and Selvaggi L. Successful establishment of pregnancy by superovulation and intrauterine insemination with sperm recovered by a modified Hotchkiss procedure from a patient with retrograde ejaculation. *Fertil Steril*. 1995;64(5):1039–42.

40. Klotz R, Joseph PA, Ravaud JF, Wiart L, and Barat M. The Tetrafigap survey on the long-term outcome of tetraplegic spinal cord injured persons: Part III. Medical complications and associated factors. *Spinal Cord*. 2002;40(9):457–67.

41. Fode M, Krogh-Jespersen S, Brackett NL, Ohl DA, Lynne CM, and Sønksen J. Male sexual dysfunction and infertility associated with neurological disorders. *Asian J Androl*. 2012;14(1):61–8.

42. Brackett NL, Lynne CM, Aballa TC, and Ferrell SM. Sperm motility from the vas deferens of spinal cord injured men is higher than from the ejaculate. *J Urol*. 2000;164(3 Pt 1):712–5.

43. Kanto S, Uto H, Toya M, Ohnuma T, Arai Y, and Kyono K. Fresh testicular sperm retrieved from men with spinal cord injury retains equal fecundity to that from men with obstructive azoospermia via intracytoplasmic sperm injection. *Fertil Steril*. 2009;92(4):1333–6.

44. Elliott SP, Orejuela F, Hirsch IH, Lipshultz LI, Lamb DJ, and Kim ED. Testis biopsy findings in the spinal cord injured patient. *J Urol*. 2000;163(3):792–5.

45. Nyboe Andersen A, Goossens V, Bhattacharya S et al. Assisted reproductive technology and intrauterine inseminations in Europe, 2005: Results generated from European registers by ESHRE: ESHRE. The European IVF Monitoring Programme (EIM), for the European Society of Human Reproduction and Embryology (ESHRE). *Hum Reprod Oxf Engl*. 2009;24(6):1267–87.

46. Chung PH, Palermo G, Schlegel PN, Veeck LL, Eid JF, and Rosenwaks Z. The use of intracytoplasmic sperm injection with electroejaculates from anejaculatory men. *Hum Reprod Oxf Engl*. 1998;13(7):1854–8.

47. Reignier A, Lammers J, Splingart C et al. Sperm cryopreservation and assisted reproductive technology outcome in patients with spinal cord injury. *Andrologia*. 2018;50(1):e12833.

48. Brackett NL, Ferrell SM, Aballa TC, Amador MJ, and Lynne CM. Semen quality in spinal cord injured men: Does it progressively decline postinjury? *Arch Phys Med Rehabil*. 1998;79(6):625–8.

49. Iremashvili V, Brackett NL, Ibrahim E, Aballa TC, and Lynne CM. Semen quality remains stable during the chronic phase of spinal cord injury: A longitudinal study. *J Urol*. 2010;184(5):2073–7.

50. Qiu Y, Wang L-G, Zhang L-H, Zhang A-D, and Wang Z-Y. Quality of sperm obtained by penile vibratory stimulation and percutaneous vasal sperm aspiration in men with spinal cord injury. *J Androl*. 2012;33(5):1036–46.

51. Rolf C, Kenkel S, and Nieschlag E. Age-related disease pattern in infertile men: Increasing incidence of infections in older patients. *Andrologia*. 2002;34(4):209–17.

52. Ku JH, Jung TY, Lee JK, Park WH, and Shim HB. Influence of bladder management on epididymo-orchitis in patients with spinal cord injury: Clean intermittent catheterization is a risk factor for epididymo-orchitis. *Spinal Cord*. 2006;44(3):165–9.

53. Mirsadraee S, Mahdavi R, Moghadam HV, Ebrahimi MA, and Patel HRH. Epididymo-orchitis risk factors in traumatic spinal cord injured patients. *Spinal Cord*. 2003;41(9):516–20.

54. Haidl G, Allam JP, and Schuppe H-C. Chronic epididymitis: Impact on semen parameters and therapeutic options. *Andrologia*. 2008;40(2):92–6.

55. Christiansen E, Tollefsrud A, and Purvis K. Sperm quality in men with chronic abacterial prostatovesiculitis verified by rectal ultrasonography. *Urology*. 1991;38(6):545–9.

56. Caremel R, Courtois F, Charvier K, Ruffion A, and Journel NM. Side effects of intradetrusor botulinum toxin injections on ejaculation and fertility in men with spinal cord injury: Preliminary findings. *BJU Int*. 2012;109(11):1698–702.

Chapter 45

PREGNANCY IN SPINAL CORD INJURY

Carlotte Kiekens

INTRODUCTION

In Western countries, traumatic spinal cord injury (SCI) is a rare condition with an incidence of 1–5 per 100 000 inhabitants per year.[1–4] The vast majority (75%–80%) of the patients are male.[1,5] There is a trend of increasing mean age at injury, cervical level of lesion, incomplete lesions, and proportion of women.[5,6] For nontraumatic SCI, mean age and percentage of women are higher.[1,3,5]

Fertility and motherhood are important issues for women with SCI. The scientific literature concerning female fertility issues, such as pregnancy rates, live births, and complications or obstetric management following SCI, mainly consists of case series and reports and opinion articles. Recently, however, some reviews and qualitative studies have been published.

MENSTRUATION, FERTILITY, AND CONTRACEPTION

Menarche has been reported to occur normally in girls who have been injured as preadolescents. When an SCI is sustained after menarche, it is usually followed by a 3- to 6-month episode of amenorrhea. Then, fertility status returns to the premorbid status.[7–10] A multicenter survey in 472 women with SCI showed that menstrual cramping is less frequent after SCI, while premenstrual syndrome increases.[8] Exacerbation of autonomic symptoms occurs at particular times in the cycle. Fewer gynecologic check-ups, mammographies, and PAP smears postinjury were reported. Menopause was induced by SCI in 14% of the subjects, but except for an increase in mood disorders, menopausal symptoms were not different.[11] Oral contraceptives may be contraindicated because of the challenged cardiovascular status and increased risk of deep venous thrombosis, especially in women who smoke or are over 35 years of age.[11] Due to sensory loss, intrauterine devices (IUDs) can be dangerous in case of complications.[4] Condoms can be used but should be latex-free in persons with spina bifida.[12]

PREGNANCY

The pregnancy rate is lower in women with SCI, independent of the level of injury, due to decreased sexual activity, decreased involvement in relationships, not wanting children, or perceived difficulty in caring for the children.[9,10]

A regular follow-up by a multidisciplinary team is mandatory: at least a general practitioner, gynecologist, and physiatrist. Ideally, also the urologist, anesthesiologist, physical therapist, occupational therapist, and midwife are involved. Moreover, Tebbet and Kennedy propose a biopsychosocial approach, and a clear need was shown for comprehensive interdisciplinary networking, starting from the preconceptual phase.[13–16,40,41] The medication scheme of the mother should be revised to avoid teratogenous effects on the fetus. A preconception renal/urologic and respiratory assessment is appropriate.[14,16] Women with spina bifida should take folic acid in a dose of 4 mg daily.[17] Psychological aspects can be discussed, particularly in women who might need assistance to care for their baby. A peer mentor system, promoting positive experiences in other women, has been experienced as very beneficial and may help to improve self-efficacy and preparation for the experience of childbirth.[13,15]

Several series and surveys on pregnancy and SCI have been published.[7,8,14,16,18–21,42] During pregnancy, weight gain can decrease mobility and independence for activities of daily living such as transfers and wheelchair propulsion. Extra help and technical aids may need to be provided. Fetal movements might not be perceived so the mother should be taught to monitor these movements by palpating the abdominal wall.

Bladder management is often disturbed: incontinence increases and more frequent intermittent catheterization may be necessary. Asymptomatic bacteriuria and urinary tract infection (UTI) increase: sufficient fluid intake should be ensured and residual volumes minimized to avoid pyelonephritis, as this may induce preterm labor and delivery. Indwelling or suprapubic catheters are contraindicated, and frequent surveillance of cultures is advised, for example every 4 weeks.[41] Some suggest to switch from "clean" to "sterile" intermittent catheterization.[9] A systematic review of 2011 confirmed that the majority of the women (64%) had at least one symptomatic UTI during pregnancy, and a weekly oral cyclic antibiotic program may be considered.[22,23] Because of a decrease in gastric motility during pregnancy, sufficient fluid (and fiber) intake and, if necessary, mild laxatives may be required to prevent constipation.[41]

The pregnant woman with SCI often shows anemia and fatigue, water retention, and edema of the lower extremities, augmented spasticity and pain, which can together with the decreased mobility cause decubitus ulcers. A larger wheelchair and change of cushion and matrass may be necessary. In case of dry skin a non-sensitizing skin moisturizer should be used.[41] Healthy diet is recommended, as well as to control weight every four weeks and then every two weeks during the last two months of pregnancy.[41] The risk for thromboembolism increases, and compression stockings as well as low-molecular-weight heparin administration from the fourth month on until the end of the postpartum period are recommended, even though a German guideline from 2019 advises it from the 28th week only.[41] In high thoracic and cervical lesions, adapted respiratory rehabilitation may be required.

Spasticity can be exacerbated, but oral baclofen can have side effects for the fetus. In five cases an intrathecal baclofen (ITB) pump was implanted before or during pregnancy, and in one case ITB was administered via an external catheter with good effect tolerance.[24,25] Attention is asked for the position of the pump, the risk for catheter problems due to the change in abdominal shape, and care not to enter the pump pocket in case of a cesarean delivery. Spinal or epidural anesthesia needles should not pierce the catheter.

The most important and dangerous complication during pregnancy (and delivery) is autonomic dysreflexia (AD).[26] This syndrome is characterized by a sudden paroxysmal hypertension known as an important, possibly life-threatening complication, for mother and baby. It is reported to occur in up to 85% of patients with an SCI at T6 or above. Any stimulus below the lesion, such as a distended bladder or bowel, UTI, pressure sore, or labor, can trigger the sympathetic nervous system (segments T1 through T5) and cause an uncontrolled increase in blood pressure due to the lack of inhibitory descending tracts, with symptoms of an infralesional vasoconstriction and supralesional vasodilatation and systemic hypertension, compensatory bradycardia, and anxiety. Above the lesion, we notice pounding headache, flushing, sweating, and, if the lesion is higher than T1, mydriasis. Below the lesion we see cool extremities and piloerection. Complications include retinal, subarachnoidal, or intracerebral hemorrhage; myocardial infarction; seizure; and death. Differential diagnosis with preeclampsia is important because the treatment is different.[11] Prevention of AD by avoiding irritations is mandatory. When treating AD, antihypertensive agents with rapid action and short duration are preferred (mostly nifedipine or captopril), but hypotension should be avoided.

LABOR AND DELIVERY

The uterus is innervated by the segments T10 through L1. Women with a lesion in T10 through L1 may present insufficient labor. When the lesion is situated in L1 or above, the onset of labor may not be perceived due to the sensory impairment. In women with lesions at T6 or higher, labor can cause AD.

Preterm labor and delivery have been reported.[16,42] Labor indicators differ greatly following SCI: supralesional or abnormal pain, ruptured membranes (which can be confused with urinary incontinence), increased spasticity, respiratory changes, symptoms of AD, or increased bladder spasms.[7,8,19]

In patients who are unable to sense contractions reliably, unattended delivery should be avoided by cervical examinations once or twice weekly after 28 weeks, and hospitalization after 36 weeks or earlier if needed.[11,18–20]

During labor and delivery, regular changes in position and skin examination should prevent pressure ulcers. Moreover, upright position may facilitate the birthing process.[41] Frequent bladder emptying by intermittent or continuous catheterization will prevent overdistention of the bladder, which could induce AD.

The following percentages of types of deliveries have been reported: spontaneous vaginal delivery between 37% and 77%, assisted vaginal 14%–31%, and cesarean from 23% up to 68%. In the series published respectively by Robertson et al and by Charlifue et al., 63% and 53% of the women had vaginal deliveries without forceps, 14 and 22% vaginal deliveries with forceps assistance, and 23 and 25% cesarean deliveries.[8,11,17,27,42] Reasons for cesarean delivery were physician choice, transverse lying twins, AD during delivery, placenta previa, prolonged labor, breech or transverse presentation, lack of progress, onset of labor 1 day postspinal fusion, a mother's request for tubal ligation, to prevent syringomyelia deterioration or emergency for obstetric indications. Crane showed a relative risk for cesarean section of 1.88.[16]

If AD can occur, an epidural anesthesia and continuous blood pressure monitoring are necessary.[14,27,40] To avoid skin breakdown, the use of nonabsorbable sutures at the episiotomy site has been recommended, especially in denervated areas.[9,28] After delivery daily wound care is needed.[41]

Women presenting a cauda equina syndrome who preserved an ability for walking often lose it at the end of the pregnancy.[28] Fetal movements as well as onset of labor will be perceived, and the abdominal muscles will help to expel the baby. However, the risk of perineal distention or even rupture is increased due to hypotonia of the pelvic floor, and a cesarean section might be indicated.

In women with lower urinary tract reconstruction, monitoring and prophylaxis of UTIs is important during pregnancy.[29–31] Elective cesarean section can be advised, although vaginal delivery has been reported with good results.[30,31] Urologic follow-up is crucial, and presence is necessary in case of a cesarean section: the augmented bladder or urinary reservoir should be moved away after a midline incision.[31]

One case report on a woman with Malone antegrade continence enema (MACE) describes an excellent fecal continence during pregnancy and an uncomplicated vaginal delivery.[32]

POSTPARTUM AND BREASTFEEDING

Patients should be assessed for bladder distention. Bladder and bowel management still require extra attention.[17,18] When extra help needs to be organized for the care of the baby, some psychological adaptation of the mother may be required. Technical aids and tips and tricks can be given by the occupational therapist. Peer groups can be very helpful in these.[15,33]

Breastfeeding is possible, but milk production might be decreased in lesions above T6 due to decreased nipple sensation, and AD may occur.[34,35,41] Infant suckling activates tactile receptors in the breast, and this signal is carried via the T4 through T6 dorsal roots to the spinal cord and hypothalamus (Figure 45.1), which releases oxytocin in the bloodstream, triggering milk ejection from the breast.[36] Cowley reported on three tetraplegic women maintaining breastfeeding for an extended period (12–54 weeks) using mental imaging and relaxation techniques. One woman needed oxytocin nasal spray to facilitate the let-down reflex. A series of 29 women who breastfed their infants reported only four with insufficient milk.[8] Additional support with breastfeeding aids, such as pillows to support the baby or adapted nursing bras with easy opening and closing, might be necessary.[26] A study on the prevalence of postpartum depression and anxiety (PPD and PPA) showed that mothers with SCI, in particular high-level SCI, may have an increased risk of PPD and PPA, that it is poorly understood and even may be underdiagnosed.[43]

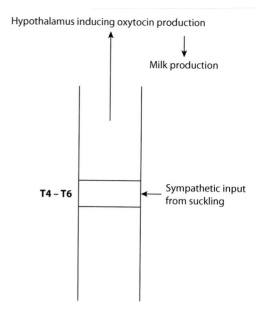

Figure 45.1 Under normal conditions, the sympathetic input from suckling enters the spinal cord at the level of T4 through T6 and from there travels up to the hypothalamus, which in turn induces oxytocin production and increases milk production. In lesions at or above T6, this normal pathway is partially or completely interrupted, which can result in a decrease of milk production.

MOTHERHOOD

Of 26 mothers with SCI with 47 children, no women felt that their family roles and the relationships between family members differed from those of other families.[37] Neither did they have the impression that their children were unable to participate in regular activities because of their SCI. The ten children who filled out the questionnaire did not perceive their mothers as different because of the SCI, and fathers did not report to have more responsibilities. In other studies, very few problems were reported by mothers with SCI except one woman who had problems going on field trips. Another woman stated that having a child provided a motivation to stay healthy.[9] In Ghidini's study, 23 out of 24 women who gave birth reported that being a parent increased their quality of life.[19]

In 2002, in a survey in 88 mothers, 46 partners, and 31 children, SCI did not appear to affect the children adversely in terms of individual adjustment, attitudes toward their parents, self-esteem, gender roles, and family functioning.[38] Mothers with SCI saw their children as being less rigid and more comfortable in adjusting to novel situations. Partners of SCI mothers seemed to enjoy more satisfying relationships with their children. The presence of maternal SCI does not predict difficulties in children's psychological adjustment, nor does it lead to problems in areas of parenting satisfaction, parenting stress, marital adjustment, or family functioning.

SUMMARY

Literature on pregnancy in SCI is scarce. However, motherhood is an important topic for women with SCI. After an episode of amenorrhea, fertility returns to the premorbid status. Contraception should be prescribed if necessary, taking into account the specific risks of each method. Pregnancy rates are lower in women with SCI. The most dangerous complication is AD, which can occur in patients with a lesion at T6 or above. Other potential complications are bladder and bowel problems, pressure sores, anemia and fatigue, increased spasticity or pain, decreased respiratory capacity, and thromboembolic events.[16,21] Extra monitoring is advised from the 28th week and hospitalization at 36 weeks to prevent preterm delivery. Delivery depends on the level of the lesion, the innervation of the uterus being situated in T10 through L1. Even though spontaneous vaginal delivery is often possible, there is an increased percentage of assisted vaginal delivery or cesarean delivery. In patients presenting a lesion at T6 or above, continuous monitoring of blood pressure and epidural anesthesia is necessary for AD. In patients with a lesion above T6, insufficient milk production may occur, but with some extra care, most of the women succeed in breastfeeding. The presence of maternal SCI does not seem to predispose for psychological adjustment problems in their children, nor does it lead to decreased parenting satisfaction or family functioning.

Pregnancy and motherhood are certainly options for women with SCI, but comprehensive interdisciplinary follow-up, for example, using the "Sexual Rehabilitation Framework" as described by Elliott, and prevention of possible complications are mandatory.[39]

REFERENCES

1. DeVivo MJ. Epidemiology of traumatic spinal cord injury: Trends and future implications. *Spinal Cord.* 2012;50:365–72.
2. Hagen EM, Eide GE, Rekand T et al. A 50-year follow-up of the incidence of traumatic spinal cord injuries in Western Norway. *Spinal Cord.* 2010;48:313–8.
3. Jain NB, Ayers GD, Peterson EN et al. Traumatic spinal cord injury in the United States, 1993–2012. *JAMA.* 2015;313:2236–43.
4. Bjørnshave Noe B, Mikkelsen EM, Hansen RM, Thygesen M, and Hagen EM. Incidence of traumatic spinal cord injury in Denmark, 1990–2012: A hospital-based study. *Spinal Cord.* 2015;53:436–40.
5. McCaughey EJ, Purcell M, McLean AN et al. Changing demographics of spinal cord injury over a 20-year period: A longitudinal population-based study in Scotland. *Spinal Cord.* 2016;54:270–6.
6. O'Connor PJ. Trends in spinal cord injury. *Accident Anal Prev.* 2006;38:71–7.
7. Jackson AB, and Wadley V. A multicenter study of women's self-reported reproductive health after spinal cord injury. *Arch Phys Med Rehabil.* 1999;80:1420–8.
8. Charlifue SW, Gerhart KA, Menter RR et al. Sexual issues of women with spinal cord injuries. *Paraplegia* 1992;30:192–9.
9. Linsenmeyer TA. Sexual function and infertility following spinal cord injury. *Phys Med Rehab Clin N Am.* 2000;11:141–56.
10. Burghi S, Shaw SJ, Mahmood G et al. Amenorrhea, pregnancy, and pregnancy outcomes in women following spinal cord injury: A retrospective cross-sectional study. *Endocr Pract.* 2008;14:437–41.
11. Cross LL, Meythaler JM, Tuel SM et al. Pregnancy, labor and delivery post spinal cord injury. *Paraplegia* 1992;30:890–902.
12. Sipski ML. Spinal cord injury and sexual function: An educational model. In: Sipski ML, and Alexander CJ, eds. *Sexual Function in People with Disability and Chronic Illness.* Gaithersburg, MD: Aspen; 1997:149–76.
13. Tebbet M and Kennedy P. The experience of childbirth for women with spinal cord injuries: An interpretative phenomenology analysis study. *Disabil Rehabil.* 2012;34:762–9.
14. Dawood R, Altanis E, Iatrikes P, Ribes-Pastor P, and Ashworth F. Pregnancy and spinal cord injury. *Obstet Gynaecol.* 2014;16:99–107.
15. Bertschy S, Geyh S, Pannek J, and Meyer T. Perceived needs and experiences with healthcare services of women with spinal cord injury during pregnancy and childbirth—A qualitative content analysis of focus groups and individual interviews. *BMC Health Serv Res.* 2015;15:234.
16. Crane DA, Doody DR, Schiff MA, and Mueller BA. Pregnancy outcomes in women with spinal cord injuries: A population-based study. *PM R.* 2019;11(8):795–806.
17. Pereira L. Obstetric management of the patient with spinal cord injury. *Obstet Gynaecol Survey.* 2003;58:678–86.
18. Baker ER and Cardenas DD. Pregnancy in spinal cord injured women. *Arch Phys Med Rehab.* 1996;77:501–7.
19. Ghidini A, Healy A, Andreani M et al. Pregnancy and women with spinal cord injuries. *Acta Obstet Gynecol Scand.* 2008;87:1006–10.
20. Skowronski E and Hartman K. Obstetric management following traumatic tetraplegia: Case series and literature review. *Aust N Z J Obstet Gynaecol.* 2008;48:485–91.
21. Chhabra HS. Chapter 39: ISCoS Textbook on Comprehensive Management of Spinal Cord Injuries. In: Biering-Sörensen F, Sipski Alexander M, Elliott S, Del Popolo G, Prévinaire JG, and Rodriguez Velez A, eds. *Sexuality and Fertility Management.* Alphen aan den Rijn, Netherlands: Wolters Kluwer; 2015:621–3.

22. Pannek J and Bertschy S. Mission impossible? Urological management of patients with spinal cord injury during pregnancy: A systematic review. *Spinal Cord.* 2011;49:1028–32.

23. Salomon J, Schnitzler A, Ville Y et al. Prevention of urinary tract infection in six spinal cord-injured women who gave birth. *Int J Infect Dis.* 2009;13:399–402.

24. Roberts AG, Graves CR, Konrad PE et al. Intrathecal baclofen pump implantation during pregnancy. *Neurology.* 2003;61:1156–7.

25. Morton CM, Rosenow J, Wong C et al. Intrathecal baclofen administration during pregnancy: A case series and focused clinical review. *PM R.* 2009;1:1025–9.

26. Krassioukov A, Rapidi CA, Wecht J, and Vogel L. Chapter 54: Autonomic Dysreflexia. In: Chhabra HS, ed. *ISCoS Textbook on Comprehensive Management of Spinal Cord Injuries.* Alphen aan den Rijn, Netherlands: Wolters Kluwer; 2015:814–24.

27. Le Liepvre H, Dinh A, Idiard-Chamois B et al. Pregnancy in spinal cord-injured women, a cohort study of 37 pregnancies in 25 women. *Spinal Cord.* 2017;55:167–71.

28. Perrouin-Verbe B and Labat JJ. Sexualité et procréation des syndromes de la queue de cheval. In: Costa P, Lopez S, and Pélissier J, eds. *Sexualité, Fertilité et Handicap.* Paris, France: Masson; 1996:81–8.

29. Greenwell TJ, Venn SN, Creighton S et al. Pregnancy after lower urinary tract reconstruction for congenital abnormalities. *BJU Int.* 2003;92:773–7.

30. Quenneville V, Beurton D, Thomas L et al. Pregnancy and vaginal delivery after augmentation cystoplasty. *BJU Int.* 2003;91:893–4.

31. Hensle TW, Bingham JB, Reiley EA et al. The urological care and outcome of pregnancy after urinary tract reconstruction. *BJU Int.* 2004;93:588–90.

32. Wren FJ, Reese CT, and Decter RM. Durability of the Malone antegrade continence enema in pregnancy. *Urology.* 2003;61:644iv.

33. Spinal cord injury and parenting. The Spinalis foundation. https://sciparenting.com/

34. Holmgren T, Lee AHX, Hocaloski S et al. The influence of spinal cord injury on breastfeeding ability and behavior. *J Hum Lact.* 2018;34:556–65.

35. Halbert LA. Breastfeeding in the woman with a compromised nervous system. *J Hum Lact.* 1998;14:327–31.

36. Cowley KC. Psychogenic and pharmacological induction of the let-down reflex can facilitate breastfeeding by tetraplegic women: A report of 3 cases. *Arch Phys Med Rehab.* 2005;86:1261–4.

37. Westgren N and Levi R. Motherhood after traumatic spinal cord injury. *Paraplegia.* 1994;32:517–23.

38. Alexander CJ, Hwang K, and Sipski M. Mothers with spinal cord injuries: Impact on marital, family, and children's adjustment. *Arch Phys Med Rehab.* 2002;83:24–30.

39. Elliott S, Hocaloski S, and Carlson M. A Multidisciplinary approach to sexual and fertility rehabilitation: The sexual rehabilitation framework. *Top Spinal Cord Inj Rehabil.* 2017;23:49–56.

40. Obstetric Management of Patients with Spinal Cord Injuries: ACOG Committee Opinion, Number 808. *Obstet Gynecol.* 2020;135(5):e230–e236.

41. Bertschy S, Schmidt M, Fiebag K, Lange U, Kues S, and Kurze I. Guideline for the management of pre-, intra-, and postpartum care of women with a spinal cord injury. *Spinal Cord.* 2020;58(4):449-458.

42. Robertson K, Dawood R, Ashworth F. Vaginal delivery is safely achieved in pregnancies complicated by spinal cord injury: a retrospective 25-year observational study of pregnancy outcomes in a national spinal injuries centre. *BMC Pregnancy Childbirth.* 2020;20(1):56.

43. Lee AHX, Wen B, Walter M et al. Prevalence of postpartum depression and anxiety among women with spinal cord injury. *J Spinal Cord Med.* 2019;1–6. doi:10.1080/10790268.2019.1666239

Part IX

PROGNOSIS AND FOLLOW-UP

Chapter 46

PROGNOSIS OF NEUROGENIC BLADDERS

Ali Alsulihem and Jacques Corcos

INTRODUCTION

Most neurologic lesions disrupt bladder-sphincter function and its central neurologic control. The long-term consequences of these dysfunctions are well elucidated. These consequences determine the patients' quality of life and mortality rates. Prognosis of neurogenic bladders is considered at two different levels: the functional and the vital. The functional level is the ability to void completely, the degree of continence as well as sexual and fertility issues. At the other end of the spectrum is the vital prognosis which includes renal function, infections, stones, and cancer.

This chapter draws in from other chapters of this book the parameters, which, put together will allow the clinician to establish a prognosis for each patient.

EVOLUTION OF THE PROGNOSIS OVER TIME

In 1927, Cushing observed that 80% of patients with SCI died within weeks after the trauma because of infections, urinary catheters, and bedsores. The acute mortality rate has improved thanks to advanced medical management. The rate has dropped from 60%–80% during World War II to 30% in the 1960s and to 6% in the 1980s.[1,2] In 50 years, the rate of death attributed to urinary complications has diminished by half in each successive decade.[3,4]

Recent data show a disease-specific yearly mortality of 8 million in Canada. However, it remains very high in developing countries such as Nigeria where it is 17.5 million.[5] This favorable evolution in the developed world is seen both in mortality and morbidity, with preventive measures and medical treatments reducing hospitalization for urologic complications.[6] Needless to say, the leading cause for rehospitalizations remains urinary complications followed by pulmonary and skin problems.[7]

FUNCTIONAL PROGNOSIS

The ability to void is an important factor in a patient's quality of life (QOL). Many are able to void spontaneously, on demand, and empty their bladder completely. This is frequently seen in patients with multiple sclerosis (MS), incomplete spinal cord injury (SCI), Parkinson's disease (PD), etc. However, in these same conditions, frequency, hesitancy, and incomplete emptying can significantly alter the patient's QOL. For instance, in MS, frequency and urgency occur in 31%–86% of cases, and incontinence and obstructive symptoms with or without urinary retention are reported in 34%–72% and 2%–49%, respectively.[8-11] The same figures are seen in SCI depending on the completeness of the cord lesion.[12]

Consequently, in patients with retention or with high postvoid residual volumes, a form of bladder drainage has to be instated. If clean intermittent catheterization (CIC) is the method of choice for bladder emptying, not all patients have the physical or the economical ability to use this sophisticated technique. Indwelling catheters are still too often used in emerging countries. They come with their complications such as infections and other mechanical complications as well their psychological, sexual, and fertility negative impact. Even in patients using CIC, QOL can be impacted by difficulty in performing catherization and the number of catheterizations necessary to ensure social continence.[13]

The degree of continence is also an important parameter of functional prognosis. One of the aims of functional management is to make the patient as continent as before the neurologic injury. Strategies to reach this high degree of continence are numerous, from oral or intravesical medication to adequate bladder drainage to electrical implants or conventional surgeries. Many of these techniques, including medications, stimulators, and artificial sphincters, are not available in most developing countries. In some of these countries, the consequences of incontinence could be devastating considering the lack of decent protections such as diapers or good-quality pads.[14]

In SCI, a large number of patients are young. Their sexuality and fertility concerns are important to consider in their functional prognosis. Various medications, injectable drugs, prostheses, and devices exist to help recover a satisfactory sexual life, but again, their accessibility in developing countries is often challenging.[15] Fertility treatments are even more technically advanced and limit their access to a few privileged patients.

VITAL PROGNOSIS

Some serious complications of neurogenic bladders are potentially fatal. On top of the list is renal failure. Others such as urinary tract infections, nephrolithiasis, and bladder cancer are potentially life threatening. These complications are compounded by the patient's general medical and nutritional status.

Several factors contribute to renal failure. Progressive deterioration of renal function is seen in recurrent infections and obstructions. Acute obstruction is typically caused by nephrolithiasis. In acute nephrolithiasis, the degree of obstruction, duration of obstruction, and presence of bacteriuria affect the severity of renal injury. Recurrent infections and obstructions compound the likelihood of upper tract damage. For example, repeated episodes of pyelonephritis or chronic pyelonephritis result in cortical and medullary scarring and loss of renal function.[16,17] Compared to chronic infections, chronic obstruction has worse outcomes. On a structural level, repeated episodes of acute, chronic, and untreated obstructions eventually result in permanent nephron loss and a decrease in glomerular filtration rate.

A more insidious etiology for renal impairment in neurogenic bladder dysfunction is the presence of chronically high detrusor pressures due to poorly controlled bladder compliance or high voiding pressures. Both conditions further increase the risk of upper tract deterioration by vesicoureteral reflux. A vicious circle settles: high pressure increases risk of reflux which increases the risk of pyelonephritis.

Urinary tract infections are common and frequent in neurogenic bladders. Many factors explain this high incidence. An important factor is the resting detrusor pressure since there is a significant difference in infection rate between patients with hypotonic bladders versus poorly compliant bladders. Other contributing factors include stones, catheters, urologic manipulations, local contamination mainly in women, and bladder and urethral diverticulum. It is sometimes difficult to control these infections because of their high recurrence/persistence rate and/or the high resistance profile of the germs.[18]

Antibiotics usage although helpful can come with its adverse effects (i.e., colitis or bacterial resistance). A thorough management of these infections is important and starts with the maintenance of a low storage bladder pressure.[19]

Bladder cancer is a serious concern mainly in the long run of bladder management. It is important to inform the patient of the long-term risk of epidermoid carcinoma (around 25% higher than in general population) and to point out the probable risk factors: smoking, infections, stones, and catheterization. Routine cytologies and cystoscopies are recommended after 10–15 years of diagnosis of neurogenic bladder.[20]

Urethral complications including strictures, diverticulum, and fistulas make catheterization difficult or impossible and are often challenging to treat, significantly impacting patients' ability to adequately manage bladder emptying.[21,22]

AGING AND COMORBIDITY

The average age of the general population is increasing. The probability of bladder functional changes is noticeable in relation with aging, hormonal status, prostatic hypertrophy, increasing cancer risk with age, and years postinjury. When there is a change in bladder function, voiding, or rate of infection, a workup needs to be considered. Adequate testing must be conducted before attributing the issue to the neurologic condition. Aging patients will present with nonneurologic health problems and concomitant medication intake. A regular medical and pharmacologic review for possible interferences with bladder management is necessary.

CONCLUSION

The prognosis of neurogenic bladder is intimately related to the prognosis of the neurologic condition (i.e., MS, PD, stroke). However, in some neurologic conditions, bladder management is at the forefront of care as it strongly impacts the patient's QOL and life expectancy. Improving QOL and minimizing morbidity and mortality are our responsibility. This difficult task requires knowledge, perseverance, a complete assessment, comprehensive treatment, and good communication of the challenges to the patient who is the active participant in his care and the final decision maker. It is only at this point of thoroughness that the patient's prognosis is optimized.

REFERENCES

1. Hartkopp A, Bronnum-Hansen H, Seidenschnur AM, and Biering-Sorensen F. Survival and cause of death after traumatic spinal cord injury. A long-term epidemiological survey from Denmark. *Spinal Cord.* 1997;35:76–85.

2. Hackler RH. A 25 years prospective mortality study in a spinal cord injured patient: Comparison with the long term living paraplegic. *J Urol.* 1977;117:486–8.

3. Whiteneck GG, Charlifue SW, Frankel HL et al. Mortality, morbidity, and psychosocial outcomes of person's spinal cord injured more than 20 years ago. *Paraplegia.* 1992;30:617–30.

4. Strauss DJ, Devivo MJ, Paculdo DR, and Shavelle RM. Trends in life expectancy after spinal cord injury. *Arch Phys Med Rehabil.* 2006;87(8):1079–85.

5. Chiu W-T, Lin HC, Lam C, Chu SF, Chiang YH, and Tsai SH. Review paper: Epidemiology of traumatic spinal cord injury: Comparisons between developed and developing countries. *Asia Pacific J Public Heal.* 2010;22:9–18.

6. Cardenas DD, Hoffman JM, Kirshblum S, and McKinley W. Etiology and incidence of rehospitalization after traumatic spinal cord injury: A multicenter analysis. *Arch Phys Med Rehabil.* 2004;85:1757–63.

7. DeJong G, Tian W, Hsieh CH et al. Rehospitalization in the first year of traumatic spinal cord injury after discharge from medical rehabilitation. *Arch Phys Med Rehabil.* 2013;94(4 Suppl).

8. Tubaro A, Puccini F, De Nunzio C et al. The treatment of lower urinary tract symptoms in patients with multiple sclerosis: A systematic review. *Curr Urol Rep.* 2012;13(5):335–42. doi:10.1007/s11934-012-0266-9

9. Schneider MP, Tornic J, Sýkora R et al. Alpha-blockers for treating neurogenic lower urinary tract dysfunction in patients with multiple sclerosis: A systematic review and meta-analysis. A report from the Neuro-Urology Promotion Committee of the International Continence Society (ICS). *Neurourol Urodyn.* 2019;38(6):1482–91. doi:10.1002/nau.24039

10. Fernández O. Mechanisms and current treatments of urogenital dysfunction in multiple sclerosis. *J Neurol.* 2002;249(1):1–8.

11. Litwiller SE, Frohman EM, and Zimmern PE. Multiple sclerosis and the urologist. *J Urol.* 1999;161(3):743–55.

12. Schops TF, Schneider MP, Steffen F, Ineichen BV, Mehnert U, and Kessler TM. Neurogenic lower urinary tract dysfunction (NLUTD) in patients with spinal cord injury: Long-term urodynamic findings. *BJU Int.* 2015;115(Suppl 6):33–8.

13. Stöhrer M, Blok B, Castro-Diaz D et al. EAU guidelines on neurogenic lower urinary tract dysfunction. *Eur Urol.* 2009;56(1):81–8.

14. Przydacz M, Denys P, and Corcos J. What do we know about neurogenic bladder prevalence and management in developing countries and emerging regions of the world? *Ann Phys Rehabil Med.* 2017;60:341–6.

15. Shridharani AN and Brant WO. The treatment of erectile dysfunction in patients with neurogenic disease. *Transl Androl Urol.* 2016;5(1):88–101.

16. Asscher AW, McLachlan MS, Jones RV et al. Screening for asymptomatic urinary-tract infection in schoolgirls. A two-centre feasibility study. *Lancet.* 1973;2(7819):1–4.

17. Styles RA, Ramsden PD, and Neal DE. Chronic retention of urine. The relationship between upper tract dilatation and bladder pressure. *Br J Urol.* 1986;58(6):647–51.

18. Waites KB, Canupp KC, and DeVivo MJ. Epidemiology and risk factors for urinary tract infection following spinal cord injury. *Arch Phys Med Rehabil.* 1993;74:691–5.

19. Alavinia SM, Omidvar M, Farahani F, Bayley M, Zee J, and Craven BC. Enhancing quality practice for prevention and diagnosis of urinary tract infection during inpatient spinal cord rehabilitation. *J Spinal Cord Med.* 2017;40:803–12.

20. Chaudhry R, Balsara ZR, Madden-Fuentes RJ, Wiener JS, Routh JC, and Seed P. Risk factors associated with recurrent urinary tract infection in neurogenic bladders managed by clean intermittent catheterization. *Urology.* 2017;102:213–8.

21. Welk B, McIntyre A, Teasell R, Potter P, and Loh E. Bladder cancer in individuals with spinal cord injuries. *Spinal Cord.* 2013;51:516–21.

22. Cornejo-Dávila V, Durán-Ortiz S, and Pacheco-Gahbler C. Incidence of urethral stricture in patients with spinal cord injury treated with clean intermittent self-catheterization. *Urology.* 2017;99:260–4.

Part X

NEUROGENIC BLADDERS IN DEVELOPING COUNTRIES

Chapter 47

CHALLENGES OF MANAGEMENT OF NEUROGENIC BLADDER IN THE DEVELOPING WORLD

Fernando Segura and Reynaldo G. Gomez

INTRODUCTION

Bladder dysfunction due to neurologic diseases, the so-called neurogenic bladder (NB), is one of the most difficult problems in urology. Analysis of international patterns of care of NB is challenging, because although NB diagnostic and management protocols are well established in developed countries, little is known about NB care in low-income countries (LIC; as defined by the World Bank, per capita incomes of or lower than USD $1,025 in 2018).[1,2] Overarching issues such as basic transportation, physical access to care, and monetary allocation are at the forefront of the discussion. The main causes of these problems in LIC are unstable economies with low per capita income, less advanced healthcare systems, poor facilities, and limited logistics.[1]

In this chapter we summarize the information on epidemiology, management, and access to the treatment of patients with NB in under-developed countries (UDCs), in order to propose future interventions and action plans.

EPIDEMIOLOGY AND ETIOLOGY

The incidence and prevalence figures for NB vary from region to region.[2,3] Not surprisingly, most systematic reviews have been carried out in developed Western countries, with only a few from Asia and other regions.[4] The epidemiology of NB in UDCs is difficult to establish because reports are scarce and may be unreliable. However, from the available information, the etiologies most frequently associated with NB are equivalent to those in developed countries: cerebrovascular accidents (CVAs), Parkinson's disease (PD), multiple sclerosis (MS), and spinal cord injury (SCI).[1]

Most of the information about NB coming from UDCs focuses on SCI; however, to some extent, it can be extrapolated to the other causes of NB.

SPINAL CORD INJURY

Spinal cord injury (SCI) occurs globally with an annual incidence ranging from 3.6 to 195.4 cases per million; however, limited information is available from UDCs.[4] In South America, Brazil and Chile are the only countries with data on SCI, with incidence from 7.8 to 71 cases per million. In Africa, the estimated SCI incidence ranges from 3.4 cases per million in Sierra Leone to 48.5 cases in South Africa[2] (Table 47.1). As can be anticipated, the majority of individuals in resource-rich countries survive the first year postinjury, but this is not the case in

Table 47.1 Incidence of Traumatic Spinal Cord Injury

Region/Country	Incidence (Per Million)
North America	
United States	27.1
Canada	42.4
Europe	
Ireland	13.1
Finland	13.8
France	19.4
Asia	
Pakistan	5.1
Thailand	5.8–23.0
China	6.7–60.6
Vietnam	13.9
Jordan	18.0
Russia	29.7–44.0
Iran	30–72.4
Africa	
Sierra Leone	3.4
Zimbabwe	11.7
South Africa	48.5
South America	
Chile	7.8
Brazil	10.1–71.0

Source: Adapted from Przydacz et al. *Ann Phys Rehabil Med.* 2017;60:341.

resource-poor environments. In one study of 24 subjects from Sierra Leone, 7 individuals died during the initial hospitalization, 8 were dead at follow-up (average 17.4 months), and 4 were lost to follow-up[5]; of the five survivors, two had incomplete injuries and were able to walk. A recent review reported a twofold difference between the highest-reported mortality rate in an UDC (17.5 annual deaths attributable to SCI per million people in Nigeria) compared to that in a developed country (8 annual deaths attributable to SCI per million people in Canada).[6]

CEREBROVASCULAR ACCIDENTS

Two-thirds of all strokes in the world occur in UDCs. In 2013, combined disability-adjusted life-years and mortality rates from ischemic and hemorrhagic stroke were significantly higher in UDCs (2189 × 100,000 inhabitants per year) than in developed nations (1022 × 100,000).[6] Cerebrovascular accidents may result in detrusor dysfunction with urinary retention soon after stroke, which can affect up to 29% of patients.[7]

PARKINSON'S DISEASE

The prevalence of PD in Western countries has been estimated at 100–150 × 100,000 people.[8] However, epidemiologic data from developing regions is variable. For example, prevalence in rural Tanzania is 20 × 100,000, whereas in China it is reported to be similar to that in developed countries.[9] Detrusor overactivity is most commonly found in urodynamic observations in patients with PD, presented in up to 93% of all such cases.[1]

MULTIPLE SCLEROSIS

The prevalence of MS is estimated to be lower in UDCs than in Western nations. The prevalence ranges from 60 to 100 × 100,000 inhabitants in Europe, Canada, and the United States but may be less than 40 × 100,000 in African and Asian countries.[10] In Latin America the prevalence is low in Ecuador, Colombia, and Panama (0.75–6.5/100,000 inhabitants) but 12–21.5 × 100,000 inhabitants in Brazil and Argentina.[1,11] The reported incidence of voiding dysfunction in patients with MS varies greatly, from 52% to 97%.[1]

ACUTE INJURY MANAGEMENT AND EARLY UROLOGIC CARE

Disparities between the capacity to deliver emergency and acute care in developing and developed worlds are evident following a SCI. In many low-resource regions, it is rare for an individual with an acute SCI to be immobilized in the field and transported by trained personnel.[3] In the setting of an unstable spine, this can lead to further neurologic damage. In one study of 83 subjects from Pakistan, none were immobilized at the accident site, and only 18 were transported by ambulance. Delays are common between injury and the beginning of specialized care, even when it is available.[12]

Appropriate bladder emptying should be provided immediately after injury, followed by early and serial neuro-urologic assessments.[13] Unfortunately, the basic principles of SCI management are usually not under the knowledge of the general practitioner and even of the general urologist, so the treatment of patients with SCI is frequently deficient away from specialized centers, which are nonexistent in most UDCs.

ACCESS TO MANAGEMENT OF NEUROGENIC BLADDER IN DEVELOPING COUNTRIES

The assessment and management of NB seems to vary markedly among countries. Paucity of information affects diagnostic and therapeutic approaches to NB patients living in less-developed regions of the world. Although some countries, like China, South Africa, and Malaysia have their own recommendations, few doctors in less-developed countries are aware of guidelines or these guidelines cannot be applied.[14,15]

Both the diagnosis process and the treatment are usually insufficient or not available to the majority of the population. As a consequence, many patients are referred late, and mainly for the treatment of complications. Due to limited access to urodynamics, serial ultrasound evaluation is performed commonly in many countries, including Malaysia and most parts of Africa.[16] However, access to ultrasound and even creatinine test may not be available for some patients, as reported in Kenya, Ethiopia, and Pakistan.[17]

Achieving adequate follow-up can also be challenging. In a report from Nigeria, only 3% of wheelchair-bound individuals kept their initial follow-up appointment after discharge, and by the second appointment, the rate had dropped further to 1.5%.[18]

NONSURGICAL UROLOGIC MANAGEMENT OF THE NEUROGENIC BLADDER

In many UDCs, the acceptance of intermittent catheterization (IC) is low, so the Credé and Valsalva maneuvers are frequent options. Low literacy and cultural resistance to IC, often brought on by fear of infertility, inability to practice obligatory ablution with Muslim prayers, and inability to marry, result in unwillingness to start or continue IC. Other reasons cited for stopping IC were mostly financial (no funds for transportation to medical clinics or for buying medical materials) and social (lack of sustainable access to basic sanitation and difficult entry into hygienic-sanitation facilities for IC).[14]

Intermittent catheterization has not been widely accepted in China, mainly because of the inconvenience or difficulty in its performance and the need for long-term bladder management.[15] The same occurs in many other countries, and as a result, the rate of serious complications, including renal failure and related death, remains high. As an example, the reported contemporary renal failure-related death rate was nearly three times higher in Nigeria than in the United States.[19]

INTERMITTENT CATHETERIZATION

Intermittent catheterization is one of the most effective and commonly used methods of bladder management for NB patients and is part of routine patient care in the larger Asian and South American countries, such as China, India, Pakistan, Iran, Turkey, Malaysia, Brazil, Mexico, and Chile.[1] However, the access to IC is limited in Kenya, Ethiopia, and Thailand.

While the use of IC appears to be widely accepted, several barriers to its wide adoption exist. Education regarding IC use may not be comprehensive or even available. Also, access to IC supplies may be inadequate, as patients in less-developed nations often rely on catheters supplied by international donors or health-promotion organizations.[3] As a result, glass and metal catheters for IC are still in use in many UDCs.[20] Because of cost constraints, disposable catheters are reused in many countries, including Thailand, India, Kenya, and Brazil, with average catheter reuse time of 3 years, as reported from Thailand.[21] Cost constraint is a major issue, and it has been shown that catheter reuse could reduce costs significantly, from USD $4722 to USD $18, over a 2-year period.[20] Interestingly, single-use catheters for IC have not been proven superior, so reuse of catheters can be safely advocated, according to a recent Cochrane review.[22]

ANTIMUSCARINICS

Antimuscarinic agents have been part of the basic treatment of NB for over 30 years in the Western world, but little is known about their use in UDCs. Although several selective anticholinergics are available in some less-developed countries, they may not necessarily be used in clinical practice because of financial issues or the absence of national recommendations. In many countries where selective anticholinergics are not yet available, other cheaper, nonselective drugs like oxyphencyclimine have been given as an alternative.[1]

SURGICAL MANAGEMENT OF THE NEUROGENIC BLADDER

When conservative management fails, surgery can provide effective treatment. Augmentation cystoplasty (AC) with or without a catheterizable channel can provide a safe, functional urine reservoir, and incontinence or intrinsic sphincter deficiency can be managed with different types of slings or the artificial urinary sphincter (AUS). Unfortunately, published literature about the use of surgical options coming from UDCs is also sparse.

Reports of AC cystoplasty for NB management have come from the largest countries of the developing world, like China, Mexico, Brazil, Iran, Pakistan, and India. In Brazil, Lima et al. concluded that bladder augmentation associated with other urologic reconstruction techniques allows protection of the upper urinary tract and contributes to a better quality of life.[23]

Other options, like acupuncture, transcutaneous tibial nerve stimulation, and intravesical onabotulinumtoxinA injections are popular in China and also in most Latin American countries. Interestingly, high-tech and high-cost techniques have been introduced recently in South America, particularly in Colombia and Chile. Sacral neuromodulation with the Interstim device for incomplete SCI NB and neurostimulation with the Brindley device have been applied in these countries with significant success.[24] Unfortunately, the complexity and high cost of these therapies prevent their more widespread use.

It is important to have these treatment alternatives, because many patients with SCI are dissatisfied with IC, and in the long-term they switch to indwelling catheterization (IDC). Predictors of switching from CIC to IDC are refractory incontinence, dependence on caregivers, spasticity, and inexistence of adequate external collection device for women.[25]

SURVEILLANCE

Avoiding complications is the primary goal of surveillance and management in NB; however, the access to diagnostic modalities to follow NB patients is variable. In Malaysia and some parts of Africa, serial bladder ultrasonography and creatinine testing are commonly performed to provide evidence of bladder and renal damage. However in Kenya, Pakistan, and Ethiopia, this is very limited.[26] Videourodynamics for the screening of voiding and storage dysfunction is widely available in developed countries, such as the United States, Canada, and the United Kingdom, and may also be available in China, but is available in only a few UDCs.[15]

A proposal for surveillance in patients with NB— the GU Health Maintenance Measures—includes the following: (1) review bladder management programs regularly; (2) investigate further if there are changes in bladder function (e.g., urinary retention, episodes of incontinence, urinary tract infections, and hematuria); (3) test renal function; (4) carry out regular imaging of the urinary tract; and (5) conduct prostate cancer screening for men.

CURRENT CHALLENGES IN DEVELOPING COUNTRIES

The first challenge is to get accurate and representative data for adequate valuation of the true incidence and prevalence of SCI NB worldwide. Centralized registers may help to improve data curation, but sociocultural issues, including distance to the closest medical center, social traditions, religious beliefs, and preference for traditional medicine, often limit access to a large number of patients and their inclusion in statistical data.

The second challenge is to organize the existing knowledge in a way that can be applied in the constrained environment of UDCs. Most guidelines developed by international societies are not fully applicable in such countries (Table 47.2). Professional societies, like the International Continence Society, the World Federation of Neurology, and others manage to produce special recommendations for UDCs in terms of organizational plans, educational programs, and also diagnosis and treatment protocols adjusted to different levels of existing capabilities and resources. With the same aim, the International Consultation for Urological Disease (ICUD) and the Societé Internationale d'Urologie (SIU) published recently a comprehensive update for the management of SCI, providing recommendations with an international perspective.[27]

The third challenge is to put those recommendations to practice. Overall in-hospital mortality of SCI patients in the high-resources settings of Canada and the United States are 11.6% and 6.1%, respectively, while in Nigeria and Sierra Leone it is 35% and 29%, respectively, with most individuals dying within a few years of injury.[28]

Table 47.2 Guidelines for Management of Spinal Cord Injury

	Organization	Observations
North America	AUA/SUFU Neurogenic Lower Urinary Tract Dysfunction Guidelines	Guidelines under development
	Consortium for Spinal Cord Medicine	Guidelines under development
	American Association of Neurologic Surgeons; Guidelines for the Management of Acute C Spine and Spinal Cord Injury	No section on bladder management
	Nutrition Guidelines for Patients with SCI	
South America	No regional guidelines	International guidelines adopted in some high-resource countries
Europe	(United Kingdom) International Spinal Cord Society (ISCoS)	
	(United Kingdom) National Guideline Clearinghouse of the National Institute of Health and Clinical Excellence (NICE)	
	(Switzerland) SwiSCI	
Asia	Chinese Urologic Association of (CUA); Neurogenic Bladder Guidelines	Original in 2011, with updates in 2014 and 2015
	Taiwanese Continence Society	
	Malaysian Pediatric Association (MPA)	
Africa	South African Spinal Cord Association; Guidelines for the Quality and Sustainable Bladder Management in the Neurogenic Bladder Patient	
Australasia	ACI State Spinal Cord Injury Service; ACI Management of the Neurogenic Bladder for Adults with Spinal Cord Injuries	

Source: Adapted from Gomelsky et al. *World J Urol*. 2018;36:1613.

Furthermore, in UDCs, the availability of quality assistive devices, such as wheelchairs, medical and rehabilitation services, and opportunities to participate in all areas of personal and social life are constrained. It is crucial to improve these services, because evidence shows that access to specialized spinal-care units (SCUs) leads to better outcomes. A study conducted in the United Kingdom demonstrated that despite having more severe injuries, the SCU-rehabilitated cohort obtained significantly improved outcomes in comparison with the non-SCU cohort.[29] Therefore, the establishment of these units should be a prime priority in the effort to improve the results.

CONCLUSIONS

There is a dearth of high-level evidence in the literature regarding international patterns of care in patients with NB. This includes registries, regional specialty centers, and protocols for acute and chronic management strategies. It is demonstrated that with these resources, the results would be better and life expectancy longer. While the situation may seem disheartening for those individuals sustaining SCI in developing countries, there are reasons to be hopeful. Ongoing epidemiologic studies will provide an accurate estimate of the incidence and prevalence of SCI in developing nations. There is also an increasing worldwide effort to disseminate the available knowledge tailored to each regional need. This information can be used to focus organizational efforts and to provide supplies and resources, and also necessary education for better diagnosis and treatment of urologic conditions after SCI.

REFERENCES

1. Przydacz M, Denys P, and Corcos J. What do we know about neurogenic bladder prevalence and management in developing countries and emerging regions of the world? *Ann Phys Rehabil Med.* 2017;60:341–6.
2. Lee BB, Cripps RA, Fitzharris M, and Wing PC. The global map for traumatic spinal cord injury epidemiology: Update 2011, global incidence rate. *Spinal Cord.* 2014;52:110–6.
3. Burns AS and O'Connell C. The challenge of spinal cord injury care in the developing world. *J Spinal Cord Med.* 2012;35:3–8.
4. Rahimi-Movaghar V, Sayyah MK, Akbari H et al. Epidemiology of traumatic spinal cord injury in developing countries: A systematic review. *Neuroepidemiology.* 2013;41:65–85.
5. Gosselin RA and Coppotelli C. A follow-up study of patients with spinal cord injury in Sierra Leone. *Int Orthop.* 2005;29:330–2.
6. Chiu WT, Lin HC, Lam C, Chu SF, Chiang YH, Tsai SH. Review paper: Epidemiology of traumatic spinal cord injury: Comparisons between developed and developing countries. *Asia Pacific J Public Heal.* 2010;22:9–18.
7. Feigin VL, Krishnamurthi RV, Parmar P et al. Update on the global burden of ischemic and hemorrhagic stroke in 1990–2013: The GBD 2013 study. *Neuroepidemiology.* 2015;45:161–76.
8. Sakakibara R, Kishi M, Ogawa E et al. Bladder, bowel, and sexual dysfunction in Parkinson's disease. *Parkinsons Dis.* 2011;2011:924605.
9. Zhang ZX, Roman GC, Hong Z et al. Parkinson's disease in China: Prevalence in Beijing, Xian, and Shanghai. *Lancet.* 2005;365:595–7.
10. Pugliatti M, Sotgiu S, and Rosati G. The worldwide prevalence of multiple sclerosis. *Clin Neurol Neurosurg.* 2002;104:182–91.
11. Corcos J. A urological challenge: Voiding dysfunction in multiple sclerosis. *Can Urol Assoc J.* 2013;7:S181–2.
12. Rathore MFA, Hanif S, Farooq F, Ahmad N, and Mansoor SN. Traumatic spinal cord injuries at a tertiary care rehabilitation institute in Pakistan. *J Pak Med Assoc.* 2008;58:53–7.
13. McIntosh PM and Dorsher PT. Neurogenic bladder. *Revista Brasileira de Medicina.* 2006;63.
14. Gomelsky A, Lemack GE, Castano Botero JC, Lee RK, Myers JB, Granitsiotis P. Current and future international patterns of care of neurogenic bladder after spinal cord injury. *World J Urol.* 2018;36:1613–9.
15. Liao L. Evaluation and management of neurogenic bladder: What is new in China? *Int J Mol Sci.* 2015;16:18580–600.
16. Engkasan JP, Ng CJ, and Low WY. Factors influencing bladder management in male patients with spinal cord injury: A qualitative study. *Spinal Cord.* 2014;52:157–62.
17. Sultan S, Hussain I, Ahmed B et al. Clean intermittent catheterization in children through a continent catheterizable channel: A developing country experience. *J Urol.* 2008;180:1852–5.
18. Nwadinigwe CU, Iloabuchi TC, and Nwabude IA. Traumatic spinal cord injuries (SCI): A study of 104 cases. *Niger J Med.* 2004;13:161–5.
19. Bowman RM, McLone DG, Grant JA, Tomita T, and Ito JA. Spina Bifida outcome: A 25-year prospective. *Pediatr Neurosurg.* 2001;34:114–20.
20. Kovindha A, Mai WNC, and Madersbacher H. Reused silicone catheter for clean intermittent catheterization (CIC): Is it safe for spinal cord-injured (SCI) men? *Spinal Cord.* 2004;42:638–42.
21. Mazzo A1, Souza-Junior VD2, Jorge BM et al. Intermittent urethral catheterization—Descriptive study at a Brazilian service. *Appl Nurs Res.* 2014;27:170–4.
22. Prieto J, Murphy CL, Moore KN, and Fader M. Intermittent catheterisation for long-term bladder management. In: Fader M, ed. *Cochrane Database of Systematic Reviews.* New York, NY: John Wiley & Sons; 2014. doi:10.1002/14651858.CD006008.pub3
23. Lima DX, Pires CR, Santos AC, Mendes RG, Fonseca CE, Zocratto OB . Quality of life evaluation of patients with neurogenic bladder submitted to reconstructive urological surgeries preserving the bladder. *Int Braz J Urol.* 2015;41:542–6.
24. Castaño-Botero JC, Ospina-Galeano IA, Gómez-Illanes R, and Lopera-Toro A. Extradural implantation of sacral anterior root stimulator in spinal cord injury patients. *Neurourol Urodyn.* 2016;35:970–4.
25. Weld KJ and Dmochowski RR. Effect of bladder management on urological complications in spinal cord injured patients. *J Urol.* 2000;163:768–72.

26. Levy LF, Makarawo S, Madzivire D, Bhebhe E, Verbeek N, Parry O. Problems, struggles and some success with spinal cord injury in Zimbabwe. *Spinal Cord*. 1998;36:213–8.

27. Gómez RG and Elliott SP. Urologic management of the spinal cord injured patient. *World J Urol*. 2018;36:1515–16.

28. Couris CM, Guilcher SJ, Munce SE et al. Characteristics of adults with incident traumatic spinal cord injury in Ontario, Canada. *Spinal Cord*. 2010;48:39–44.

29. New PW, Simmonds F, and Stevermuer T. Comparison of patients managed in specialised spinal rehabilitation units with those managed in non-specialised rehabilitation units. *Spinal Cord*. 2011;49:909–16.

Part XI

REFERENCES FOR REPORTS AND GUIDELINES

Chapter 48

REPORTS AND GUIDELINES IN RELATION TO NEUROGENIC BLADDER DYSFUNCTION
A Selection

Floriane Michel and Gilles Karsenty

INTRODUCTION

The modern history of guidelines began almost 30 years ago in the early 1990s.[1,2] By these three decades, a rigorous process to identify, evaluate research evidence and adapt it appropriately, in a transparent manner with effective management of conflict of interests during the guideline development process, was found to be critical for a guideline to be able to provide a meaningful framework against which medical quality of care can be measured and important health systems' decisions be based on.[2]

Reports, guidelines, and recommendations in relation to neurogenic bladder dysfunction are published by different health organizations, mainly national or international urologic and rehabilitation medicine associations. Most of them are available online, and some are updated on a regular basis. Some are directed at urologists, others at rehabilitation physicians or general practitioners, and some also to patients. In this chapter, we propose a selection of these documents presented as a repertoire to allow the reader to easily consult their last versions. Main selection criteria were evidence-based development, English language, update frequency, completeness, or disease specificity.

GUIDELINES FOR GENERAL MANAGEMENT OF NEUROGENIC BLADDER

The *International Consultation on Incontinence* (ICI) held every third year offers through 23 chapters and a 2549-page book (last issue 2017 Tokyo) the most comprehensive state-of-the-art series on all forms of urinary and fecal incontinence. For the specific field of neurogenic bladder, this book offers a chapter on the *neural control of the lower urinary tract* (Birder L [coordinator], Blok B, Burnstock G, Cruz F, Griffiths D, Kuo HC, Yoshimura N, Fry C, Thor K) and another one on *neurologic urinary and fecal incontinence* (Apostolidis A, Drake MJ, [coordinator], Emmanuel A, Gajewski J, Hamid R, Heesakkers J, Kessler T, Madersbacher H, Mangera A, Panicker J, Radziszewski P, Sakakibara R, Sievert K-D, Wyndaele J-J).

Additionally, two evidence-based summaries on *neurologic urinary incontinence management* and *fecal incontinence in neurologic patients* are provided; the ICI book is available via the ICS website: https://www.ics.org

The *European Association of Urology* (EAU) proposes complete and regularly updated guidelines on neuro-urology. EAU guidelines, updated yearly, provide since 2006 evidence-based information for clinical practitioners on incidence, definitions, diagnosis, therapy, and follow-up of neuro-urological disorders, regardless of the underlying neurologic disease. They are downloadable for free at https://uroweb.org/guideline/neuro-urology/ in a full-text comprehensive version including bibliography as well as a summarized pocket version focused on recommendations. The last update (2019) is authored by Blok B, Castro-Diaz D, Del Popolo G, Groen J, Hamid R, Karsenty G, Kessler TM, Pannek J, Ecclestone H, Musco S, Padilla-Fernández B, Phé V, Sartori A, and 't Hoen L.

The *Canadian Urological Association* proposed in 2019 their first general guidelines on neurogenic bladder entitled: "Diagnosis, management, and surveillance of neurogenic lower urinary tract dysfunction" (Kavanagh A, Baverstock R, Campeau L, Carlson K, Cox A, Hickling D, Nadeau G, Stothers L, Welk B). This bilingual (English/French) document offers practice recommendations graded according to level of evidence at the end of each section (of particular interest is a strategy flowchart based on an upper urinary tract impairment risk stratification). It is published as a summary in *the Canadian Urological*

Association Journal (2019;13[6]:156–65) and as a full-text version at https://www.cua.org/en/guidelines.

The *National Institute for Health and Care Excellence* (NICE) published in 2012, the National Clinical Guideline Centre [Internet], "Urinary incontinence in neurological disease: management of lower urinary tract dysfunction in neurological disease." This guideline covers assessing and managing urinary incontinence in children, young people, and adults with neurologic disease: https://www.nice.org.uk/guidance/cg148/evidence/full-guideline-188123437; https://pathways.nice.org.uk/pathways/urinary-incontinence-in-neurological-disease#path=view%3A/pathways/urinary-incontinence-in-neurological-disease/urinary-incontinence-in-neurological-disease-overview.xml&content=view-index

TERMINOLOGY AND ASSESSMENT OF NEUROGENIC BLADDER

The *International Continence Society* (ICS) and its standardization committee offer reports on several domains directly related to neurogenic bladder. All reports are available on the ICS website (free-access https://www.ics.org/folder/standardisation). A new valuable tool is available on the ICS website: the glossary (https://www.ics.org/glossary), made to find any standardized term and its actual definition.

The report on standardization of lower urinary tract terminology (published in 2002) is one of the first reports of this series and is widely accepted in the urologic community; it covers normal function of the lower urinary tract as well as main symptoms, signs, and urodynamic observations associated with lower urinary tract dysfunction: https://www.ics.org/folder/standardisation/current-ics-standardisations/lower-urinary-tract-function/d/the-standardisation-of-terminology-of-lower-urinary-tract-function-report-from-the-standardisation-sub-committee-of-the-ics

Several other terminology reports are more specific and come to refine this first general report on standardization of lower urinary tract terminology. The most specific and relevant of the neurogenic bladder subjects is entitled "An International Continence Society (ICS) report on the terminology for adult neurogenic lower urinary tract dysfunction (ANLUTD)" and was published in 2017 (authors: Gajewski JB, Schurch B, Hamid R, Averbeck M, Sakakibara R, Agrò EF, Dickinson T, Payne CK, Drake MJ, Haylen BT): https://www.ics.org/folder/standardisation/current-ics-standardisations/d/ics-report-on-the-terminology-for-adult-neurogenic-lower-urinary-tract-dysfunction-anlutd-2017

Since urodynamics studies are recommended and widely performed in the assessment of neurogenic bladder, the ICS standardization committee has pursued constant efforts to promote reproducible, reliable, and high-quality urodynamic practice through four reports from 2004 to 2014: https://www.ics.org/folder/standardisation/current-ics-standardisations/urodynamics-and-diagnostics

- *Ambulatory urodynamic monitoring*, van Waalwijk van Doorn E, Anders K, Khullar V, Kulseng Hansen S, Pesce F, Robertson A, Rosario D, Schafer W. *Neurourology and Urodynamics* (2000;19:113–25).
- *Good urodynamic practices: Uroflowmetry, filling cystometry, and pressure-flow studies*, Schafer W, Abrams P, Liao L, Mattiasson A, Pesce F, Spangberg A, Sterling AM, Zinner NR, van Kerrebroeck P. *Neurourology and Urodynamics* (2002;21[3]:261–74).
- *Standardisation of urethral pressure measurement*, Lose G, Griffiths D, Hosker G, Kulseng-Hanssen S, Perucchini D, Schaefer W, Thind P, Versi E. *Neurourology and Urodynamics* (2002;21:258–60).
- *International Continence Society Guidelines on Urodynamic Equipment Performance*, Gammie A, Clarkson B, Constantinou C, Damaser M, Drinnan M, Geleijnse G, Griffiths D, Rosier P, Schafer W, Van Mastrigt R. *Neurourology and Urodynamics* (2014;33[4]:370–9).

Additionally, the ICS provides since 2016 through a section named the "ICS education" teaching modules on urodynamic testing practice (basic and advanced) in adult and children. *The ICS Education Module* includes a three-part format: official ICS-consensus PowerPoint available for download, a studio-quality video (hosted on the ICS website), and a peer-reviewed published article published in Neurourology and Urodynamics (NAU). ICS Education Modules are available online on the ICS website (https://www.ics.org/education/icsstandardoperatingprocedures/publicationsops).

SPECIFIC GUIDELINES AND RECOMMENDATIONS

PATIENT WITH SPINAL CORD INJURY

The *International Consultation on Urologic Disease* (ICUD) and *Société Internationale d'Urologie* (SIU) provided in 2016 comprehensive evidence-based recommendations for the urologic management of the patient with spinal cord injury: *Urologic Management of the Spinal Cord Injured Patient (2016)*, authors: Sean Elliott and Reynaldo Gómez.

Eleven committees cover epidemiology, early neurologic and urologic care, surveillance and urologic complications, nonsurgical and surgical management, fertility and sexuality, bowel management, children and aging specificities, and comparison of current and future patterns of care after spinal cord injury. An e-book is available on the SIU website (https://www.siu-urology.org/society/siu-icud#ICUD), and a summary has been published in a special issue of the *World Journal of Urology* (https://link.springer.com/journal/345/36/10/page/).

The *Paralyzed Veterans of America* (https://pva.org) proposes evidence-based comprehensive clinical practice guidelines for adults with spinal cord injury. Among the 12 domains covered, 3 are in the scope of neurogenic pelvic dysfunctions: *Sexuality and Reproductive Health in Adults with Spinal Cord Injury* (2010); *Bladder Management for Adults with Spinal Cord Injury* (2008); and *Neurogenic Bowel Management in Adults with Spinal Cord Injury* (1998). The frequency of updates is not clear.

The *International Spinal Cord Society* (ISCOS) developed in 2015 a framework to bring together the broad skills and competencies that a trainee would need to develop to work as a medical practitioner looking after people with spinal cord impairment: *Recommended Knowledge and Skills Framework for Spinal Cord Medicine*. It includes specific sections on neurogenic bladder, sexual dysfunction, and fertility neurogenic bowel: https://www.iscos.org.uk/uploads/sitefiles/Knowledge%20and%20Skills%20Framework/ISCoS_Framework_SCI_Medicine_Dec.pdf

The mission of the *Spinal Cord Outcomes Partnership Endeavour* (SCOPE) is to enhance the development of clinical trial and clinical practice protocols that will accurately validate therapeutic interventions for spinal cord injury (SCI) leading to the adoption of improved best practices. On the SCOPE website (http://scope-sci.org/), a monthly updated list of all the current SCI clinical trials of drug, cell, rehabilitation, or surgical interventions and technology to improve neurologic and related functional outcomes is available.

PATIENTS WITH MULTIPLE SCLEROSIS

Despite the fact that MS is responsible for frequent and severe neurogenic lower urinary tract dysfunction, there is still no widely accepted clinical practice guideline on the management of neurogenic bladder due to MS.

However, two publications are of interest in this field:

- *Consensus guidelines on the neurologist's role in the management of neurogenic lower urinary tract dysfunction in multiple sclerosis*, De Ridder D et al. *Clinical Neurology and Neurosurgery* (2013;115[10]:2033–40).
- *The neurogenic bladder in multiple sclerosis: Review of the literature and proposal of*

management guidelines. De Sèze M et al. and GENULF. *Multiple Sclerosis Journal* (2007;13[7]:915–28). Review.

PATIENTS WITH SPINAL DYSRAPHISM AND NEUROGENIC BLADDER: CHILDREN AND ADOLESCENTS

The *International Children's Continence Society* (ICCS) provides standardized terminology for lower urinary tract function in children and adolescents as well as recommendations for children with congenital neuropathic bladder. These recommendations are not available on the ICCS website (http://i-c-c-s.org/). Summaries have been published in NAU.

- *The standardization of terminology of lower urinary tract function in children and adolescents: Update report from the standardization committee of the International Children's Continence Society*. Austin PF, Bauer SB, Bower W, Chase J, Franco I, Hoebeke P, Rittig S, Walle JV, von Gontard A, Wright A, Yang SS, Nevéus T. *Neurourology and Urodynamics* (2016;35[4]:471–81).
- *International Children's Continence Society standardization report on urodynamic studies of the lower urinary tract in children*. Bauer SB, Nijman RJ, Drzewiecki BA, Sillen U, Hoebeke P; International Children's Continence Society Standardization Subcommittee. *Neurourology and Urodynamics* (2015;34[7]:640–7).
- *International Children's Continence Society's recommendations for initial diagnostic evaluation and follow-up in congenital neuropathic bladder and bowel dysfunction in children*. Bauer SB, Austin PF, Rawashdeh YF, de Jong TP, Franco I, Siggard C, Jorgensen TM; International Children's Continence Society. *Neurourology and Urodynamics* (2012;31[5]:610–4).
- *International Children's Continence Society's recommendations for therapeutic intervention in congenital neuropathic bladder and bowel dysfunction in children*. Rawashdeh YF, Austin P, Siggaard C, Bauer SB, Franco I, de Jong TP, Jorgensen TM; International Children's Continence Society. *Neurourology and Urodynamics* (2012;31[5]:615–20).

The *European Association of Urology* (EAU) in collaboration with the *European Society of Pediatric Urology* (ESPU) provides yearly updated recommendations on pediatric urology including a chapter on neurogenic bladder management (https://uroweb.org/wp-content/uploads/EAU-Guidelines-on-Paediatric-Urology-2018-large-text.pdf).

The *International Consultation on Urologic Disease* (ICUD) and the *Société Internationale d'Urologie* (SIU) held in October 2019 in Athens a consensus meeting on Congenital Lifelong Urology. Chaired by Hadley Wood and Dan Wood, the six committees of this consultation focused on the most salient issues that arise when patients with congenital urologic disease move from pediatric care to adult care and will cover spinal dysraphisms (from minor dysraphism to myelomeningocele): https://www.siu-urology.org/siu-news/coming-soon-the-joint-siu-icud-2019-on-congenital-lifelong-urology-pu

SEXUAL DYSFUNCTION, FERTILITY AND BOWEL DYSFUNCTION IN NEUROLOGIC PATIENT

The only general guidelines to cover both sexual dysfunction and fertility in males and females with recommendations, although limited, are the *EAU guidelines* as previously cited.

The *sixth ICI book* is the only one to provide a specific chapter on neurogenic bowel dysfunction with recommendations.

The *ICUD/SIU 2016* report and the *Paralyzed Veterans of America guidelines* offer more comprehensive, though disease-specific (specific of spinal cord injured patients) chapters on bowel management, male fertility, and male sexual dysfunction.

The *Spina Bifida Association* (https://www.spinabifidaassociation.org) proposes evidence-based *clinical guidelines for bowel management in patients with spinal dysraphism from birth to adulthood* (authors: Beierwaltes P [Chair], Ambartsumyan L, Baillie S, Shurch P, Dicker J, Gordon T, Liebold S): https://www.spinabifidaassociation.orgappuploads

CONCLUSION

In 2018 Jaggi et al. compared the three main clinical guidelines for neurogenic lower urinary tract dysfunction in two papers and concluded:[3,4]

In the absence of high-quality clinical evidence, many of the recommendations made across all three guidelines are based on expert opinion. NICE, the EAU and ICI have similarities but they place differing emphasis on costs and expert opinion, which translated in notably different recommendations. It is evident that increased research efforts, possibly in the form of prospective registries, pragmatic trials, and resource utilization studies, are necessary to improve the underlying evidence base for NLUTD, and subsequently the strength and concordance of recommendations across guidelines. Better collaboration between the ICI, NICE, and EAU could improve the quality and consistency between NLUTD clinical guidelines and ultimately improve health outcomes for this important patient group.

We fully agree and emphasize the need for national and supranational prospective neuro-urology registries on which more precise and condition-specific clinical guidelines and recommendations will be based.

REFERENCES

1. Field MJ and Lohr KN, eds.*Clinical Practice Guidelines: Directions for a New Program.* Marilyn JF, and Kathleen NL (eds.). Washington, DC: National Academies Press; 1990. Institute of Medicine (US). Committee to Advise the Public Health Service on Clinical Practice Guidelines.
2. Soumyadeep B. Use of evidence for clinical practice guideline development. *Trop Parasitol.* 2017;7(2):65–71.
3. Jaggi A, Drake M, Siddiqui E, and Fatoye F. A comparison of the treatment recommendations for neurogenic lower urinary tract dysfunction in the national institute for health and care excellence, European Association of Urology and international consultations on incontinence guidelines. *Neurourol Urodyn.* 2018;37(7):2273–80.
4. Jaggi A, Drake M, Siddiqui E, Nazir J, Giagos V, and Fatoye F. A critical appraisal of the principal guidelines for neurogenic lower urinary tract dysfunction using the AGREE II instrument. *Neurourol Urodyn.* 2018;37(8):2945–50.

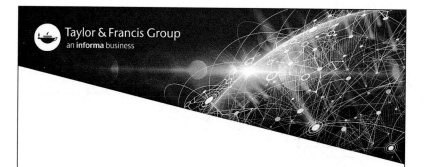